Medical Management
of Long-Term Disability

Medical Management of Long-Term Disability

Second Edition

Rehabilitation Institute of Chicago

Edited by

David Green, M.D., Ph.D.

Professor of Medicine, Northwestern University Medical School, Chicago;
Attending Physician, Departments of Medicine and Physical Medicine and
Rehabilitation, Northwestern Memorial Hospital, Rehabilitation Institute of
Chicago, and Veterans Administration Lakeside Medical Center, Chicago, Illinois

Publications Coordinator, Rehabilitation Institute of Chicago
Don A. Olson, Ph.D.
Associate Professor of Physical Medicine and Rehabilitation and Neurology,
Northwestern University Medical School, Chicago; Director, Education and
Training Center, Rehabilitation Institute of Chicago, Illinois

With a foreword by
Henry B. Betts, M.D.
Professor, Department of Physical Medicine and Rehabilitation, Northwestern
University Medical School, Chicago; Chief Executive Officer,
Rehabilitation Institute of Chicago, Illinois

Butterworth-Heinemann
Boston Oxford Johannesburg Melbourne New Delhi Singapore

Copyright © 1996 by Butterworth–Heinemann

 A member of the Reed Elsevier group

Every effort has been made to ensure that the drug dosage schedules within this text are accurate and conform to standards accepted at time of publication. However, as treatment recommendations vary in the light of continuing research and clinical experience, the reader is advised to verify drug dosage schedules herein with information found on product information sheets. This is especially true in cases of new or infrequently used drugs.

Recognizing the importance of preserving what has been written, Butterworth–Heinemann prints its books on acid-free paper whenever possible.

Library of Congress Cataloging-in-Publication Data
Medical management of long-term disability / edited by David Green ;
    publications coordinator, Rehabilitation Institute of Chicago, Don A.
    Olson ; with a foreword by Henry B. Betts. — 2nd ed.
       p. cm.
    Includes bibliographical references and index.
    ISBN 0-7506-9604-4 (alk. paper)
    1. Chronically ill—Rehabilitation.   I. Green, David, 1934–
    [DNLM: 1. Disabled.   2. Rehabilitation.   3. Chronic Disease–
  –rehabilitation.   WB 320 M4888 1996]
    RC108.M43 1996
    617'.06—dc20
    DNLM/DLC
    for Library of Congress 96-26646
      CIP

British Library Cataloguing-in-Publication Data
A catalogue record for this book is available from the British Library.

The publisher offers special discounts on bulk orders of this book.
For information, please contact:
Manager of Special Sales
Butterworth–Heinemann
313 Washington Street
Newton, MA 02158–1626

Tel: 617-928-2500
Fax: 617-928-2620

For information on all medical publications available, contact our World Wide Web home page at:
http://www.bh.com/med/

10 9 8 7 6 5 4 3 2 1

Printed in the United States of America

Contents

Contributing Authors

Rowland W. Chang, M.D., M.P.H.
Associate Professor of Medicine and Physical Medicine and Rehabilitation, Northwestern University Medical School, Chicago; Attending Physician and Co-Director, Arthritis Center, Rehabilitation Institute of Chicago; Attending Physician, Northwestern Memorial Hospital, Chicago, Illinois

David Chen, M.D.
Assistant Professor of Physical Medicine and Rehabilitation, Northwestern University Medical School, Chicago; Director, Spinal Cord Injury Program, Rehabilitation Institute of Chicago, Illinois

Gene Z. Chiao, M.D.
Assistant Professor of Medicine, Indiana University School of Medicine, Indianapolis; Attending Physician, Department of Medicine, Indiana University Medical Center, Indianapolis, Indiana

James I. Couser, Jr., M.D.
Clinical Assistant Professor of Medicine, University of Wisconsin Medical School, Madison; Staff Physician, Departments of Pulmonary Medicine and Critical Care, St. Marys Hospital Medical Center, Madison, Wisconsin

Robert M. Craig, M.D.
Chief, Division of Gastroenterology, Department of Medicine, Northwestern University Medical School and Northwestern Memorial Hospital, Chicago, Illinois

James C. Erickson III, M.D., M.Sc.
Professor of Anesthesia, Northwestern University Medical School, Chicago; Attending Staff Physician, Department of Anesthesia, Northwestern Memorial Hospital, Chicago, Illinois

Benjamin T. Esparaz, M.D.
Medical Oncologist/Hematologist, Department of Internal Medicine, Decatur Memorial Hospital, Decatur, Illinois

David Green, M.D., Ph.D.
Professor of Medicine, Northwestern University Medical School, Chicago; Attending Physician, Departments of Medicine and Physical Medicine and Rehabilitation, Northwestern Memorial Hospital, Rehabilitation Institute of Chicago, and Veterans Administration Lakeside Medical Center, Chicago, Illinois

Peter J. Kahrilas, M.D.
Professor of Medicine, Northwestern University Medical School, Chicago; Medical Director, Gastrointestinal Diagnostic Laboratory, Department of Medicine, Northwestern Memorial Hospital, Chicago, Illinois

Frank A. Krumlovsky, M.D.
Associate Professor of Medicine, Northwestern University Medical School, Chicago; Attending Physician, Department of Medicine, Northwestern Memorial Hospital, Chicago, Illinois

Santosh Lal, M.D., M.M.
Former Assistant Professor of Physical Medicine and Rehabilitation, Northwestern University Medical School, Chicago, Illinois; Consultant Physiatrist, Department of Internal Medicine, Gottlieb Memorial Hospital, Melrose Park, and Holy Family Hospital, Des Plaines, Illinois

Przemyslaw Lastowiecki, M.D.
Attending Physician, Department of Medicine, Holy Cross Hospital, Chicago, Illinois

Victor L. Lewis, Jr., M.D.
Professor of Clinical Surgery, Division of Plastic Surgery, Northwestern University Medical School and Northwestern Memorial Hospital, Chicago, Illinois

Christina Marciniak, M.D.
Assistant Professor of Physical Medicine and Rehabilitation, Northwestern University Medical School, Chicago; Attending Physician, Department of Physical Medicine and Rehabilitation, Rehabilitation Institute of Chicago, Chicago, Illinois

John R. McGuire, M.D.
Instructor in Physical Medicine and Rehabilitation, Northwestern University Medical School, Chicago; Attending Physician, Department of Physical Medicine and Rehabilitation, Rehabilitation Institute of Chicago, Chicago, Illinois

Mark E. Molitch, M.D.
Professor of Medicine, Northwestern University Medical School, Chicago, Illinois

Salim Mujais, M.D.
Associate Professor of Medicine and Nephrology, Northwestern University Medical School, Chicago; Staff Physician, Department of Medicine, Northwestern Memorial Hospital, Chicago, Illinois

John B. Nanninga, M.D.
Associate Professor of Urology, Northwestern University Medical School, Chicago; Attending Urologist, Northwestern Memorial Hospital, Chicago, Illinois

Peter Pertel, M.D.
Clinical Instructor in Medicine and Research Associate in Microbiology/Immunology, Northwestern University Medical School, Chicago, Illinois

Elliot J. Roth, M.D.
Professor and Chairman, Department of Physical Medicine and Rehabilitation, Northwestern University Medical School, Chicago; Medical Director, Rehabilitation Institute of Chicago, Chicago, Illinois

William Z. Rymer, M.D., Ph.D.
Professor of Physiology, Physical Medicine and Rehabilitation, and Biomedical Engineering, Northwestern University Medical School, Chicago; John G. Searle Chair in Rehabilitation Research and Director, Department of Research, Rehabilitation Institute of Chicago, Chicago, Illinois

Mahmoud Salem, M.D.
Assistant Professor of Medicine, Division of Nephrology, University of Mississippi Medical Center, Jackson

George E. Shambaugh III, M.D.
Professor of Medicine, Division of Endocrinology, Northwestern University Medical School, Chicago; Chief, Endocrinology and Metabolic Section, Department of Medicine, Veterans Administration Lakeside Medical Center, Chicago, Illinois

James Sliwa, D.O.
Associate Professor of Physical Medicine and Rehabilitation, Northwestern University Medical School, Chicago; Program Director, Department of General Rehabilitation, Rehabilitation Institute of Chicago, Chicago, Illinois

Michele Till, M.D.
Assistant Professor of Medicine, Northwestern University Medical School, Chicago, Illinois

Mark T. Upton, M.D.
Assistant Professor of Medicine, Northwestern University Medical School, Chicago; Associate Attending Physician, Department of Medicine, Northwestern Memorial Hospital, Chicago, Illinois

Yeongchi Wu, M.D.
Associate Professor of Physical Medicine and Rehabilitation, Northwestern University Medical School, Chicago; Attending Physician, Department of Physical Medicine and Rehabilitation, Rehabilitation Institute of Chicago, Chicago, Illinois

Foreword

Patients benefit the most and outcomes are most positive when rehabilitation begins soon after the onset of disability or chronic illness. Without early intervention, secondary complications arise: patients wonder about what next steps are practicable, depression can be exacerbated, and families and other concerned parties may be less motivated to help.

A goal of physical medicine and rehabilitation has always been to bring together, as expediently as possible, an array of experts to deal with the complexity of disability and the issues involving loss of function. Specialists in physical medicine and rehabilitation have been leaders in the development of the dynamics of interdisciplinary medicine and, in order to implement comprehensive rehabilitation, established teams consisting of professionals from nursing, physical therapy, occupational therapy, vocational counseling, social work, chaplaincy, speech, psychology, and therapeutic recreation.

Early in the history of rehabilitation medicine, patients were sent to centers long after the diagnosis of functional loss. In many instances, "medical" problems were solved before rehabilitation began. In recent years, probably because of diagnosis-related groups (DRGs), patients have begun arriving much earlier and with concomitant problems beyond neuromuscular and orthopedic deficits. Therefore, at the Rehabilitation Institute of Chicago, an internal medicine service with sections on general medicine, arthritis, hematology, infectious disease, and pulmonary medicine was established to manage these medical problems. In addition to providing patient care, this structure has enhanced the capability for interdisciplinary teaching of residents, medical students, and allied health personnel.

Dr. David Green, Chief of Medicine, and his associates from Northwestern University Medical School offer this immediate and comprehensive service to their patients. The information provided in this book, which expands on their experiences in dealing with the major medical problems of the rehabilitation population, will be invaluable to health care professionals who are confronted daily with the illnesses of the chronically disabled.

Henry B. Betts, M.D.

Preface

This book grew out of our recognition that chronically disabled persons are vulnerable to certain specific medical problems and that the knowledge required to manage these problems constitutes a particular body of information. Because this material did not appear to reside in any one source, we brought together internists, physiatrists, and surgical subspecialists to create this volume.

The subject matter addressed within these pages is diagrammed in Figure 1. Each disorder listed is the theme of a specific chapter, and the chapters are grouped under the principal medical specialties. For example, swallowing disorders, abnormal bowel motility, and weight loss are found in Section IV, Gastroenterology. For many of the topics, a team comprising a physiatrist and an internist or surgeon has prepared the text.

In the five years since the publication of the first edition, there has been a major change in the provision of health care to disabled persons. It has shifted from specialist physicians to primary caregivers, including family practitioners, general internists, skilled nurses, and physician assistants. These health workers have been given major responsibility for the long-term management of patients with strokes, amputations, spinal cord injuries, and other disabling conditions and are required to become knowledgeable about the treatment of such problems as spasticity, autonomic dysreflexia, and pressure sores as well as osteoporosis, anemia, and abnormal bowel motility.

To meet this need, the current edition has been extensively revised and expanded. New chapters on spasticity and autonomic dysreflexia as well as scholarly treatises on heart failure, diabetes, and blood pressure control have been added. The chapters on nutrition, infectious diseases, pulmonary disorders, and drug usage have been rewritten to be more directly applicable to clinical practice and to reflect newer knowledge in these areas. Finally, appended to several chapters are case management studies, which allow the reader to work through clinical problems with the guidance of an expert. In summary, it is my hope that this volume will help to improve the care of those with chronic disabilities by strengthening the information base of their caregivers.

I thank all of the contributors to this volume for their cooperation and diligence and the entire staff of the Rehabilitation Institute of Chicago, whose skill and exper-

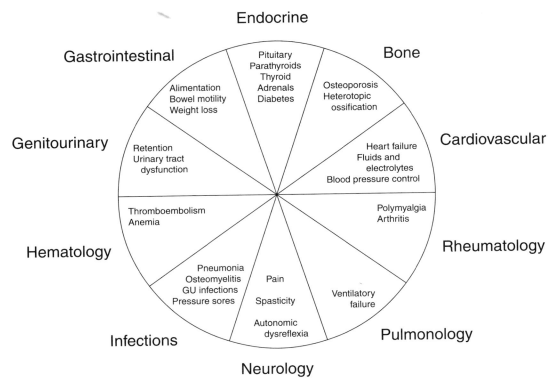

Figure 1. The scope of the medical problems of chronically disabled patients that are addressed in this book.

tise has taught us much about the management of disabled patients. Last, I acknowledge my wife, Theodora, without whose inspiration and encouragement this project could not have been brought to fruition.

David Green

Part I

Renal and Cardiovascular Disorders

Chapter 1

Disorders of Body Fluids and Electrolytes

Elliot J. Roth and Frank A. Krumlovsky

The physiologic mechanisms that normally function to maintain the homeostasis of body fluids and electrolytes in able-bodied persons often are absent or altered in persons with chronic disability. A number of pathogenetic factors may contribute to these metabolic abnormalities in this patient group. Mechanical effects, humoral responses, and autonomic alterations, resulting from several conditions, including prolonged recumbency, muscle paralysis, and neurogenic dysfunction, can predispose persons with chronic disease or disability to fluid shifts and electrolyte imbalances. The clinical implications of these disorders are variable. Although some patients may be asymptomatic, common manifestations of fluid and electrolyte abnormalities include chronic dependent edema, dehydration, orthostatic hypotension, and chronic renal failure. Hyponatremia, hypernatremia, metabolic acidosis, and metabolic alkalosis also are frequent clinical problems. These disorders and other effects of abnormal handling of body water and salt occur frequently in certain chronically disabled groups. By impeding rehabilitation efforts, limiting functional capabilities, and adversely affecting quality of life, these clinical problems often serve to complicate further an already difficult living situation imposed by the disabling condition.

Unfortunately, studies of fluid and electrolyte responses to disabling illness and injury are few and limited in scope. Most experiments have focused primarily on the direct effects of a few specific clinical conditions: prolonged immobilization, spinal cord injury, acute brain injury, and stroke. Although

it is likely that other disabling conditions affect the body's handling of fluid and electrolytes, reports of the effects of these diseases are sparse. However, generalizations based on the application of physiologic and pathophysiologic processes, as well as empirical findings derived from investigation of immobilized and paralyzed persons, provide a basis for understanding some of the metabolic effects of chronic disability and their methods of management.

Overview of Fluid and Electrolyte Disorders

Disorders of Serum Sodium

Hyponatremia

Hyponatremia [1] can be defined as a serum sodium below 135 mEq/liter. Hyponatremia is best classified clinically into dilutional hyponatremia (excess total body water with total body sodium level normal or increased), depletional hyponatremia (absolute total body sodium and water depletion), syndrome of inappropriate antidiuretic hormone secretion (SIADH), and factitious hyponatremia.

Pathophysiology
DILUTIONAL HYPONATREMIA. In an adult with normal renal function, approximately 150 liters of glomerular filtrate is formed every 24 hours. Normally, approximately 60% of this filtrate is reabsorbed isosmotically in the proximal convoluted tubule. The remainder is delivered to Henle's loop.

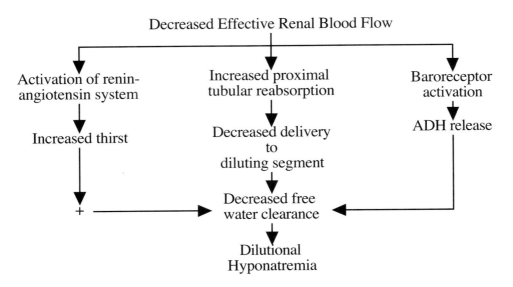

Figure 1-1. Pathophysiology of dilutional hyponatremia.

As filtrate traverses the ascending limb of Henle's loop and the cortical diluting segment of the nephron, salt is actively reabsorbed but water is not, leading to progressive dilution of the urine. By the time the urine leaves the cortical diluting segment, it is maximally dilute, with a osmolality of approximately 50 mOsm/kg. The remainder of the nephron is impermeable to water in the absence of antidiuretic hormone (ADH). A normal adult can excrete a maximum of 10–15% of the glomerular filtration rate in the form of dilute urine, representing a normal free water excretion capacity of 15–20 liters per 24 hours. It would thus be extremely rare to develop hyponatremia solely as a consequence of excess water ingestion. For dilutional hyponatremia to develop, one or more of the following renal abnormalities will usually be present:

1. Reduced glomerular filtration rate.
2. Increased isosmotic proximal tubular reabsorption of salt and water. Either reduced glomerular filtration rate or increased proximal tubular reabsorption will decrease delivery of filtrate to the diluting segment of the nephron.
3. Impairment of salt reabsorption in the cortical diluting segment.

4. Increased levels of ADH, resulting in excessive reabsorption of free water.

Precise regulation of plasma levels of ADH is necessary to regulate urine osmolality, maintain body fluid balance, and prevent dilutional hyponatremia. Normally, plasma osmolality is precisely maintained between 280 and 290 mOsm/kg. Secretion of ADH is almost totally suppressed at serum osmolalities below 280 mOsm/kg, resulting in maximal urinary dilution. When plasma osmolality increases above 280 mOsm/kg, secretion of ADH increases rapidly in a linear manner. At a serum osmolality of 290 mOsm/kg, a high level of ADH is present, which results in near maximal urinary concentration. ADH release is also controlled by baroreceptors located in the left atrium, aortic arch, and carotid sinus. These baroreceptors respond to changes in extracellular fluid volume. An important point to remember is that baroreceptor response will generally predominate over osmoreceptor response.

Dilutional hyponatremia (Figure 1-1) is seen primarily in association with decreased effective intravascular volume and decreased effective renal blood flow. In congestive heart failure, the most common cause of dilutional hyponatremia, the baroreceptors interpret low cardiac output as a sign of intravascular volume depletion. Low cardiac output also decreases effective renal blood flow. In patients with the nephrotic syndrome or hepatic failure, hypoalbuminemia also decreases effective intravascular volume and renal blood flow and stimulates baroreceptors. In all of these conditions, decreased effective renal blood flow results in both decreased formation of glomerular filtrate and increased proximal tubular reabsorption of filtrate. These cause a decrease in the delivery of filtrate to the diluting segment of the nephron, impairing the ability to excrete ingested free water. Concurrently, the increased baroreceptor stimulation results in increased release of ADH and a concentrated urine, which also impairs renal water excretion. This is considered "appropriate" release of ADH, because it occurs as a result of normal physiologic mechanisms, and is to be distinguished from the syndrome of inappropriate ADH secretion, which is discussed later. The decreased effective renal blood flow also stimulates the renin-angiotensin-aldosterone axis. The increased angiotensin production stimulates thirst, which in turn increases the free water intake. Thus, free water is ingested in excess of the kidneys' capacity to excrete it, resulting in a surplus of free water and dilutional hyponatremia. In the case of renal failure, the primary problem is decreased glomerular filtration. In conditions associated with severe dilutional hyponatremia, the maximal ability to excrete free water may be reduced to as little as 1 or 2 liters/day or even less. It is easy to see how these patients may develop dilutional hyponatremia with normal fluid intake, and why fluid restriction becomes such an important part of their management (Figure 1-1).

DEPLETIONAL HYPONATREMIA. Patients with depletional hyponatremia are depleted of total body salt and water, salt more than water, as a consequence of gastrointestinal or renal losses of both salt and water (Table 1-1). Gastrointestinal losses may be due to vomiting, diarrhea, nasogastric suction, or ileostomy losses. Renal losses are typically a consequence of adrenal insufficiency or a salt-wasting nephropathy. In addition to the actual salt and water losses from the gastrointestinal tract or kidneys, the associated intravascular hypovolemia again decreases effective renal blood flow, reduces the glomerular filtration rate, increases proximal tubular reabsorption, and decreases filtrate delivery to the diluting segment, resulting in decreased free water

Table 1-1. Causes of Depletional Hyponatremia

Gastrointestinal losses
  Diarrhea
  Vomiting
  Nasogastric suction
  Ileostomy
  Sequestration of sodium
    Peritonitis
    Pancreatitis
Renal losses
  Salt-wasting nephropathy
    Nonoliguric acute tubular necrosis
    Polyuric phase of acute tubular necrosis
    Postobstructive diuresis
    Chronic interstitial nephritis
  Diuretic administration
  Osmotic diuresis
    Hyperglycemia
    Mannitol
    Adrenal insufficiency
Skin losses
  Heat exposure
  Burns

excretion. The intravascular hypovolemia also stimulates baroreceptors and the renin-angiotensin-aldosterone axis, again impairing free water excretion and increasing thirst. Repletion of intravascular volume with normal saline will usually correct both the total body salt and water deficit as well as the pathophysiologic condition leading to ongoing free water retention.

SYNDROME OF INAPPROPRIATE ANTIDIURETIC HORMONE RELEASE. In the syndrome of inappropriate antidiuretic hormone release (SIADH), ADH release is inappropriate to both the volume and osmolar status of the patient. This process occurs in contradistinction to the "appropriate" release of ADH discussed previously, in which ADH is released in response to an appropriate baroreceptor stimulus. SIADH may be seen in a variety of clinical conditions, including intracranial pathologic states that affect the hypothalamic-pituitary axis regulating ADH release; malignancies that result in ectopic production of ADH-like hormones; pulmonary disease that may increase ADH production as a consequence of hypoxemia, hypercarbia, or reduced left atrial filling pressures; or as a consequence of use of a variety of drugs that either cause increased release of ADH (nicotine, morphine, bar-

Table 1-2. Syndrome of Inappropriate Antidiuretic Hormone Secretion

Disorders of central nervous system
  Head injury
  Brain tumors
  Meningitis
  Encephalitis
  Cerebral vascular accident
  Pain
  Schizophrenia or other psychoses
  Anxiety
  Brain abscess
  Guillain-Barré syndrome
Pulmonary diseases
  Carcinoma
  Pneumonia
  Emphysema
  Tuberculosis
  Respiratory failure
  Abscess
  Asthma
Malignancies
  Lymphoma
  Lung
  Others
Drugs
  Cyclophosphamide
  Vincristine
  Nonsteroidal anti-inflammatory drugs
  Chlorpropamide
  Tolbutamide
  Carbamazepine
  Oxytocin
  Clofibrate
  Colchicine
  Amitriptyline
  Thioridazine
  Nicotine
  Morphine
  Barbiturates
  Isoproterenol
  Sulfonylureas

biturates, vincristine, cyclophosphamide, clofibrate, isoproterenol) or potentiate its action on the kidney (chlorpropamide, cyclophosphamide, nonsteroidal anti-inflammatory drugs) (Table 1-2). In addition, inappropriate ADH release has been associated with hypothyroidism and glucocorticoid deficiency, as well as certain psychiatric disorders; mechanisms of SIADH in these conditions are poorly understood (see also Chapter 6).

FACTITIOUS HYPONATREMIA. Factitious hyponatremia, which can be defined as hyponatremia associated with normal serum osmolarity, may be due to one of two mechanisms. Pseudohyponatremia is seen in the face of severe hyperlipidemia or hyperproteinemia, such as in the presence of large quantities of paraproteins. In this condition, the volume of serum occupied by the lipids or proteins is so great that when a serum sample is analyzed, the sodium concentration per milliliter of serum is abnormal; however, the sodium concentration in the lipid-free or protein-free aqueous phase of serum would be entirely normal. In the case of hyperosmolar states, such as severe hyperglycemia or after mannitol, ethanol, ethylene glycol, or glycerine administration, the osmotic effect of the glucose or mannitol will pull free water from the intracellular to the extracellular space, thus diluting the serum sodium concentration by approximately 1.6 mEq/liter for each 100 mg/dl increase in serum glucose or mannitol concentration.

DIURETIC-ASSOCIATED HYPONATREMIA. Diuretic-associated hyponatremia is not a separate entity, but merely represents a combination of factors already discussed. Most patients receiving diuretics have either congestive heart failure, nephrotic syndrome, liver disease, or renal failure, conditions that produce hyponatremia independent of diuretic therapy by mechanisms already discussed. In addition, diuretics cause a modest initial natriuresis and diuresis, resulting in mild intravascular volume depletion. This hypovolemia may decrease glomerular filtration rate, increase proximal reabsorption, decrease distal tubular delivery, and lead to free water retention. The mild volume depletion also has the potential for baroreceptor stimulation, further increasing free water retention through nonosmolar stimulation of ADH secretion, as well as for stimulation of the renin-angiotensin-aldosterone axis, stimulating thirst. In addition, the natriuretic action of the diuretic itself may decrease sodium reabsorption in the diluting segment of the nephron, resulting in a primary impairment of diluting ability. This is especially true of the thiazide diuretics. In addition, the hypokalemia induced by diuretics may potentially shift sodium into cells, contributing to the hyponatremia. Finally, there is evidence that severe potassium depletion may increase the sensitivity of osmoreceptors, resulting in ADH release at inappropriately low osmolalities.

Diuretic-induced hyponatremia is seen most frequently in patients older than age 55 years, and it has been suggested that there is increased baroreceptor sensitivity with age, predisposing this population to hyponatremia on the basis of barore-ceptor-mediated ADH release.

RESET OSMOSTAT. Finally, the so-called reset os-mostat phenomenon should be mentioned. In some conditions, osmoreceptors appear to reset so that in-stead of maintaining plasma osmolality in the nor-mal range of 280–290 mOsm/kg, plasma osmolality may be maintained in a lower range, from 260–275 mOsm/kg, and plasma ADH responses to changes in plasma osmolality are reset to this lower set point. The mechanism of resetting is unknown. This condition is seen most frequently in severe ill-nesses, typically those associated with severe cachexia and malignancy, especially carcinoma of the lung. No therapy for this condition is required, because regulation remains intact and severe levels of hyponatremia typically do not occur.

Differential Diagnosis. A careful history is essen-tial, looking in particular for evidence of any of the conditions typically associated with dilutional hy-ponatremia (congestive heart failure, nephrotic syn-drome, diuretic administration, liver disease, or renal failure), depletional hyponatremia (vomiting, diarrhea, nasogastric suction, ileostomy losses, adrenal insufficiency, or salt wasting nephropathy), SIADH (central nervous system pathologic states, malignancy, pulmonary disease, or ingestion of any of the drugs associated with SIADH), and for evi-dence of severe hyperlipidemia, hyperproteinemia, or hyperglycemia, which may be associated with factitious hyponatremia.

Usually, however, the diagnosis of the type of hyponatremia can be made on physical examina-tion. In dilutional hyponatremia, even though the effective intravascular volume is reduced, there will be increased total body salt and water and in-creased total extracellular volume, manifested most typically by the presence of edema or ascites or pleural effusion, frequently associated with pul-monary rales or increased jugular venous disten-tion. These patients will thus usually appear "wet." In contrast, patients with depletional hyponatremia appear "dry"; they typically will not exhibit edema, ascites, pleural effusion, rales, or jugular venous distention, but rather dry mucous mem-

Table 1-3. Signs and Symptoms of Hyponatremia

Lethargy
Confusion
Personality changes
Irritability
Delirium
Seizures
Coma
Headache
Muscle weakness
Cramps
Nausea, vomiting
Asterixis
Myoclonus
Anorexia

branes, orthostatic hypotension, or orthostatic tachycardia, as well as an increased blood urea ni-trogen (BUN)-to-creatinine ratio, suggestive of volume depletion. Patients with SIADH typically appear euvolemic, with no evidence on physical examination of either volume excess or volume depletion. This is because these patients have in-trinsically normal hearts and kidneys, so that al-though the excess ADH initially promotes free water retention, they can "escape" from the fluid-retaining effect of ADH. This surplus fluid in-creases glomerular filtration rate, decreases proximal tubular reabsorption, increases delivery of filtrate to the diluting segment of the nephron, and results in an increased free water clearance that compensates for the increase in ADH present, resulting in a stabilization of fluid status only 1–2 kg above normal total body water, an excess unde-tectable on physical examination. Patients with factitious hyponatremia also appear euvolemic on physical examination.

Hyponatremia itself, independent of etiology, may be associated with characteristic signs and symptoms (Table 1-3). These are typically seen only with moderate to severe hyponatremia (serum sodium less than 130 mEq/liter). Laboratory exam-ination may be helpful in revealing the presence of hyperlipidemia or severe hyperglycemia, consistent with factitious hyponatremia. Laboratory evaluation may reveal a picture of hypokalemic hypochloremic metabolic alkalosis that would be typical of di-uretic-induced hyponatremia. An increased BUN-to-creatinine ratio may suggest dehydration and therefore depletional hyponatremia, although this picture may also be seen with the decreased effective intravascular volume associated with dilutional hyponatremia. The urine sodium value may be quite helpful; the urine sodium concentration will typically be low in dilutional hyponatremia, because of the decreased glomerular filtration rate, increased proximal tubular reabsorption, and increased distal tubular reabsorption of sodium resulting from the secondary hyperaldosteronism almost invariably present in this condition. This may be masked by concurrently administered diuretics, as well as by the presence of metabolic alkalosis, which tends to increase urine sodium concentration even in the face of intravascular volume depletion. A low urine chloride concentration is a useful clue to help detect the presence of intravascular hypovolemia associated with metabolic alkalosis. In depletional hyponatremia, the urine sodium may be high if salt-wasting nephropathy or adrenal insufficiency is present, but will be low, representing appropriate renal conservation, if gastrointestinal losses represent the etiologic factor.

Laboratory tests are perhaps most helpful in making the diagnosis of SIADH. In this condition, the urine osmolality will be inappropriately concentrated for the reduced serum osmolality and volume status of the patient. Typically, the urine osmolality will be greater than the serum osmolality, although any urine osmolality greater than maximally dilute urine (50–100 mOsm/kg) in the face of serum hypoosmolality is consistent with SIADH. In addition, the BUN will typically be low (less than 10 mg/dl) and the serum uric acid level will also typically be low (less than 5 mg/dl). This is because the increased effective intravascular volume associated with SIADH results in increased effective renal blood flow and a hypernormal glomerular filtration rate, resulting in increased renal clearance of urea, creatinine, and uric acid. Continued renal salt wasting is also typical of SIADH. In spite of severe hyponatremia, urine sodium concentration will typically be in the range of 70–80 mEq/liter. This renal salt wasting is again a consequence of increased effective intravascular volume, increased effective renal blood flow, decreased proximal tubular reabsorption of salt and water, and suppression of the renin-angiotensin-aldosterone axis because of the expanded intravascular volume; thus sodium re-

absorption is inhibited in both the proximal and distal tubules, and ongoing renal salt wasting will ensue. If there is uncertainty whether hyponatremia is depletional or caused by SIADH, the administration of 1.0–1.5 liters of normal saline solution may help clarify the issue. In depletional hyponatremia, urine sodium concentration typically will not increase significantly; in SIADH, the urine sodium concentration, elevated before the infusion, will usually double or triple within 1–2 hours after saline administration, reflecting the already expanded intravascular volume before saline administration.

Treatment. The underlying condition that has caused the hyponatremia should be addressed and corrected to the extent possible. The cornerstone of management of dilutional hyponatremia is restriction of free water intake. Because the primary defect of these patients is a limited ability to excrete free water, the hyponatremia can always be corrected by restricting free water intake to a quantity that the patient is capable of excreting. Sodium administration is almost always contraindicated in these patients, because total body sodium already is elevated, and additional sodium intake will only further expand the already increased extracellular fluid volume. If the serum sodium concentration is less than 115 mEq/liter or major neurologic manifestations of hyponatremia are present, and if the patient is not in pulmonary edema, cautious administration of 3% saline in small quantities accompanied by a furosemide diuresis should be attempted. Hypertonic saline should be administered only in sufficient quantity to raise the serum sodium value to a level of 118–120 mEq/liter. The use of angiotensin-converting enzyme inhibitors such as captopril or enalapril may be of particular benefit. By providing afterload reduction, they may increase cardiac output and increase effective renal blood flow, improving the ability of the kidneys to excrete free water. Also, these agents inhibit the synthesis of angiotensin II, which is a potent stimulator of thirst. Thus, the patients experience less thirst and are more readily able to limit their free water intake. The combination of angiotensin-converting enzyme inhibitor and a loop diuretic appears to be especially effective in the management of dilutional hyponatremia. Angiotensin-converting enzyme inhibitors must be used with particular caution and may be contraindicated in the presence of renal insufficiency, where their use may lead to a worsening of renal function as well as to the development of hyperkalemia. Patients with depletional hyponatremia may be effectively treated simply by administration of an isotonic saline solution.

Patients with SIADH present a unique therapeutic challenge. If the serum sodium value is greater than 115 mEq/liter and the patient is asymptomatic, SIADH is usually best managed simply with fluid restriction, initially placing the patient on a rigid limit of perhaps 800 ml per 24 hours; this may be liberalized as the serum sodium level improves. A serum sodium concentration below 115 mEq/liter or symptomatic hyponatremia (see Table 1-3) (especially central nervous system manifestations such as seizures, lethargy, confusion, irritability, and headache) represent medical emergencies requiring immediate therapy. Fluid restriction should be instituted, but faster acting measures must be implemented concurrently. Administration of 3% saline solution intravenously to correct the serum sodium to a level of approximately 118–120 mEq/liter is usually effective. Infusion at a rate of 50–100 ml/hour is usually optimal and seldom will more than 200–400 ml of 3% saline be required to correct the serum sodium concentration to a level of 118–120 mEq/liter or to control neurologic symptoms. Hypertonic saline may be combined with a loop diuretic, resulting in even more rapid correction. Extreme caution must be used to avoid correcting the hyponatremia too rapidly, because this may result in central pontine myelinolysis, a destruction of myelin in the central nervous system that may result in death. This seems to occur primarily when serum sodium is corrected at a rate more rapid than 0.5–1.0 mEq/liter per hour, or when it is corrected to normal levels too rapidly. On the other hand, if one delays excessively in correction of severe hyponatremia, the risk of ongoing seizures and irreversible central nervous system damage may increase. We advise correcting the serum sodium concentration to a level of approximately 120 mEq/liter at a rate no greater than 0.5–1.0 mEq/liter per hour using 3% saline solution with or without furosemide. Once the serum sodium has been corrected to this level, the risk of serious central nervous system manifestations is greatly reduced. The serum sodium concentration may then be corrected more gradually to a level of 130–135 mEq/liter over the next 48–72 hours by restricting free water intake (both oral and intravenous).

Long-term management of SIADH may present a problem if it is not possible to effectively treat the primary underlying disorder. In such cases, therapy with demeclocycline in doses of 900–1,200 mg/day has been effective in some cases. However, this drug should be used with great caution or avoided in patients with known cardiac, hepatic, or renal disease.

Hypernatremia

Pathophysiology. Hypernatremia [1, 2] is most frequently the result of excessive losses of hypotonic fluids, occasionally from the gastrointestinal tract or skin, but most commonly via the kidneys. Diabetes insipidus, either central or nephrogenic, causes impaired renal concentrating ability, excessive free water losses, and hypernatremia. Drugs that interfere either with ADH release, such as phenytoin or ethanol, or with the renal response to ADH, such as demeclocycline, lithium, and amphotericin, may also cause excessive free water losses and hypernatremia. A solute diuresis, which may occur during diabetic ketoacidosis, during the recovery phase of acute tubular necrosis, after mannitol administration, or after relief of urinary tract obstruction, may cause urinary losses of water greater than salt and also result in hypernatremia. A patient who is deprived of access to free water may develop hypernatremia as a manifestation of severe dehydration, because there would be obligate urinary losses of water accompanying metabolic solutes.

Much more rarely, hypernatremia may be due to an excessive intake of sodium. This occurs most commonly via iatrogenic mechanisms such as administration of excessive amounts of sodium bicarbonate after cardiopulmonary resuscitation or via inappropriate administration of isotonic saline solution to patients excreting hypotonic urine.

Differential Diagnosis. The differential diagnosis of hypernatremia is usually not difficult if the pathophysiologic mechanisms of the disorder are kept in mind.

Treatment. If the patient is severely volume depleted, isotonic saline should be administered until evidence of overt circulatory insufficiency is eliminated. In patients who are severely hyperglycemic but without circulatory failure, fluids that contain some sodium, such as 0.45% normal saline, usually should be the initial intravenous fluid since correction of hyperglycemia will result in shifts of water back into the cells, potentially precipitating intravascular volume depletion.

In patients without evidence of circulatory insufficiency, the defect is one of free water loss, and thus administration of 5% dextrose in water or 5% dextrose in 0.2% or 0.45% normal saline is usually appropriate. Slow correction of the hypernatremia, with a goal of correcting 50% of the estimated free water deficit in the first 24 hours and the remainder over the succeeding 36 hours, is usually appropriate. Excessively rapid administration of free water and rapid correction of hypernatremia may be associated with a worsening neurologic status and seizures as a result of cerebral edema. This is believed to be caused by generation of so-called idiogenic osmols within the central nervous system in response to prolonged hyperosmolality, causing cerebral edema as free water is administered. To prevent this, slow correction of the hypernatremia is preferable, permitting time for dissipation of the idiogenic osmols.

Acute Renal Failure

Acute renal failure [3, 4] is best defined as an abrupt decline in the pre-existing level of renal function. Acute renal failure may develop in patients with normal renal function or in those with pre-existing chronic renal disease. Any increase in the rate of decline of renal function in a patient with known chronic renal disease should prompt a search for acute factors that may be superimposed on the chronic underlying disease.

Acute renal failure may be anuric, oliguric, or nonoliguric. A totally normal urine volume does not exclude the presence of acute renal failure.

Acute renal failure is best classified into three major categories: prerenal, postrenal, and intrarenal (Table 1-4). Prerenal failure is caused by renal hypoperfusion. Postrenal acute renal failure is caused by obstruction anywhere along the urinary tract. Intrarenal causes of acute renal failure may be subdivided into glomerular, vascular, and tubulointerstitial; the latter may be further subdivided into acute tubular necrosis (ischemic or nephrotoxic) and acute interstitial nephritis.

Pathophysiology

Prerenal acute renal failure is due entirely to renal hypoperfusion. If renal perfusion is restored, renal function will immediately return to its previous baseline level. There is no anatomic or histologic abnormality of the kidney itself in prerenal azotemia.

Postrenal azotemia is caused by obstruction of the urinary tract anywhere along its course. If obstruction is brief (hours to days), renal function may revert to the previous baseline level after relief of obstruction. If obstruction is prolonged, irreversible renal damage may occur.

There is a continuous spectrum between prerenal azotemia and ischemic acute tubular necrosis (ATN). Any condition that causes renal hypoperfusion may progress to ischemic ATN. Whether a given insult so progresses depends on the severity and duration of the insult and varies from patient to patient. It is this potential progression from totally reversible prerenal azotemia to potential irreversible ischemic ATN that makes it so important to identify and attempt to reverse potential etiologic factors as rapidly as possible, before this progression can occur.

Nephrotoxic ATN may be caused by a large variety of agents (Table 1-4). Iodinated contrast media are a common cause of nephrotoxic ATN. Exposure to these agents may occur as a result of computed tomographic scans, angiography, or intravenous pyelography. Risk of contrast nephrotoxicity is increased in states of intravascular volume depletion, pre-existing renal insufficiency, or with exposure to multiple sequential studies. Other risk factors predisposing a patient to contrast nephropathy include diabetes mellitus, especially diabetes with pre-existing renal insufficiency, multiple myeloma, and increased age.

Nephrotoxicity from aminoglycoside antibiotics is dose related, and toxicity can be minimized by careful monitoring of blood levels. Nephrotoxicity due to amphotericin B is cumulatively dose related.

Acute interstitial nephritis has been described in association with a large number of drugs (Table 1-4). In contrast to nephrotoxic ATN, acute interstitial nephritis is not dose related, but rather represents an allergic or hypersensitivity reaction. Thus, even exposure to small doses of drug over a relatively short period of time may result in acute interstitial nephritis.

Nonsteroidal anti-inflammatory drugs may cause acute renal failure, both by causing acute al-

Table 1-4. Classification of Acute Renal Failure

Prerenal
  Intravascular volume depletion
    Gastrointestinal losses
      Vomiting
      Diarrhea
      Nasogastric suction
      Ileostomy
    Renal losses
      Osmotic diuresis
        Hyperglycemia
        Mannitol
      Diuretic administration
      Postobstructive diuresis
      Polyuric phase of acute tubular necrosis
      Chronic interstitial nephritis
    Adrenal insufficiency
    Skin losses
      Burns
      Diaphoresis
    Hypoalbuminemia
    Hemorrhage
    Anaphylaxis
    Sepsis
    Anesthesia
    Antihypertensive medications
    Third spacing
      Ascites
      Peritonitis
      Pancreatitis
      Burns
      Tissue traumas
      Ischemic limb
      Mesenteric ischemia
  Decreased cardiac output
    Congestive heart failure
    Constrictive pericarditis
    Cardiomyopathy
    Pulmonary embolus
  Renal vascular disease
    Renal artery stenosis
    Renal artery emboli
    Atheroemboli
    Systemic vasculitis
Postrenal (obstructive)
  Urethral
    Prostatic hypertrophy or malignancy
    Urethral stricture
    Cervical carcinoma
  Bladder
    Tumor
    Neurogenic bladder
  Ureteral
    Stones
    Tumor
    Stricture

    Blood clots
    Sloughed papilla
    Uric acid crystals
    Retroperitoneal fibrosis
    Inadvertent surgical ligation
Intrarenal
  Glomerular, vascular
    Glomerulonephritis
    Bacterial endocarditis
    Systemic vasculitis
    Scleroderma
    Atheroemboli
    Malignant hypertension
    Thrombotic thrombocytopenia purpura
    Hemolytic-uremic syndrome
    Disseminated intravascular coagulation
    Systemic lupus erythematosis
    Hepatorenal syndrome
  Tubular (acute tubular necrosis)
    Ischemic
      Intravascular volume depletion
      Hypotension
    Toxins
      Drugs
        Iodinated contrast agents
        Antibiotics
          Aminoglycosides
          Amphotericin B
        Chemotherapeutic agents
          Cisplatin
          Methotrexate
          Streptozocin
        Anesthetic agents
          Methoxyflurane
          Enflurane
      Endogenous toxins
        Myoglobin
        Hemoglobin
        Myeloma light chains
        Urate nephropathy
        Hypercalcemia
      Exogenous toxins
        Carbon tetrachloride
        Ethylene glycol
        Tetrachloroethylene
        Mercury
        Arsenic
        Bismuth
        Cadmium
        Lead
        Paraquat
  Tubulointerstitial (acute interstitial nephritis)
    Nonsteroidal anti-inflammatory drugs
    Antibiotics
      Penicillins

Table 1-4. (*continued*)

    Cephalosporins
    Sulfonamides
    Rifampin
    Trimethoprim
    Polymyxin
  Diuretics
    Furosemide
    Thiazides
  Other drugs
    Allopurinol
    Cimetidine
    Phenytoin
    Carbamazepine
    Clofibrate
    Sulfinpyrazone
    Phenindione
  Systemic diseases
    Infectious mononucleosis
    Legionnaires' disease
    Toxoplasmosis
    Leptospirosis
    Measles
    Brucellosis
    Mucormycosis
    Syphilis

lergic interstitial nephritis and by a prerenal mechanism in which decreased synthesis of vasodilatory prostaglandins results in decreased effective renal blood flow. These agents also inhibit the renin-angiotensin-aldosterone axis and thus may cause hyporeninemic hypoaldosteronism with hyperkalemia and a picture analogous to type IV renal tubular acidosis. Patients with pre-existing renal hypoperfusion, such as in congestive heart failure, nephrotic syndrome, liver disease with ascites, chronic renal insufficiency, or systemic vasculitis, or patients receiving diuretics, are especially susceptible to acute renal failure from nonsteroidal anti-inflammatory drugs, because with pre-existing borderline renal perfusion, inhibition of synthesis of vasodilatory prostaglandins can result in a marked decrease in renal perfusion.

Diagnosis and Differential Diagnosis

Acute renal failure is best diagnosed by the detection of an acute increase in levels of BUN, creatinine, or both from pre-existing baseline levels. As noted previously, oliguria is an unreliable guide to the presence of acute renal failure. Even acute renal failure resulting from obstructive uropathy may present with entirely normal urine output, since the renal failure from incomplete obstruction reflects a decreased urinary concentration of waste products.

A careful history and physical examination focusing on the clinical conditions usually associated with prerenal, postrenal, and intrarenal causes of acute renal failure should be the initial step in evaluation. A careful review of exposure to drugs or toxins is also of critical importance, since, as noted previously, many cases of acute renal failure are drug-related.

In prerenal and postrenal azotemia, the urinalysis tends to be bland, although patients with some postrenal causes of acute renal failure may exhibit red blood cells or crystals in the urine. The presence of red blood cells or red blood cell casts suggests glomerulonephritis or vasculitis. The presence of white blood cells or white blood cell casts is most typical of acute interstitial nephritis. Urinary eosinophils are suggestive of drug-induced acute interstitial nephritis.

The urinary indices (Table 1-5) may be helpful in evaluation of acute renal failure. In patients with prerenal azotemia, the problem is renal hypoperfusion. Tubular function will be normal and will respond appropriately to renal hypoperfusion, resulting in a concentrated urine with low urine sodium concentration. Conversely, in ATN, tubular function is impaired, resulting in an isosmotic urine, with osmolality approaching serum osmolality, and a high urine sodium concentration. This is a result of renal salt wasting from tubular damage. In general, indices in acute glomerulonephritis or systemic vasculitis most closely resemble those of prerenal azotemia, and indices in obstructive uropathy most closely resemble those seen with ATN. However, in very early obstruction, indices may resemble those in prerenal azotemia.

The fractional excretion of sodium, defined as

$$\frac{\text{urine sodium/plasma sodium}}{\text{urine creatinine/plasma creatinine}} \times 100$$

may be especially helpful in differentiating prerenal azotemia from ATN. The fractional excretion of sodium will typically be less than 1% in prerenal

Table 1-5. Urinary Indices in Acute Renal Failure

Indices	Prerenal	Acute Tubular Necrosis
Urine sodium concentration (mEq/liter)	<30	>40
Urine osmolality	>400	<400
Fractional excretion of sodium	<1%	>1%
Urine: Plasma creatinine ratio	>40	<20
Urine: Plasma osmolality ratio	>1.2	<1.1
Blood urea nitrogen-to-creatinine ratio	>15:1	<15:1

azotemia and acute glomerulonephritis, and will typically be greater than 1% in ATN. Exceptions to this rule include contrast nephropathy and pigment nephropathy, which are both associated with low fractional excretion of sodium. Both urine sodium concentration and fractional excretion of sodium may be increased by diuretic therapy or by the presence of metabolic alkalosis, which obligates urinary sodium excretion. Conversely, the urine sodium and fractional excretion of sodium may be low, even in the presence of ATN, if there is a superimposed severe prerenal process concurrently present, such as hepatorenal syndrome or severe intravascular volume depletion. The urine chloride may be especially helpful in evaluating patients with metabolic alkalosis, since urine chloride will remain low in prerenal states even in the presence of metabolic alkalosis.

It is critical to rule out obstruction in any case of acute renal failure in which the cause is not immediately clear or that does not resolve after a few days of appropriate intervention. As noted previously, oliguria need not occur in acute renal failure secondary to obstructive uropathy. All patients with acute renal failure in which the cause is not immediately obvious or that does not promptly reverse with appropriate therapy, should first have a urethral catheter inserted to rule out lower tract obstruction. If obstruction is not present, a renal ultrasound study should be done promptly. This is a noninvasive and highly sensitive test for urinary tract obstruction. False-negative studies may occasionally be seen if ultrasound examination is done early in the course of obstruction or occasionally in the presence of infiltrative or fibrotic renal disease. If the initial ultrasound result is negative, and suspicion of obstruction persists, a repeat ultrasound examination should be done a few days later. If the result is still negative and suspicion of obstruction is

strong, antegrade or retrograde pyelography should be performed.

Acute interstitial nephritis is classically associated with allergic manifestations such as fever, rash, eosinophilia, arthralgias, and eosinophiliuria. Presence of any of these findings in a patient with acute renal failure who is taking a drug that may be associated with acute interstitial nephritis usually is sufficient reason to stop administration of that drug immediately. Unfortunately, drug-induced acute interstitial nephritis may and frequently does occur in the absence of any or all of these manifestations. Thus, a high index of suspicion must be maintained, and if a patient develops acute renal failure without a clearly evident cause, serious consideration must be given to immediate withdrawal of all drugs that may potentially cause this entity and replacement with alternate agents as appropriate. The acute interstitial nephritis secondary to nonsteroidal anti-inflammatory drugs is atypical in that it usually is not associated with fever, rash, arthralgias, eosinophilia, or eosinophiliuria, but frequently is associated with the nephrotic syndrome.

Prevention and Treatment

Prophylactic measures may prevent some forms of acute renal failure. Patients scheduled to receive iodinated contrast material should be aggressively hydrated, as their volume and cardiovascular status permit, beginning the evening before the study. We routinely administer 5% dextrose in 0.45% normal saline at the rate of 100 ml/hour, beginning the evening before the study and continuing until the evening after the study. If metabolic acidosis is present, we administer 5% dextrose in 0.2% normal saline with 50 mEq sodium bicarbonate per liter added at the same rate. If the patient is volume depleted, a higher rate of infusion may be necessary, and conversely in the face of volume overload or congestive heart failure, a reduced rate of fluid administration may be required. If the patient can take adequate fluid by mouth, this may be a satisfactory substitute, although we favor intravenous hydration in all high-risk patients. Potassium may need to be added to the hydration fluid. All pre-existing volume depletion should be corrected before administration of the contrast medium, and the patient should be undergoing a solute diuresis at the time the contrast medium is given. Calcium channel blockers have recently been demonstrated to have a prophylactic benefit in the prevention of contrast nephropathy, and administration of a calcium channel blocker prior to contrast administration should be considered in high-risk patients in whom their use is not otherwise contraindicated. Dopaminergic doses of dopamine (1–2 μg/kg per minute) may also be of value in the prophylaxis of contrast nephropathy in high-risk nondiabetic patients.

Intravenous hydration with normal or 0.45% normal saline before each dose of amphotericin B appears to have a substantial prophylactic benefit. Hydration with or without mannitol may also be of prophylactic benefit in patients receiving cisplatin or with pigment nephropathy (acute hemoglobinuria or myoglobinuria). Pretreatment with hydration and mannitol may also be of benefit in patients subjected to a potential ischemic insult, such as a major surgical procedure. This is especially true for high-risk patients (elderly, diabetic, or with pre-existing renal insufficiency).

In patients with prerenal azotemia, every effort should be made to correct the etiologic factors as rapidly as possible to prevent progression to ischemic ATN. Prompt intravascular volume repletion is essential. If the patient remains hypotensive and continues to exhibit findings consistent with prerenal azotemia after appropriate measures to optimize intravascular volume status and cardiac output, introduction of dopaminergic doses of dopamine (1–2 μg/kg per minute) may improve renal perfusion to a more satisfactory level.

Administration of loop diuretics may convert oliguric acute renal failure to nonoliguric acute renal failure, but this has not been shown to speed recovery or to alter the ultimate outcome. These agents may facilitate management, because fluid and electrolyte management is easier in a nonoliguric patient than in an oliguric patient; however, care must be used to avoid administering these agents to patients who already have intravascular volume depletion, because this may worsen any element of prerenal azotemia that is already present. The combination of dopaminergic doses of dopamine with furosemide may be especially effective in inducing a diuresis, but again there is no clear evidence that this beneficially affects the ultimate outcome of the renal failure.

In patients with acute allergic interstitial nephritis, all drugs that can potentially be incriminated should be stopped immediately if possible. There is some evidence that acute administration of corticosteroids in the form of prednisone, 40–60 mg/day for 5–7 days, may hasten resolution of the process and may even improve the ultimate level of renal function achieved after recovery. If there is no contraindication to their use, we believe that this is a reasonable intervention.

Once acute renal failure has developed, its management is relatively straightforward. A loop diuretic may be used in an attempt to induce a diuresis and convert oliguric to nonoliguric renal failure. If reasonable doses (furosemide, 80–120 mg) have failed to produce a diuresis, we recommend withdrawal of these agents for 24 hours and then another trial, rather than continued administration. If the patient is oliguric, salt and water intake must be appropriately restricted. Hyperkalemia is a major risk in these patients and serum potassium must be closely monitored. Administration of exogenous potassium, either in the diet or intravenous fluids, should be avoided in most cases. If hyperkalemia develops, it should be treated at its early stages (i.e., when serum potassium value reaches approximately 5 mEq/liter) rather than waiting for more severe hyperkalemia to occur. Hyperkalemia can usually best be treated by administration of sodium polystyrene sulfonate (Kayexalate), either orally or rectally as needed. Acute hyperkalemia can also be treated by intravenous administration of 50–100 mEq sodium bicarbonate as well as by infusions of glucose and insulin (10 units of regular insulin together with 50 g intravenous glucose). The latter measures merely shift potassium from the extracellular to the intracellular spaces, but do not remove potassium from the body as does Kayexalate. If there are electrocardiographic conduction defects consistent with hyperkalemia (broadening of the QRS complex), the hyperkalemia can be treated with intravenous calcium gluconate, 10 ml of 10% solution, while other therapeutic measures are being instituted. Metabolic acidosis may develop as a consequence of acute renal failure and can be treated with intravenous administration of sodium bicarbonate as volume and cardiovascular status permit.

Patients with acute renal failure are at high risk for the development of gastrointestinal bleeding and infection. Histamine receptor blockers or aluminum hydroxide prophylaxis against peptic ulcer disease may be appropriate. Foley catheters should not be left in place in patients who are severely oliguric or anuric, because they then become a source of infection. Nutritional support is extremely important in acute renal failure because these patients are frequently postoperative or septic and thus highly catabolic (see Chapter 7). Enteral or parenteral nutrition may be indicated as appropriate. Obviously, particularly careful attention must be given to fluid, electrolyte, and acid-base status when undertaking nutritional support in patients with renal failure.

Patients who develop hyperkalemia, volume overload, or metabolic acidosis unresponsive to conservative management outlined previously, or who develop a pericardial friction rub consistent with uremic pericarditis, or in whom the BUN level increases above 100 mg/dl, should be promptly referred for consideration of institution of dialysis.

It is important that appropriate dosage adjustments be made in all drugs administered to patients with renal failure. A comprehensive review of dosage adjustments appropriate in renal failure is readily available [5].

Acid-Base Abnormalities

Pathophysiology

There are four major primary acid-base disturbances [6]: metabolic acidosis, metabolic alkalosis, respiratory acidosis, and respiratory alkalosis. The focus of this chapter is on the metabolic disorders; respiratory disorders are addressed in Chapter 17 of this text.

Acid-base disorders may occur as either simple disorders, with appropriate compensation, or mixed disorders, in which compensation is inappropriate, indicating the presence of a second or even third primary disorder. Normally metabolic acidosis is compensated by hyperventilation and consequent hypocarbia (respiratory alkalosis), metabolic alkalosis by hypoventilation and hypercarbia (respiratory

Table 1-6. Causes of Metabolic Acidosis

Normal anion gap (hyperchloremic)
  Loss of bicarbonate
    Renal losses
      Proximal renal tubular acidosis (type II)
      Acetazolamide (Diamox)
    Extrarenal losses
      Diarrhea
      Ureterosigmoidostomy
  Addition or retention of hydrogen ion
    Distal renal tubular acidosis (type I)
    Type IV renal tubular acidosis (hyporeninemic hypoaldosteronism)
    Ammonium chloride administration
High anion gap
  Diabetic ketoacidosis
  Lactic acidosis
  Alcoholic ketoacidosis
  Starvation ketosis
  Exogenous toxins
    Salicylates
    Methanol
    Ethylene glycol
    Paraldehyde
  Renal failure

acidosis), respiratory acidosis by renal generation of a metabolic alkalosis, and respiratory alkalosis by renal generation of a metabolic acidosis. If compensation is inappropriate, this defines the presence of a primary disorder of the compensating mechanism as well.

Differential Diagnosis

Metabolic Acidosis. Metabolic acidosis is best approached by first determining the anion gap (serum sodium – [chloride + bicarbonate]). The anion gap is normally 10–12 mEq/liter and normally includes phosphates, sulfates, proteins, and organic anions. If the anion gap is increased in the presence of metabolic acidosis, this provides a major clue to the cause of the acidosis (Table 1-6). If high anion gap metabolic acidosis is identified, determination of the nature of the unmeasured anion will in almost all cases provide the diagnosis of the cause of the acidosis.

Normal anion gap (hyperchloremic) metabolic acidosis on the other hand is normally caused by loss of bicarbonate or addition of hydrogen ion, neither of which affect the anion gap (Table 1-6).

Table 1-7. Causes of Metabolic Alkalosis

Loss of hydrogen ion
  Renal
    Diuretics (loop diuretics; thiazides)
    Mineralocorticoid excess
      Cushing's syndrome
      Primary hyperaldosteronism
      Licorice ingestion
    Bartter's syndrome
    Posthypercapnia
    Hypokalemia
  Gastrointestinal
    Vomiting
    Nasogastric suction
Gain of bicarbonate
  Sodium bicarbonate administration
  Postlactic acidosis
  Postketoacidosis
  Acetate administration
  Citrate administration
Contraction alkalosis

Metabolic Alkalosis. When considering the diagnosis of metabolic alkalosis, it is important to identify mechanisms that have generated the alkalosis and then mechanisms that are maintaining the alkalosis, because metabolic alkalosis may persist long after mechanisms that have generated it have ceased to operate or have been corrected, owing to the body's inability to eliminate the retained bicarbonate.

Metabolic alkalosis is generated in a manner analogous to a mirror image of normal anion gap metabolic acidosis, by loss of hydrogen ion or gain of bicarbonate (Table 1-7). Loss of hydrogen ion may occur from the gastrointestinal tract (in particular, loss of gastric contents by vomiting or nasogastric suction) or from the kidney, via diuretic administration (loop diuretics or thiazides) or in the presence of hypermineralocorticoid states such as hyperaldosteronism and Cushing's syndrome. Metabolic alkalosis may also be generated via gain of exogenous base, in particular by sodium bicarbonate administration, as well as lactate, acetate, or citrate administration or accumulation, all of which may be readily metabolized to bicarbonate.

Once generated, metabolic alkalosis is maintained by the presence of intravascular hypovolemia, hypochloremia, hypokalemia, hypercarbia, or renal failure. All of these mechanisms interfere with renal excretion of the excess bicarbonate. In the case of renal failure, glomerular filtration rate is reduced and the kidneys' ability to filter and eliminate excess bicarbonate is impaired. In the presence of intravascular hypovolemia, renal filtration of bicarbonate is impaired and proximal tubular reabsorption is increased. Also, secondary hyperaldosteronism will be present, so that any sodium reaching the distal tubule will tend to be exchanged for hydrogen ion, perpetuating the metabolic alkalosis. Hypochloremia is usually associated with hypovolemia, and this may be its major mechanism of maintaining metabolic alkalosis. Also, chloride is the only other readily reabsorbable anion besides bicarbonate, so that hypochloremia will tend to result in increased bicarbonate reabsorption. Hypokalemia facilitates proximal tubular bicarbonate reabsorption and also facilitates increased distal exchange of sodium for hydrogen ion in conditions associated with secondary hyperaldosteronism, such as volume depletion. Hypercarbia facilitates proximal tubular bicarbonate reabsorption. Any or all of these mechanisms may cause persistence (maintenance) of metabolic alkalosis.

Thus, we must first ask what generated the metabolic alkalosis, and then what is maintaining it. A careful history and physical examination accompanied by determination of serum electrolytes and arterial blood gases will usually permit ready determination both of factors that generated and that may be maintaining the metabolic alkalosis. Determination of the urine chloride concentration may be helpful. Most cases of metabolic alkalosis will be responsive to chloride and will be associated with a low urine chloride concentration, usually less than 10 mEq/liter. In patients with low urine chloride, the metabolic alkalosis is almost invariably maintained by a combination of hypovolemia and hypochloremia, and correction of the volume and chloride deficit with normal saline solution will generally permit renal bicarbonate excretion and correction of the alkalosis. If the urine chloride concentration is high, greater than 20 mEq/liter, this may indicate the presence of chloride-resistant metabolic alkalosis. This is typically caused by mineralocorticoid excess states such as primary hyperaldosteronism or Cushing's disease, or occasionally by Bartter's syndrome. These patients will not respond to volume or chloride repletion.

Treatment

Metabolic Acidosis. In patients with normal anion gap (hyperchloremic) metabolic acidosis, treatment is usually relatively simple. Patients with distal renal tubular acidosis require relatively small amounts of sodium bicarbonate, generally in the range of 1 mEq/kg per day to completely correct their acidosis and prevent major long-term side effects such as bone demineralization, renal stone formation, and possibly renal failure. In patients with proximal renal tubular acidosis, administration of larger amounts of sodium bicarbonate may be required, and even this will not normally fully correct the acidosis but may exacerbate renal potassium wasting and worsen hypokalemia; thus, only partial correction is generally attempted. In the case of gastrointestinal causes, therapy is generally either not required or readily accomplished with modest doses of bicarbonate.

Treatment of high anion gap metabolic acidosis, especially ketoacidosis and lactic acidosis is much more controversial, largely because ketones and lactate are ultimately metabolized to bicarbonate. Thus, aggressive initial attempts to treat the acidosis with bicarbonate may result in an overshoot alkalosis as ketones or lactate are subsequently metabolized to bicarbonate. Also, because of delayed equilibration between blood and the central nervous system, rapid correction of acidosis may result in a diminution of respiratory compensation while severe residual central nervous system acidosis persists.

On the other hand, not treating the acidosis also presents dangers. As the arterial pH decreases below 7.20, adverse cardiovascular effects occur, including arteriolar vasodilatation, hypotension, myocardial depression, and increased sensitization of the myocardium to arrhythmias. Also, as acidosis becomes severe, respiratory compensation reaches its physiologic limits, and a small further decrement in serum bicarbonate may result in a marked life-threatening decrease in pH, since further respiratory compensation is no longer possible. For these reasons, we recommend administration of sodium bicarbonate in quantities sufficient to raise the pH to a level of approximately 7.15–7.20. This reduces cardiovascular risks of severe acidosis, minimizes the risk of development of overshoot alkalosis, and provides sufficient buffering reserve to reduce the risk of a severe decrease in pH should respiratory compensation falter.

Metabolic Alkalosis. Initial treatment consists of identifying and attempting to remove factors that are responsible for generating or maintaining the metabolic alkalosis. In the great majority of cases the metabolic alkalosis will be chloride-dependent and thus can be readily corrected by administration of sodium chloride solution. This expands intravascular volume and facilitates renal bicarbonate excretion. Potassium chloride administration will almost invariably be required as well, because these patients are usually hypokalemic to begin with, and administration of large amounts of saline will increase renal potassium excretion. If saline administration is contraindicated, as for example in patients with congestive heart failure, renal bicarbonate excretion can be increased by administration of acetazolamide (Diamox), which blocks renal bicarbonate resorption and facilitates renal bicarbonate excretion.

In patients with chloride-resistant metabolic alkalosis, medical management usually includes administration of spironolactone (Aldactone) or triamterene. Sodium restriction also tends to reduce renal bicarbonate excretion in these patients. Supplemental potassium administration is usually also required.

In patients with severe metabolic alkalosis, especially if renal failure is present concurrently (thereby preventing ready renal bicarbonate excretion), the metabolic alkalosis may be treated more directly by intravenous administration of dilute hydrochloric acid solution or arginine hydrochloride, or by oral administration of ammonium chloride. These measures are seldom required.

In patients in whom vomiting or ongoing nasogastric suction cannot be readily eliminated, administration of H_2-receptor antagonists such as cimetidine or ranitidine reduces hydrogen ion losses and prevents further worsening of the metabolic alkalosis.

Fluid and Electrolyte Disorders in Specific Clinical Situations

Immobilization

Persons who have chronic disabilities frequently suffer the effects of prolonged immobilization and inactivity. These effects contribute further to the medical morbidity that complicates the natural history of the disabling illness. Chronically disabled persons may experience the complications of prolonged inactivity and bed rest either as a direct result of paralysis and the disabling condition itself, or because of the use of immobilization as a treatment modality. Regardless of its cause, recumbency alters the orientation of the body in relation to the direction of the pull of gravity. Together with inactivity, this postural change results in shifts of water and salt into, out of, and between the body space compartments.

The body's responses to bed rest were studied first by Campbell and Webster [7] in 1921 and by Cuthbertson [8] in 1929, and later by Dietrick et al. [9] in 1948 and by Taylor and associates [10] in 1949. These reports heralded the beginning of the modern era of immobilization studies. More than 160 clinical studies have been conducted since that time, documenting metabolic and physiologic responses to bed rest in almost 2,000 normal healthy volunteer subjects of both sexes, with a variety of ages, prestudy activity levels, and lifestyles [11–16]. Several excellent reviews exist that summarize the findings from these studies [16–19].

Many of the early studies were limited by their failure both to report specific details of their protocols for immobilization and to maintain appropriate bed rest consistently among all subjects throughout the entire course of the studies. Fortunately, the more recent investigations have addressed these deficiencies; they report specifically their methods, durations, and variables of study [11,14,16]. In general, these studies call for maintenance of the body in a horizontal position in bed without a break for days, weeks, or even months, with the maximum period of bed rest reported at over 7 months. Early studies allowed variable bathroom use, but recent investigations specifically deny use of the bathroom, even during the longer durations of recumbency. In most reports, the subjects are allowed to rise up only on one elbow to eat, and then only for a period of 20–30 minutes three times a day. By carefully controlling environmental conditions, these studies have yielded more reliable findings than otherwise would have been possible.

Pathophysiologic Mechanisms

Gravity forces fluids downward. Normal upright posture results in pooling of body fluids into the intravascular and interstitial spaces of the lower extremities. Assumption of the supine position, as occurs with bed rest, essentially causes withdrawal of the effects of gravity and results in a headward shift of body fluids.

This cephalad volume redistribution causes expansion of the central circulating blood volume, which in turn increases intrathoracic fluid pressure. Elevated central venous pressure stimulates three groups of specialized baroreceptors in the chest, which sense filling of the chest cavity, heart, and pulmonary and systemic arteries. The response of the system to stimulation of these receptors is both an inhibition of three major mechanisms—i.e., sympathetic nervous system, renin-angiotensin-aldosterone axis, and ADH release—and also an excitation of two other mechanisms—i.e., prostaglandin and natriuretic hormone synthesis and release. Suppression of ADH accompanied by activation of atrial natriuretic peptide release probably account for much of the observed natriuresis and diuresis [16, 20, 21].

The net consequence of these physiologic mechanisms is an early and striking diuresis, resulting in a reduction of blood volume [15, 22]. A natriuresis and subsequent loss of total body sodium generally accompany this loss of total body water. These mechanisms, shown schematically in Figure 1-2, help to explain the increased urinary excretion of water and salt that is a universal finding of studies conducted during the first few days of bed rest [16].

Alterations of Body Fluid Volumes

Total body water consists of intracellular and extracellular fluids. The normal volume of water in the average lean young adult man is approximately 42 liters, made up of approximately 23 liters (55%) intracellular fluid and approximately 19 liters (45%) extracellular fluid. The extracellular fluids consist of plasma (3 liters; 40 ml/kg; 7.5% of total body water), interstitial fluid (9 liters; 20% of total body water), and other fluids (7 liters; 17.5% of total body water) [23–26]. These volumes depend on the amount of body fat; obesity, advancing age, and female sex tend to reduce the amount of total body water.

The actual magnitudes of shifts in fluid volumes that occur with recumbency have been measured empirically at various stages of bed rest. On assumption of the horizontal position, an initial redis-

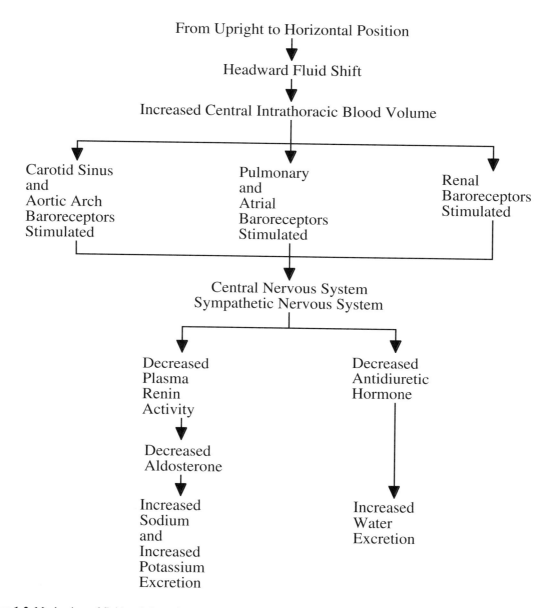

Figure 1-2. Mechanism of fluid and electrolyte regulation following position change to recumbency.

tribution occurs of approximately 500–700 ml of blood toward the head, resulting in an expected reduction of lower extremity fluid volume. Using tracer and isotope marker techniques, it has been shown that about one-half of the fluid that is transferred in the cephalad direction comes from the vascular spaces of the pelvis, thighs, and lower legs, with the remainder coming from the extravascular spaces [27]. As a consequence, the volume of the thighs and upper legs decreases by 6%, the volume of the lower legs by 5%, and the circumference of the calves by 3% [27, 28].

By elevating central venous pressure, this headward fluid shift sets into motion the mechanisms listed previously, resulting in diuresis. A hallmark of the physiologic responses to bed rest, this early loss of fluid causes a negative water balance. By the second day of bed rest, total body water decreases by about 600 ml [29]. Initially, both intracellular and extracellular volumes are affected, with extracellular losses accounting for the majority of the diuresis. By the fourth day of bed rest, extracellular volume has decreased by about 400 ml from baseline levels, with plasma volume reduced by about 440 ml [12]. By 12–14 days, total body water has decreased by about 1,480 ml. During this time, the extracellular fluid volume has returned to its normal baseline level, plasma volume is reduced by only about 500 ml (a value that is roughly similar to the plasma volume loss noted after only the first 4 days), and interstitial volume has increased by about 300–400 ml (an amount that is approximately equal to the decrease in plasma volume) [29–31].

The finding of reduced total body water in the presence of normal extracellular fluid volumes at the end of the second week suggests that most of the volume losses ultimately must have come from intracellular fluids. This demonstrates that homeostatic mechanisms serve to preserve extracellular fluid volume primarily, giving maintenance of extracellular fluids precedence over preservation of other fluid compartment volumes [27]. Because of the loss of plasma volume in the face of normal extracellular fluid volume, interstitial fluid appears to be the controlling factor, serving as a buffer by supplying the most readily available exchangeable fluids.

More studies have evaluated the magnitude and pattern of loss of plasma volume than of any other fluid variable. The diuresis of bed rest causes an early and rapid loss of plasma volume, even as early as the first day [15, 22]. In a series of elegantly designed investigations, Greenleaf and associates [27–33] found that plasma volume decreased by approximately 5–10% (150–300 ml) within the first 24 hours of horizontal bed rest, 15–20% over the first 2–4 weeks, and 30% if bed rest is maintained as long as 100–200 days [33]. Many other studies have confirmed these findings [31, 34–47]. By accumulating and analyzing serial plasma volume data among the multiple studies of bed rested subjects, Greenleaf and colleagues [31] were able to determine a mathematical model to estimate the amount of plasma volume loss at each day of bed rest as follows:

Plasma volume loss (ml) = (bed rest days/–0.11) + (–0.0013 × bed rest days)

Changes in cardiac stroke volume, and therefore cardiac output, parallel changes in fluid volumes. The initial headward movement of fluids on the assumption of bed rest causes an increase in intrathoracic volume, causing initial elevations in ventricular filling pressure, stroke volume, and cardiac output. As bed rest continues, the low pressure baroreceptors and volume receptors react by the several mechanisms noted previously to restore central volumes to normal levels via diuresis. These reflex changes tend to return stroke volume and cardiac output toward normal levels within the first 2 or 3 days following onset of bed rest. However, prolonged inactivity results in positional adaptations that cause continued decreases in stroke volume and cardiac output, eventually stabilizing at levels that are significantly lower than normal [16].

Electrolyte Changes

The initial diuresis of bed rest is associated with a natriuresis, resulting in marked losses of body sodium and a negative sodium balance during the first few days of recumbency. Increased urinary excretion of potassium becomes significant toward the end of the first week of bed rest and continues thereafter. Despite these changes in electrolyte excretion, plasma sodium and potassium concentrations generally remain unchanged, even with prolonged bed rest.

Hormonal Changes

There are prompt and sustained decreases in ADH concentration, plasma renin activity, and aldosterone concentration over the first 8 hours of enforced bed rest [48]. Plasma renin activity returns to normal by 24 hours, but aldosterone levels remain depressed. Beyond the first day of bed rest, plasma renin activity increases, probably as a response to continued sodium loss [30, 48–51]. However, there is an uncoupling of the effect of plasma renin activity on aldosterone concentration during bed rest, such that plasma aldosterone levels are either unchanged or decreased despite the presence of elevated plasma renin activity. Atrial natriuretic factor is increased in these patients, which may explain the failure of aldosterone to increase in proportion to the increase in renin. However, both plasma renin activity and aldosterone continue to respond appropriately to changes in volume. Additionally, the sensitivity of adrenal aldosterone secretion in response to adrenocorticotropin appears to be unchanged [48] and renal sensitivity in response to endogenously secreted aldosterone also is unchanged. Postural variation in aldosterone secretion is also retained. Normally, aldosterone secretion is three times lower at night during sleep (in the supine position) than during the day (in the upright position). However, during prolonged bed rest, nighttime secretion increases so that the differences between daytime and nighttime aldosterone secretion disappear [30]. Plasma aldosterone levels also vary with blood volume [52]. As central blood volume increases, aldosterone secretion is decreased by the low-pressure volume receptor reflex. However, these physiologic fluctuations of aldosterone secretion have little effect on sodium and potassium excretion among bed rested individuals.

Spinal Cord Injury

Spinal cord injuries, described as the most devastating calamity of human existence, occur with an incidence of 8,000–10,000 new injuries per year in the United States. With a prevalence of 200,000–400,000 persons with spinal cord injuries alive today in the United States, spinal cord injury is a major cause of chronic disability. Neuronal trauma causes not only motor and sensory disability, but also autonomic dysfunction and accompanying complications. The physiologic effects of prolonged bed rest and paralysis are compounded by both the loss of sympathetic control and the presence of neurohumoral alterations associated with spinal cord injury. As such, spinal cord injury serves as an excellent model to study the multiple physiologic mechanisms of water and salt handling in persons with paralysis. Important clinical phenomena include not only alterations in fluids and electrolytes, but also hormonal changes, dependent edema, and renal failure.

Body Fluid and Electrolyte Changes

As noted in noninjured immobilized subjects, there are strongly negative fluid balances during the first month after spinal cord injury [53]. Brown and associates [54] and Sitprija and associates [55] were among the first authors to report the appearance of "abnormal polyuria" among patients with spinal

cord injuries, especially those with cervical level injuries resulting in quadriplegia. More recent investigations [56–58] and extensive clinical experience have continued to verify the existence of this early diuresis. Kooner and colleagues [58] observed that quadriplegic subjects experience a diuresis during recumbency whereas paraplegic and nonparalyzed subjects do not. Upright tilt and long duration following injury may limit the fluid losses [59, 60].

Although serial evaluations have shown that fluid compartment volumes of quadriplegic subjects are generally within the normal range, there is a relative (less than 10%) increase in the extracellular fluid volume compared with the intracellular fluid volume [61]. Additionally, fluid balances in individuals with spinal cord injuries tend to be positive in the morning and negative at night [60]. These diurnal variations are similar to those for healthy subjects. In contrast, there is both a temporary deletion of daily rhythms of electrolyte excretion and a permanent deletion of the effect of posture on aldosterone excretion [62].

Immediately after the onset of spinal cord trauma, cell injury causes a loss of intracellular fluid and solute, resulting in relatively large urinary potassium excretion in the early stages [53, 63, 64]. As a consequence of this kaliuresis, there is a statistically significantly reduced exchangeable potassium level early and a relatively low or normal serum potassium level later. Urinary potassium excretion is greater in the early postinjury stages (less than 8 weeks) than in the chronic stages (over 8 months), but mean urinary potassium values have consistently been found to be within the normal range [53, 64–66].

Changes in sodium regulation are similar to those observed for potassium. In early spinal cord injury, there usually is a low normal serum sodium level [53, 64]. The initial muscle tissue injury is associated with a statistically significant elevation in exchangeable sodium, perhaps as a consequence of concurrent hyperaldosteronism. This sodium is probably stored in the relatively increased extracellular fluid space. In chronically injured patients (over 8 months), serum sodium is normal. Likewise, although urinary sodium excretion is at a level that is similar to control values, more sodium is excreted in the early stages (when serum sodium is in the low normal range) than in the later stages (when serum sodium is in the middle of the normal range) [53, 64–67].

To summarize the changes [68], it should be noted that paralysis generally leads to muscle tissue loss, and therefore to relatively high urine potassium in the early postinjury period. Ultimately, there is a decrease in exchangeable potassium and an increase in exchangeable sodium within the extracellular intravascular space. There also is a substantial increase in the volume of extracellular fluid containing the excess sodium. Although serum electrolytes may be normal [67], serial urinary electrolyte measurements may demonstrate changes over time, specifically in the excretion of sodium [69]. Homeostatic mechanisms act to maintain stable serum electrolyte levels by altering amounts of electrolytes excreted in the urine.

Management of fluid and potassium deficits in the early period following injury requires intensive therapy. Up to 300 mEq potassium may be required in a 24-hour period [56]. Appropriate fluid and electrolyte replacement regimens should be directed toward replacement of gastrointestinal, urinary, and insensible losses and should be adjusted according to results obtained during ongoing diagnostic monitoring of fluid and electrolyte levels.

Hormonal Changes

Removal of the descending inhibition of the sympathetic nervous system on the renal apparatus, which synthesizes and releases renin, causes sustained stimulation of renin release. Increased plasma renin activity ensues, stimulating angiotensin II formation, and thereby promoting synthesis of aldosterone. The effects of increased aldosterone are to promote sodium reabsorption and potassium excretion by the kidneys, both of which are observed in new quadriplegic patients. Moreover, the enhanced sodium reabsorption induces the water retention noted earlier [70].

Thus, multiple studies of plasma renin activity levels in quadriplegic subjects have found elevated values under a variety of conditions, including supine positioning [64, 71], head-up tilt positioning [57, 64, 71–74], wheelchair activity [64, 71, 72], sodium deprivation, and thiazide diuretic intake [64].

Likewise, aldosterone levels are elevated in quadriplegic subjects under a number of conditions, including during rest, tilt, wheelchair use [57, 64], thiazide diuretic intake [64], a cold pressor test [75], and daily stress [60, 62]. As a consequence of the effects of aldosterone on the kidneys' handling of salt and water, there is an initial low urinary sodium output [60, 61, 64, 65, 69], an increase in exchangeable body sodium, and a late increase in potassium excretion [71]. Results of multiple investigations of fluid, electrolyte, and hormonal alterations and their physiologic mechanisms in individuals with quadriplegia have been accumulated and summarized extensively by Claus-Walker and Halstead [68, 70], and this review should be consulted for additional background information on physiologic and metabolic changes in persons with spinal cord injuries.

Supine plasma renin activity levels have been found to range from 3.45 to 4.19 ng/ml per hour in quadriplegic patients, values that are significantly greater than the 1.04 ng/ml per hour recorded in healthy subjects [64]. Supine plasma aldosterone levels have been found to be 111–123 pg/ml in quadriplegic subjects, compared with 54 pg/ml in healthy control subjects [64]. Urinary aldosterone levels are also greater in quadriplegic persons than healthy control subjects [62]. The elevated values of plasma renin activity and aldosterone in quadriplegic patients have been confirmed in a number of studies [57, 62, 72]. An appreciation of the magnitude and rapidity of the increase in serum aldosterone is important because it illustrates that it is not only paralysis and prolonged recumbency that alter body water and salt in these patients [70], but also deafferentation of the regulatory system for fluids and electrolytes that contributes to the observed fluid and electrolyte changes.

In a study of one female patient by Claus-Walker and associates [64], for example, plasma renin activity was noted to increase during the first 5 days after injury, with most of that increase occurring within the first day after injury. In a more extensive investigation of 42 traumatic quadriplegic patients, Claus-Walker and associates [64] found that supine plasma renin activity and aldosterone levels were increased, the elevations in these values were greatest in the early postinjury stages, bed rest increased the levels more than did wheelchair activity, upright values were greater than supine values, and neither upright nor supine values of aldosterone or plasma renin activity were influenced by urinary output.

In a related investigation by Najenson and associates [74], individuals with spinal cord injuries demonstrated high plasma renin values, normal responses to changes in dietary sodium intake, and elevations in plasma renin activity following 45-degree upright tilt for quadriplegic patients, but not paraplegic patients. Similar findings have been noted by Mathias and coworkers [57, 58, 72].

The role of ADH in the regulation of blood pressure and fluid volume in quadriplegic subjects during head-up tilting has been the subject of some recent investigation. ADH has been found to be involved in the orthostatic reflex in animals [77–82], and Vallbona et al. [59] suggested that ADH release might be increased among quadriplegic persons in the head-up tilt position.

In a study of six quadriplegic subjects and six healthy control subjects, Sved and associates [83] found that quadriplegic patients experienced a four-fold increase in ADH during rapid tilt and a similar but less dramatic elevation in plasma ADH level after gradual tilt. In contrast, no change in ADH concentration occurred in normal subjects during either rapid or gradual tilt. These data suggest that ADH is actively involved in the maintenance of blood pressure for quadriplegic subjects in the head-up position. Because orthostatic hypotension, loss of vasomotor control, and lower extremity venous pooling in quadriplegic patients create a loss of effective blood volume, and because hypovolemia is a potent stimulus of ADH release [84, 85], the observations of both elevated ADH levels and enhanced responsiveness to ADH in quadriplegic patients [86, 87] are not surprising. Indeed, although basal levels of ADH in quadriplegic subjects may be normal [83, 88], this hormone may play a major role in fluid regulation in quadriplegic subjects when they assume the upright wheelchair sitting position. A recent study of hormonal changes in patients with spinal cord injuries by Naftchi [89] confirmed impairments in the hypothalamic-hypophyseal-sympathetic functioning.

Chronic Dependent Edema

Dependent edema is a common and clinically significant complication in patients with chronic disability secondary to spinal cord injury. Usually occurring in the lower extremities, the edema is relatively symmetric, tends to be most severe in the distal portion of the limbs, can occur in the upper extremities or trunk as well, and is most prominent in the dorsal surfaces of the lower and upper extremities (pretibial leg, dorsal foot, extensor forearm, and extensor hand). Ranging from mild swelling of small portions of limbs to massive edema with pitting present on deep finger palpation, the dependent edema probably results from prolonged sitting in an upright position with the lower extremities in a downward dependent position. For this reason, it is common not only among chronic spinal cord injured patients but also among individuals with other causes of paralysis or limb immobilization, including Guillain-Barré syndrome, multiple sclerosis, other neuromuscular diseases, orthopedic disorders, and autonomic dysfunction.

Unfortunately, reports in the medical literature of formal studies or even casual observation of the incidence, clinical characteristics, diagnostic features, pathophysiology, and treatment of this problem are extremely limited [90]. Nonetheless, the impact that this common problem may have on the medical or functional outcome and on the quality of life of paralyzed persons is great. Problems that may arise from lower extremity swelling include pressure sores, contractures, wheelchair seating challenges, practical difficulties experienced during shoe fitting, and unsightly appearance. Of course, other causes of lower extremity swelling, including deep venous thrombosis, heterotopic ossification, cellulitis, intramuscular hemorrhage, or other medical complications should be ruled out. Generally, however, the timing, symmetry, appearance, and clinical setting of these problems are different from those of dependent edema.

One of the causes of the swelling is the pooling of fluid and blood in the veins and interstitial spaces of the lower extremities, which are frequently placed in the dependent position by most paraplegic and quadriplegic persons. An additional factor is lower extremity muscle paralysis. The accompanying reduction of muscle pumping action causes a loss of the normal propulsion of fluid and blood in a cephalad direction against gravity. Finally, the loss of autonomic nervous system control over vascular smooth muscle tone and venous valve activity, which normally provide a continuous upward flow of blood and fluid, provides an additional etiologic factor for the genesis of dependent edema. In the absence of these normal mechanisms, the effects of gravity are to increase the net

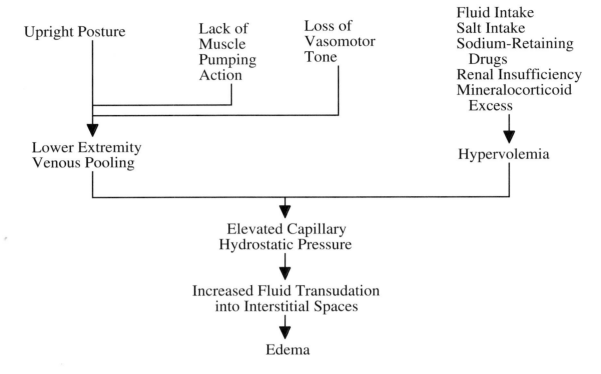

Figure 1-3. Mechanism of dependent edema formation.

flow of fluid downward. The results are venous and interstitial fluid pooling in the lower extremities, dependent edema, and enlarged lower extremity volume. The mechanism of edema formation is illustrated in Figure 1-3.

The best treatment of dependent edema is preventive in nature. Elevation of the lower extremities and avoidance of the dependent position as much as possible are advisable. This often requires the use of elevating leg rests attached to the wheelchair. Antiembolism stockings, such as TED Hose (Kendall Health Care Products, Mansfield, MA) or Jobst compression stockings (Jobst and Co., Toledo, OH) are useful to prevent soft tissue swelling of the lower extremities. Thigh-high stockings are most beneficial in reducing the amount of edema. Although knee-high stockings are often better tolerated by patients, they have the drawback that their elastic band may constrict and impair venous return. Regular use of appropriate stockings is important.

A salt-restricted diet may help to reduce the amount of fluid retention, and in rare instances of extremely severe and refractory edema, mild diuretics may be used. Special attention should be given to the possibility of electrolyte abnormality (e.g., hypokalemia and hyponatremia) secondary to diuretic use, and appropriate corrective measures should be taken in the event of such changes. Furthermore, the findings of the study by Claus-Walker and associates [64] should be borne in mind, demonstrating the metabolic effects of sodium restriction and thiazide diuretic use in quadriplegic patients. In that study, both treatments caused an inappropriately rapid and excessive diuresis, resulting in hemoconcentration, orthostatic intolerance, electrolyte imbalance, and excessive dehydration. Therefore, because of their potential risks, thiazide diuretic agents may be considered beneficial but should be used with extreme caution in quadriplegic persons with dependent edema and reserved for only severe situations.

Hyponatremia

Hyponatremia is not an uncommon problem among individuals with spinal cord injuries [91]. Usually it is relatively mild and of little clinical consequence. Frequently, the hyponatremia is caused by the greater retention of water compared with salt, resulting from enhanced ADH levels accompanied by ongoing free water intake after the initial diuresis. Sica and associates [92] have identified a deficiency of prostaglandin E_2 (PGE_2) excretion in some patients with spinal cord injuries. Because PGE_2 normally opposes ADH activity, a lack of PGE_2 in spinal cord–injured persons would cause increased fluid retention. In other patients with spinal cord injuries, concomitant head injury may cause SIADH. Medication use and fluid intake may be involved as well. It should be kept in mind that in most clinical settings, excessive free water intake remains the major cause of hyponatremia. Although the water ingestion may occur by oral intake, it is quite common among those patients who receive alternative forms of enteral feeding. The use of water to dilute nasogastric or gastrostomy tube feedings may cause the hyponatremia, and changing the diluting medium to saline may correct the problem.

In a recent study conducted by Peruzzi and colleagues at the Midwest Regional Spinal Cord Injury Care System [93], hyponatremia was found to occur in approximately one-third of 282 consecutive patients with acute traumatic spinal cord injuries. The incidence is greater than that in the general medical-surgical population of patients without spinal cord injuries. In the study, hyponatremia generally occurred within the first week after injury. Multiple logistic regression analysis demonstrated that completeness of injury was a highly significant predictor of hyponatremia, whereas level of injury was not; patients with complete sensorimotor spinal cord injury had a 62% incidence of hyponatremia, whereas incidence figures among those with incomplete sensory function, incomplete nonfunctional motor activity, incomplete functional motor activity, and neurologically intact patients were 48%, 41%, 23%, and 16%, respectively.

Another recent study [94] found that hyponatremia in patients with spinal cord injuries usually could be attributed to uncontrolled fluid intake in the presence of an acute or semiacute illness. Patients generally recovered uneventfully from their hyponatremic episodes.

Renal Failure in Spinal Cord Injury

Historically, renal failure was the most common cause of death among persons with spinal cord injuries. Even when nonfatal, renal disorders were major contributing factors to long-term morbidity in these patients. Recent advances in antibiotic use to treat urinary tract infections, institution of aggressive management of urinary tract stones, careful attention to urinary drainage methods to manage the neurogenic bladder, and rigorous and meticulous follow-up of the renal status after injury have decreased greatly the extent and severity with which renal failure alters the length and quality of life of persons with spinal cord injury.

Factors that contribute to the incidence of renal disease among patients with spinal cord injuries are chronic or recurrent urinary tract infections, urinary tract stones, chronic bladder retention, vesicoureteral reflux, chronic pyelonephritis, hydronephrosis, amyloidosis, and others. In a classic study by Dietrick and Russi [95], the autopsy results of 55 persons with traumatic and nontraumatic spinal cord injury were documented. The most common primary pathologic diagnosis at death was renal disease, which included infection, obstruction, and amyloidosis, and accounted for 20% of the deaths. In addition to the primary diagnosis, 90% had some genitourinary disorder.

Freed and coworkers [96] found a renal death incidence of 26% among their spinal cord injured patients. Nyquist and Bors [97] found that renal failure accounted for 33% of 258 deaths in their sample of 1,852 traumatic spinal cord–injured patients between 1946 and 1965, and that the incidence of renal deaths declined sharply in patients who survived 15 years or more after injury. Hackler [98] observed that 43% of individuals with spinal cord injury died of renal failure, and that the incidence of renal deaths decreased with increasing years postinjury. In a major series of long-term longitudinal studies, Geisler and colleagues [99, 100] found that renal failure caused 30% of deaths in 1977 and only 15% of deaths in 1983, representing a drop in rank order of frequency from first to fourth most common. Le and Price [101] also found that renal causes of death ranked fourth in another series of patients with spinal cord injury. Another more recent study [102] has verified that the incidence of renal disease is declining. It is reasonable to conjecture that closer attention to proper urinary drainage and routine follow-up of renal and bladder status might account for this favorable secular mortality trend.

Even when nonfatal, renal failure affects the nature of survival with a spinal cord injury. The advent of hemodialysis has extended the life of individuals with end-stage renal disease, including those who also have spinal cord injury. Although the incidence of treatable end-stage renal disease among patients with spinal cord injuries has not been clearly determined, estimates place the frequency at approximately one new end-stage renal disease patient per 2,000 patients with spinal cord injuries per year, or about four times the incidence in the general population [91, 103].

Mitchell [104] was among the first to report the use of hemodialysis in spinal cord–injured patients; since that time, numerous reports have appeared and extensive clinical experience has been accrued. These reports suggest that the patient with spinal cord injury with end-stage renal disease can be successfully managed by dialysis, with most patients achieving a level of function near that experienced before the onset of dialysis [91, 103, 105, 106]. Even peritoneal and home dialysis programs, despite their accompanying high frequencies of potential problems, such as peritonitis, atelectasis, and mechanical dialysis malfunction, may be used successfully in patients with spinal cord injuries, with acceptable complication rates and good control of uremia [91, 107, 108].

It should be noted, however, that there are some differences between spinal cord–injured patients on dialysis and ambulatory patients on dialysis. Prognosis differs between patients with spinal cord injuries and noninjured individuals on dialysis. Vaziri and associates [108–110] reported a 60% 1-year survival for patients with spinal cord injuries, compared with an 80% 1-year survival rate for patients without spinal cord injuries. Other studies [91, 103, 111] have confirmed these findings. Sepsis, other bacterial infections, and amyloidosis were the main causes of death among spinal cord–injured patients on dialysis, whereas cardiovascular diseases were the leading causes of mortality among patients without spinal injuries [91, 111–113].

Barton and coworkers [112] have described the renal pathologic entities found at autopsy of 21 patients with spinal cord injuries and end-stage renal disease. Chronic pyelonephritis was a common finding

in these patients and was found less frequently among control subjects. Amyloidosis occurred in 81% of patients with spinal cord injuries and 5% of the control subjects. The primary cause of death in the patients with spinal cord injuries on dialysis was gram-negative sepsis, present in 62%. In patients without spinal injuries, the primary cause of death was myocardial infarction. Other common findings present in patients with spinal cord injuries with end-stage renal disease include coronary atherosclerosis [114], elevated serum triglyceride levels, lower high-density lipoprotein levels [115], moderate to severe anemia [116], chronic active urinary tract infection [117], endocrine gland amyloidosis [118], gastrointestinal tract amyloidosis [119], and protein-calorie malnutrition [105]. Although not universally experienced, these problems can further complicate an already difficult course for patients with spinal cord injury.

Because the risk of renal diseases is great and their potential impact on morbidity and mortality after spinal cord injury is significant, it is essential that routine periodic assessment of renal function and urinary tract anatomy be performed [91, 120]. By carrying out urologic evaluation on a regular basis (usually yearly), kidney abnormalities may be recognized and treated early, potentially reversible destructive problems of the kidneys may be corrected, and further loss of renal function may be prevented. Usually, urinary tract ultrasonography is performed [121]. Intravenous pyelography is used less often today than in the past, but is still widely employed as a screening test. It carries the risk of contrast nephropathy, especially in the setting of intravascular volume depletion. Voiding cystourethrography and cystoscopy are used in many patients for better anatomic definition. Radioisotope studies, using iodine 131 orthoiodohippurate renal scintillation, can determine changes in renal function, as reflected by the estimated renal plasma flow [122]. Standard determinations of BUN, serum creatinine, and 24-hour urinary creatinine clearance may be performed, although serum creatinine is not sensitive and does not reflect accurately the changes in renal function in patients with spinal cord injuries [123, 124], and creatinine clearance formulas for normal persons are not applicable for these patients [105, 125, 126]. Two major clinically useful diagnostic tools for renal function follow-up are a high index of suspicion for renal abnormality and a rigorous disciplined approach to long-term monitoring of kidney function.

Head Trauma

Alterations of body fluids and electrolytes in patients who sustain disability from head trauma are similar to those that occur among patients with trauma elsewhere in the body [127]. Immediately after injury, there is retention of sodium and water and excretion of potassium. Proportionally more water than salt is retained, however, so that a mild hyponatremia to a level of 130–135 mEq/liter is common. It should be noted that despite this hyponatremia, total body sodium is not deficient or depleted; rather, there is actually salt retention. Aldosterone is responsible for the sodium retention and ADH for the water retention. The potassium loss observed in the early stages after injury results both from the effects of aldosterone and from the release of potassium from injured cells [128].

Steinbok and Thompson [129] studied a series of patients with head injuries and found an increase of blood osmolality on admission that paralleled blood alcohol levels. Both hyponatremia and hypernatremia occurred with approximately equal frequency. Electrolyte abnormalities were found in about one-third of patients whose head injuries were severe enough to cause loss of consciousness for 1 hour and in about two-thirds of patients whose head injuries were severe enough to cause loss of consciousness for 1 day.

Extreme hyponatremia in the patient with a head injury usually results from excessive fluid intake. In most clinical situations, restriction of fluid intake is adequate treatment [128]. However, some patients, especially those with basal skull fractures, are hyponatremic as a result of SIADH. Hyponatremia may also result from mechanical ventilation and from severe sepsis in these patients [128]. Hyponatremia may cause secondary damage to the already injured brain or contribute to misdiagnosis of an intracranial complication related to the head injury. Because severe hyponatremia can impair cerebral functioning, it may cause lethargy, stupor, coma, hallucinations, seizures, and other mental status changes that mimic the symptoms of the head trauma itself.

Hypernatremia usually results from inadequate fluid intake. A common clinical presentation is that of a brain-damaged patient who is conscious but confused, uncooperative, and combative, who refuses to or is unable to take adequate oral food or fluid, and who does not tolerate nasogastric feeding tubes. Another cause of hypernatremia in patients with head trauma is excessive use of osmotic diuretic agents for the control of elevated intracranial pressure [128]. Finally, approximately 1 in 200 patients with severe head trauma develops diabetes insipidus as a consequence of hypothalamic involvement by the original trauma. The lack of ADH in this syndrome causes excessive free water loss and therefore hypernatremia. Presenting signs and symptoms are usually transient, and consist of polyuria, polydipsia, and a persistent low urinary specific gravity. Occasionally, exogenous intranasal administration of ADH (desmopressin) is needed [128, 130].

Most of the alterations of body fluids and electrolytes that accompany head trauma are temporary and occur only during the acute phase of management. However, even individuals who sustain chronic disability from head trauma may experience these problems. Altered thirst mechanisms, prolonged reliance on gastric or nasogastric tube feedings, paralysis, recumbency, and neuroendocrine factors may contribute to long-term shifts in salt and water in these patients.

Stroke

One Japanese study of 196 patients with acute cerebral infarction and 56 patients with acute cerebral hemorrhage found that the incidence figures for hypernatremia, hyponatremia, hyperkalemia, and hypokalemia were higher in patients with hemorrhagic stroke (18%, 7%, 13%, and 14%, respectively) than in those with cerebral infarction (5%, 5%, 11%, and 6%, respectively) and were also higher in patients with cortical lesions than in those with deep cerebral strokes [131]. Among those with hemorrhagic strokes, location in the brain stem and large size of stroke were associated with an increased risk of hypernatremia. In addition, hypernatremia was found to be associated with a greater risk of early death.

Conclusion

A multiplicity of metabolic and endocrine changes occur among patients with various forms of disabling illnesses or injuries. Although some of the

Table 1-8. Summary of Fluid and Electrolyte Responses to Disabling Conditions

---

Effects of immobilization
  Early diuresis
  Natriuresis
  Decreased fluid volumes
    Total body water
    Intracellular fluid volume
    Plasma volume (5–10% day 1; 15–20% day 14;
      30% day 100)
  Early increase in ventricular filling and output
    volumes, later return to normal
  Decreased antidiuretic hormone levels
  Early suppression of plasma renin activity, later
    return to normal
  Persistent decrease in aldosterone
Effects of spinal cord injury
  Early diuresis
  Natriuresis
  Kaliuresis
  Early mild hyponatremia, later return to normal
  Mild increase in extracellular volume
  Increased exchangeable sodium
  Decreased exchangeable potassium
  Normal serum electrolyte concentrations
  Increased plasma renin activity
  Increased aldosterone
  Marked increase in antidiuretic hormone
  Dependent edema possible
  Chronic renal failure possible
Effects of head injury
  Water retention
  Mild salt retention
  Mild hyponatremia
  Kaliuresis
  Severe hyponatremia possible
  Syndrome of inappropriate antidiuretic hormone
    possible
  Diabetes insipidus possible
Effects of stroke
  Hypernatremia
  Hyponatremia
  Hyperkalemia
  Hypokalemia

---

problems are related to the primary disease process itself, other complications derive from the institution of certain treatment regimens (e.g., recumbency, erect posture, medications, fluid intake). A significant proportion of the changes in body fluids and electrolytes occur early after onset of the disability; diuresis and natriuresis [132], with relative

hyponatremia and hyperkalemia, are examples. However, other changes, including dehydration, hypernatremia, metabolic alkalosis or acidosis, dependent edema, and renal failure may occur at any time after onset of disease or disability and indeed are more common in the chronic phase. Knowledge of the mechanical and hormonal processes involved in fluid and salt regulation and an understanding of the pathophysiologic events that accompany disabling conditions are critical, both for determining the actual effects that these clinical problems will impose on chronically disabled individuals (Table 1-8) and for directing preventive and therapeutic interventions for these complications.

Case Management Study

Case Presentation

A 57-year-old man fell approximately 30 feet to the ground while at work on a construction project. He sustained a closed head injury with a subdural hematoma and multiple temporal contusions, as well as multiple rib fractures and internal injuries. He underwent evacuation of the subdural hematoma approximately 48 hours after his injury. Approximately 2 weeks after admission, his serum sodium was noted to be 132 mEq/liter, potassium was 4.2 mEq/liter, BUN was 8 mg/dl, creatinine was 0.8 mg/dl, and uric acid was 2.5 mg/dl. He was placed on carbamazepine as seizure prophylaxis and shortly thereafter was transferred to the Rehabilitation Institute of Chicago. Shortly after admission, his serum sodium was noted to be 128 mEq/liter and BUN was 7 mg/dl. Urine sodium was 65 mEq/liter and urine osmolality was 450 mOsm/liter. The patient was thought to have SIADH and was placed on mild fluid restriction, with an increase in his serum sodium to 134 mEq/liter.

The patient remained in stable condition for approximately 6 weeks, when he was noted to acutely develop a temperature of 104.4°F, a pulse of 130, respirations of 24, and blood pressure of 112/72. On examination, the neck veins were not distended and there was no edema. There were findings of consolidation in the right lower lobe, and a chest film revealed a right lower lobe pneumonitis. The patient was transferred to Northwestern Memorial Hospital for acute care. At the time of admission, the white blood count was 14,000, serum sodium was 118 mEq/liter, BUN was 10 mg/dl, uric acid was 3.5 mg/dl, and urine sodium was 70 mEq/liter. The patient appeared euvolemic on examination. The patient was started on appropriate antibiotics for his pneumonia and received aggressive hydration with normal and half normal saline because of his high fever and poor oral intake. Two days later, his serum sodium was noted to be 112 mEq/liter, and he was somewhat confused. At that point a diagnosis of SIADH was made, and he was started on fluid restriction. His serum sodium subsequently rose to 132, and his pneumonia resolved. His carbamazepine was subsequently discontinued, and his serum sodium rose further to 138 mEq/liter.

Case Discussion

This patient represents a classic case of SIADH. Several factors can be implicated in the etiology of the syndrome in this patient. Virtually any central nervous system pathologic state, including subdural hematoma and brain injury, in this case presumably related to his multiple temporal contusions, can be implicated in the etiology of his initial hyponatremia. A low serum sodium level in association with low BUN, creatinine, and uric acid levels, as well as high urine sodium concentration and high urine osmolality, are all classic for SIADH. The patient initially develops intravascular volume expansion as a result of excessive production of ADH. In patients with normal cardiac status, as in this patient, this will result in an increased cardiac output and increased renal perfusion with increased glomerular filtration rate. This in turn results in low to low normal values for BUN, creatinine, and uric acid. The urine sodium will tend to be high as a result of decreased proximal tubular resorption of sodium secondary to the renal hyperperfusion and to a suppression of aldosterone because of the intravascular hypervolemia. The patient will appear euvolemic because the increased renal perfusion and glomerular filtration rate will result in a partial escape from the salt- and water-retaining effects of inappropriate levels of ADH, so that clinical evidence of fluid overload, such as jugular venous distention and peripheral edema will not develop. The patient was subsequently begun on the carbamazepine, one of many drugs known to be associated with the development of SIADH.

Subsequently, the patient developed pneumonia. Virtually any pulmonary process, including pneumonia and atelectasis, can be associated with the development of SIADH. Thus, at the time of his admission to the acute care hospital, the patient had SIADH as a consequence of at least three potential causes, namely residual central nervous system scarring from his initial head trauma, effects of the carbamazepine, and his superimposed acute pneumonitis. Again, his low values of serum sodium, BUN, creatinine, and uric acid, in association with high urine sodium and urine osmolality, were a classic presentation for SIADH in a euvolemic patient. Unfortunately, this was not recognized and he was hydrated with fluids including half normal saline, which contains substantial amounts of free water. This resulted in a further decrease of his serum sodium to a level that may be associated with central nervous system manifestations. His SIADH was finally recognized and treated with fluid restriction. His pneumonia resolved and the carbamazepine was discontinued. His serum sodium rose to a stable level of 138mEq/liter, still somewhat low, probably as a result of residual mild SIADH from scarring related to his initial head trauma. His serum sodium could, however, at this point be well controlled simply with mild ongoing fluid restriction.

As stated in the text of the chapter, SIADH is usually associated with central nervous system pathologic states, malignancy, pulmonary pathologic entities, or one of a number of drugs. This patient illustrates three of the four primary causes of SIADH. SIADH can easily be distinguished from dilutional hyponatremia, in which case the patient almost always demonstrates evidence of volume overload in the form of edema, jugular venous distention, pleural effusion, rales, or ascites. Also, in dilutional hyponatremia, the BUN will generally be elevated or at the upper limits of normal, and the creatinine and uric acid levels will be normal to elevated. The urine sodium will generally be low. In depletional hyponatremia, the patient will generally appear volume depleted, with orthostatic hypotension or orthostatic tachycardia, flat neck veins, and no evidence of edema. The urine sodium will generally be low unless a salt-wasting nephropathy is present, in which case it may be elevated. These patients are usually best managed with administration of normal saline.

The treatment of SIADH generally involves restriction of free water intake and treatment of underlying etiologic conditions. In this case, treatment of the underlying pneumonia and removal of the offending drug carbamazepine resulted in substantial improvement. If the serum sodium is markedly reduced, usually below 116–118 mEq/liter, small amounts of 3% saline may be administered in conjunction with restriction of free water intake.

Serum sodium should not be allowed to increase at a rate faster than 0.5 mEq per hour, as this may result in central nervous system damage. Small amounts of furosemide may also be administered in conjunction with saline, as this will impair renal concentrating ability and facilitate free water excretion. Chronic SIADH, such as that caused by residual central nervous system injury, can generally be best managed with chronic mild fluid restriction. Chronic administration of demeclocycline may be indicated in such cases, but because of its potential toxicity this is generally best avoided if possible.

References

1. Robertson GL, Berl T. Pathophysiology of Water Metabolism. In BM Brenner (ed), The Kidney. Philadelphia: Saunders, 1996;898.
2. Palevsky PM, Bhagrath R, Greenberg A. Hypernatremia in hospitalized patients. Ann Intern Med 1996;124:197.
3. Brady HR, Brenner BM, Lieberthal W. Acute Renal Failure. In BM Brenner (ed), The Kidney. Philadelphia: Saunders, 1996;1200.
4. Davda RK, Guzman NJ. Acute renal failure. Postgrad Med 1994;96:89.
5. Bennett WM, Aronoff GR, Golper TA, et al. Drug Prescribing in Renal Failure. Philadelphia: American College of Physicians, 1987.
6. Du Bose TD Jr, Cogan MG, Rector FC Jr. Acid-Base Disorders. In BM Brenner (ed), The Kidney. Philadelphia: Saunders, 1996;929.
7. Campbell JA, Webster PA. Day and night urine during complete rest, laboratory routine, light muscular work and oxygen administration. Biochem J 1921;15:660.
8. Cuthbertson DP. The influence of prolonged muscular rest on metabolism. Biochem J 1929;23:1328.
9. Dietrick JR, Wheden GD, Shorr E. Effects of immobilization upon various metabolic and physiologic functions of normal man. Am J Med 1948;4:3.
10. Taylor HL, Henschel J, Brozek J, Keys A. Effects of bed rest on cardiovascular function and work performance. J Appl Physiol 1949;2:223.
11. Goldwater DJ, Convertino V, Sandler H. 1981 Preprint. Aerosp Med Assoc Preprints 1981;179.
12. Greenleaf JE, Kozlowki S. Physiological Consequences of Reduced Physical Activity During Bed Rest. In RA Terjung (ed), Exercise and Sport Sciences Review (Vol 10). Philadelphia: Franklin Institute Press, 1982;84.
13. Nicogossian AE, Sandler H, Whyte AA, et al. Chronological summaries of United States, European, and Soviet bed rest studies. NASA 1979;SP-377. Washington, DC: National Aeronautics and Space Administration, 1979.
14. Sandler H, Goldwater D, Rositano S, et al. 1979 Preprint. Aerosp Med Assoc Preprints 1979; 43.
15. Sandler H. Heart and Heart-like Organs (Vol 2). New York: Academic, 1980; 435.
16. Sandler H, Vernikos J (eds). Inactivity: Physiological Effects. Orlando: Academic, 1986.
17. Browse NL. The Physiology and Pathology of Bed Rest. Springfield, IL: Thomas, 1965.
18. Spencer WA, Vollbona C, Carter RE. Physiologic concepts of immobilization. Arch Phys Med Rehabil 1965;46:89.
19. Steinberg FU. The Immobilized Patient—Functional Pathology and Management. New York: Plenum, 1980.
20. Gauer OH, Henry JP, Behn C. The regulation of extracellular fluid volume. Ann Rev Physiol 1970;32:547.
21. Gauer OH, Henry JP. Neurohormonal Control of Plasma Volume. In AC Guyton, AW Crowley (eds), International Review of Physiology. Cardiovascular Physiology (Vol 9, Sect II). Baltimore: University Park Press, 1976;145.
22. Taylor HL, Erickson L, Henschel A, Kayes A. The effect of bed rest on the blood volume of normal young men. Am J Physiol 1945;144:227.
23. Gamble JL. Chemical Anatomy, Physiology and Pathology of Extracellular Fluid (7th ed). Cambridge: Harvard University Press, 1958.
24. Edelman IS, Leibman J. Anatomy of body water and electrolytes. Am J Med 1959;27:256.
25. Guyton AC. Textbook of Medical Physiology (5th ed). Philadelphia: Saunders, 1976.
26. Selkurt EE (ed). Physiology (4th ed). Boston: Little, Brown, 1976.
27. Greenleaf JE. Physiological responses to prolonged bed rest and fluid immersion in humans. J Appl Physiol 1984;57:619.
28. Blomquist CG, Nixon JV, Johnson RJ, Mitchell JH. Early cardiovascular adaptation to zero gravity simulated by head-down tilt. Acta Astronautica 1980;7:543.
29. Jacobson LB, Hyatt KH, Sullivan RW, et al. Evaluation of +GZ Tolerance Following Simulated Weightlessness (Bed Rest). NASA TMX-62311. Washington, DC: National Aeronautics and Space Administration, 1973;1.
30. Melada GA, Goldman RH, Luetscher JA, Zager PG. Hemodynamics, renal function, plasma renin, and aldosterone in man after 5 to 14 days of bed rest. Aviat Space Environ Med 1975;46:1049.

31. Greenleaf JE, Bernauer EM, Young HL, et al. Fluid and electrolyte shifts during bed rest with isometric and isotonic exercise. J Appl Physiol 1977;42:59.

32. Greenleaf JE, Silverstein L, Bliss J, et al. Physiological Responses to Prolonged Bed Rest in Man: A Compendium of Research. NASA TM-81324. Washington, DC: National Aeronautics and Space Administration, 1982.

33. Greenleaf JE. In J Garcia, M Guerin, C Laverlochere (eds), Space Physiology. Toulouse: Toulouse Cepaudes Edit., 1983;335.

34. Miller PB, Johnson RL, Lamb LE. Effects of four weeks of absolute bed rest on circulatory functions in man. Aerospace Med 1964;35:1194.

35. Stevens RM, Miller PB, Gilbert CA, et al. Influence of long-term lower body negative pressure on the circulatory functions of man during prolonged bed rest. Aerospace Med 1966;37:257.

36. Stevens RM, Lynch TN. Effects of 9-alpha fluorohydro-cortisone on dehydration due to prolonged bed rest. Aerospace Med 1966;37:1049.

37. Vogt FB, Mack PB, Johnson PC. Tilt table response and blood volume changes associated with thirty days of recumbency. Aerospace Med 1966;37:771.

38. Vogt FB, Mack PB, Johnson PC, Wade L. Tilt table response and blood volume changes associated with fourteen days of recumbency. Aerospace Med 1967;38:43.

39. White PD, Nyberg IW, Finney LM, White WJ. A Comparative Study of the Physiological Effects of Immersion and Bed Rest. Report DAC-59226. St. Louis: Douglas Aircraft Co., 1966.

40. Vogt FB, Johnson PC. Plasma volume and extracellular fluid volume change associated with 10 days of bed recumbency. Aerospace Med 1967;38:21.

41. Saltin B, Blomqvist G, Mitchell JH, et al. Response to exercise after bed rest and after training. Circulation 1968;38(Suppl 7):1.

42. Donaldson CL, Hulley SB, McMillan DE, et al. The Effects of Prolonged Simulated Non-gravitational Environment on Mineral Balance in the Adult Male. NASA Contract Reports 108314. Washington, DC: National Aeronautics and Space Administration, 1969.

43. Hyatt KH, Kamenetsky LG, Smith WM. Extravascular dehydration as an etiologic factor in post-recumbency orthostatism. Aerospace Med 1969;40:644.

44. Bohnn BJ, Hyatt KH, Kamenetsky LG, et al. Prevention of bedrest induced orthostatism by 9-alpha fluorohydrocortisone. Aerospace Med 1970;41:495.

45. Johnson PC, Driscoll TB, Carpentier WR. Vascular and extravascular fluid changes during six days of bedrest. Aerospace Med 1971;42:875.

46. Leach CS, Johnson PC, Driscoll TB. Effects of bedrest and centrifugation of humans on serum thyroid function tests. Aerospace Med 1972;43:400.

47. Jacobson LB, Hyatt KH, Sandler HA. Effects of simulated weightlessness on responses of untrained men to +GZ acceleration. J Appl Physiol 1974;36:745.

48. Dallman MF, Vernikos J, Keil LC. Hormonal, Fluid, and Electrolyte Responses to 6 Hours of Anti-orthostatic Bed Rest in Healthy Male Subjects. In E Usdin, J Kretansky, J Axelrod (eds), Stress: The Role of Catecholamines and Other Neurotransmitters (Vol II). London: Gordon and Beach, 1984.

49. Volicer L, Jean-Charles R, Chobianan AV. Effects of head-down tilt on fluid and electrolyte balance. Aviat Space Environ Med 1976;47:1065.

50. Chavarri M, Ganguly A, Luetscher JA, Zager PG. Effect of bed rest in circadian rhythms of plasma renin, aldosterone, and cortisol. Aviat Space Environ Med 1977;48:633.

51. Hargens AG, Tipton CM, Gollnick PD, et al. Fluid shifts and muscle function in humans during acute simulated weightlessness. J Appl Physiol 1983;54:1003.

52. Wolff H, Torbica M. Determination of plasma aldosterone. Lancet 1963;1:1346.

53. Claus-Walker J, Carter RE, DiFerrante NM, Singh J. Immediate endocrine and metabolic consequences of traumatic quadriplegia in a young woman. Paraplegia 1977–78;15:202.

54. Brown M, Pyzik S, Kinkle JR. Causes of polyuria and polydipsia in patients with injuries of the cervical spinal cord. Neurology 1959;9:877.

55. Sitprija V, Pochanugool C, Benyajati C, Suwanwela C. Polydipsia and polyuria associated with quadriplegia. Ann Intern Med 1966;65:62.

56. Burke DC, Murray DD. Handbook of Spinal Cord Medicine. New York: Raven, 1975.

57. Mathias CJ, Fosbraey P, De Costa DF, et al. The effect of desmopressin on nocturnal polyuria, overnight weight loss, and morning postural hypotension in patients with autonomic failure. BMJ 1986;293:353.

58. Kooner JS, Frankel HL, Mirando N, et al. Haemodynamic, hormonal and urinary responses to postural changes in tetraplegia and paraplegic man. Paraplegia 1988;26:233.

59. Vallbona C, Lipscomb HS, Carter RE. Endocrine responses to orthostatic hypotension in quadriplegia. Arch Phys Med Rehabil 1966;47:412.

60. Claus-Walker J, Vallbona C, Carter RE, Lipscomb HS. Resting and stimulated endocrine function in human subjects with cervical spinal cord transection. J Chronic Dis 1971;24:193.

61. Cardus D, Spencer WA, McTaggert WG. Study of Gross Composition of Body of Patients with Extensive Muscular Paralysis. Social and Rehabilitation Services Project RD 1871-M, Final Report. Houston: Baylor College of Medicine, 1969.

62. Claus-Walker J, Carter RE, Lipscomb HS, Vallbona C. Daily rhythms of electrolytes and aldosterone excretion in men with cervical spinal cord section. J Clin Endocrinol Metab 1969;29:300.

63. O'Connell FH, Gardner WJ. Metabolism in paraplegia. JAMA 1953;153:706.

64. Claus-Walker J, Spencer WA, Carter RE, Halstead LS. Electrolytes and renin-angiotensin-aldosterone axis in

traumatic quadriplegia. Arch Phys Med Rehabil 1977;58:283.

65. Cardus D, McTaggert WG. Total <u>creatine</u> in patients with extensive muscular paralysis estimated by radioisotope tracer method. Social and Rehabilitation Services Project R122—Project Report 11. Houston: Baylor College of Medicine, 1972.

66. Claus-Walker J, Cardus D, Griffith D, Halstead LS. Metabolic effects of sodium restriction and thiazides in tetraplegic patients. Paraplegia 1977–78;15:3.

67. Sinton EB, Taylor TN, Jackson RR, et al. Hematological and biochemical findings in the spinal cord injured man. In RJ Vinken, GW Bruyn (eds), Handbook of Clinical Neurology (Vol 26). Amsterdam: North-Holland, 1971;377.

68. Claus-Walker J, Halstead LS. Metabolic and endocrine changes in spinal cord injury: I. The nervous system before and after transection of the spinal cord. Arch Phys Med Rehabil 1981;62:595.

69. Claus-Walker J, Campos RJ, Carter RE, et al. Longitudinal analysis of daily excretory rhythms in men with tetraplegia due to cervical spinal cord transection. Paraplegia 1972;10:142.

70. Claus-Walker J, Halstead LS. Metabolic and endocrine changes in spinal cord injury: II (Section 2). Partial decentralization of the autonomic nervous system. Arch Phys Med Rehabil 1982;63:576.

71. Kamelhar DL, Steele JM, Schacht RG. Plasma renin and serum dopamine-beta-hydroxylase during orthostatic hypotension in quadriplegic man. Arch Phys Med Rehabil 1978;59:212.

72. Johnson RH, Park DM, Frankel HL. Orthostatic hypotension and renin-angiotensin system in paraplegia. Paraplegia 1971–72;9:146.

73. Mendelsohn FA, Johnson CI. Renin release in chronic paraplegia. Aust N Z J Med 1971;4:393.

74. Najenson T, Rosenfeld JB, Aloof S, et al. Plasma renin studies in patients with traumatic spinal cord injuries. Isr J Med Sci 1973;9:587.

75. Claus-Walker J, Halstead LS, Carter RE, et al. Biochemical responses to intense local cooling in healthy subjects and in subjects with cervical spinal cord injury. Arch Phys Med Rehabil 1976;57:50.

76. McCarthy DP, Wilmot CB. Renal sodium and water conservation in acute paraplegia. Paraplegia 1970;8:186.

77. Doba N, Reis DJ. Cerebellum: Role in reflex cardiovascular adjustments in posture. Brain Res 1972;39:495.

78. Doba N, Reis DJ. Changes in regional blood flow and cardiodynamics evoked by electrical stimulation of the fastigial nucleus in the cat and their similarity to orthostatic reflexes. J Physiol (Lond) 1972;227:729.

79. Doba N, Reis DJ. Role of the cerebellum and the vestibular apparatus in regulation of orthostatic reflexes in the cat. Circ Res 1974;34:9.

80. Huang TF, Carpenter MB, Wang SC. Fastigial nucleus and orthostatic reflex in cat and monkey. Am J Physiol 1977;232:H676.

81. Cowley AW. Vasopressin and Cardiovascular Regulation. In AC Guyton, JE Hall (eds), International Review of Physiology. Baltimore: University Park Press, 1982;26:189.

82. Del Bo A, Sved AF, Reis DJ. Fastigial stimulation releases vasopressin amounts that elevate arterial pressure. Am J Physiol 1983;244:H687.

83. Sved AF, McDowell FH, Blessing WW. Release of antidiuretic hormone in quadriplegic subjects in response to head-up tilt. Neurology 1985;35:78.

84. Robertson GL. The regulation of vasopressin function in health and disease. Recent Prog Horm Res 1977;23:333.

85. Schrier RW, Bert T, Anderson RJ. Osmotic and nonosmotic control of vasopressin release. Am J Physiol 1979;236:F321.

86. Wagner HN, Braunwald E. The pressor effect of the antidiuretic principle of the posterior pituitary in orthostatic hypotension. J Clin Invest 1956;35:1412.

87. Mohring J, Glanzer K, Maciel JA, et al. Greatly enhanced pressor response to antidiuretic hormone in patients with impaired cardiovascular reflexes due to idiopathic orthostatic hypotension. J Cardiovasc Pharmacol 1980;2:367.

88. DiPette D, DePette P, North W, et al. Plasma vasopressin response to hyperosmotic solution (Renografin) and its effect on blood pressure in quadriplegic patients. Clin Res 1982;30:510A.

89. Naftchi NE. Alterations of neuroendocrine functions in spinal cord injury. Peptides 1985;6(Suppl 1):85.

90. Trieschmann RB. Aging with a disability. New York: Demos, 1987.

91. Stacy WK, Midha M. The Kidney in the Spinal Cord Injury Patient. In MN Ozer, JK Schmitt (eds), Physical Medicine and Rehabilitation State of the Art Reviews—Medical Complications of Spinal Cord Injury 1987;1:415.

92. Sica DA, Midha M, Zawada ET, et al. Prostaglandin E_2 excretion in spinal cord injury patients. J Am Paraplegia Soc 1984;7:27.

93. Peruzzi WT, Shapiro BA, Meyer PR, et al. Hyponatremia in acute spinal cord injury. Crit Care Med 1994;22:252.

94. Sica DA, Midha M, Zawada ET, et al. Hyponatremia in spinal cord injury. J Am Paraplegia Soc 1990;13:78.

95. Dietrick R, Russi S. Tabulation and review of autopsy findings in fifty-five paraplegics. JAMA 1958;166:41.

96. Freed M, Bakst H, Barrie D. Life expectancy, survival rates, and causes of death in civilian patients with spinal cord trauma. Arch Phys Med Rehabil 1966;47:457.

97. Nyquist R, Bors E. Mortality and survival in traumatic myelopathy during nineteen years, from 1946 to 1965. Paraplegia 1967;5:22.

98. Hackler R. A 25-year prospective mortality study in the spinal cord injured patient: Comparison with the long-term living paraplegic. J Urol 1977;117:486.

99. Geisler W, Jousse A, Wynne-Jones M. Survival in traumatic transverse myelitis. Paraplegia 1977;14:262.

100. Geisler W, Jousse A, Wynne-Jones M, Breithaupt D. Survival in traumatic spinal cord injury. Paraplegia 1983;21:364.

101. Le C, Price M. Survival from spinal cord injury. J Chronic Dis 1982;35:487.

102. Frisbie JH, Kache A. Increasing survival and changing causes of death in myelopathy patients. J Am Paraplegia Soc 1983;6:51.

103. Stacy WK, Falls WF, Hussey RW. Chronic hemodialysis in spinal cord injury patients. J Am Paraplegia Soc 1983;6:7.

104. Mitchell G. The use of haemodialysis in renal failure complicating paraplegia—A report of five cases. Paraplegia 1986;24:254.

105. Mirahmadi MK, Byrne C, Barton C, et al. Prediction of creatinine clearance from serum creatinine in spinal cord injury patients. Paraplegia 1983;21:23.

106. Vaziri ND, Bruno A, Byrne C, et al. Maintenance hemodialysis in end-stage renal disease associated with spinal cord injury. Artif Organs 1982;6:13.

107. Smith B, Sica DA, Stacy WK. Peritoneal dialysis in spinal cord injury. Nephron 1986;44:245.

108. Vaziri ND, Lopez G, Nikakhtar B, et al. Peritoneal dialysis in renal failure associated with spinal cord injury. J Am Paraplegia Soc 1984;7:63.

109. Vaziri N. Chronic hemodialysis in end stage renal disease associated with paraplegia. Int J Artif Organs 1984;7:111.

110. Vaziri ND. Long-term haemodialysis in spinal cord injured patients. Paraplegia 1984;22:110.

111. Mirahmadi MK, Vaziri ND, Ghobadi M, et al. Survival on maintenance dialysis in patients with chronic renal failure associated with paraplegia and quadriplegia. Paraplegia 1982;20:43.

112. Barton CH, Vaziri ND, Gordon S, Tillis S. Renal pathology in end-stage renal disease associated with paraplegia. Paraplegia 1984;22:31.

113. Vaziri ND, Mirahmadi MK, Burton CH, et al. Clinicopathological characteristics of dialysis patients with spinal cord injury. J Am Paraplegia Soc 1983;6:3.

114. Pahl M, Vaziri N, Gordon S, Tuero S. Cardiovascular pathology in dialysis patients with spinal cord injury. Artif Organs 1983;7:416.

115. Vaziri ND, Gordon S, Nikokhtar B. Lipid abnormalities in chronic renal failure associated with spinal cord injury. Paraplegia 1982;20:183.

116. Vaziri N, Byrne C, Mirahmadi M, et al. Hematologic features of chronic renal failure associated with spinal cord injury. Artif Organs 1982;6:69.

117. Vaziri N, Cesario T, Mootoo K, et al. Bacterial infection in patients with chronic renal failure: Occurrence with spinal cord injury. Arch Intern Med 1982;142:1273.

118. Barton CH, Vaziri ND, Gordon S, Eltorai I. Endocrine pathology in spinal cord injured patients on maintenance dialysis. Paraplegia 1984;22:7.

119. Meshkinpour H, Vaziri N, Gordon S. Gastrointestinal pathology in patients with chronic renal failure associated with spinal cord injury. Am J Gastroenterol 1982;77:562.

120. Graham SD. Present urological treatment of spinal cord injury patients. J Urol 1981;126:1.

121. Rao KG, Hackler RH, Woodlief RM, et al. Real-time renal sonography in spinal cord injury patients: Prospective comparison with excretory urography. Urological neurology and urodynamics. J Urol 1986;135:72.

122. Lloyd KL, Dubovsky EV, Bueschen AJ, et al. Comprehensive renal scintillation procedures in spinal cord injury: Comparison with excretory urography. J Urol 1981;126:10.

123. Kuhlemeier KV, McEachran AB, Lloyd LK, et al. Serum creatinine as an indicator of renal function after spinal cord injury. Arch Phys Med Rehabil 1984;65:694.

124. Price M, Kottke FK. Comparison of glomerular filtration rate, blood urea nitrogen and serum creatinine in patients with chronic urinary tract disease. Minn Med 1980;63:781.

125. Mohler JL, Barton SD, Blouin RA, et al. The evaluation of creatinine clearance in spinal cord injury patients. J Urol 1986;136:366.

126. Sawyer WT, Hutchins K. Assessment and predictability of renal function in spinal cord injury patients. Urology 1982;19:377.

127. McLaurin RL, King LR. Metabolic effects of head injury. In Vinken, Bruyn (eds), Handbook of Clinical Neurology (Vol 24). Amsterdam: North Holland, 1976;109.

128. Jennett B, Teasdale G. Management of Head Injuries. Philadelphia: FA Davis, 1982.

129. Steinbok P, Thompson GB. Metabolic disturbance after head injury. Abnormalities of sodium and water balance with special reference to the effects of alcohol intoxication. Neurosurgery 1978;3:9.

130. Berrol S. Medical assessment. In M Rosenthal, ER Griffith, MR Bond, JD Miller (eds), Rehabilitation of the Head Injured Adult. Philadelphia: FA Davis, 1985;231.

131. Kusuda K, Daku Y, Sadoshima S, et al. Disturbances of fluid and electrolyte balance in patients with acute stroke. (Nippon Ronan Igakkai Zasshi) Jpn J Geriatr 1989;26:223.

132. Vallbona C. Bodily responses to immobilization. In FJ Kottke, GK Stillwell, JF Lehmann (eds), Krusen's Handbook of Physical Medicine and Rehabilitation (3rd ed). Philadelphia: Saunders, 1982;963.

Chapter 2
Unique Aspects of Blood Pressure Control in Disability

Mahmoud Salem and Salim Mujais

Hypertension is a major cause of disability: It is the single most potent, common, and remediable risk factor for cerebrovascular disease, congestive heart failure, and coronary heart disease in individuals older than 60 years of age [1]. The preponderance of elderly patients in rehabilitation programs makes the management of hypertension a recurring theme. The peculiarities of this population of patients require a well-tailored treatment strategy. Regrettably, there is a dearth of data on the unique aspects of hypertension in the disabled. The present review is an attempt to fill this gap and direct the attention of the practicing physician to some of the special aspects and potential pitfalls. Because an increasing proportion of patients using rehabilitation centers are elderly, special attention is paid to this subgroup of the disabled. This chapter is divided into three sections: (1) an overview of the general characteristics of disabled patients that are pertinent to the management of hypertension; (2) a discussion of the pitfalls in the diagnosis of hypertension that are particularly important for disabled and elderly patients; and (3) peculiar aspects of treatment, both nonpharmacologic and pharmacologic, in disabled and elderly patients.

Disability Characteristics Pertinent to Hypertension Management

The approach to hypertension management is increasingly focused on individualized care, with particular emphasis on the peculiarities that may occur in the individual patient. Nowhere is this more important than in the chronically disabled patient. A list of the more common aspects of the management of hypertension in chronically disabled patients is presented in Table 2-1.

A unique aspect is the increasing number of hypertensive disabled patients referred for rehabilitation after the occurrence of what were once previously fatal hypertensive complications (e.g., cerebral hemorrhage and strokes). In these subjects, serious hypertensive end-organ damage has already developed, and antihypertensive therapy must be tailored to the resultant frequently precarious state. Treatment must prevent any recurrence of hypertensive complications without furthering damage or delaying recovery. Closely related is the increasing preponderance of the elderly among the chronically disabled, reflecting the overall increased survival of the population. Many of these patients have multiple organ involvement and receive a number of drugs that may interact with or affect their blood pressure (BP) management (nonsteroidal anti-inflammatory drugs) [2].

The chronic disability state introduces some particular aspects in addition to those shared with the general population. Limited activity or even prolonged bed rest are prominent features of the clinical status of some of these patients. This is reflected in frequent obesity and deconditioning with propensity to postural hypotension. Psychosocial stress, panic attacks, and depression are more common in these patients than in the general population; invasive

Table 2-1. Peculiar Aspects of Blood
Pressure Control in the Disabled Patient

Pre-existing complicated hypertension
Preponderance of elderly
Restricted activity
Obesity
Multiple organ dysfunction
Multiple pharmacopeia
Substance abuse
Frequent invasive diagnostic and therapeutic interventions
Absence of normal physiologic mechanisms

Table 2-2. Causes of Lability of Blood Pressure

Orthostatic hypotension ± supine hypertension
Postprandial hypotension
Sleep apnea
Hypoglycemia
Mild volume depletion
Stress syndrome
Spinal cord injury
Anesthesia
Substance abuse
Silent myocardial ischemia
Pulmonary hypertension

studies, anesthesia, and surgeries are experienced more frequently, and postoperative hypertension can be particularly severe. Some of these patients may be totally dependent on the medical team for nutrient and fluid intake because of bypassing or absence of the normal mechanisms (e.g., the quadriplegic, artificially ventilated patient with a stomach tube, or the elderly patient with a defective thirst mechanism). The amount and type of fluid administered may affect the hypertension status.

Postural hypotension is common in this patient population, particularly in spinal cord injury patients, and can be worsened by antihypertensive therapy. Also of note is the association of idiopathic postural hypotension, commonly seen in the elderly and disabled, with supine episodic hypertension [3]. This may require a differential diagnosis from pheochromocytoma (see Chapter 6), labile hypertension, or other diseases or conditions (porphyria, paraplegia) in which marked spontaneous fluctuations of arterial pressure may occur. Postural hypotension also makes evaluation of treatment options difficult. Finally, patients enrolled in rehabilitation programs for substance abuse may suffer from hypertension owing to the abused substance (e.g., alcohol) or during withdrawal.

Diagnostic Pitfalls

Safe and proper management of hypertensive states requires careful attention to pitfalls in the diagnosis of elevated BP and in monitoring of therapeutic response (Table 2-2).

Pseudohypertension

Pseudohypertension is a cuff reading above 140/90 mm Hg in the absence of true elevation of the BP as determined by an intra-arterial recording. The most common cause is a cuff artifact from hardened arteries (arteriosclerosis). It leads to overestimation of diastolic and underestimation of systolic pressures [4] and frequently results in overtreatment. This condition should be suspected when a discrepancy between the severity of hypertension and end-organ damage is found. In a study by Spence et al., half the patients with a discrepancy between severity and duration of hypertension (as measured by cuff) and lack of end-organ damage showed a 30-mm average cuff overestimation of diastolic pressure [5] when compared with intra-arterial measurement. A positive Osler's sign is diagnostic. This sign refers to a palpable brachial or radial artery (pipe stem arteries) after inflation of the cuff above systolic pressure as determined by pulse disappearance. Intra-arterial pressure measurement confirms this discrepancy and may provide a guide to future management by determining the difference between cuff pressures and true intra-arterial pressure. This helps the physician avoid hazards of excessive treatment that include postural hypotension, dizziness, falls, cerebral hypoperfusion leading to transient ischemic attacks, general weakness, lack of compliance, and possibly excess cardiac events.

Pseudohypertension should not be confused with the isolated elevation of systolic BP resulting from indistensible hard arteries. This is a true elevation of the BP and is discussed later. Excessive vascular reactivity is another cause of pseudohypertension. This may be reflected in elevated BP during anxiety attacks and depression. Another example is office hypertension (white coat syndrome), where the simple act of BP measurement by a physician may increase the BP as much as 75/40 mm Hg [6]. BP monitoring at home may be more reflective of the true BP and has a psychological benefit, because it involves the patient in managing his or her own disease. A hand grip during BP measurement may give a falsely high reading in a subset of patients with increased vascular reactivity. Finally, an important cause of pseudohypertension is obesity [7]. A large cuff ameliorates but does not eliminate the overestimated diastolic pressure in obese individuals. This may be as high as 23 mm Hg [7]. This is important to recognize because obesity is more common in disabled patients than in the general population.

Pseudonormotension

Pseudonormotension is a normal BP reading in the presence of true elevation of the BP. It is usually suspected when blood pressures are normal in the presence of hypertensive end-organ damage. Some of the causes of pseudonormotension are:

1. Subclavian artery stenosis, which is more commonly found in elderly disabled than in the general population.
2. A discrepancy between intermittent BP measurement in the clinic and ambulatory BP recordings. High ambulatory pressures identify more accurately (more sensitively) the patients who have end-organ disease related to increased BP [8], despite normal BP recorded in the office (office pseudonormotension). Increased left ventricular mass on echocardiography is another sensitive method of detecting these patients' conditions [9].
3. An auscultatory gap, which occurs in severe vascular disease and leads to underestimation of the systolic BP. Adequate inflation of the cuff well above the systolic pressure determined by palpation will eliminate this cause of pseudonormotension.

Lability of Blood Pressure

BP variability is a ubiquitous finding in both normotensive and hypertensive individuals. The absolute variability is higher in hypertensive patients [10]. Older patients have an even higher variability, possibly because of decreased vascular compliance and diminished baroreflex function [11, 12]. This variability has to be taken into account when devising or adjusting the treatment schedule and timing of doses. Home measurements, with simple charting of activity, meals, and time of medicine intake, will help clarify some of these variations, thus avoiding overtreatment and its attendant morbidity.

BP tends to be highest in the morning, gradually decreases over the course of the day, and is lowest during the night [13]. A mildly hypertensive patient with a resting systolic pressure of 140 mm Hg might be expected to reach a level of 240 mm Hg during exercise and 120 mm Hg during sleep [14].

In elderly persons, the lability is mainly in the direction of orthostatic hypotension. A postprandial decrease in BP is common in the elderly and may continue for up to 3 hours [15, 16]. This may result from splanchnic vasodilatation in individuals who exhibit some degree of abnormal baroreflex function, vascular volume depletion, and diminished cardiac function.

In sleep apnea, daytime hypertension may be accompanied by either nocturnal hypotension or hypertension, more commonly the latter. It may be important to look for this in bedridden patients with paralysis because of the potential for partial airway obstruction during the night. If found and treated, hypertension may resolve [17].

Patients with autonomic neuropathy or idiopathic orthostatic hypotension may exhibit orthostatic hypotension during the day and supine hypertension during the night [18], thus avoiding detection if BP is measured only during the day. This is a particularly difficult condition to manage but important to recognize because autonomic neuropathy may be a common feature of patients with disability secondary to advanced neuropathy, whether degenerative, related to a spinal cord injury, or related to a cerebrovascular accident.

A variety of other causes can be associated with paroxysmal alteration in BP. Hypoglycemia, through activation of the sympathoadrenal system, can cause severe elevation of BP [19]. Mild volume depletion can also be associated with paroxysmal hypertension. During periods of psychological crises, which are common before the patient adapts to the disability, the elevated BP may be a manifestation of the underlying stress syndrome [20] and can be difficult to control. Panic attacks can precipitate paroxysmal hypertension [21].

Another form of labile episodic hypertension may occur in patients with spinal cord injuries, especially in association with procedures (e.g., bladder catheterization) and volume depletion [22]. Stresses of anesthesia and surgery, to which the disabled are frequently exposed, often result in postoperative paroxysmal hypertension. The most severe cases occur after cardiopulmonary bypass [23] and other vascular and neurosurgical procedures [24]. Intravenous methyldopa or labetalol are particularly useful in these situations.

Another cause of lability of BP is commonly seen in rehabilitation programs for alcohol and substance abuse. Withdrawal hypertension is clearly related to excess sympathetic discharge and can be treated by clonidine [25].

Silent myocardial ischemia may present as paroxysmal elevation of the BP [26]. Patients with pulmonary hypertension may have associated systemic paroxysmal hypertension [27].

Isolated Systolic Hypertension

Systolic BP is a significant risk factor and is closely correlated with morbidity [28]. It is a common finding in the elderly [29] and is related to loss of elasticity of major blood vessels [30]. When coinciding with diastolic normotension, the decision to treat and the determination of target BP level are difficult. A mean arterial pressure above 110 mm Hg warrants treatment [31], and this level can be used as a therapeutic goal (mean arterial pressure = diastolic + ⅓ pulse pressure).

The beneficial and safe aspects of the treatment of systolic hypertension have been recently confirmed in the final report of the Systolic Hypertension in the Elderly Program Cooperative Research Group [32]. The absolute benefit in terms of stroke reduction at 5 years of treatment was estimated at 30 events per 1,000 participants. This result was observed even though 35% of those assigned to placebo took known antihypertensives during the study. The incidence of non-fatal myocardial infarction plus coronary death was 27% lower in the active treatment group. For all cardiovascular events, the reduction in incidence was 32% for the active treatment group. This translates into an absolute benefit of 55 events per 1,000 participants at 5 years. There was a low-order excess of adverse effects in the treatment group, but no increased incidence of depression or dementia.

The Elderly Hypertensive Disabled Patient

In industrialized societies BP increases with age. Hypertension is ubiquitous in the elderly population, ranging from 40% to 68% in different studies [33]. The gradient of risk for each increment in BP becomes steeper with advancing age [34]. The contribution of hypertension to disability in the elderly is clear when its relationship to strokes is considered. Forty-two percent of strokes in elderly men and 70% of strokes in elderly women are caused by hypertension [35]. Hypertension also contributes to the vascular dementias, which make up 10-20% of the dementias in the elderly [36]. The definition of hypertension in the elderly needs to be formulated in functional terms. It can best be defined as that level of BP at which the benefits of therapy exceed the risks and costs of no treatment. Therefore, even though BP above 140/90 mm Hg is diagnostic in the young, the diagnosis of hypertension in the elderly is frequently made at 160/90 mm Hg or higher pressures.

Hypertension in the elderly is characterized by increased vascular resistance and decreased cardiac output and intravascular volume [37]. Baroreceptor sensitivity is decreased, making (together with decreased intravascular volume) wide fluctuations in the BP the rule rather than the exception, and predisposing patients to postural hypotension in response to treatment (as high as 40% in one study) [38].

In above-the-knee amputees, the risk of aortic aneurysms is five times higher [39]. This may be related to asymmetric blood flow at the aortic bifurcation. Hypertension in these patients aggravates the aneurysmal dilatation and should be treated aggressively.

Considerations in Treatment

Physical Exercise

Physical therapy entailing general exercise activity is frequently an integral part of rehabilitation of the disabled. Both dynamic (endurance or isotonic) and isometric (strength or static) training lead to an acute increase in the BP, the latter more than the former [40]. Hypertension per se adversely affects maximal exercise capacity [41], and hypertensive middle-aged and older patients run a higher risk of sudden death during exercise than the general population [42]. It has also been found that if the BP exceeds 230/90 mm Hg during moderate activity, cardiovascular risk increases more than twofold, even when the basal BP is normal [43]. For the previously mentioned reasons, BP should be controlled before embarking on a vigorous exercise program. However, in the long run, dynamic exercise helps reduce BP an average of 11 and 6 mm Hg for systolic and diastolic pressures, respectively [31]. This can be a significant advantage when combined with other nonpharmacologic measures (e.g., weight reduction, alcohol restriction, behavioral therapy, and a low salt diet). It should be noted, however, that this antihypertensive effect of exercise was observed with three-times-weekly sessions in which the patients achieved at least 60% of their maximal capacity for a minimum duration of 30 minutes.

The beneficial effects of exercise disappeared after stopping. The underlying hemodynamic alterations that lead to such a salutary effect are not well defined. Another important factor to be taken into consideration when designing an exercise program is end-organ damage in a hypertensive patient. The type of antihypertensive drug used may also profoundly affect exercise endurance. Diuretics limit exercise capability [44]. Beta blockers, especially the nonselective ones, have the same effect plus decreasing the maximal heart rate [31]. Angiotensin-converting enzyme (ACE) inhibitors and calcium blockers do not alter exercise tolerance [31] and are probably the drugs of choice for patients wishing to exercise regularly up to their maximal potential. Treadmill exercise testing is recommended before embarking on an exercise program in hypertensive subjects. In disabled patients without the ability to cooperate in a treadmill test, a 24-hour Holter monitor to detect episodes of silent ischemia may be worthwhile. In stroke patients, there is a high incidence of ischemic heart disease that can be worsened by vigorous rehabilitation efforts [45, 46].

Principles of Pharmacologic Treatment

The following general guidelines can be offered for the management of hypertension in the chronically disabled. Before the initiation of drug treatment, an empirical trial of nonpharmacologic therapy is warranted in mild and moderate cases of hypertension.

Start low and go slow. Unless a hypertensive emergency is at hand, there is rarely an urgency to lower BP rapidly. Considering the time required for chronic autoregulation and the delay in resetting of baroreceptors after a reduction in BP, a deliberate and slowly progressive regimen is recommended [47]. This is especially true in cerebrovascular accidents. Only in subarachnoid bleeding is rapid control of the BP the goal, and even then, no more than a 25% reduction of BP should be sought. Transient ischemic attacks may be caused by hemodynamic disturbances precipitated by treatment and not by thromboembolic disease. Patients with antecedent cerebrovascular complications have a greater incidence of side effects from antihypertensives with a site of action in the central nervous system—e.g., clonidine and alpha-methyldopa. However, in the absence of a cerebrovascular accident, these drugs are excellent choices in the elderly provided they are given in small doses and not combined with other sedatives (haloperidol plus alpha-methyldopa may cause dementia). In general, these cerebrovascular accident patients need less medicine to control their BP after the stroke than they used before the stroke. This may be related to bed rest, dietary changes, and some deconditioning process.

The elderly need smaller doses of most drugs because clearance is diminished. Thiazide diuretics in small doses are of proven benefit in the elderly, are generally well tolerated, are low in cost, and have no adverse effects on the central nervous system. At these small doses, postural hypotension is not prominent. Thiazides should be avoided in elderly patients with diabetes, gout, renal failure, previous myocardial infarction, arrhythmias, and impotence. Large doses of potent diuretics (e.g., furosemide) should be avoided. Methyldopa and clonidine, if given in small doses at bedtime, can give excellent control with minimal daytime sedation. Beta blockers are less effective than in the young and can cause fatigue and decreased functional capacity, which is a most undesirable side effect in an elderly disabled patient. Calcium channel blockers and ACE inhibitors have several advantages. They do not cause postural hypotension or metabolic abnormalities and have no sedative side effects. Attempts at gradual withdrawal of antihypertensive drugs (step-down therapy) after establishing good control for 10 or more months have been successful in at least 25% of patients [48].

Use small doses of two drugs rather than large doses of a single drug. This will help reduce side effects and may be therapeutically beneficial if the agents chosen for the combination have synergistic antihypertensive effects.

Postural hypotension during the day with nocturnal supine hypertension presents a complex therapeutic challenge. Some useful approaches include nighttime administration of antihypertensives; avoidance of potent diuretics; use of direct vasodilators (e.g., hydralazine), which encourage some water retention and thus avoid hypovolemia-related orthostasis; elevation of the head of the bed; slow assumption of the upright position; elastic stockings during the day; and, finally, early activation of the disabled patient. In one study of stroke patients [49], early assumption of the standing position with the help of nurses was associated with a lower increase in heart rate during tilting and a lower incidence of severe cardiovascular disability. During rehabilitation, use of tilt-table conditioning to reverse the deconditioning of bed rest has been used with benefit [50].

Associated conditions may benefit from a specific antihypertensive. Examples include beta blockers in patients with ischemic heart disease and ACE inhibitors in patients with congestive heart failure (see Chapter 3) or diabetic renal disease. Clonidine may have the additional benefit of relieving spasticity in paraplegics and quadriplegics [51]. Alpha$_1$-adrenoreceptor blockers such as prazosin and terazosin may be appropriate for elderly patients with benign prostatic hypertrophy and hypertension because they improve urine flow [52]. Other conditions may be worsened by a specific antihypertensive—e.g., beta blockers and peripheral vascular disease.

The multiplicity of medical conditions prevalent in elderly and chronically disabled patients frequently lead to multiple pharmacopeia. Drug interactions are therefore likely. Nonsteroidal anti-inflammatory drugs interfere with the antihypertensive effect of treatment [2]. This blunting effect is least marked with clonidine, methyldopa, and calcium channel blockers.

Antacids may interfere with the absorption of most antihypertensives if given concomitantly. The clinical significance of this interaction is usually small. Sympathomimetics in nasal decongestants may increase BP. Combined use of verapamil and beta blockers may cause severe negative inotropic and chronotropic actions, leading to heart failure and bradycardia or heart block.

Addition of ACE inhibitors to a diuretic is an effective combination but may cause severe hypotension [53]. Initiation of ACE inhibitors in diuretic-treated patients should be done carefully. Verapamil should probably be avoided in disabled bedridden patients with a propensity to constipation because it inhibits the smooth muscles of the gut. Verapamil also increases digoxin and quinidine levels.

Propranolol and methyldopa in combination have been reported to result in a hypertensive reaction [54]. Amitriptyline antagonizes the antihypertensive effect of methyldopa [55]. Methyldopa plus haloperidol may result in a reversible dementia [56].

Case Management Study

A 31-year-old woman had insulin-dependent diabetes mellitus (IDDM) of 25 years' duration complicated by multiple organ disease including nephropathy, retinopathy, and severe peripheral vascular disease. The patient's hypertension was controlled with a combination of ACE inhibitor and diuretics until shortly before she was seen, at which point she had developed hyperkalemia necessitating the discontinuation of the ACE inhibitor and substitution of a calcium channel blocker. She developed progressive gangrene of the toes that initially was treated conservatively. However, a fungal superinfection in the gangrenous area required surgical intervention, and bilateral below-knee amputations were performed. The patient recovered uneventfully and was referred for rehabilitation.

The patient's blood pressure was noted to be quite variable, with periods of adequate control followed by episodic hypertension, which was sometimes severe. As an outpatient, these periods of loss of control were ascribed to lack of compliance and, occasionally, hypoglycemia. While in the Rehabilitation Institute, however, the patient was compliant and her blood sugar control was stable and adequate. On interview, she was found to be suffering from recurrent vomiting, a feeling of prolonged fullness after meals, and persistent mild nausea. A workup revealed gastroparesis that was likely related to her diabetes mellitus and impaired emptying of her stomach. This was thought to have impaired absorption of antihypertensive medications. The patient was switched from oral medications to a transdermal delivery system with a sympatholytic and her blood pressure stabilized.

Discussion

This case illustrates the dilemma that faces the physician whose patient has a complex medical history. The case study illustrates the necessity of tailoring antihypertensive therapy to the changing medical condition of the patient: the ACE inhibitor had to be discontinued because of her hyperkalemia, which is a known complication with this category of drugs in patients with renal insufficiency and hyporeninemic-hypoaldosteronism from diabetes mellitus. Further, beta blockers could not be used because of the history of hypoglycemic episodes. Calcium channel blockers provided good control of the blood pressure initially, but subsequently the patient had erratic responses because of the development of yet another complication of her diabetes, namely, gastroparesis. While lack of compliance should always be considered as a first cause for apparently erratic control, a search for alternate explanations may be necessary in patients with complex renal problems.

References

1. Kannel WB, Gordon T. Evaluation of cardiovascular risk in the elderly: The Framingham study. Bull NY Acad Med 1978;54:573.
2. Sahloul M, al-Kiek R, Ivanovich P, Mujais SK: Nonsteroidal anti-inflammatory drugs and antihypertensives. Nephron 1990;56:345.
3. Niarchos AP, Magrini F, Tarazi RC, et al. Mechanism of spontaneous supine blood pressure variations in chronic autonomic insufficiency. Am J Med 1978;65:547.
4. Messerli FH, Ventura HO, Amodeo C. Osler's maneuver and pseudohypertension. N Engl Med J 1985;312:1548.
5. Spence JD, Sibbald WJ, Cape RD. Direct, indirect and mean blood pressures in hypertensive patients: The problem of cuff artefact due to arterial wall stiffness and a partial solution. Clin Invest Med 1980;2:165.
6. Mancia G, Ferrari A, Gregorini L. Blood pressure and heart rate variabilities in normotensive and hypertensive human beings. Circ Res 1983;53:96.
7. Porter R, Rangno R. Hypertension in obesity: Measurement error and effect of weight loss. [Abstract.] Clin Invest Med 1987;10(Suppl):B88.
8. Floras JS, Jones JV, Hassan MO, et al. Cuff and ambulatory blood pressure in patients with essential hypertension. Lancet 1981;2:107.
9. Simone GD, Devereux RB, Roman MJ, et al. Echocardiographic left ventricular mass and electrolyte intake predict arterial hypertension. Ann Intern Med 1991;114:202.
10. Mancia G. Blood pressure variability at normal and high blood pressure. Chest 1983;83:317.
11. Rowe JW. Clinical consequences of age-related impairments in vascular compliance. Am J Cardiol 1987;60:68G.
12. Watson RDS, Stallard TJS, Flinn RM, et al. Factors determining direct arterial pressure and its variability in hypertensive man. Hypertension 1980;2:333.
13. Clark LA, Denby L, Pregibon D, et al. The effects of activity and time of the day on the diurnal variations of the blood pressure. J Chronic Dis 1987;40:671-681.
14. Watson RDS, Hamilton CA, Reid JL, et al. Changes in plasma norepinephrine, blood pressure and heart rate during physical activity in hypertensive man. Hypertension 1979;1:341.
15. Fagan TC, Conrad KA, Mar HJ, et al. Effect of meals on hemodynamics: Implications for antihypertensive drug studies. Clin Pharmacol Ther 1986;39:255.
16. Lipsitz LA, Nuquist RP Jr, Wei JY, et al. Postprandial reduction in the blood pressure in the elderly. N Engl J Med 1983;309:81.
17. Hoffstein V, Chan CK, Slutsky AS. Sleep apnea and systemic hypertension: A causal association review. Am J Med 1991;91:190.
18. Mann S, Altman DG, Raftery EB, et al. Circadian variation of blood pressure during autonomic failure. Circulation 1983;68:477.
19. Farr MJ. Diazoxide, glipizide, hypertension and hypoglycemia. Lancet 1976;2:1138.
20. Schneider RH, Egan BM, Johnson EH, et al. Anger and anxiety in borderline hypertension. Psychosom Med 1986;48:242.
21. White WB, Baker LH. Episodic hypertension secondary to panic disorder. Arch Intern Med 1986;146:1129.

22. Naftch NE, Demeny M, Lowman EW, et al. Hypertensive crises in quadriplegic patients. Changes in cardiac output, blood volume, serum dopamine-betahydroxylate activity, and arterial prostaglandin PGE2. Circulation 1978;57:336.

23. Estanfous FG, Tarazi RC, et al. Systemic arterial hypertension associated with cardiac surgery. Am J Cardiol 1980;46:685.

24. Caplan LR, Skillman J, Ojemann R, et al. Intracerebral hemorrhage following carotid endarterectomy: A hypertensive complication? Stroke 1978;9:457.

25. Abrams WB. In summary: Satellite symposium on central alpha adrenergic blood pressure regulating mechanisms. Hypertension 1984;6(Suppl II):II87.

26. Rozanski A, Bairey CN, Krantz DS, et al. Mental stress and the induction of silent myocardial ischemia in patients with coronary artery disease. N Engl J Med 1988;318:1005.

27. Steissman KE, Simon JI, Wasserman K. Pulmonary hypertension presenting as a panic disorder. Chest 1987;91:910.

28. Kannel WB. Role of blood pressure in cardiovascular morbidity and mortality. Prog Cardiovasc Dis 1974;17:5.

29. Vogt TM, Ireland CC, Black D, et al. Recruitment of elderly volunteers for a multicenter clinical trial: The SHEP pilot study. Controlled Clin Trials 1986;7:118.

30. Koch-Wesser J. Correlation of pathophysiology and pharmacology in primary hypertension. Am J Cardiol 1973;32:499.

31. Fagard R, Bielen E, Hespel P, et al. Physical Exercise in Hypertension. In JH Laragh, BM Brenner (eds), Hypertension: Pathophysiology, Diagnosis, and Management. New York: Raven, 1990;1985.

32. SHEP Cooperative Research Group. Prevention of stroke by antihypertensive drug treatment in older persons with isolated systolic hypertension: Final results of the systolic hypertension in the elderly program (SHEP). JAMA 1991;265:3255.

33. Hulley SB, Furberg CD, Gurland B, et al. The systolic hypertension in the elderly program (SHEP): Antihypertensive efficacy of chlorthalidone. Am J Cardiol 1985;56:913.

34. Kannel WB. Some lessons in cardiovascular epidemiology from Framingham. Am J Cardiol 1976;37:269.

35. Appelgate WB. Hypertension in the elderly. Generations 1987;(Fall):16.

36. Forette F, Boller F. Hypertension and the risk of dementia in the elderly. Am J Med 1991;90:14S

37. Messerli FH, Ventura HO, Glade LB, et al. Essential hypertension in the elderly: Hemodynamics, intravascular volume, plasma renin activity, and circulating catecholamine levels. Lancet 1983;2:983.

38. Caird FI, Andrews GR, Kennedy RD. Effects of posture on blood pressure in the elderly. Br Heart J 1973;35:527.

39. Vollmar JF, Paes E, Pauschinger P, et al. Aortic aneurysms as late sequelae of above-knee amputation. Lancet 1989;2(8667):834.

40. Asmussen E. Similarities and dissimilarities between static and dynamic exercise. Circ Res 1981;48(Suppl I):I3.

41. Fagard R, Staessen J, Amery A. Maximal aerobic power in essential hypertension. J Hypertens 1988;6:859.

42. Vermani R, Robinwitz M, McAllister HA. Non-traumatic death in joggers. Am J Med 1982;72:874.

43. Sowers JR, Mohanty PK. Effect of advancing age on cardiopulmonary baroreceptor function in hypertensive men. Hypertension 1987;10:274.

44. Nielsen B, Kubica R, Bonnesen A, et al. Physical work capacity after dehydration and hyperthermia. Scand J Sports Sci 1981;3:2.

45. Kaplan MS, Pratley R, Hawkins W. Silent myocardial ischemia during rehabilitation for cerebrovascular disease. Arch Phys Med Rehabil 1991;72:59.

46. Roth EJ, Weisner S, Green D, et al. Amputee rehabilitation: The value of cardiovascular monitoring during physical therapy. Arch Phys Med Rehabil 1987;68:582.

47. Strandgaard S. Autoregulation of cerebral blood flow in hypertensive patients. The modifying influence of prolonged antihypertensive treatment on the tolerance to acute drug induced hypotension. Circulation 1976;53:720.

48. Herman KJ, Eisalo A. Possibility of reduction of antihypertensive therapy in hypertension. [Abstract.] In Proceedings, Seventh Scientific Meeting of the International Society of Hypertension. New Orleans, 1980;136.

49. Asberg KH. Orthostatic tolerance training of stroke patients in general medical wards. An experimental study. Scand J Rehabil Med 1989;21:179.

50. Hoeldtke RD, Cavanaugh ST, Hughes JD. Treatment of orthostatic hypotension: Interaction of pressor drugs and tilt table conditioning. Arch Phys Med Rehabil 1988;69:895.

51. Donovan WH, Carter RE, Rossi CD, et al. Clonidine effect on spasticity: A clinical trial. Arch Phys Med Rehabil 1988;69:193.

52. Ramsay JWA, Scott GI, Whitefield HN. A double-blind controlled trial of a new alpha-1-blocking drug in the treatment of bladder outflow obstruction. Br J Urol 1985;57:657.

53. Cleland JGF, Dargie HJ, McAlpine H, et al. Severe hypotension after first dose of enalapril in heart failure. Br Med J 1985;291:1309.

54. Nies AS, Shand DG. Hypertensive response to propranolol in a patient treated with methyldopa: A proposed mechanism. Clin Pharmacol Ther 1973;14:823.

55. White AG. Methyldopa and amitriptyline. Lancet 1965;2:441.

56. Thornton WE. Dementia induced by methyldopa with haloperidol. N Engl J Med 1976;294:1222.

Chapter 3

Heart Failure

Mark T. Upton

This discussion begins with a brief review of the pathophysiology and treatment of heart failure. Unique problems in the management of chronically disabled patients with heart failure then are described. Last, case histories of patients seen at the Rehabilitation Institute of Chicago are presented for illustrative purposes.

Definition

Congestive heart failure can be defined as a condition in which the heart is unable to pump a sufficient quantity of blood to meet the demands of the peripheral tissues. Congestive heart failure should be distinguished from situations in which there is fluid overload in the *absence* of myocardial failure. The latter syndrome, termed the *congested state*, may result from abnormal salt and water retention in association with renal failure or massive intravenous infusions.

Underlying Causes of Heart Failure

It is important to identify not only the underlying but also the precipitating causes of heart failure. Almost all major categories of congenital and acquired heart disease can result in heart failure. The most common causes include coronary artery disease, valvular heart disease, hypertensive heart disease, congenital heart disease, cardiomyopathies, pericardial disease, and high output states (Table 3-1).

Precipitating Causes of Heart Failure

Over half of all heart failure episodes are secondary to a precipitating cause. The underlying cardiac abnormality may persist for years, producing little if any disability, and only when an additional burden is placed on the myocardium does the heart decompensate. Identifying the precipitating cause is of critical importance because prompt alleviation may be lifesaving. Some of the common precipitating causes of heart failure include inappropriate reduction or discontinuation of a drug regimen, increased salt or fluid intake, excessive physical or emotional stress, systemic infection, pulmonary embolism, arrhythmias, hypertension, myocardial ischemia, renal failure, and onset of high output states (hyperthyroidism, pregnancy) (Table 3-1).

Categories of Heart Failure

Heart failure may be described as acute versus chronic, left versus right, backward versus forward, systolic versus diastolic, and low output versus high output. Although these terms may be useful in the clinical setting, they are purely descriptive and do not represent fundamentally different disease states (Table 3-2).

Acute Versus Chronic Heart Failure

Acute heart failure develops precipitously with a massive myocardial infarction or sudden rupture

Table 3-1. Causes of Heart Failure

Underlying Causes	Precipitating Causes
Coronary artery disease	Excessive stress
Valvular heart disease	Increased salt intake
Hypertensive heart disease	Reduction of drug therapy
Congenital heart disease	Systemic infection
Pericardial disease	Pulmonary embolism
High output states	Arrhythmia
	Hypertension
	Myocardial ischemia

Table 3-2. Categories of Heart Failure

Acute versus chronic
Left versus right
Backward versus forward
Systolic versus diastolic
Low versus high output

of an aortic valve leaflet. On the other hand, chronic heart failure may have an insidious onset and be present for years in a compensated state. Frequently, there is no significant distinction between these two conditions. For example, a patient with long-standing hypertensive heart disease may have minimal symptoms of congestive heart failure until an acute precipitating episode, such as a small myocardial infarction or arrhythmia, causes the subject to decompensate abruptly.

Left Versus Right Heart Failure

Although heart disease commonly affects the entire myocardium, with rare exceptions, one ventricle fails before the other. In left heart failure, the left ventricle is unable to handle the blood returning from the lungs. This results in pulmonary congestion and a low cardiac output. In right heart failure, the right ventricle cannot accommodate blood returning from the systemic circulation. As a result, there is elevated venous pressure, with engorgement of the liver and peripheral edema.

Backward Versus Forward Failure

Backward failure refers to the damming up of blood in the veins proximal to the failing ventricle, resulting in systemic venous congestion (in right heart failure) and pulmonary congestion (in left heart failure). In forward heart failure, the heart is unable to pump a sufficient amount of blood forward into the arterial system, resulting in underperfusion of the vital organs. The distinction between backward and forward failure is artificial, because in a closed circuit the inability of the heart to sustain its forward output must eventually result in backward venous pooling.

Systolic Versus Diastolic Failure

Although systolic dysfunction with reduced pump function is the predominant cause of heart failure, diastolic dysfunction with impaired ventricular filling also occurs, especially in the presence of left ventricular hypertrophy and acute myocardial ischemia. The principal clinical manifestations of systolic failure result from an inadequate forward output, whereas the major consequences of diastolic failure relate to the elevated ventricular filling pressure causing pulmonary or systemic venous congestion.

Low Versus High Output Failure

The common causes of heart failure—atherosclerosis, hypertension, cardiomyopathies, and valvular heart disease—tend to be low output states. These are characterized by a reduced stroke volume and pulse pressure, peripheral vasoconstriction, and a widened arteriovenous oxygen difference. Heart failure may also result from several high output states such as thyrotoxicosis, severe anemia, and arteriovenous fistula. High output failure is associated with an increased stroke volume, widened pulse pressure, peripheral vasodilatation, and a reduced arteriovenous oxygen difference. Nevertheless, the heart fails to meet the increased metabolic demands imposed by these high output conditions.

Assessment of Cardiac Performance

The performance of the heart is dependent on four determinants: preload, afterload, contractility, and

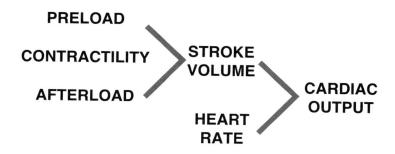

Figure 3-1. Determinants of cardiac output.

heart rate. The relationship among these factors is not fixed; they can play greater or lesser roles, depending on the state of the heart (Figure 3-1).

Preload

According to the Frank-Starling mechanism, an increase in end-diastolic volume (preload) is followed by a more forceful contraction that improves ventricular emptying.

Afterload

The afterload of the heart may be defined as the tension or stress developed in the ventricle during ejection. The primary determinant of afterload is blood pressure.

Contractility

Contractility refers to the intrinsic force that the myocardium develops as the heart beats. Contractility can be enhanced without a corresponding increase in preload or a reduction in afterload. Contractility does not limit the performance of the normal heart, but cardiac pump function is depressed in the failing heart.

Heart Rate

The cardiac output is determined by the heart rate and the stroke volume. During exercise and in many

Table 3-3. Compensatory Mechanisms

Increased sympathetic activity
Dilation
Hypertrophy
Tachycardia

disease states, the heart rate plays the primary role in mediating an increase in cardiac output.

Compensatory Mechanisms

In the presence of chronic heart failure, the heart depends on four compensatory mechanisms for maintaining pump function: increased contractility resulting from sympathetic activity, dilation, hypertrophy, and tachycardia (Table 3-3). The clinical manifestations of heart failure may be lessened or delayed by operation of these compensatory mechanisms. However, each has a limit beyond which cardiac performance deteriorates.

Sympathetic Activity

The essential feature of heart failure is depression of myocardial contractility. To support the failing heart, there is an increase in catecholamines released by sympathetic cardiac nerves and the adrenal medulla, which enhance myocardial contractility. This generalized increase in sympathetic activity is frequently more of a burden than a blessing because it can be associated with a marked in-

Table 3-4. Left Heart Failure

Symptoms	Signs
Fatigue	Cardiomegaly
Weakness	Ventricular gallop
Dyspnea	Pulmonary rales
Orthopnea	Holosystolic murmur
Paroxysmal nocturnal dyspnea	

crease in afterload without contributing appreciably to the contractile state of the failing heart.

Dilation

For a long time, dilation may serve as a compensatory mechanism, increasing contractility by means of the Frank-Starling principle. However, as heart failure progresses, the increase in ventricular performance in response to cardiac dilation diminishes. Furthermore, this increase in end-diastolic volume (preload) eventually results in pulmonary and systemic congestion.

Hypertrophy

Chronic exposure to abnormal pressure and volume loads leads to myocardial hypertrophy. This increase in muscle mass initially is beneficial because it reduces ventricular wall stress. Excessive hypertrophy, however, reduces diastolic compliance and interferes with normal filling.

Tachycardia

Because the stroke volume is usually small and fixed in heart failure, an increase in cardiac output is accomplished primarily by an increase in heart rate. Excessive tachycardia, however, leaves insufficient time for ventricular filling. In addition, the energy cost of marked tachycardia is high.

In the early stages of heart failure the compensatory mechanisms may sustain the circulatory needs of the body. Eventually, however, as myocardial failure progresses, the compensatory mecha-

nisms can no longer maintain the pump function of the heart, and the clinical manifestations of congestive heart failure emerge.

Clinical Manifestations of Heart Failure

The symptoms and physical findings of congestive heart failure depend on the severity of heart failure and whether left or right heart failure predominates.

Left Heart Failure

The major symptoms of left ventricular failure include fatigue, weakness, exertional dyspnea, orthopnea, and paroxysmal nocturnal dyspnea. As heart failure progresses, dyspnea at rest may develop. On physical examination, the heart is enlarged, a ventricular gallop is frequently heard, and pulmonary rales or frank pulmonary edema is usually present. Occasionally, a systolic murmur is present at the apex consistent with mitral regurgitation (Table 3-4).

Right Heart Failure

Isolated right heart failure is uncommon and is generally a consequence of cor pulmonale secondary to chronic obstructive lung disease or pulmonary embolism. More often, right heart failure is a sequel of left heart failure. Symptoms of predominantly right heart failure include anorexia and nausea caused by congestion of the liver and mesentery and right upper quadrant pain caused by stretching of the hepatic capsule. Physical findings are a consequence of the elevated systemic venous pressure. These include jugular venous distention, hepatojugular reflux, hepatomegaly, ascites, and peripheral edema (Table 3-5).

Laboratory Testing in Heart Failure

Electrocardiography

The electrocardiogram may occasionally identify an unsuspected myocardial infarction or left ventricular hypertrophy.

Table 3-5. Right Heart Failure

Symptoms	Signs
Anorexia	Jugular venous distention
Nausea and vomiting	Hepatojugular reflux
Epigastric pain	Hepatomegaly
	Ascites
	Edema

Table 3-6. Treatment of Heart Failure

General measures
  Correction of underlying cause
  Avoidance of precipitating factors
  Rest
  Salt restriction
Drug therapy
  Digitalis (contractility)
  Diuretics (preload)
  Vasodilators (afterload)

Holter Monitoring

Ambulatory electrocardiographic monitoring may be useful in detecting paroxysmal arrhythmias and silent ischemia that might precipitate heart failure.

Chest Radiography

A chest x-ray film can be exceedingly helpful in the diagnosis of left heart failure. Typically, there is enlargement of the cardiac silhouette and pulmonary vascular congestion.

Echocardiography

Echocardiography can assess cardiac size, wall thickness and wall motion, and, when used in combination with Doppler techniques, can quantitate the severity of valvular lesions.

Radionuclide Angiography

The noninvasive technique of radionuclide angiography permits analysis of regional and global wall motion and provides a measurement of the left ventricular ejection fraction both at rest and during exercise.

Treadmill Stress Testing

Exercise testing is used to detect myocardial ischemia, screen for arrhythmias, and determine the extent of functional impairment, but often it is not feasible in the management of disabled patients.

Cardiac Catheterization

Although the presence of heart failure can usually be established by noninvasive testing, cardiac catheterization may be necessary to determine the underlying cause and severity of the heart disease.

Treatment of Heart Failure

General measures in the treatment of chronic congestive heart failure include correction, if possible, of the underlying cause, avoidance of the precipitating factors, rest, and salt restriction. Drug therapy is used to enhance contractility (digitalis), to control excessive fluid retention (diuretics), and to reduce afterload (vasodilators). Most physicians initiate drug therapy with digitalis. If digitalis is insufficient in controlling the symptoms of heart failure, then a diuretic is added. Vasodilators are usually reserved for more severe heart failure. However, there has recently been a tendency to add vasodilators earlier, especially the angiotensin-converting enzyme inhibitors, because of studies demonstrating their ability to reduce mortality in chronic congestive heart failure (Table 3-6).

Digitalis

Digitalis improves the contractility of the heart. Its exact mechanism of action is still not completely understood, but it involves an increase in the intracellular concentration of calcium. As a consequence of the increased contractility, cardiac output increases, end-diastolic pressure and volume decrease, and systemic vascular resistance diminishes. Digitalis is particularly helpful when congestive heart failure is associated with atrial fibrillation because of its ability to slow the ventricular response. Although there are many digitalis compounds, the one that is almost exclusively used is digoxin, which can be given in both intravenous and oral forms.

The use of digitalis is limited to a large extent by its narrow toxic-to-therapeutic range and its adverse and potentially fatal side effects. Common signs of toxicity include gastrointestinal distress (anorexia, nausea, and vomiting), neurologic symptoms (drowsiness, disorientation, and confusion), and visual disturbances (scotomas, halos, and changes in color perception). Cardiac toxicity to digitalis is manifested by arrhythmias, including ventricular premature beats, ventricular tachycardia, and fibrillation; high-degree atrioventricular (AV) block; and supraventricular tachycardia, especially in association with AV block. Serum digoxin levels can be helpful in diagnosing digitalis toxicity, especially in the presence of renal failure, when dosing may be difficult. The mainstay for treating digitalis toxicity is to stop the medication. If hypokalemia is present, it should be corrected. Lidocaine, procainamide, and propranolol are helpful in controlling ventricular arrhythmias. Digoxin-specific antibodies are occasionally used in the presence of refractory ventricular tachycardia and fibrillation.

Diuretics

Retention of sodium and water by the kidneys with resulting pulmonary and systemic congestion is a common manifestation of congestive heart failure and is responsible for many of the symptoms. Diuretics increase the excretion of sodium and water by inhibiting the reabsorption of sodium at various sites along the nephron. Less water in the vascular system improves congestive symptoms and reduces ventricular preload.

Thiazides

Thiazide diuretics act in the distal tubule, where they inhibit sodium reabsorption. They are helpful in mild heart failure but less effective in severe heart failure and in the presence of marked renal failure. Because of their long duration of action, hypokalemia frequently occurs with the chronic use of thiazide diuretics.

Loop Diuretics

Furosemide, ethacrynic acid, and bumetanide act primarily on the ascending limb of the loop of Henle where they inhibit the reabsorption of sodium and chloride. They are extremely potent diuretics that can be given both intravenously and orally and are effective when renal function is impaired. Volume depletion, hypotension, hyponatremia, and hypokalemia are among the most frequently seen problems. Patients on these diuretics should be monitored closely for symptoms such as fatigue, confusion, and nausea, which may indicate the presence of drug-induced fluid and electrolyte imbalance.

Aldosterone Antagonists

A characteristic feature of congestive heart failure is high circulating levels of renin and aldosterone. Aldosterone enhances sodium reabsorption and increases potassium excretion. Aldosterone antagonists interfere with these actions, causing sodium excretion and potassium retention. Three agents are available: spironolactone, triamterene, and amiloride. All three act by competing for receptor sites in the distal tubule. They are relatively mild diuretics but have the advantage of preventing hypokalemia. They are frequently used for this purpose in combination with a thiazide or loop diuretic.

Vasodilator Therapy

In patients with congestive heart failure, the arterial and venous beds are often inappropriately constricted. Venoconstriction tends to displace blood into the chest, causing pulmonary congestion, while arteriolar constriction increases left ventricular afterload. In choosing the proper vasodilator, a clinical decision has to be made whether the patient would benefit most from reduction in preload (venous), afterload (arteriolar), or both.

Venodilators

Venous dilators reduce systemic venous tone and increase the capacity of the systemic venous bed. In patients with chronic pulmonary congestion and edema resulting from elevated left atrial pressures, systemic venodilators provide considerable symptomatic relief so long as the decrease in preload does not significantly lower cardiac output. The prototype venodilator is nitroglycerin.

Arteriodilators

Arterial dilators are intended to relieve the intense systemic arteriolar vasoconstriction that characterizes left ventricular failure and to promote the normal distribution of cardiac output. They reduce afterload or impedance to ejection by reducing systemic arteriolar tone. As a result, cardiac output increases and distribution of blood flow to the vital organs (brain, kidney, and heart) improves. Because of the increase in cardiac output, systemic arterial blood pressure usually does not decrease. The prototype of this group is hydralazine.

Combined Venous and Arterial Dilators

The most popular combined vasodilators are the angiotensin-converting enzyme inhibitors. Multiple drugs are now currently available including captopril, enalapril, and lisinopril. The renin-angiotensin system is invariably activated in congestive heart failure. Angiotensin-converting enzyme inhibitors block the enzyme that converts angiotensin I to angiotensin II. Angiotensin II is a potent vasoconstrictor that also stimulates aldosterone secretion from the adrenal cortex. Aldosterone increases renal sodium reabsorption, leading to fluid retention. By inhibiting the formation of angiotensin II, these drugs reduce peripheral vasoconstriction and thereby decrease left ventricular afterload. Furthermore, inhibition of aldosterone secretion diminishes salt and water retention, which is beneficial in congestive heart failure. Consequently, angiotensin-converting enzyme inhibitors may decrease cardiac workload in congestive heart failure by reducing both afterload (prevention of vasoconstriction by angiotensin II) and preload (by inhibiting aldosterone secretion).

Serious side effects with angiotensin-converting enzyme inhibitors are rare and drug tolerance or attenuation of response, as occurs with other vasodilators such as prazosin, is rarely seen.

Special Concerns in Rehabilitation Patients

Rehabilitation programs must be adjusted to accommodate the unique requirements of patients with heart failure. Furthermore, patients in rehabilitation programs may be stable on presentation but develop heart failure during the course of their therapy. Because the recognition of heart failure in these patients may be difficult, noninvasive testing is frequently required. Chronically disabled patients are particularly susceptible to the side effects and toxicity of cardiovascular drug therapy.

Rehabilitation Strategies in Patients with Known Heart Failure

Many patients with complex cardiac disease are referred for rehabilitation, often after large myocardial infarctions or complicated open heart operations. These patients are too debilitated to go home or to participate in routine outpatient cardiac rehabilitation programs. Many have confirmed heart failure. These patients have a different set of expectations than the usual cardiac patients recovering from uncomplicated myocardial infarctions or coronary artery bypass surgery. Most have had prolonged hospitalizations and are frequently depressed by the long-standing ordeal of their cardiac disease and their marked limitations.

Nevertheless, rehabilitation has well-documented benefits in heart failure patients. Modified exercise programs and physical therapy help heart failure patients increase their functional capacity and may substantially enhance the quality of their lives. Indeed, successful therapy in these patients may mean the difference between living independently or in a chronic care facility.

If at all possible, these patients should have low-level stress tests before beginning exercise programs, both to assess their functional capacity and to aid in designing individualized rehabilitation programs to meet their specific needs. Patients with decompensated heart failure, unstable angina, or complex, potentially fatal arrhythmias are not candidates for rehabilitation. The target heart rate should be adjusted to 10 beats per minute below any significant endpoints of exercise such as a decrease in blood pressure, serious arrhythmia, or onset of severe dyspnea, angina, or ST-segment de-

Table 3-7. Important Types of Noninvasive Testing

Electrocardiogram
Holter monitoring
Echocardiography
Radionuclide angiography
Treadmill stress testing
Dipyridamole-thallium stress testing

pression. The heart rate, blood pressure, and weight should be monitored regularly. Telemetry may be required during the exercise sessions in patients with exercise-induced myocardial ischemia or complex arrhythmias.

Dynamic muscle strengthening exercises are preferable to isometrics. Warm-up and cool-down periods are desirable. Patients with heart failure can accommodate only limited workloads. Overzealous exercise or therapy may result in prolonged fatigue for hours or days after the session. The staff must be trained to recognize and meet the special needs of patients with heart failure.

Recognition of Heart Failure in Chronically Disabled Patients

Many patients in rehabilitation programs are old and have generalized atherosclerosis. Because of their sedentary life-style, manifestations of heart failure may be masked until they are revealed by the increased physical demands of therapy. Furthermore, because the activity levels of many disabled patients are reduced, symptoms of heart failure frequently do not retain their usual activity-precipitated characteristics. Unfortunately, the history and physical examination have limitations in diagnosing heart failure in rehabilitation patients. Many have altered mental acuity or cognitive disturbances related to illness or stroke. Obtaining an accurate history or evaluating symptoms may be extremely difficult. Confirmatory data must frequently be obtained from old medical records or family members. The coexistence of multiple diseases and depression also hinders the accurate evaluation of symptoms. Some of the traditional symptoms used to diagnose heart failure may be obscured in rehabilitation patients. Rales may be a result of pulmonary disease and ankle edema a result of venous insufficiency rather than heart failure.

The Importance of Noninvasive Testing

Because of the difficulties in obtaining an accurate history and evaluating physical findings, noninvasive tests assume greater importance (Table 3-7). The resting electrocardiogram may be useful in diagnosing an acute myocardial infarction as the cause of heart failure in an aphasic patient. Holter monitoring may reveal unsuspected paroxysmal atrial fibrillation in a patient with critical aortic stenosis who is experiencing intermittent heart failure. Echocardiography, especially in conjunction with Doppler imaging, can help determine the significance of heart murmurs. The left ventricular ejection fraction can be measured by radionuclide angiography, quantitating the degree of left ventricular impairment caused by a dilated cardiomyopathy. Treadmill stress testing can give an objective assessment of functional impairment in a patient with heart failure caused by long-standing hypertensive heart disease. A dipyridamole-thallium stress test may unmask the presence of silent myocardial ischemia in patients unable to exercise because of marked deconditioning, stroke, amputation, arthritis, severe pulmonary disease, or intermittent claudication.

Cardiovascular Drug Therapy in the Chronically Disabled

Drug therapy in rehabilitation patients is limited by toxicity and side effects. Physicians, nurses, and therapists should be aware of potential complications caused by the various cardiac medications. Multiple drugs and concomitant multisystem chronic diseases make patients more susceptible to problems with medications. Noncompliance or errors in taking drugs is frequent and is often related to visual or cognitive impairment.

Digitalis

Digitalis toxicity is common and accentuated by the limited volume of distribution and decline in renal excretion (even with a normal creatinine clearance) in elderly patients with heart failure. As a general

Table 3-8. Principles of Drug Therapy

Initiate at a low dose
Increase gradually
Simplify regimen
Periodic reassessment
Discontinue unnecessary medications

rule, the maintenance dose of digoxin should be cut in half in this population. Frequently, digitalis can be discontinued without clinical deterioration in many chronically disabled patients who are in sinus rhythm and without overt heart failure.

Diuretics

Aggressive diuretic therapy may result in dehydration, especially in patients who are not able to regulate fluid intake. Excessive fatigue and weakness may be early signs of fluid and electrolyte imbalance.

Vasodilators

Vasodilators often cause hypotension, and postural hypotension can be a major problem in patients with strokes or spinal cord injuries. Therapeutic modalities that produce systemic vasodilation, such as exercise and whirlpool baths, should be used cautiously in patients on vasodilators. Also, angiotensin-converting enzyme inhibitors have the capacity to cause severe renal failure and hyperkalemia, especially in patients with underlying renal vascular disease.

General Outline for Drug Therapy

In general, drug therapy should be initiated at a low dose and gradually increased, if necessary, in chronically disabled patients with heart failure. The drug regimen should be as simple as possible. Whenever possible, medications should be given once a day rather than in split doses, in order to increase compliance. There should be periodic reassessment of drug therapy, and unnecessary drugs should be discontinued (Table 3-8).

Case Management Studies

Patient with Previous Coronary Artery Bypass Surgery

Brief History

A 79-year-old retired lawyer with a long history of exertional angina underwent emergency coronary artery bypass surgery for unstable angina after an acute myocardial infarction. He had a protracted postoperative course complicated by congestive heart failure and persistent atrial fibrillation. He was eventually transferred to a rehabilitation facility to improve his overall cardiovascular fitness before returning home. His medications included digoxin, 0.375 mg qd, and furosemide, 80 mg qd.

Problem

Initially, the patient was alert, cooperative, and enthusiastic about initiating therapy. However, by the end of the first week, there was a distinct change in his demeanor. He became confused and lethargic, with poor oral intake. His pulse, which had been irregular, became slow and regular.

Evaluation

After the patient was evaluated, digitalis toxicity was suspected. This was confirmed by a digoxin level of 3.6 ng/ml. In addition, the blood urea nitrogen level, which had been in the normal range on transfer, was 48 mg/dl, and the potassium level was 3.0 mEq/liter. His electrocardiogram demonstrated atrial fibrillation with atrioventricular dissociation and a slow, regular junctional escape rhythm.

Solution

The digoxin and furosemide were withheld, intravenous fluids were begun, and the hypokalemia corrected. The next day he was noted to have ventricular bigeminy. This resolved promptly with additional potassium administration. The patient soon returned to his previous pleasant state. The digoxin dose was reduced to 0.125 mg qd, and a thiazide diuretic in combination with spironolactone was used instead of furosemide to help prevent dehydration and potassium depletion.

Discussion

Digitalis toxicity occurs frequently in elderly people in whom the classic manifestations may not be present. In this case, the large dose of furosemide led to dehydration with decreased renal perfusion. This, in turn, resulted in reduced renal clearance of digoxin and the subsequently elevated blood level. Furthermore, the hypokalemia exacerbated the cardiac toxicity of digitalis.

Patient with Acute Myocardial Infarction

Brief History

A 68-year-old woman had insulin-dependent diabetes since age 11 years. She had long-standing hypertension and a previous non–Q wave myocardial infarction with mild, compensated heart failure. She was transferred to a rehabilitation facility after undergoing a right, below-the-knee amputation for a nonhealing ischemic ulcer on her foot.

Problem

Several weeks after her admission, she was noted to be excessively fatigued and short of breath during physical therapy. She had subtle personality changes and a decrease in appetite. She became dyspneic when lying flat and had to sleep with her head propped up on pillows. At no time did she complain of chest pain.

Evaluation

On examination she had findings of congestive heart failure with a ventricular gallop, bibasilar rales, neck vein engorgement, hepatomegaly, and pedal edema. As part of her evaluation an electrocardiogram was obtained that demonstrated a new anterior myocardial infarction.

Solution

She was transferred back to an acute care facility for monitoring and treatment of the heart failure.

Discussion

In this case, the precipitating factor for heart failure was a silent myocardial infarction. In elderly patients, especially with diabetes, chest pain may not occur with myocardial infarctions. Atypical manifestations of acute myocardial infarction are frequent in these patients and include personality changes, excessive fatigue, alterations in eating patterns, and the exacerbation of heart failure.

Patient with a Stroke and Heart Murmur

Brief History

A 56-year-old man had a large dominant hemisphere stroke with hemiplegia and expressive aphasia. He had a significant past history of hypertensive heart disease and an ill-defined heart murmur thought to be caused by mitral regurgitation. On transfer to a rehabilitation facility, he was taking digoxin, 0.125 mg qd, furosemide, 40 mg qd, and captopril, 25 mg tid.

Problem

Shortly after admission, he was found agitated and acutely short of breath.

Evaluation

On examination, he had a rapid irregular pulse of 140 beats per minute, a blood pressure of 86/52 mm Hg, a loud holosystolic murmur at the apex, and bibasilar rales. An electrocardiogram demonstrated atrial flutter with left ventricular hypertrophy, and a chest x-ray film showed cardiomegaly with vascular congestion.

Solution

He was stabilized and rapidly moved to an acute care facility. An emergency echocardiogram demonstrated a hypertrophic cardiomyopathy with a large left ventricular outflow gradient. The digoxin, furosemide, and captopril were discontinued, and he was begun on beta-blocker therapy, with rapid clinical improvement. The next day he spontaneously converted back to sinus rhythm.

Since his stroke was thought to be embolic, antico-agulants were given.

Discussion

Hypertrophic cardiomyopathy is commonly misdi-agnosed in elderly patients. An incorrect diagnosis, with resultant inappropriate drug therapy (e.g., dig-italis, excessive diuretics, and vasodilators), may exacerbate the outflow obstruction and result in se-rious complications. Atrial fibrillation or flutter with the loss of an atrial kick is poorly tolerated in these patients and may result in acute heart failure. This case illustrates how important it is to define the cause of the underlying heart disease in rehabilita-tion patients in order to prevent an acute precipitat-ing illnesses.

Suggested Reading

Brammel HL. Rehabilitation of the Cardiac Patient. In JA DeLisa (ed), Rehabilitation Medicine: Principles and Practice. Philadelphia: Lippincott, 1988;671.

Braunwald E, Grossman W. Clinical Aspects of Heart Fail-ure. In E Braunwald (ed), Heart Disease: A Text Book of Cardiovascular Medicine (4th ed). Philadelphia: Saunders, 1992;444.

Coats AJS, Adamopoulos S, Meyer TE, et al. Effects of phys-ical training in chronic heart failure. Lancet 1990;335:63.

Lowenthal DT, Affrime MB. Cardiovascular drugs for the geriatric patient. Cardiology 1981;36:65.

Smith TW, Braunwald E, Kelly RA. The Management of Heart Failure. In E Braunwald (ed), Heart Disease: A Text Book of Cardiovascular Medicine (4th ed). Philadelphia: Saunders, 1992;464.

Stevenson LW, Perloff JK. The limited reliability of physi-cal signs for estimating hemodynamics in chronic heart failure. JAMA 1989;261:884.

Sullivan MJ, Higginbotham MB, Cobb FR. Exercise train-ing in patients with chronic heart failure delays ventila-tory anaerobic threshold and improves submaximal exercise performance. Circulation 1989;79:324.

Upton MT. Laboratory Methods in the Diagnosis of Chest Pain due to Ischemic Heart Disease. In AJ Miller (ed), Diagnosis of Chest Pain. New York: Raven, 1988;195.

Wenger NK. Rehabilitation of the Patient with Coronary Heart Disease. In RC Schlant, RW Alexander (eds), Hurst's The Heart: Arteries and Veins (8th ed). New York: McGraw-Hill, 1994;1223.

Part II
Disorders of Bone

Chapter 4

Prevention and Treatment of Osteoporosis

George E. Shambaugh III and Christina Marciniak

Osteoporosis can be defined as an absolute decrease in the amount of bone. This decrease is gradual and painless until minimal trauma results in fracture [1–3]. Osteoporosis has been identified as the world's most common skeletal disorder, producing symptomatic disease in over 15 million women in the United States alone [4]. This disease affects both sexes during aging, and the increasing life expectancy (from 47 years in 1900 to 73 years in 1985) ensures a continuing increase in the magnitude of this problem [1]. It has been estimated that by age 65 years, 25% of all women suffer from osteoporosis, and that a 50-year-old woman has a 54% chance of sustaining a hip, vertebral, or Colles' fracture during her remaining life span [5].

Osteoporosis is more prevalent in the disabled population. This is because of a lack of local stresses on bone resulting from paralysis as well as generalized immobilization. It has been found that bone mineral loss occurs even in healthy volunteers placed at bed rest [6], and for a disabled person confined to a wheelchair such problems may continue over a lifetime. In addition to a general increase in the prevalence of osteoporosis in the disabled population, some subgroups have skeletal regions where osteoporosis manifests a selective intensity. Thus, in patients with polio, bone loss has been seen primarily in weight-bearing bones, whereas hemiplegic patients who have had cerebrovascular accidents show a reduction in cortical thickness, bone mineral content, and bone mineral density on the involved side compared with the uninvolved side [7]. This difference in bone mineral content is more dramatic in the upper than the lower limbs [8]. The osteoporosis that results from hemiplegia significantly increases the risk of fracture. Eighty-two percent of femoral neck fractures occurred on the hemiplegic side in a prospective study of patients with previous cerebrovascular accidents [9]. Osteoporosis is almost always present after a spinal cord injury. Fractures may be seen after trivial trauma, and in a retrospective study of fractures in one group, 12 of 27 patients had no known cause for the fracture [10]. Disabled patients are also more likely to have some of the other risk factors for osteoporosis, including chronic kidney disease, use of corticosteroids, or the use of phenytoin.

Although osteoporosis is common in the disabled population, fractures resulting from osteoporosis in a previously nondisabled group continually add these patients to the ranks of the disabled. Three sites that are especially vulnerable to fracture include the lumbar vertebrae, distal radius, and femoral neck. Fractures of the femoral neck are accompanied not only by the greatest morbidity but by a 10% mortality within 3 months of fracture because of complications during and after surgical fixation [11]. The cost of caring for such patients per year is close to $1 billion [12], and because femoral neck and vertebral fractures were found to increase by 40% in the decade from 1975 to 1985, it has been estimated that acute health care costs for hip fracture could be greater than $5 billion by the end of the century [1]. This was extended by Cummings et al. [13], who estimated that with the increasing population of elderly men and

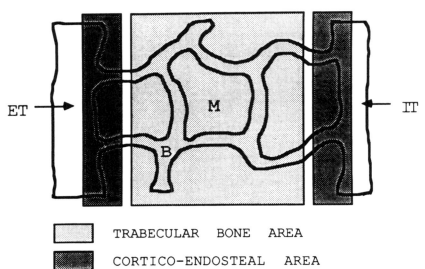

ET

IT

TRABECULAR BONE AREA

CORTICO-ENDOSTEAL AREA

Figure 4-1. Bone regions in an iliac crest bone biopsy specimen. Cortical bone is identified by heavily shaded region. ET and IT refer to the external cortex and internal cortex. The lightly shaded area identifies the medullary space (M) and the bony trabeculae crossing this space are identified as B. (Reprinted with permission from JP Brown, PD Delmas, M Arlot, et al. Active bone turnover of the corticoendosteal envelope in postmenopausal osteoporosis. J Clin Endocrinol Metab 1987;64:954. Copyright 1987 by The Endocrine Society.)

women, the total number of hip fractures will increase from 238,000 in 1990 to 512,000 in 2040. If the average cost per fracture were fixed at $29,800, the resulting cost would be $15.21 billion. The economic drain, combined with a progressive strain on the limited nursing home and rehabilitation facilities that are currently available, attest to the magnitude of this ever-increasing worldwide problem [12]. Such costs are probably underestimated because they do not include the indefinite requirement for medical care of younger disabled persons with fractures and osteoporosis. In this chapter, osteoporosis is discussed through a consideration of our present knowledge of the pathophysiology of this entity, the diagnostic tools available, and the modalities for prevention and treatment.

Natural History of Bone Formation and the Etiology of Osteoporosis

Bone formation begins during fetal life and continues throughout the life of the host. Although remodeling is most extensive during the first 2 years of life, it continues even into adult life, with approximately 5% of cortical bone being remodeled each year [14]. The changes in bone mass during life have been divided by Parfitt [15] into three periods: the first, extending from prenatal develop-

ment to epiphyseal closure, is characterized by an increase in bone volume in both the trabecular and cortical bone. Trabecular bone is formed by ossification of a cartilaginous template (endochondral ossification) and cortical bone is formed by periosteal and endosteal apposition of osseous tissue. This phase is followed by a period of consolidation during adolescence wherein cortical bones that have been formed become more dense. The peak of adult bone mass is reached in trabecular bone soon after epiphyseal closure, but consolidation of cortical bone representing 5–10% of the peak mass is reached at age 35–40 years. Men have a 25–30% greater peak bone mass than women and blacks about 10% greater than whites [16]. Bone loss, the third stage, begins a few years after attaining the peak bone mass [15]. Bone formation and bone breakdown are coupled, but a true equilibrium exists only between ages 25 and 40 years. Before 25 years of age, bone formation predominates and after ages 30–40 years, bone loss predominates. Bone contains cortical and trabecular regions, and the relationship between cortical and trabecular bone is indicated in Figure 4-1. The relative abundance of cortical and trabecular elements varies with different bones. Cortical bone, which makes up the shafts of long bones and the cortical shell of vertebrae, ribs, and pelvis, is much denser than trabecular bone. Cortical bone represents 85% of the total skeleton and accounts for the weight-bearing capability of individual bones [17]. Thus, the thin cortical bone of vertebrae accounts for 45–75% of their strength [18]. Cortical bone loss begins around age 40 years in both sexes at an initial rate of 0.3–0.5% per year and increases with aging. Eventually it results in a decrease of 35% in bone mass [2, 19]. In postmenopausal women an additional rate of bone loss of 2–3% per year is superimposed on the previously described pattern [20]. Trabecular bone predominates in flat bones, including the pelvis, ribs, vertebrae, and the ends of long bones. Trabecular bone consists of a series of plates that are interlinked and serve as struts to support the structure. An electron photomicrograph of trabecular bone [21] is shown in Figure 4-2. The large surface area provides a ready response to alterations in mineral homeostasis. Trabecular bone losses begin in women at age 30 years; the rates of loss (0.6% per year) are somewhat greater than that for cortical bone and continue progressively into old age, resulting in an eventual loss of 50% of the bone mass. The accelerated postmenopausal phase of trabecular bone loss was found to have an initial rate that was greater, and a duration that was shorter, than cortical bone loss [2]. The relative contributions of age and menopause were analyzed by Nordin et al. [22] in 485 patients whose age at menopause could be established. Serial scans of the forearm using single photon densitometry were carried out, and their data, shown in Figure 4-3, defined two curves. The first was a linear curve that began at age 55 years and continued to decline at a rate of 1% per year through the study (age 75 years); the second was a curvilinear decrease that accounted for 11% of bone loss in the first 5 years after menopause and a further 5% in the next 20 years [23]. The decrease in bone loss was supported by iliac bone biopsy specimens obtained from women with postmenopausal osteoporosis. These were shown to have a significant increase in bone formation and resorption at the corticomedullary interface when compared with biopsy specimens similarly obtained from age-matched women without osteoporosis [24]. To clarify these findings, a concept of bone remodeling was formulated in 1987 by Frost [25] to represent the action of a "mechanostat." In the presence of diminished estrogen, the mechanostat set point would be raised and the perceived excess of bone would result in a

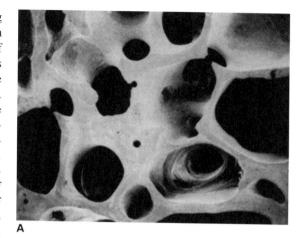

A

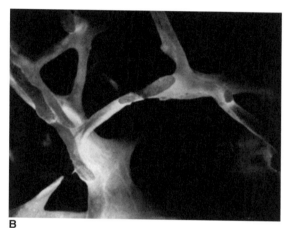

B

Figure 4-2. Low-power scanning electron micrographs of biopsy specimens of normal and osteoporotic bone from the iliac crest. A. Trabecular plate in a 75-year-old woman. B. Trabecular region from a 47-year-old woman with multiple compression fractures. Note the conversion of intact plates to discontinuous spicules. (Reprinted with permission from DW Dempster, E Shane, W Horbert, et al. A simple method for correlative light and scanning EM of human iliac crest biopsies: Qualitative observations in normal and osteoporotic subjects. J Bone Mineral Res 1986;1:15. Copyright 1986 by Mary Ann Liebert, Inc.)

heightened remodeling and a decrease in bone mass. The weight bearing on the decreased bone mass would be registered as a strain that would lower the set point of the mechanostat. The remodeling would now cease, and bone turnover would stabilize at a new equilibrium. Such a concept applies well to menopausal changes but less well to

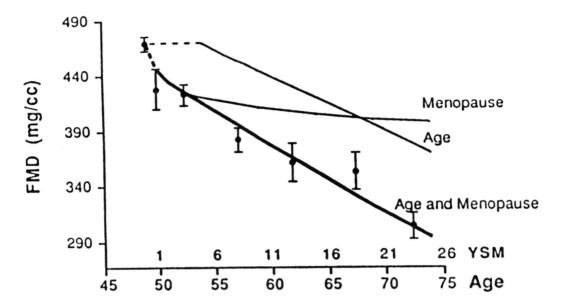

Figure 4-3. Calculated mean forearm mineral density (FMD) as a function of age and years since menopause (YSM), separately and together assuming a menopausal age of 49 years. The lower line is the sum of the upper two lines. (Reprinted with permission from BEC Nordin, AG Need, BE Chatterton, et al. The relative contributions of age and years since menopause to postmenopausal bone loss. J Clin Endocrinol Metab 1990;70:83. Copyright 1990 by the Endocrine Society.)

aging, where there is an obligatory loss of bone that is constant.

When bone mineral density is plotted as a function of age, the increase in bone density peaks between ages 20 and 40 years and then decreases progressively (Figure 4-4). When bone mineral density in the lumbar spine is measured, women with vertebral compression fractures have a generally lower density than normal, with some overlap (Figure 4-5). By contrast, when the values for women with vertebral compression fractures are superimposed on a curve of a normal age regression of bone mineral density in the distal radius (containing both cortical and trabecular bone), the values largely overlap (see Figure 4-4). When the bone mineral density of the proximal femur was plotted as a function of age, a linear decrease was seen between 20 and 100 years of age. Bone mineral density in patients with hip fractures fell into a normal range, similar to what was seen in patients with fractures of the distal radius. In men, the decrease in bone mineral density of the proximal femur was two-

thirds of that in women, whereas the decrease in the lumbar spine was only one-fourth of that found in women [19]. Thus, although women have twice as many hip fractures as men, they have eight times as many vertebral fractures [26].

The diagnosis of osteoporosis has been established by generalized radiolucency on spinal radiographs and one or more vertebral compression fractures occurring with trivial activities such as bending, coughing, or lying quietly in bed [27]. When bone mineral density measurements are made, fractures are found to occur when the bone mineral density decreases to 1 g/cm^2 [2]. The greater initial bone density in blacks [28] and a genetically determined variation in bone density may explain, in part, the lower incidence of osteoporosis in blacks and the higher incidence in some families [29]. The progressive decrease in bone density with age and the sexual differences in these changes, when combined with the greater frequency of vertebral fractures in women, prompted Riggs and Melton [30] to identify two clinical groups of osteoporosis, an idea

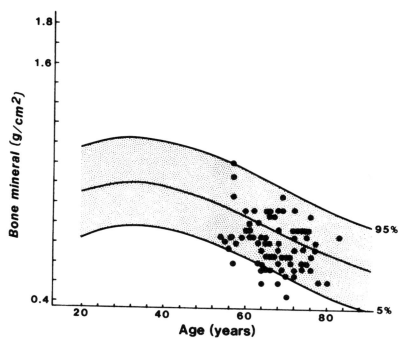

Figure 4-4. Individual values for bone mineral density of the distal radius in 76 osteoporotic women, with one or more vertebral compression fractures shown by the solid circles. These values are superimposed on a regression line drawn for normal women. The shaded area represents the 90% confidence limits. Bone mineral density in grams per square centimeter is shown on the ordinate and age in years is shown on the abscissa. (Reprinted with permission from BL Riggs, HW Wahner, WL Dunn, et al. Differential changes in bone mineral density of the appendicular and axial skeleton with aging: Relationship to spinal osteoporosis. J Clin Invest 1981;67:328. Copyright 1981 The American Society for Clinical Investigation.)

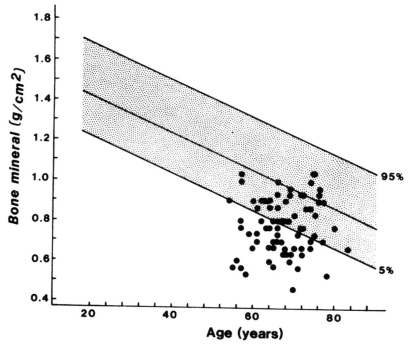

Figure 4-5. Individual values for bone mineral density of the lumbar spine of 76 osteoporotic women with one or more vertebral compression fractures shown by the solid circles. These values are superimposed on the regression line shown for normal women, with the 90% confidence limit identified by the shaded area. Bone mineral density in grams per square centimeter is shown on the ordinate and age in years is shown on the abscissa. (Reprinted with permission from BL Riggs, HW Wahner, WL Dunn, et al. Differential changes in bone mineral density of the appendicular and axial skeleton with aging: Relationship to spinal osteoporosis. J Clin Invest 1981;67:328. Copyright 1981 The American Society for Clinical Investigation.)

Table 4-1. Two Types of Involutional Osteoporosis

	Type I	Type II
Age (yr)	51–75	>70
Sex ratio (F:M)	6:1	2:1
Type of bone loss	Mainly trabecular	Trabecular and cortical
Rate of bone loss	Accelerated	Not accelerated
Fracture sites	Vertebrae (crush) and distal radius	Vertebrae (multiple wedge) and hip
Parathyroid function	Decreased	Increased
Calcium absorption	Decreased	Decreased
Metabolism of 25-hydroxyvitamin D to 1, 25 dihydroxyvitamin D	Secondary decrease	Primary decrease
Main causes	Factors related to menopause	Factors related to aging

Source: Reprinted with permission from BL Riggs, LJ Melton. Involutional osteoporosis. N Engl J Med 1986;314:1676. Copyright 1986 by Massachusetts Medical Society.

proposed by Albright 36 years before but never widely accepted. The two types, identified as types I and II, are shown in Table 4-1. The pathophysiologic mechanisms underlying types I and II osteoporosis are different. In type I, the loss of bone is related to the menopause and is characterized by an accelerated loss of bone with a release of calcium, heightened calcitonin level, diminished secretion of parathyroid hormones, and secondary decrease in 25-hydroxyvitamin D_3 1-alpha-hydroxylase activity. This results in a diminished production of 1,25-dihydroxyvitamin D_3, and consequently a diminished calcium absorption. These events are self-limited and are largely over by age 75 years. The clinical manifestations include Colles' fracture of the distal forearm, painful, deforming vertebral fracture [2], and loss of teeth [31]. Type II osteoporosis appears at a later age than type I and is associated with an equal rate in both trabecular and cortical bone loss. This type of osteoporosis is the culmination of a steady rate of bone loss from the age of 40 years in both sexes at approximately 3% per decade. The clinical manifestations are wedging of the thoracic vertebrae, producing a "dowager's hump." The pathogenesis of type II osteoporosis is related in part to decreased osteoblast function and in part to impaired production of 1,25-dihydroxyvitamin D_3, resulting in decreased calcium absorption. Parathyroid hormone in these patients is increased. The syndrome of type II osteoporosis is more common in women. Although rates of bone loss in 75-year-old

women are similar to rates in age-matched men, women have already suffered an accelerated bone loss between ages 45 and 75 years that brings the total rate of bone decrease to 9% per decade during this period [20].

A mechanistic classification with relevance for therapeutic approaches has been presented by Parfitt [15] and is shown in Table 4-2. Here type I is classified as osteoclast mediated and type II as osteoblast mediated. The differences in remodeling of the bone structural unit include the initial step of lining cell activation with greater osteoclast activity in the former and diminished activation and the recruitment of fewer osteoblasts in the latter. The results of these changes on bone wall thickness are shown in Figure 4-6. The consequences of osteoclast-mediated resorption are shown in Figure 4-7. The rapid resorption results in a heightened excavation on either side of a trabecular plate and perforation. Because the slow bone loss characterized by diminished osteoblast recruitment continues apace, a postmenopausal woman with a decreased initial bone mass is at heightened risk for fracture. The increased prevalence of vertebral fractures and the increased incidence of proximal femoral fractures seen at a bone mineral density of less than 1 g/cm^2 is shown in Figure 4-8. A higher incidence of fractures could also be seen if the rapid bone loss were perpetuated in thyrotoxicosis, alcohol abuse, cigarette smoking, and hyperparathyroidism (Table 4-3).

Table 4-2. Comparison of Two Morphologic Types of Bone Loss

Characteristic	Osteoclast-Mediated	Osteoblast-Mediated
Cellular defect	Lack of restraint	Lack of number
Remodeling mechanism	Deeper resorption	Shallower formation
Structure		
Trabecular	Perforation and disconnection	Simple thinning
Cortical	Subendosteal cavitation	Simple thinning
Reduction in strength	More than predicted*	As predicted*
Timing	Early	Late
Rate	Rapid	Slow
Magnitude	Usually greater	Usually less
Activation	Often increased	Often decreased

*From reduction in mass or mineral content.
Source: Reprinted with permission from AM Parfitt. Bone Remodeling: Relationship and Prevention of Fractures. In BL Riggs, LJ Melton (eds), Osteoporosis: Etiology, Diagnosis, and Management. New York: Raven, 1988;45.

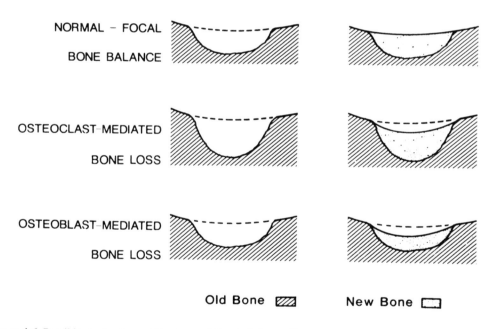

Figure 4-6. Possible mechanisms of focal remodeling imbalance. The upper panel shows a normal depth resorption cavity (left) that is completely filled with new bone (right). The middle panel shows osteoclast-mediated bone loss, which is characterized by a resorption cavity of excessive depth that is incompletely filled with the same quantity of new bone as shown in the top panel on the right. The bottom panel shows an osteoblast-mediated bone loss. Here the resorption cavity (left) is of normal depth, but the quantity of new bone is subnormal (right). The net bone loss is similar in magnitude to that resulting from osteoclast-mediated resorption but has been caused by a different cell mechanism. (Reprinted with permission from AM Parfitt. Bone Remodeling: Relationship to the Amount and Structure of Bone, and the Pathogenesis and Prevention of Fractures. In BL Riggs, LJ Melton III [eds], Osteoporosis: Etiology, Diagnosis, and Management. New York: Raven, 1988:45.)

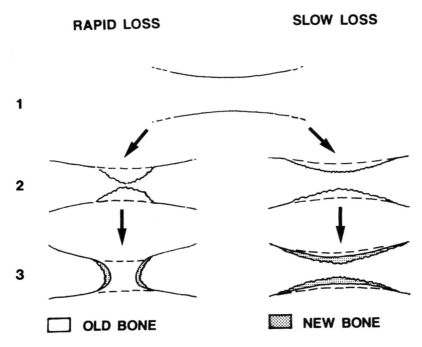

RAPID LOSS   **SLOW LOSS**

1

2

3

☐ **OLD BONE**   ▨ **NEW BONE**

Figure 4-7. Rapid and slow loss of trabecular bone. The effects of rapid bone loss characterizing osteoclast-mediated resorption is shown on the left. Here the deep resorption cavities have resulted in perforation. The new bone is apposed on either side, but does not bridge the gap. On the right is shown the effects of slow bone loss characterizing osteoblast-mediated resorption. Here the resorption cavity is not deep enough to perforate, but the reduced quantity of bone results in reduced wall thickness. (Reprinted with permission from AM Parfitt. Bone Remodeling: Relationship to the Amount and Structure of Bone, and the Pathogenesis and Prevention of Fractures. In BL Riggs, LJ Melton III [eds], Osteoporosis: Etiology, Diagnosis, and Management. New York: Raven, 1988:45.)

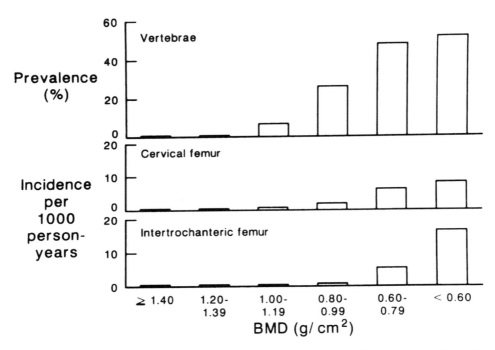

Figure 4-8. Occurrence of vertebral and proximal femoral fractures, both cervical and intertrochanteric, in a random sample of women in Rochester, Minnesota. Prevalence of vertebral fractures and incidence of femoral fractures are shown on the ordinate. Bone mineral density (BMD) in grams per square centimeter is identified on the abscissa. (Reprinted with permission from BL Riggs, LJ Melton. Involutional osteoporosis. N Engl J Med 1986;314:1676. Copyright 1986 by Massachusetts Medical Society.)

Table 4-3. Possible Discriminatory
Historical Risk Factors

Postmenopausal (within 20 years after menopause)
White or Asian
Premature menopause
Positive family history
Short stature and small bones
Leanness
Low calcium intake
Inactivity
Nulliparity
Gastric or small bowel resection
Long-term glucocorticoid therapy
Long-term use of anticonvulsants
Hyperparathyroidism
Thyrotoxicosis
Smoking
Heavy alcohol use

Source: Reprinted with permission from BL Riggs. Practical
Management of the Patient with Osteoporosis. In BL Riggs, LJ
Melton III (eds), Osteoporosis: Etiology, Diagnosis, and Man-
agement. New York: Raven, 1988;481.

Diminished mineralization of the skeleton occurs
with immobilization, bed rest, and weightlessness.
The first detailed study in humans was carried out
in healthy young men immobilized in plaster body
casts for 6–7 weeks [32]. In these subjects a loss of
calcium, phosphorus, and nitrogen in the urine continued as long as bed rest was maintained. Studies
in rodents in space flights indicated a complete cessation of bone growth at periosteal and endosteal
surfaces [33]. The inhibition of periosteal bone formation during space flight was not seen during the
postflight recovery period [34]. The greatest alterations during space flight have been recorded in the
appendicular skeleton, but changes have also been
seen in non–weight-bearing bone, including the
mandibles, teeth, and ribs [35]. Changes in
non–weight-bearing bones were fully corrected by a
29-day recovery period. By contrast, trabecular
bone mass in the proximal tibia remained abnormal
[36], suggesting that additional systemic factors
played a role in the problem of weightlessness. The
data in humans reviewed by Whedon [37] indicated
a mineral loss similar to that seen in patients with
recent paralytic polio. The loss of muscle mass and
bone mineral content persisted in astronauts' legs
despite a vigorously executed exercise regimen

while in space. In healthy men on prolonged bed
rest (30–36 weeks), large losses of mineral were observed in the os calcis, but these losses were rectified after ambulation. Mineral gain during
ambulation occurred at a rate similar to the rate of
mineral loss observed during bed rest [5].

In the disabled population, accelerated osteoporosis may be seen in selective regions, depending
on the type of disability. The type of bone dissolution after spinal cord injury has been characterized
by a loss of trabecular bone but a lack of change in
cortical bone [38]. Although bone loss is seen in the
axial skeleton acutely after spinal cord injury, it returns to near normal levels [39], and bone mineral
density at the lumbar spine has been found to be
near that of an able-bodied control group an average of 5.6 years after spinal cord injury [40]. This
may explain the observation that spontaneous fractures of long bones occur in 2–6% of paraplegic patients, whereas vertebral fractures in such patients
are seen less often [10, 41]. Despite the use of their
arms to propel themselves, paraplegic patients lose
trabecular bone in the upper extremities as well. In
hemiplegic patients, a smaller degree of cortical
thinning was observed with better voluntary muscle function [7]. Indeed, in a current review, the
severity of osteoporosis in patients with spinal cord
injury was found to be less after the institution of
mobilization [42]. In addition, hypercalcemia in incomplete tetraplegic patients could be diminished
by tilt-table exercises. The effectiveness of such a
program was greater when the exercises were instituted within 6 months of the injury [14]. The metabolic response to spinal cord injury, whether it
results in paraplegia or quadriplegia, is characterized by an initial rapid urinary loss of hydroxyproline, calcium, and phosphorus during the first 7
weeks, followed in turn by a slower phase from 7
to 16 weeks [43]. By 8 weeks after injury, urinary
phosphorus and magnesium levels had returned to
normal, whereas calcium levels remained elevated
and hydroxyproline levels were elevated in quadriplegic but not in paraplegic patients. In addition to
collagen, several minerals, including calcium, magnesium, and zinc, are excreted in larger than normal
amounts in patients with spinal cord injury [44, 45].
Although bone loss can be attenuated in postmenopausal women by exercise programs [46],
such programs, unless selectively carried out, can
increase the number of fractures in a susceptible

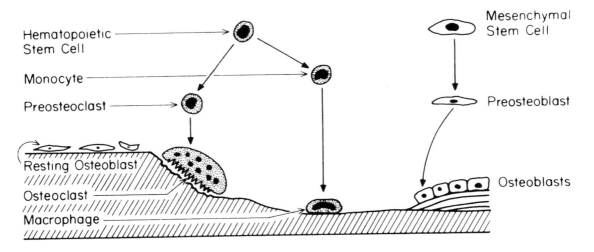

Figure 4-9. Schematic representation of trabecular bone remodeling. Trabecular bone remodeling is shown to occur in four stages. In the first stage pre-osteoclasts are activated to form a multinucleated mature osteoclast. In the resorption phase, the osteoclast walls off an area that is demineralized by hydrogen ions and the matrix is degraded by lysosomal enzymes. In the third or reversal stage, the osteoclasts are replaced by macrophages. In the fourth stage, pre-osteoblasts differentiate into osteoblasts and new bone matrix is laid down. This matrix is subsequently mineralized. (Reprinted with permission from LG Raisz. Local and systemic factors in the pathogenesis of osteoporosis. N Engl J Med 1988:318:818. Copyright 1988 by Massachusetts Medical Society.)

population [47]. Indeed, after spinal cord injury the incidence of lower extremity fractures is greater in paraplegic patients than in quadriplegic patients. This was thought to be related to the greater level of activity in the former [10]. In addition to exercise, another potential therapeutic modality is electrical stimulation, which has been shown to reverse osteoporosis in the extremity of a sciatic-denervated rat [48]. Results of this modality have so far been disappointing in humans, and in a small number of quadraplegic men who underwent 6 months of electrical stimulation via bicycle ergometry training no increase in femoral bone mineral density could be clearly demonstrated [49].

Pathogenesis

To gain insight into the cellular mechanisms of osteoporosis, a quantum concept of bone remodeling was first proposed by Frost in the 1960s and updated in 1985 [50]. This concept was extended by Parfitt [51] and Eriksen [52]. Here the skeleton is conceptualized as a brick structure, each brick representing a bone structural unit. These units are remodeled in a sequence that has been illustrated by Raisz [53] and is shown in Figure 4-9. The remodeling begins with activation of a quiescent bone surface covered by lining cells that are connected by cell processes to the inner osteocytes that can serve as sensors for the effects of mechanical stresses. During the activation step, the lining cells release proteolytic enzymes that uncover mineralized bone. Bone resorption then supervenes as the second stage, which involves osteoclast differentiation from a hematopoietic stem cell precursor. The preosteoclasts subsequently fuse to form multinucleated osteoclasts [54]. The osteoclast then walls off an area for resorption. In cortical bone, this area is known as a cutting cone and in trabecular bone as a Howship's lacunae [55]. Into this region lysosomal enzymes and hydrogen ions are secreted to degrade bone matrix and dissolve minerals [56]. The next stage has been identified as a reversal stage. The osteoclasts disappear and macrophages line the resorption cavity. This precedes the fourth stage, which is bone formation. Bone formation occurs in two phases: matrix formation and mineralization. Raisz [53] has suggested that the rate of new matrix formation is dependent on four factors: (1) unresorbed bone at the remodeling site to serve as a template for osteoblasts; (2) release of factors needed for osteoblast renewal; (3) the ability of mesenchymal precursor to differentiate into osteoblasts; and (4) the capability of the osteoblasts to produce normal matrix. In the second phase of bone formation, mineralization of the newly formed matrix slowly occurs, a process that is dependent in part on the availability of calcium and phosphorus. The timing between bone replacement phases is markedly different. It has been estimated that one new bone remodeling unit appears and one structural unit is completed every 10 seconds in a skeleton, with an average turnover rate of 10% per year [15]. Within each replacement unit, osteoclastic activity requires 10 days to form an appropriate cavity, and osteoblast function with mineralization to form new bone requires 100 days.

Although bone resorption and formation are coupled, a decline in bone mass begins as soon as a peak bone mass is attained. In osteoblast-mediated bone resorption, the lacuna scooped out by osteoblasts is never filled completely, as shown on the right side in Figure 4-6. The mechanism is unclear, but it appears to be more closely related to diminished numbers of osteoblasts rather than a decline in individual capabilities [57]. Present evidence suggests that osteoblasts may activate bone resorption. This has been reviewed in detail by Peck and Woods [58]. In osteoclast-mediated bone resorption, it has been suggested that the greater depth of penetration consequent to heightened osteoclast activity leads to perforation of the trabecular plates [15]. The same events cause erosion of the cortex, resulting in conversion of cortical to trabecular bone. A diagrammatic representation of these events is provided in Figures 4-10 and 4-11. The result of the perforations is shown in scanning photomicrographs (see Figure 4-2). Here the plates have been reduced to a series of rods and spicules, with little if any capability of supporting skeletal structure. Once the trabeculae have been disrupted, new bone does not bridge the gap. The three-dimensional structure of iliac trabecular bone has been compared in postmenopausal women with and without vertebral fractures [59]. These investigators found a heightened mean trabecular plate thickness but a significantly greater mean plate separation in the group with fractures. The mean plate density decreased progressively between ages 50 and 80 years. The subjects with fracture had an age-related decrease in mean plate density that paralleled rates seen in control subjects but at lower levels. The increased plate thickness may have been a potential consequence of continued stress and heightened remodeling, but greater mean plate separation probably indicates a failure to generate new trabecular connections [60]. These findings indicate that adding bone to existing surfaces may be insufficient to repair structural damage [55].

The identification of exogenous and endogenous factors in the pathogenesis of osteoporosis is a direct extension from the observations that bone remodeling is a continuous process throughout life and that regeneration is essential for repair. Some historic risk factors are listed in Table 4-3 and have been reviewed in detail by Melton and Riggs [61]. The genetic factors include racial factors that include not only differences in skeletal mass [28] but also alterations in parathyroid hormone levels and in circulating 1,25-dihydroxyvitamin D_3 [62]. When these genetic factors are combined with environmental or additional hormonal factors, the stage is set for developing osteoporosis [29, 63, 64]. The question of a hereditary role in osteoporosis was addressed in a retrospective epidemiologic study from Sweden [65], and the results showed no greater incidence of vertebral fractures in daughters of osteoporotic women than in daughters of nonosteoporotic women. On the other hand, Australian investigators carried out bone mineral content measurements in 25 postmenopausal women with osteoporotic compression fractures and in their daughters [66]. They found that daughters of osteoporotic women had lower bone content in the lumbar spine, femoral neck, and femoral midshaft. A study of 84 premenopausal women from St. Louis was carefully controlled for physical activity, sunlight exposure, dietary calcium and vitamin D intake, physical activity, age, parity, and lactation. None of these factors were related to changes in vertebral bone density measured by quantitative computed tomographic scans of T12 to L3. Premenopausal estrogen exposure was significantly related to changes in vertebral bone density, and these authors concluded

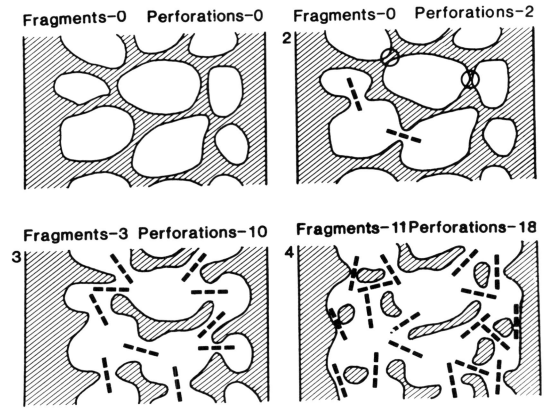

Figure 4-10. Microstructure of trabecular bone loss. The plate that bridges the medullary space between the internal and external cortex is shown at the upper left. Two perforations are shown at the upper right. Continuing perforations, shown on the lower left, cause reduction of the plate into discontinuous spicules, shown at the lower right. (Reprinted with permission from AM Parfitt. Bone Remodeling: Relationship to the Amount and Structure of Bone, and the Pathogenesis and Prevention of Fractures. In BL Riggs, LJ Melton III [eds], Osteoporosis: Etiology, Diagnosis, and Management. New York: Raven, 1988:45.)

that lifelong estrogen and genetic rather than environmental factors were the major determinants of osteoporosis [67]. Of the four hormonal factors (thyroid, glucocorticoids, testosterone, estrogen), estrogen deficiency is the one hormonal deficit that is unequivocally related to the development of osteoporosis. This has been reviewed extensively [30, 68–72]. Even before the cessation of their menses, women with irregular periods and elevated follicle-stimulating hormone levels have a decreased vertebral bone mass correlating with a decrease in estrogen production [73]. A potential impact of estrogen deficiency has been reported in the diminished vertebral bone mass in elite women distance runners [74] and in oligomenorrheic college athletes [75].

These observations and the reported inhibition of estrogens on rates of bone loss [1, 76] implicate a major role for this hormone. In an elderly man with an increased bone resorption, a positive linear correlation has been found between the relative area of cortical bone and circulating levels of testosterone and aldosterone [77]. Osteoporosis in men is less common than in women, and in a recent clinical review, causal factors were identified in 64% [78]. In a recent review of glucocorticoid-induced osteoporosis [79], the incidence of glucocorticoid-induced osteoporosis was estimated to be 30–50% in patients receiving steroids. The amount of bone replaced in each remodeling cycle was reduced by 30%, largely because of a shortening of the osteoblast life span

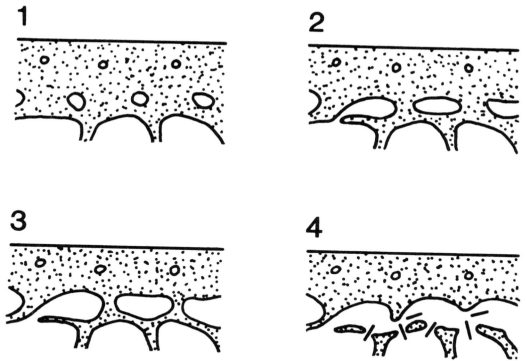

Figure 4-11. Microscopic evolution of cortical bone loss. Successive stages in osteoclast-dependent thinning of cortical bone. (1) Normal adult cortex with larger haversian canals closer to the inner cortical surface. (2) Enlargement of subendosteal spaces and communication with the marrow cavity. (3) Further enlargement and conversion of the inner third of the cortex to a structure that topologically resembles trabecular bone, with expansion of the marrow cavity. (4) Perforation and disconnection of the new trabecular structures. (Reprinted with permission from AM Parfitt. Bone Remodeling: Relationship to the Amount and Structure of Bone, and the Pathogenesis and Prevention of Fractures. In BL Riggs, LJ Melton III [eds], Osteoporosis: Etiology, Diagnosis, and Management. New York: Raven, 1988:45.)

and function, although osteoclastic bone resorption was also stimulated by glucocorticoids. Although an inhibition of osteoblast formation represents the principal effect of glucocorticoids [80], the action of these hormones is complex. Thus glucocorticoids have been shown to inhibit bone resorption in vitro but can antagonize the effect of vitamin D on calcium absorption and can produce a secondary hyperparathyroidism with bone resorption in vivo. Thyroid hormones stimulate bone resorption directly via local factors, including interleukins or osteoclast-activating factors [81]. The calcium released from bone resorption shuts off parathyroid hormone. A decline in parathyroid hormone not only diminishes 1,25-dihydroxyvitamin D_3 formation, which results secondarily in decreased intestinal calcium absorption, but diminishes renal calcium absorption as well [81].

The availability of sensitive thyroid-stimulating hormone (TSH) assays to monitor hyperthyroid states makes thyroid disease an uncommon cause of osteoporosis. Whether TSH-suppressive doses of thyroxine given to patients with thyroid carcinoma are deleterious to bone mass remains controversial at present [82].

Anticonvulsant agents have been shown to produce bone changes in patients given these drugs longterm [83]. The radiographic changes include a decrease in trabecular structure of the femur and some thinning of cortical bone and were associated with low serum calcium concentration, but were unrelated either to duration of therapy or to fracture increase. In other studies [84], the radiologic appearance in children was that of osteomalacia. Osteomalacia developing in patients on phenytoin has been improved by simply switching to another medication [85]. The hypocalcemia and hypophosphatemia seen with phenytoin or phenobarbital have been accompanied by normal levels of 1,25-dihydroxyvitamin D_3 but lower levels of 25-hydroxyvitamin D (25-OH-D) [86]. Heparin osteoporosis, first reported in a 15-year-old boy [87], has resulted in multiple vertebral compression fractures in pregnancy [88]. The mechanisms have been reviewed by Avioli [89] and involve complexing with calcium ions, direct resorption of bone, and functioning as a co-factor in parathyroid hormone-mediated bone resorption.

In adult men, the environment may play a greater role in the pathogenesis of osteoporosis than hormonal or genetic factors [78]. Strong correlations in rates of bone loss in mid-life were identified in male twin pairs followed for 16 years. The bone loss in identical twin pairs was only slightly greater than that in fraternal twins [90]. The investigators concluded that environmental factors within the family predominated over genetic factors. A major environmental factor is excessive ethanol ingestion. Ethanol diminishes osteoid matrix and delays mineralization in drinkers [91]. Heavy alcohol and cigarette consumption both result in osteoporosis, and the effects are additive [92]. The mechanism of alcohol has been studied in rodents, and a decreased trabecular bone volume has been seen despite normal rates of mineralization. These findings have been interpreted to indicate an enhanced resorption as the principal effect of alcohol [93]. In vitro studies in embryonic chick tibia exposed to 0.3% ethanol have shown an inhibition of bone formation, whereas lower ethanol concentrations (0.03%) have resulted in an increased bone cell proliferation [94]. The effects of ethanol on chick embryonic bone were found to parallel the effects of other agents that increased membrane fluidity. In addition to effects on bone, chronic ethanol ingestion in rats results in decreased duodenal calcium transport [95]. In the Nurses Health Study, 84,484 women aged 34–59 years completed a questionnaire regarding daily caffeine (greater than 2 cups of coffee) and alcohol (greater than 1 oz) ingestion and were followed for 6 years by Hernandez-Avila et al. [96]. Their results, reported in 1991, showed that excess caffeine consumption was associated with a 2.95-fold greater risk for hip fractures, and excess alcohol consumption carried a 2.33-fold greater risk for hip fracture and a 1.38-fold greater

risk for forearm fractures. Smoking was found to exacerbate osteoporosis in thin postmenopausal women [97], and early loss of teeth in women smokers paralleled the presence of osteoporosis [31]. In both smokers and nonsmokers obesity conferred some protection against osteoporosis [97]. Cigarette smoking has been shown to decrease serum estradiol and serum placental protein levels and to blunt the effect of estrogen replacement therapy on the endometrium in postmenopausal women [98].

In addition to hormones and drugs, exercise has important significant relevance as an exogenous factor acting to prevent bone mineral loss in aging women [99]. Inactivity has been shown to heighten osteoporosis, whereas regular exercise (1 hour three times a week) significantly increases calcium balance of postmenopausal women [46]. Exercises designed to strengthen muscles have a potentially critical role in preventing falls. Falls have been found to be a key determinant of hip fractures in elderly persons [100]. Although patients with hip fractures have a lower bone mass than in age-matched controls, the differences are small. Similar findings have been reported in other studies [101]. In a prospective study of femoral neck fractures in 200 women after minor trauma, bone mass measurements were similar to a control population not having fractures [102]. It was concluded that postural instability was the major cause for femoral neck fracture. Recently, bone density measurements have provided a quantitative assessment of the type of femoral neck fracture to expect. As shown in Figure 4-8, fractures were found to be uncommon with a femoral bone density greater than 1 g/cm^2, but at cervical femur densities of less than 0.6 g/cm^2, fracture occurred in 8.3 per 1,000 person-years, and at intertrochanteric femur densities of less than 0.6 g/cm^2, fracture occurred in 16.6 per 1,000 person-years [70]. These data extended previous observations that trochanteric fractures were more common in severely osteoporotic women, whereas cervical fractures predominated in those who were not osteoporotic [102].

The impact of nutrition on osteoporosis in postmenopausal women is unclear. Bone mineral density measurements across a wide range of calcium intake (0.260–2.035 g/day) showed no significant correlation when such measurements were made either at the midradius or lumbar spine [103]. By contrast, women with a calcium intake of less than 0.40 g/day for 7 months lost density of the lumbar vertebrae (L2 to L4) at a greater rate than women taking 0.78 g/day [104]. In women given oral calcium (2 g/day) for 2 years a slower loss of bone mineral content was observed in the proximal forearm (compact bone) but not in the distal forearm or lumbar spine (trabecular bone). Total body mineral content was modestly increased in the calcium-supplemented group [105]. In addition to calcium, 1,25-dihydroxyvitamin D_3 levels are lower in the elderly [106] and respond subnormally to parathyroid hormone infusion [107]. Thus the elderly (73±4 years of age) who take in a limited calcium diet may be at a greater risk for mineral deficiency than younger persons consuming a similar calcium content. A lack of sunlight exposure combined with a low dietary intake of vitamin D has resulted in low serum levels of 25-OH-D in elderly patients confined to bed rest [63]. In patients who are periodically exposed to sunlight, serum levels of 25-OH-D fluctuate with the seasons (highest levels in the fall and lowest in the spring). Lactase-deficient women may represent a special group at risk for mineral deficiency because of their avoidance of calcium-containing foods [108]. The calciuretic effects of dietary protein have been well documented [109], but the long-term impact on mineral metabolism requires documentation. A recent study of 980 postmenopausal women by Barrett-Connor et al. [110] examined an association between lifetime intake of caffeinated coffee and regular milk intake on decreasing bone density at the hip and lumbar spine. A significant association between decreasing bone density was observed in women 50–98 years of age who drank 2 cups of coffee a day. This was not seen in those who drank coffee and a glass of milk a day. These data are consistent with a calciuretic effect of caffeine. The potential risk of osteoporosis is less in younger women, in whom calcium supplementation results in increased intestinal calcium absorption, but older women are less able to compensate for the calcium losses [111]. Finally, Rigotti et al. noted that in women with anorexia nervosa the density of bone mass in the radial shaft was inversely related to the duration of amenorrhea [112]. These investigators noted that reductions in bone density were not rapidly reversed in these women despite attaining 80% of ideal weight and resuming menses. Thus anorexia nervosa in youth may ad-

versely affect bone mass in adulthood and place one at risk for osteoporosis, with the accompanying susceptibility to fractures.

Immobilization hypercalciuria is a self-limited clinical response to immobilization after injury. The renal excretion of calcium usually acts as a safety valve against hypercalcemia, but when dehydration, chronic renal failure, or the administration of thiazide diuretics supervenes, the stage is set for hypercalcemia. Immobilization hypercalcemia is usually seen in patients under 21 year of age who have been very active before injury. In persons with spinal cord injuries, those at greatest risk have high cervical and complete injuries and prolonged immobilization [113]. Immobilization hypercalcemia after this type of injury suggests that body weight may not be the major mechanical load on either the lower extremities or the spine. The levers represented by the spine and lower extremities are so inefficient that muscle forces exert 2–10 times body weight to move the body mass in earth's gravity [25, 114, 115]. A relaxation of these muscles after a high cervical injury is registered by the skeletal "mechanostat" [25] as a relative overabundance of bone, and the bone mass diminishes until the strain imposed by the remaining functioning muscle groups results in a new equilibrium at this diminished bone mass. The decrease in bone mass is accompanied by hypercalcemia, which is self-limited, beginning at the fourth week of immobilization, reaching a maximum at 16 weeks, and returning to normal by 18 months [116]. The bone density as determined by radiography is reduced by 30% at this time [117]. A similar state is seen in astronauts when gravity diminishes [34, 118]. The hypercalcemia of hyperparathyroidism can be unmasked in immobilization and some critically ill surgical patients have developed a hyperparathyroid state [119]. The heightened bone remodeling that characterizes Paget's disease also produces hypercalcemia during immobilization. Other conditions that predispose persons to hypercalcemia during immobilization include multiple myeloma, metastatic carcinoma, the milk-alkali syndrome, and heightened vitamin D states [113]. Hypervitaminosis A is an uncommon cause of hypercalcemia.

Endogenous paracrine and autocrine factors play a key role in bone physiology. Bone undergoes continuous remodeling in response to external stresses. To coordinate the impact of these environmental perturbations, the osteocytes on the surface of bone communicate with the interior by cell processes [53]. The relationships between cells, autocrine and paracrine factors, and circulating hormones have been reviewed by Peck and Woods [60]. The present thinking is that osteocytes transmit mechanical stress or electrical signals to resting osteoblasts that have become bone lining cells. The transmitter(s) of these signals is unknown, but these authors have suggested adenosine as a candidate. The lining cells then release prostaglandins to assist in the contraction of the lining membrane to expose the mineralized surface [60]. The response to stressing of fetal rat embryonic bone has been tested by allowing bone cultures to become confluent in plastic Petri dishes, then deforming the dish mechanically. The cultures have responded by producing prostaglandin E_2 (PGE_2) and secondarily, cyclic adenosine monophosphate [120]. The incorporation of thymidine into DNA was heightened 24 hours after the stress had been instituted. Indomethacin, a prostaglandin inhibitor, prevented the enhanced incorporation. A bone morphogenic protein derived from demineralized bone matrix of several mammals, including humans, has produced bone when placed in muscle pouches or in bone defects [121]. This non–collagen-containing protein is growth hormone dependent and declines in quantity in the bone matrix from aging animals [122]. It is unknown at present whether epithelial cells secrete bone morphogenic protein or whether they induce mesenchymal cells to secrete such a protein. The protein, however, induces an entire developmental program [121]. A second protein, called bone-derived growth factor, acts as a local or paracrine or autocrine growth factor and stimulates proliferative growth and metabolic activities similar to the somatomedins. Other factors include multifunctional cytokines produced by human lymphocytes and monocytes when stimulated by mitogens. These cytokines, called tumor necrosis factors β and α, function as osteoclast-activating factors and have been shown to resorb bone and to inhibit collagen synthesis [123]. Interleukin-1 can be produced by thymocytes that have been exposed to phytohemagglutinin. In low doses this monokine stimulated DNA, collagen, and noncollagen protein synthesis in rat calvaria, but with either high doses or prolonged exposure time from 24–96 hours, interleukin-1 inhibited collagen synthesis [124]. Unlike interleukin-1, lymphotoxin and tumor

necrosis factor stimulated thymidine incorporation, whereas lymphokine interferon-gamma inhibited thymidine incorporation into DNA in fetal rat calvariae. Interferon-gamma also inhibited osteoclast resorption stimulated by lymphotoxin tumor necrosis factor and interleukin-1 [125]. Because these factors are produced by cells contained in marrow, it has been suggested that conditions may exist in vivo for a local action of these factors on bone [53]. The role of prostaglandins in bone formation and absorption had been reviewed [126, 127], and their contribution to bone resorption remains to be determined. The inhibition of collagen synthesis by lymphotoxin and tumor necrosis factor is blocked, in part by indomethacin, suggesting that prostaglandin may in fact have a regulatory role. The early increase in bone resorption following immobilization can be reversed by indomethacin [128] and is an effect consistent with such a role. In addition to prostaglandins, bone cells produce both insulin-like growth factors I and II (IGF-I and -II). IGF-I production in embryonic rat tibia has been demonstrated following incubation with growth hormone [129]. Estradiol has been shown to stimulate production of both IGF-I and -II by a rat osteosarcoma cell line [130]. Estradiol also stimulates transforming growth factor β production in mouse osteoblasts, and ovariectomy reduces transforming growth factor β in rat tibia [131]. Finally, estradiol stimulates production of both mRNA and the peptide transforming growth factor β in human bone cells [132]. Bone cells cultured from osteoporotic postmenopausal women have shown a lower production of PGE_2, interleukin-1, and tumor necrosis factor that parallels heightened proliferative growth when compared with bone cells from nonosteoporotic women [133]. 1,25-dihydroxyvitamin D_3 increased PGE_2 levels to normal in cells with a high proliferation rate but lowered PGE_2 production in cells with a low proliferation rate, indicating that the response was also dependent on the stage of maturation. Because the vitamin-K dependent protein osteocalcin is synthesized by osteoblasts and is responsive to 1,25-dihydroxy D_3 [134], levels of 25-OH-D, IGF-I, and osteocalcin have been examined in osteoporotic patients [135]. A correlation between serum 25-OH-D, osteocalcin, and IGF-I was found, and in patients with spine fractures, IGF-I levels were lower. Men with symptomatic osteoporosis have diminished plasma IGF-I levels that correlate with diminished bone densities [136]. Finally, circulating IGF and IGF binding protein 3 have been shown to be decreased in patients with osteoporosis [137]. As these and other authors have pointed out [60], more work needs to be done to define the regulation of bone turnover [138] and the relationship between changes in circulating hormones and their effects on hormonal responses in the bone [139].

Diagnosis of Osteoporosis

The diagnosis of osteoporosis has traditionally been made by a combination of radiographs showing less dense bone and a history of a fracture, particularly of the vertebral bodies, proximal femur, and distal radius [1, 2, 53]. Concepts of bone physiology have expanded to include structural fatigue over time, with microscopic deterioration of cortical and trabecular bone [140]. While these alterations can be identified by cement lines on histologic examination of a biopsy specimen, the current measurements of bone mineral density are too insensitive to identify these very early changes in bone fragility and porosity. To diagnose these conditions is not clinically possible with the available tools. The standard radiograph will identify bone loss only when 30% of the skeleton has been demineralized. Local bone lesions can, however, be excluded.

The cortical thickness measurement uses the standard radiograph to estimate the combined cortical thickness as a fraction of the total thickness of a long bone, usually the midshaft of the second metacarpal. A nonosteopenic bone is taken as one in which the cortical thickness is greater than one-half of the total bone width. This method detects only excessive osteopenia and gives no estimation of the density of the cortex. Wishart et al. modified this technique to include the use of needle calipers for measurement of cortical to total area (metacarpal morphometry) and found that the information attained was comparable to single and dual photon absorptiometry [141]. Other methods for evaluating bone density include dual x-ray absorptiometry and quantitative computed tomography. These techniques have recently been reviewed by Genant [142]. The single photon beam absorptiometry (SPA) records the interference by the shaft of an appendicular bone (wrist or hand) when the extremity is placed in the path of a source of radiation [143]. The measurement requires a constant soft

tissue path length, requiring that the bone to be measured be immersed in water. This limits measurements to the radius or to the os calcis. The reproducibility of SPA is very good, but the bone measured contains 25% cortical and 75% trabecular bone at the distal end of the radius and does not reflect changes in the hip [143]. Similarly, when vertebral or hip fractures occur, the bone density may not be diminished in the wrist [19]. The os calcis, which consists of 20% cortical and 80% trabecular bone, has been used as an index of trabecular bone to be measured with single photon beam absorption but the correlation with density in the lumbar spine is too low for this technique to be used as a means of prediction [2, 144]. Not unexpectedly, the bone density of the femoral neck was shown to be a better predictor of hip fracture than density of the calcaneous [145]. SPA cannot be used for femoral neck measurements and the dual photon absorptiometry (DPA) technique must be used. The DPA technique uses an isotope source gadolinium 153 with two energy peaks (44 and 100 keV) that permit bone density to be measured independently of soft-tissue thickness and composition. This method can be used for both vertebrae and femur. DPA measures the entire vertebrae, is reproducible with a precision of 3–5%, and delivers only a slightly greater (three- to sixfold) radiation dose than the single photon beam, and one-tenth the radiation of a chest film [142]. The vertebra contain only 70% trabecular bone [2], and estimates of bone density are inaccurate when vertebra are wedged or accompanied by calcified ligaments or bony spurs. Despite these drawbacks, DPA makes possible an estimate of bone mineral density, which in male and female patients with osteoporosis and vertebral fractures was 0.965 g/cm^2 [19]. Dual x-ray absorptiometry (DEXA) uses the simulation of the dual energy peaks of gadolinium using x-ray tubes. The results are comparable with DPA but with a precision of 0.5–1.0% and a radiation exposure comparable with the SPA measurements. DEXA delivers a greater radiation flux, allowing for greater precision and a shorter scan time. DEXA is generally superior to DPA [146].

Quantitative computed tomography (QCT) can also be used to measure trabecular bone in the vertebral body. Indeed, QCT can measure trabecular and cortical bone at any skeletal site [142]. Dual radiation is used to avoid inaccuracies from vertebral fat, but the result so far has been a high radiation exposure (equivalent to a chest film), and an accuracy that is less than with DPA [143, 147]. For estimation of strength at the spine and in the femoral neck, QCT has shown the best sensitivity and specificity for discriminating between normal and osteoporotic bone followed by DEXA, DPA, and SPA. For appendicular fractures SPA is superior to QCT [142].

At present, the disabled patient can best be monitored by SPA for the appendicular skeleton and DPA or DEXA for the axial skeleton, measured at 12-month intervals [143, 148, 149]. Because the rate of bone loss averages 1–2% per year after the menopause and the precision of the techniques varies from 2–5%, more frequent measurements to follow mineral loss or response to therapy would not be helpful. In nondisabled persons who are not at high risk for developing osteoporosis, densitometry should not currently be used for general screening to assess risk for fractures [149, 150].

Ultrasound is a newly adopted technique for assessment of bone fragility and fatigue and has an advantage over the established methods of bone mass analysis described above [151]. Early reports have indicated that ultrasound is just as effective as DEXA but much less expensive [152].

Biochemical markers of bone turnover can be classified as markers of bone formation and bone resorption. The former group includes serum alkaline phosphatase and osteocalcin or bone Gla protein as the principal markers. The latter group includes urinary hydroxyproline, which correlates poorly with bone breakdown, because the majority of hydroxyproline is metabolized by the liver [153]. Two nonreducible pyridinium cross-links are a part of interchain stabilization of the collagen molecule. Deoxypyridinoline has been found only in type I collagen in bone [154] and is not metabolized. Thus urinary excretion has been used as a marker for bone resorption. Christiansen et al. [155] have used a prospective technique using a combination of SPA, a determination of body fat mass, urinary calcium, and hydroxyproline, and serum alkaline phosphatase repeated every 3 months for 2 years. Using these biochemical markers they formulated a regression equation that correlated closely with the directly measured bone mineral content. This group has gone on to identify women at risk for osteoporosis using one bone mass measurement and one combined biochemical assessment of future bone loss [156]. Although such assessments represent a promising application of biochemical markers and

bone densitometry, their value is limited by the inadequacy of present biochemical markers and by the fact that they represent events happening throughout the skeleton and not in a specific but crucial bone—e.g., the femoral neck.

A bone biopsy specimen from the iliac crest provides an accurate assessment of a specific region and is useful when a question of osteomalacia arises. The iliac crest bone may not, however, be representative of osteopenia, the status of osseous remodeling, or the hematopoietic state in other bones, such as the femoral neck [157]. Bone biopsy may be useful in young adults with idiopathic osteoporosis, to exclude osteomalacia and to evaluate patients not responding to therapy [158]. Tetracycline double labeling should be used concurrently to assess both mineralization and turnover.

Treatment

A variety of therapeutic modalities have been evaluated for use in either preventing osteoporosis or halting progression of the disease. Minerals, vitamins, hormones, and exercise have all been studied, but few have been shown to decrease the incidence of fractures in susceptible groups.

Calcium

Despite its widespread use, the value of calcium supplementation, once osteoporosis has occurred, remains controversial [159]. Calcium may, however, have a role in the prevention of the disease. Bone density continues to increase until about age 30 years [160], and more calcium taken during the adolescent growth spurt can result in a heavier and denser skeleton. Comparative studies of calcium balance in adolescent females (11–14 years old) compared with young adults (19–32 years old) have shown a positive balance only within the first 12 years after menarche. Thereafter calcium balance was negative [161]. Epidemiologic studies have demonstrated that higher calcium ingestion by women correlates with denser bones and fewer hip fractures [162], whereas an increased incidence of osteoporosis has been found in lactase-deficient women who have avoided dairy products [108]. Acute calcium supplementation at doses of 1 g/day in adults results in a decrease in the hydroxyproline-creatinine ratio as well as in the alkaline phosphatase values [163, 164]. These findings indicate that calcium acts to produce a biochemical decrease in bone resorption. Horsman and colleagues [165] found that calcium supplements given to postmenopausal women could slow bone loss in the forearm. More recent studies do not support these observations. Thus Riis and associates [105], using DPA, found that calcium supplements produced only slight changes in cortical bone loss, whereas no effect was seen on trabecular bone. Others have found that calcium alone does not prevent bone loss as measured by QCT of the vertebrae or appendicular cortical skeleton [166]. In a longitudinal study made over a period of 4.1 years, Riggs and associates [103] reported that the rates of change in bone mineral density of the midradius and lumbar spine were not different in women taking 0.260 g/day of calcium when compared with those taking 2.035 g mg. When bone density has been controlled for, there has been no apparent relationship between vertebral fractures and dietary calcium [158]. Dawson-Hughes to the contrary noted the prevention of bone loss at the femoral neck, radius, and spine in patients supplemented with 500 mg of calcium citrate malate for 2 years, whereas patients receiving the same dose of calcium carbonate maintained their bone density only in the femoral neck and radius [167]. Since calcium absorption from calcium carbonate is impaired in achlorhydria and this condition is common in older persons or in patients after a total gastrectomy, calcium citrate would provide better calcium bioavailability than calcium carbonate [168]. Calcium, 1,200 mg, plus 20 mg of vitamin D was found by Chapuy et al., not only to prevent bone loss, but also to significantly reduce the frequency of fractures in elderly women [169]. The results of these and other studies that have identified a positive effect of calcium supplementation have been reviewed by Heaney [170]. He summarized the disparate findings by making the point that a high calcium intake *will* prevent a calcium deficiency bone loss, and that the differences in timing of the supplementation in relation to menopause, the degree of investigator control of calcium intake, or both in these various studies may explain the inconsistent results, i.e., in the first 3–5 years after menopause, hormonal factors may predominate over the effects of calcium. The *real* question that

should be addressed in prospective studies is the relationship between bone fragility and the magnitude of calcium deficiency bone loss [170].

Recent studies have focused on the time of life when calcium supplementation is begun [161]. Eighteen months of calcium supplementation supplied as 500 mg of calcium citrate malate produced a significant increase in total body and spinal bone density in adolescent girls as compared with those taking placebo [171]. Similarly, supplementation of calcium over a 3-year duration in preadolescent children produced a significant increase in bone mass over those children who were not supplemented [172]. These studies suggest that the recommended daily allowance during this period may not be sufficient to bring about maximal bone deposition [173]. The administration of 1 or 2 g calcium to perimenopausal Dutch women has been carried out in a controlled trial within the first years of menopause. A significant decrease in bone loss in lumbar vertebrae but not appendicular cortical bone was observed. This effect was greater in the group supplemented with 2 g calcium [174]. In a second study, women from New England, who were 3–5 years postmenopause, were divided into two groups, one with a calcium intake of less than 400 mg/day of calcium and a second whose intake ranged from 400 to 650 mg/day [167]. In both groups bone loss from the spine was rapid and unaffected by calcium supplements. When women with a low baseline calcium intake had been postmenopausal for 6 years or more, bone loss was less at the femoral neck, radius, and spine in those receiving calcium supplements. The effect was less pronounced in the group with the higher baseline intake of calcium [167]. A study of New Zealand women who ingested 750 mg/day calcium and who were 3 years postmenopause was carried out by Reid et al., who used DPA measurements of lumbar spine and proximal femur every 6 months for 2 years [175]. In this study women were given calcium supplements, 1 g/day for 2 years, or a placebo. The loss of bone mineral density seen in the placebo group was decreased by 35% in the legs, 67% in the femoral neck, and eliminated in the trunk in those receiving calcium supplements.

The average American diet exclusive of dairy products contains about 500 mg calcium per day. Doses of 1,500 mg are currently recommended for postmenopausal and pregnant women [176], because a daily intake of 2,000 mg calcium has been shown to slow the loss of compact bone [105]. Eight hundred to 1,200 mg is required for growing children and improved absorption can be achieved when calcium is combined with vitamin D, citric acid, or lactose [176]. Foods that contain high concentrations of oxalate, phosphate, or phytate have poorer calcium bioavailability.

Calcium supplementation has not been shown to be effective in slowing the accelerated osteoporosis seen in the disabled. Furthermore, calcium should be used with caution in patients at risk for the development of immobilization hypercalcemia, renal function impairment, and kidney stone.

Estrogen

Estrogens have been studied extensively in women with postmenopausal osteoporosis, and their effect on the inhibition of bone resorption has been documented. Estrogen given to postmenopausal women decreases the fracture rate in the hip and lower forearm [177], as well as the vertebrae [178]. In their study, Riggs and coworkers found that the incidence of postmenopausal vertebral fractures in patients receiving estrogens as well as calcium and vitamin D was approximately half that of the group receiving only calcium and vitamin D. This improvement was related to maintenance of bone mass. In a longitudinal study, Ettinger and colleagues [166] found an insignificant loss of bone mass in 73 women receiving a combination of estrogen plus calcium, whereas patients receiving no supplementation, or treated with calcium alone, had a decreased trabecular bone mineral content. These studies were extended by Felson et al. [179], who examined the effect of estrogen in the postmenopausal age groups less than 75 and greater than 75 years of age. In the former group, taking estrogens for at least 7 years produced significantly higher bone mineral density than that of those who had never taken estrogens. In the latter group significant differences were found only in the shaft of the radius. Similar findings were present in women treated for 10 years. Lindsay and Tohme gave estrogen to women for 2 years at varying times following menopause. They found a significant increase in bone mineral density in women begun on estrogens as late as 35 years after the menopause [180]. In addition to their ef-

fect on bone, estrogens increase the cardioprotective high density lipoprotein and high density lipoprotein 2 and decrease the low density lipoproteins, and have reduced the risk of coronary artery disease by 30–50% [181].

Doses of 0.625 mg of conjugated estrogens a day have been shown to be effective in preventing bone loss. A higher estrogen dose is not more effective and increases the risk of complications [182, 183]. The complications of estrogen therapy at the antiresorptive dose (0.625 mg conjugated estrogens) include breast and uterine cancer. These have been reviewed by Cummings [184]. Although current users of estrogen had a 40% increased risk for breast cancer, 5-year mortality in these women was lower than rates from breast cancer in nonusers. Because a 50-year-old woman is 10 times more likely to die of heart disease than either breast cancer or hip fracture and 30 times more likely to die of heart disease than endometrial cancer, the benefits of estrogen replacement far outweigh the risk [185]. Women who have had their ovaries removed before age 50 years should receive cyclic estrogen and progesterone treatment if no contraindications exist. For example, 0.625 mg conjugated estrogen could be taken orally on days 1 through 25 each month and 5–10 mg medroxyprogesterone acetate taken on days 16 through 25 each month. Patients should have annual Papanicolaou smears, and an endometrial biopsy should be considered if breakthrough bleeding occurs. In persons who fall into the high-risk groups for osteoporosis, cyclic estrogen and progesterone treatment should be initiated soon after menopause, provided that there are no contraindications and that the patient understands the risks.

The addition of a progestational agent decreases the risk of uterine cancer, but it is not clear whether this subsequently impairs the effectiveness of estrogen in the treatment of osteoporosis. One study suggests that it does not, because alkaline phosphatase and bone Gla protein were found to increase with the use of both estrogen plus progesterone, whereas urinary calcium and hydroxyproline excretion decreased [186]. The duration of estrogen treatment should be at least 5–10 years [160].

Because the oral route of estrogen administration has resulted in cholelithiasis, thrombophlebitis, and pulmonary embolization [187], transdermal estrogen therapy has been used to avoid high concentrations in the portal system seen after oral administration.

This route of administration decreased bone turnover and the risk of vertebral fracture but had minimal effect on low density or high density lipoprotein cholesterol [188, 189]. Because the administration of estrogens to postmenopausal women aged 47–75 years has resulted in a diminished bone turnover and a diminished fracture rate [189], it has been suggested that estrogens should continue to be regarded as an effective therapeutic agent in those postmenopausal women with established osteoporosis [190].

Bisphosphonates

Bisphosphonates are synthetic analogues of pyrophosphate but contain a carbon in lieu of oxygen interposed between the phosphates and are not capable of being hydrolyzed. Absorption of bisphosphonates is poor from the gastrointestinal tract. Only 4% of an oral dose of etidronate is absorbed [191]. Alendronate is 500–1,000 times more potent than elidronate in inhibiting bone resorption and acts by inhibiting osteoclast activity. As is the case with etidronate, the gastroinstestinal absorption of alendronate is low. Only 1% of the administered dose is absorbed in the absence of food and even less in the presence of food. The properties of the bisphosphonates have been recently reviewed [192]. Once absorbed, 20–50% goes to bone, where the biphosphonates are adsorbed onto the surface of hydroxyapatite crystals at sites of new bone formation and remodeling. The effect of diphosphonates is to diminish activation. This results in limited resorption, which is followed in turn by diminished formation of new bone. The apparent increase in bone mass is simply the result of a nonequilibrium state where a decline in bone formation is delayed [193]. Two studies have been carried out using etidronate in women with postmenopausal osteoporosis. Watts et al. [194] and Storm et al. [195] have used a cyclic course of 400 mg/day oral etidronate followed by 13 weeks of calcium. The rationale for this dosing schedule was formulated from biochemical indicators obtained in etidronate-treated patients with Paget's disease [191]. In these people, 2 weeks of treatment suppressed bone resorption (estimated by urinary hydroxyproline) without affecting bone formation (estimated by serum alkaline phosphatase levels).

The 13 weeks was based on normal bone remodeling times. At the end of 2 years in Watts's group and 3 years in Storm's group, etidronate-treated patients had small but significant increases in spinal bone density and a marked decrease in fractures [194, 195]. The disproportionate decrease in fractures relative to small increases in bone mass implicates maintenance of intact trabecula. These studies were criticized by Parfitt [193], who thought that they were of insufficient duration and thereby avoided the potential long-term consequences of cyclic etidronate in lowering osteoblastic activity. Harris et al. [196] recently reported on an extension of the previous 2-year trial to a third year of blinded treatment with intermittent cyclic etidronate followed by 1 year of open therapy. At year 3, no significant difference was noted in vertebral fracture rate except for patients with low bone mass and a higher initial number of fractures, and the value of cyclic etidronate therapy has been questioned [197]. A third bisphosphonate, pamidronate, has a similar mechanism of action to etidronate but its half-life in bone is about 300 days, compared with the 90-day half-life of etidronate. Studies using pamidronate have resulted in a plateau in bone mineral gain after 2–5 years in one study, but a continuing increase in mineral content after 4 years in another [193]. An increase in mineral density has been observed 9 months after two 6-week courses of 20 or 40 mg alendronate given orally. Because bone turnover is slow and an increase in mineralization for up to 2 years may not be sustained beyond that time, longer periods of study must be conducted to evaluate the potential advantages of this bisphosphonate [192]. The biphosphates are generally free of toxic effects except for nausea and diarrhea when high doses are used and have been used successfully to control the hypercalcemias of malignancy and immobilization [116].

Calcitonin

Calcitonin is a polypeptide hormone that is bound to osteoclasts by specific receptors. Their actions reduce the life span of osteoclasts and inhibit their endocytotic activity that is needed for bone resorption. Calcitonin is produced by mammals and fish, and the latter calcitonins are 50- to 100-fold more potent than mammalian calcitonins [198]. The use of calcitonin for Paget's disease, summarized by Avioli [199], has resulted in reversal of osteolytic bone disease, reversal of nerve entrapment, and a halt in hearing losses experienced by these patients. Over 75% of patients treated for the hypercalcemia of malignancy or Paget's disease have also had a relief of pain, a direct effect on pain threshold centers in the central nervous system. Calcitonin is most effective in patients with rapidly turning over bone and is apparently as effective as estrogens in preventing bone loss in postmenopausal osteoporosis [200]. Problems attending calcitonin therapy include flushing and nausea after subcutaneous injection of the drug and the problems of self-administered daily subcutaneous infections, which have resulted in poor compliance [198]. In addition, a loss of hormone activity has been observed in patients given daily calcitonin injections of 50–100 international units (IU)/day. A loss of activity has been seen less commonly in patients given lower doses of calcitonin, i.e., less than 50 IU/day. These observations suggest that osteoclast receptors might not be saturated and might not be downregulated at these doses. Limiting daily doses to 5 days out of 7 might further allow time for recovery of osteoclast responsiveness [198]. Hypersensitivity reactions manifested by bronchospasm have been reported in a few patients treated with salmon calcitonin, and one anaphylactic death has been reported [201]. Patients should be queried about a history of drug allergies or asthma, and, if positive, skin testing should be considered. Skin hypersensitivity reactions have been reported to occur in 5% of patients and local pruritis at the site of injection in 10%, but these have been mild and have been ameliorated by 50 mg diphenhydramine hydrochloride (Benadryl) given daily 20–30 minutes before the injection [199]. The skin reactions diminish with continued subcutaneous infections. Epigastric fullness consequent to the inhibition of free acid production can be minimized if calcitonin is administered at bedtime or 4–5 hours after eating [199]. The dosing schedule of calcitonin given to patients for 1 year on and 1 year off has resulted in a gain in bone mass in both the appendicular skeleton and spine compared with a placebo group treated similarly [202]. The problems attending subcutaneous administration of calcitonin have prompted trials with an intranasal preparation and with a rectal suppository preparation. Both were equally effective, although plasma levels obtained were different [203]. Intranasal calcitonin has been shown to prevent bone loss in the spine of early postmenopausal women as well as in women with established osteoporosis. Unlike the side effects accompanying subcutaneous injection, intranasal administration had no side effects, and only one patient had mild nausea after using a repeated calcitonin suppository [203]. The use of 100 IU of calcitonin intranasally every other day has prevented glucocorticoid-induced osteoporosis in nephrotic children [204], and 100–200 IU daily have been given to adults with established osteoporosis to prevent bone loss [205]. Because vitamin D deficiency blunts the effect of calcitonin, it has been recommended that measurements of 25-hydroxycholecalciferol (25-OH-D or calcifediol) levels be obtained and that replacement be instituted before beginning calcitonin therapy in calcifediol-deficient patients [199].

In immobilization hypercalcemia, Meythaler et al. [116] have used a combination of calcitonin and etidronate. This represented an extension of the observation of Thiebaud et al. [206], who showed an initial depression of tubular reabsorption of calcium that was self-limited to 3 days when calcitonin was given. The combined therapy was successful in normalizing calcium levels within 3 days. In the patients with immobilization hypercalcemia, Meythaler's group recommends calcitonin, 100 IU subcutaneously twice a day, and etidronate, 800 mg twice a day. When serum calcium decreases to normal, they taper calcitonin to 100 IU subcutaneously every day and after 3 more days of normal levels they discontinue the calcitonin. Etidronate, 800 mg twice a day, is continued for 14 days then tapered to 800 mg every day until 3 months, a time when maximal anticipated hypercalcemia has passed [116]. In addition to calcitonin and etidronate, a major correctable condition in immobilization hypercalcemia is dehydration, and rehydrating such patients is a top priority. Saline therapy will not only assist renal excretion but sodium will compete with proximal tubular reabsorption of calcium. Furosemide will help calcium excretion only in the presence of adequate hydration with saline. Whether treatment of immobilization hypercalcemia in the disabled population acutely after injury will prevent or reduce the incidence of longer term osteoporosis is not known.

Fluorides

Unlike the estrogens, biphosphonates, and calcitonin, which act primarily to inhibit bone resorption, fluorides produce an intense osteoblastic response. The replacement of osteoclasts by osteoblasts bypasses the coupling of resorption and new bone formation, and the newly formed bone contains osteocytes in areas of diminished mineralization [15, 207]. In addition, fluorides are substituted in the mineral structure of bone to form fluorohydroxyapatite, which decreases osteoclastic resorption [208]. This new bone has a microscopic picture of osteomalacia, but unlike the usual forms, incompletely mineralized bone is added to mineralized bone. The mineralization defect can be diminished by providing calcium supplements of 1 g/day [208], which increase the uncoupling and diminish the secondary hyperparathyroidism that occurs in the presence of fluoride. The result is to enhance bone mass. Vitamin D, a usual treatment for osteomalacia, has been of questionable value in fluorotic bone. An impairment of mineralization has been seen when doses of fluoride have exceeded 75 or 80 mg/day, but with doses less than 40–45 mg, bone formation does not occur. Thus, the therapeutic window is narrow. The effects of fluoride on bone formation are seen in 2–6 months, and during a 4-year trial, bone density in the lumbar spine increased steadily, as well as in the femoral neck and trochanter [209]. Bone mineral density in the radius, however, declined. Women given 75 mg/day had three times as many gastrointestinal side effects of nausea, epigastric pain, or vomiting as women given placebos, and 10 times greater symptoms of lower extremity pain. Half of the women with lower extremity pain had incomplete or stress fractures. These healed within 6–8 weeks of stopping the drug [209]. Because calcium balance in patients given fluorides has shown no change despite the increase in spinal bone mass, it has been suggested that fluorides cause an increase in vertebral trabecular mass at the expense of appendicular cortical bone. A review of the four prospective placebo-controlled trials has shown that fluoride did not diminish the vertebral fracture rates [207]. Thus, new bone was either mechanically incompetent or mineral was not deposited in a region that could protect against fracture, e.g., increasing mineralization on either side of a broken trabecula without bridging the gap [15].

These problems combined with heightened bone fragility that predispose fluoride-treated patients to fracture of the femoral neck and long bone fractures [210]. These complications have prompted the suggestion that fluoride therapy be limited to 30 months [211]. Indeed, patients receiving 80 mg/day fluoride had 2.9 new fractures per year, whereas untreated control subjects had 0.3 fractures per year in the first year of a prospective study [212]. In the second and third years, however, no difference in fracture rates could be detected between the groups. Recently, Pak et al. reviewed their series of patients given slow-release sodium fluoride, 25 mg twice daily, in repeated cycles of 12 months on and 2 months off the medication. All patients received 400 mg of calcium as calcium citrate twice daily. In patients carried through two cycles, the fluoride group had a lower new vertebral fracture rate, no microfractures or hip fractures, and no change in radial bone density [213]. These studies were reviewed by Heaney who compared the results of these studies with others and suggested further trials with the correct dose and slow-release preparations of fluoride [214]. He also re-emphasized the importance of co-therapy with adequate calcium supplements when this osteogenic drug was used. Finally, although the quality of bone as woven bone is not as strong as lamellar bone, the former apposed on the latter may act to preserve existing lamellar bone mass. In a study using minipigs, one year's treatment with sodium fluoride increased bone volume but not bone strength, whereas in minipigs given alendronate, bone strength and bone volume were directly correlated [215].

Parathyroid Hormone

The effect of parathyroid hormone (PTH) on bone may be twofold, a resorptive effect when given by intravenous infusion and an osteoblastic effect when given by daily subcutaneous injections [216]. The enhancement of collagen synthesis by transient PTH administration to rat calvaria cultures has been accompanied by a local production of IGF-I. Anti-IGF-I added to the culture medium inhibited this enhancement [217]. In clinical studies the effects of PTH are complex. Treatment with low doses of PTH has improved calcium balance and with high doses has worsened it. Despite little change in calcium balance, the cancellous bone of iliac biopsy specimens was increased by 70% after PTH treatment [218]. In other studies reviewed by Riggs [208], the combination of PTH and 1,25-dihydroxyvitamin D_3 resulted in an increase in vertebral density over 6–12 months, which was followed by a decrease. The cortical bone of the radius was progressively decreased, similar to the response to fluoride. The effects of these changes on fracture rate have not been reported. Daily doses of PTH (40 μg given subcutaneously) have prevented bone loss in young women (20–44 years old) with estrogen deficiency [219]. In crossover studies in estrogen-deficient rats, PTH increased bone mass and mechanical strength. Estrogen alone could maintain these anabolic effects of PTH. Osteopenic rats maintained on the antiresorptive doses of estrogen responded to the anabolic effects of PTH when this hormone was given at a later time [220].

Vitamin D Therapy

In elderly subjects serum 25-hydroxyvitamin D decreases in part because of dietary deficiency and in part because of diminished exposure to sunlight. In addition, nearly 50–60% of patients with postmenopausal osteoporosis have calcium malabsorption and reduced levels of 1,25-dihydroxy D_3 [221]. A trial with vitamin D in nursing homes in France has resulted in a halving of fracture rates in control subjects [222]. In studies with 1,25-dihydroxyvitamin D_3, vertebral fracture rates were decreased by 50% after 1 year [221]. Studies from New Zealand have shown a decreased vertebral fracture rate in patients given vitamin D but not calcium [223], and vitamin D analogues have been shown to reduce vertebral fracture rates in Japanese women [224]. By contrast, investigators from the University of Washington [225] showed no effect of calcitriol in a 2-year study conducted in postmenopausal women and concluded that this hormone was no more effective than calcium alone. Two problems may have been a slightly lower dose of calcitriol and the adequate patient serum levels of 25-OH-D (26.3 ng/ml). The average serum 25-OH-D in the European studies was 10 ng/ml, a level that may cause secondary hyperparathyroidism [221]. The studies to date therefore suggest that vitamin D analogues may be most effective in those osteoporotic patients who are vitamin D deficient. Their use in patients who have normal 25-OH-D levels is still open to question.

Treatment of Complications

Fractures are the primary complication of osteoporosis, producing both pain and functional impairment. In the patient with postmenopausal osteoporosis, fractures occur most commonly in the distal radius, femoral neck, and lumbar vertebrae. In the population with spinal cord injuries, fractures may be seen with little or no trauma. Supracondylar fractures are more frequent (33%), with femoral (30%) and tibial (15%) next [10]. Callus formation generally occurs quickly and may be seen sooner than expected in a nonparalyzed person [226]. Whether treatment with either pillow splinting or casting is used, caution needs to be exercised to prevent the development of pressure sores [10].

Postmenopausal osteoporotic compression fractures of the vertebrae are seen primarily in the weight-bearing vertebrae at the T7 level and lower, with fractures at T12 to L2 being the most common. Fractures about T6 are rarely a result of osteoporosis [227]. After a compression fracture, spasm of the erector spinae produces a compensatory lumbar lordosis, with an increased anteroposterior curvature. Continued pain is probably the result of the abnormal stresses on the ligaments, muscles, and apophyseal joints from the change in posture. If vertebral wedging results in severe kyphosis, pressure of the ribs on the iliac crest can cause pain [227]. In a study examining quality of life issues in women with such fractures, pain, particularly with standing, and increased difficulty with lifting and carrying objects were the most frequently reported problems [228]. Patients often feel more comfortable lying supine with a small pillow under the head and a regular thickness pillow under the knees. Alternatively, some patients prefer lying on their sides, with the hips and knees flexed [229].

For an acute compression fracture, bed rest is generally prescribed for several days up to 2 weeks, but this should be minimized. Ice applied intermittently to the erector spinae or other painful areas may decrease the pain and muscle spasm. Other patients may find that heat is more effective. Muscle relaxants can be helpful but should be used judiciously in the older population and especially if used in combination with a narcotic. Pain control can often be achieved by maximizing the dose of salicylates or nonsteroidal anti-inflammatory drugs. Transcutaneous electrical nerve simulators may be helpful for controlling both acute and chronic pain.

Once the acute pain has decreased, the patient should be instructed in isometric abdominal strengthening exercises and spinal extension exercises to improve spine support (Figure 4-12). Extension exercises along with those to decrease lumbar lordosis will improve posture. Pectoral and intercostal muscle stretching may be required in patients with significant kyphosis. Active trunk flexion exercises should be avoided, as explained in the section on prevention [47].

For patients with acute back pain, immobilization of the spine with a rigid polypropylene brace may afford some relief when they are upright. The Jewett brace is also used for this purpose. Those patients unable to tolerate these braces may be helped by a thoracolumbar brace with rigid stays [229]. For the patient with chronic postural deformities or pain, an abdominal binder may increase intra-abdominal pressure and reduce pain. The cross anterior spine hyperextension orthosis has been used in this setting by Lal [230]. Sinaki recently described the results of a trial using the posture training support, a thoracolumbar support with a weighted pouch posteriorly below the scapulae. In this trial, significant relief of back pain was noted by 17 of 23 patients, whereas improvements in posture were noted by 19 [231].

Prevention of Osteoporosis

Osteoporosis results in 15 million fractures each year in the United States [232], and 25% of these fractures occur in white women older than 60 years who are osteoporotic. In his review, Levin mentioned that 20% of women died of complications consequent to hip fracture and of the 80% who survived, only 15% could walk across a room and only 6% could walk half a mile, whereas 86% and 41%, respectively, could do these activities before the fracture. This type of information underscores the need for prevention.

Risk factors for osteoporosis include inadequate nutrition from dairy products, especially in the preadolescent and premenopausal years. Matkovic and Heaney [233] reviewed 519 calcium balance studies in infants (0–1 year old), children (2–8 years old), adolescents (9–17 years old), and young adults (18–30 years old). Their study clearly showed the existence of an intake threshold where calcium balance ceased to be a function of intake and remained constant and independent of intake. The threshold was 1 g/day for infants and young adults and 1.5 g/day for children and adolescents. Sentipal et al. reported that the intakes for 67% of young girls 8–10 years of age was 800 mg calcium, but that only 16% of adolescent girls took in the recommended 1,200 mg calcium [234]. In their study the vertebral bone mineral density (BMD) was related to age, sexual maturity rating, and calcium intake. Thus, during the sexual maturity rating of Tanner stage 2–4, increasing the intake of calcium can increase vertebral BMD. These data indicated that an adequate calcium intake maintained during adolescence is crucial to acquiring a normal bone mass [234]. Indeed, it has been shown in carefully controlled studies that a positive calcium balance is lost within 12 years after menarche [161]. The obligatory urinary loss of calcium is independent of calcium intake, and calcium is not retained by the skeleton until 800 mg/day is ingested [235]. This is important because by the age of 16 years, daughters have accumulated 90–97% of the bone mass of their premenopausal mothers. Unfortunately, 29% of adolescent girls consumed less than 850 mg calcium, thereby compromising their skeletal mass [235]. Although a logical area of prevention is nutrition education during adolescence, supplementation of an 800-mg calcium diet with low-fat dairy products containing 500–600 mg calcium has also resulted in a decrease in vertebral bone loss in women aged 30–42 years [236]. Thus dietary supplements can be a preventive measure against osteoporosis in both adolescent and premenopausal adults.

In addition to calcium, trace minerals may also play a role in the maintenance of BMD. A 2-year study of BMD in the lumbar vertebrae, using DEXA, was recently carried out in women 10 years postmenopause given daily supplements of calcium (1 g) with and without a trace mineral supplement containing copper (5 mg), manganese (2.5 mg), and zinc (15 mg). The BMD decreased by 3% in the placebo controls, 2% with trace minerals alone, and 1.5% with calcium, but the BMD remained stable

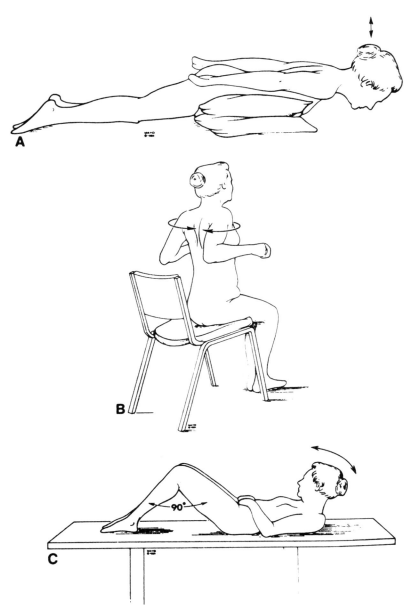

Figure 4-12. Exercises for patients with postmenopausal spinal osteoporosis. A, B. Examples of back extension exercises. C. Isometric abdominal muscle-strengthening exercises. (Reprinted with permission from M Sinaki, BA Mikkelsen. Postmenopausal spinal osteoporosis: Flexion versus extension exercises. Arch Phys Med Rehabil 1984:65:593. Copyright 1984 by American Congress of Rehabilitation Medicine.)

in women taking both calcium and the trace mineral supplements [237]. In healthy women 36–85 years of age, an elevated urinary zinc excretion was associated with a 90% chance of having osteoporosis. In such women, urinary hydroxyproline excretion correlated with zinc excretion, suggesting that heightened excretion of zinc may reflect heightened bone resorption [238]. In premenopausal women,

iron, magnesium, and zinc intake were correlated positively with bone mineral content in the forearm, suggesting that bone mass had been influenced by dietary factors other than calcium [239].

The second area of prevention is modification of environmental factors known to contribute to osteoporotic changes. These include giving up tobacco, restricting caffeine to 2 cups of coffee a day, and re-

Table 4-4. Targeted Interventions in a Study of Frailty and Injuries

Risk Factor Identified	Specific Interventions
Postural hypotension	Behavioral recommendations (e.g., hand clenching, ankle pumps–dorsiflexion/plantar flexion)
	Elevate head of bed
Use of benzodiazepines or other sedative–hypnotics	Education on proper medication use
	Nonpharmacologic treatment of sleep disorders
	Medication tapered and discontinued
Use of four or more prescription drugs	Medication review with primary physician
Environmental hazards raising risk of tripping or falling	Environmental manipulations (e.g., hazard removal, safer furniture, grab bars, handrails)
Unsafe tub and toilet transfers	Transfer training
	Environmental manipulations (e.g., grab bars, raised toilet seats)
Any transfer or balance impairment	Transfer training
	Balance exercises
	Environmental manipulations

stricting alcohol to one ounce a day. Medications known to enhance osteoporosis must be monitored. Because TSH levels are logarithmically related to serum levels of l-thyroxine, TSH levels should be used to monitor adequacy of thyroid hormone replacement [82]. Anticonvulsant agents may produce an osteomalacia-like picture, and 25-OH-D levels should be monitored [84–86]. In patients given glucocorticoids, 25-OH-D levels should also be monitored and vitamin D replaced if needed. In patients given long-term pharmacologic doses of glucocorticoids, such as in the treatment of childhood nephrosis, the use of calcitonin should be considered [204].

The third area of prevention should focus on avoidance of fractures in osteoporotic falls. Factors that increase the risk of falling include gait and mobility impairments—i.e., foot and balance dysfunction and medication use [240]. Postural dizziness on standing was also found to be more important than postural hypotension as a cause of falling [241]. The most common association was with anxiety or sleeping medications. The diagnosis of postural dizziness can be made when a patient reports dizziness 1 minute after assuming the standing position after lying supine for 5 minutes [241]. Because 98% of femoral neck fractures are the result of falls, a prevention program should also include an assessment of safety with mobility and within the home. Areas of attention would include providing appro-

priate assistive devices for ambulation or transfers, eliminating throw rugs in the home, and adapting bathroom fixtures including bathtub rails, bath seats, and raised height of toilet seats. Identification of risk factors and their specific intervention is shown in Table 4-4. A trial is currently underway to assess the impact of just such intervention strategies on the incidence of falls in the elderly [242].

Because bone loss occurs with bed rest, this type of immobilization should be minimized in the treatment of acute illness or at the onset of disability caused by injury. Regular forms of weight-bearing exercise, such as walking, appear to be helpful. Postmenopausal women walking approximately 1 mile per day have a greater mean bone density than those walking less [243]. Aloia and colleagues studied 18 postmenopausal women, half of whom exercised three times per week for 1 year [46]. Total body calcium increased in the exercise group and decreased in the sedentary group, but no difference between the groups was found in the bone mineral content measured at the distal radius. Smith and coworkers did find an improvement in bone mineral content at the distal radius, but only after the first year of a 3-year study [99]. Weight-bearing exercises performed three times per week by postmenopausal women have led to an increase in bone mineral content of the vertebrae, but improvement was not sustained and mineral content decreased after exercises were discontinued [244]. Although weight-bearing exercises are most effective in preventing osteoporosis, tilt-table exercises in patients with incomplete spinal cord injuries reduce the hypercalciuria seen acutely after injury and thus may be helpful in delaying osteoporosis [14].

Limburg et al. developed a back isometric dynamometer and showed that aging resulted in a progressive reduction in back extensor strength [245]. For osteoporosis involving the vertebrae, back extension exercises should be prescribed and trunk flexion avoided (see Figure 4-12). In a retrospective, nonrandomized study, Sinaki and Mikkelsen [47] found significantly fewer vertebral fractures in osteoporotic women who performed extension exercises as opposed to flexion exercises (16% versus 89%, respectively). Those doing both flexion and extension exercises had an intermediate rate of further fractures of 53%, whereas of those prescribed no exercises, 67% were found to have further fractures 1 year later. In healthy, estrogen-deficient women, back extensor exercises have improved muscle strength and decreased dorsal kyphosis [246]. Nonloading back extension exercises do not prevent postmenopausal vertebral bone loss [247], although bicycle exercise over an 8-month period was shown to increase spinal but not femoral bone density [248].

Women with greater bone mass have fewer problems with osteoporosis [28]. Vertebral postmenopausal bone loss is reduced in overweight women. This effect has been ascribed to heightened production of androgens from the adrenals and to heightened conversion of adrenal precursors to estrogens by the adipose tissue [249]. Such women can have serious disability from obesity, and osteoporosis is replaced by osteoarthritis and gout, which can be equally disabling [250]. Although bone mass may in part be racially determined, denser bones have been reported in women ingesting greater quantities of dietary calcium during the adolescent growth spurt and early adult life [162]. These observations indicate that dietary prevention of osteoporosis in the elderly should optimally be instituted in childhood. Young et al. have reviewed the literature regarding acquisition and losses of body calcium and have emphasized that total body calcium increases from 25–30 g at birth to 1,000 g by late adolescence, a magnitude that is twofold greater than the estimated 600-g loss seen with the menopause and aging [251]. These investigators also studied the effects of vigorous exercise in oligomenorrheic 17-year-old ballet dancers, and using DEXA measurements they showed that cortical bone mineral density in the femoral neck, trochanter, and lumbar spine was increased when dancers were compared with nonathletic age-matched oligomenorrheic women with comparable total body fat. Unlike the weight-bearing bones, mineral densities in the non–weight-bearing bones, including ribs, arms, and skull, were similar in both groups. These studies indicated that vigorous weight-bearing exercises may offset the effects of hypogonadism in weight-bearing bones [251]. Thus, in addition to nutrition and gonadal hormones, exercise per se can make a substantial contribution toward maximizing the acquisition of bone mass during adolescence and can thereby assist to further diminish the future prospects of osteoporosis and its attendant morbidity during aging.

Case Management Studies

Case 1

A 59-year-old woman slipped on a newly waxed floor and fractured her right hip. After traction and orthopedic placement of a pin, she was admitted to the Rehabilitation Institute for further care. On admission, a thorough history revealed that she was white, 5 feet, 2 inches tall, and weighed 106 pounds. She ceased having regular menstrual periods at age 45 years and her menses ceased completely at age 49 years. Because her best friend died of a stroke several years earlier while taking estrogen for menopausal symptoms, she avoided estrogens. She had been intermittently sexually active in her twenties and thirties, but in the years since her menopause had not dated and gradually lost her sexual drive. She had, however, recently had a problem of intermittent vaginal itching. She had smoked since she was 16 years old and enjoyed wine with her meals.

Questions

1. Is the history complete?
2. What further diagnostic studies should be done?
3. What treatment would your provide for her?
4. What social changes might you advise?
5. What might have caused the vaginal itching?

Case 2

A 14-year-old boy was involved in an automobile collision and suffered injuries to his extremities and his pelvis. He was treated for several weeks in a body cast and was transferred to the Rehabilitation Institute.

On admission, a family history indicated that milk was not commonly drunk because it resulted in diarrhea in his mother and his siblings and caused him to have excessive flatulence. At one point he drank Diet Cokes and coffee, but recently the gang to which he belonged considered it "uncool" not to drink beer. He was teased because cigar smoking made him sick, but recently his fellow gang members had given him menthol mild cigarettes, which he not only tolerated but had begun to enjoy. His favorite pastime was watching television quiz shows and sports events, but recently he had begun to date and was showing off for some female pedestrians when he hit a utility pole with his friend's car. On physical examination he was found to be 5 feet, 11 inches tall with an arm span of 74 inches and a pubis-to-crown height of 34 inches. He was noted to have small, firm testes and a small penis.

Questions

1. Could osteoporosis be a future problem?
2. What caused the flatulence?
3. What treatment should he receive?
4. What would you, as a physician, recommend for changes in his life style?

Case 3

A 19-year-old man suffered a fracture of C4-5 in a diving accident. He was transferred to the Rehabilitation Institute with normal chemistries and with physical therapy but developed a fever and pyuria, which resulted in cessation of physical therapy and a return to bed rest. He was begun on a sulfa drug but became anorectic and vomited. A blood chemistry analysis showed a blood urea nitrogen of 25 mg/dl, creatinine of 1.5 mg/dl, sodium of 148 mmol/liter, bicarbonate of 35 mmol/liter, chloride of 90 mmol/liter, potassium of 4.5 mmol/liter, calcium of 13 mg/dl, and phosphorus of 3.0 mg/dl. He was hydrated with 5% dextrose in water and placed NPO. However, he vomited and aspirated coffee ground material, which was hema-

test positive, and was aspirated. He developed chills and fever and was found to have a right lower lobe infiltrate. A nasogastric tube was placed, and the patient was treated with broad spectrum antibiotics. Because the patient developed abdominal distention, an emergency x-ray film was obtained, which showed a large bowel obstruction. On rectal examination, very hard stools were palpated, and after several enemas the impaction was reduced. The stool was black.

Questions

1. What caused the vomiting?
2. Was the type of hydration appropriate?
3. What caused the melena?
4. Was it related to the constipation?
5. What should be done now?
6. Can this be avoided in the future?

Case 4

A 55-year-old woman fractured both legs in a skiing accident and developed chronic back pain. An x-ray film showed a wedge compression fracture of one of her lumbar vertebrae. While at the rehabilitation center she complained of feeling hot at night and sweating. Her temperature was never elevated, although her pillow had in fact been wet, and she also noted increasing irritability and depression, which was atttributed to menopausal symptoms. She had not gained muscle strength despite continuing physical therapy, and after she exercised she felt very fatigued. The nursing staff noted that her resting pulse very often was over 100 and that she had not gained weight despite the fact that she ate well. She had a family history of diabetes and hypertension. A blood chemistry analysis showed a serum calcium of 11.5 mg/dl, phosphorus 3.0 mg/dl, and uric acid 9.0 mg/dl.

Questions

1. What are the likely causes of the sweating?
2. What tests might be helpful?
3. How would you treat her back pain acutely and chronically?
4. Are wedge compression fractures a common ski injury? Why?
5. Why is appropriate treatment important?

Discussion of Cases

Case 1—Summary Statement

The patient in case 1 is a small-boned, white, menopausal woman who smokes. She is a candidate for osteoporosis, so our goal should be to treat her and to educate her regarding prevention. Because she is afraid of estrogen therapy, you must update her regarding present-day concepts [184, 185]; most women would be interested in hormone replacement once informed [252]. Bone densitometry would not be particularly helpful from a therapeutic standpoint but may be useful in convincing her to begin therapy [253].

Answers to questions:

1. The history is not complete. (a) Has she had previous fractures? (b) What is her family history of fractures? (c) Is there breast cancer in the family?
2. She should have a bone density DPA or DEXA study, which will show bone findings relative to normal individuals. A finding of low bone density may help you convince her to begin estrogens.
3. Estrogens would be important to maximize loss of bone mass. She should also have a pelvic examination with vaginal smears for estrogen effects.
4. Social changes would be to give up smoking and to restrict alcohol to one drink a day. Implementing these changes will decrease bone loss.
5. Vaginal itching may be consequent to infection but is probably related to estrogen deficiency.

Case 2—Summary Statement

This young man has two genetic and two environmental factors that may contribute to osteoporosis: Klinefelter's Syndrome and Lactase deficiency [108], alcohol [91], and cigarettes [90]. He also has eunuchoid measurements, and the small firm testes suggest that he has hypogonadism. This should be evaluated with determinations of serum testosterone and gonadotropins FSH and LH. If in fact he is hypogonadal, bone densitometry should be carried out and the results compared with those for normal 14-year-olds if possible. Since he is accumulating bone mass at this stage, he should be treated for the hypogonadism [254].

Answers to questions:

1. This black male is using two agents that will enhance osteoporosis: tobacco and alcohol. On the other hand, he is black and the effects may be less devastating than in a white male.
2. The flatulence is a consequence of lactase deficiency. This can result in a lifelong avoidance of dairy products.
3. The treatment would be lactase-containing diet supplements such as yogurt.
4. Changes in life style would be participating in aerobic exercise and athletics when possible, giving up smoking, and limiting alcohol.

Case 3—Summary Statement

The patient in case 3 has hypercalcemia of immobilization. The natural history of this condition was nicely summarized by Maynard [113] and Meythaler et al. [116]. The course of this hypercalcemia is self-limited to 14 months, and the challenge is to ride out the storm. Remember that the kidney is a calcium escape valve, but dehydration not only diminishes renal clearance but heightens proximal tubular resorption of calcium. Normal saline is the treatment of choice to maximize renal clearance. It is important to keep in mind that calcitonin may produce a transient inhibition of calcium reabsorption [206].

Answers to questions:

1. This is a problem of immobilization hypercalcemia, and the vomiting was related to gastric irritability, peptic ulcers, or both, which may be seen in hypercalcemic states.
2. The hydration should have been normal saline. This will restore plasma volume and will competitively inhibit renal calcium absorption.
3. Melena was related to a bleeding ulcer.
4. Constipation is seen in hypercalcemic states.
5. The patient should be hydrated with saline and if calcium values continue to be elevated, consider adding calcitonin and etidronate.
6. Immobilization hypercalcemia is self-limited and physical therapy may result in normalizing calcium.

Case 4—Summary Statement

The patient in case 4 has two problems that may contribute to osteoporosis. The first is a hypermetabolic state, which may be a manifestation of thyrotoxicosis, cancer, infection, or even a rare pheochromocytoma. The elevated calcium level is disturbing and should be evaluated from the standpoint of hyperparathyroidism. It turns out that she did have an elevated PTH level. A thorough physical examination and a pelvic examination revealed a cervical erosion, but a Pap smear showed no malignant cells. Estrogen therapy would be an important consideration, not only for treatment of osteoporosis but also for a protection against the bone resorbing effects of parathyroid hormone [255].

Answers to questions:

1. Although this woman may have menopausal symptoms, she may have a chronic infection such as tuberculosis of brucellosis or a bone metastasis from breast cancer.
2. Tests should include x-ray films of the chest and back with bone detail, serum TSH, FTI titers for *Brucella,* PPD skin test, physical examination of the neck, generalized muscle wasting, reflexes, skin texture, breast examination.
3. Bed rest is indicated for acute pain, then extension exercises to strengthen back muscles.
4. Wedge compression fractures are not a common ski injury. The legs are vulnerable to ski injury. Compression fractures may be consequent to local bone damage or osteoporosis. Incidentally, the majority of compression fractures in osteoporotic women aged 60–80 years occur spontaneously or after trivial strain [27].
5. If thyrotoxicosis is found and is not treated, she may be at increased risk for osteoporosis. Untreated infection can be a continuing source of morbidity and will interfere with healing of her fractures. An undiagnosed breast cancer may cause severe incapacitation.

Acknowledgments

This work was supported in part by a merit review grant from the Research Service, VA Central Office. The patient secretarial support of June Pedersen is gratefully acknowledged.

References

1. Lindsay R, Dempster DW. Osteoporosis: Current concepts. Bull NY Acad Med 1985; 61:307.
2. Riggs BL, Melton LJ III. Involutional osteoporosis. N Engl J Med 1986; 314:1676.
3. Smith DM, Khairi MRA, Johnston CC Jr. The loss of bone mineral with aging and its relationship to risk of fracture. J Clin Invest 1975;56:311.
4. Kaplan FS. Osteoporosis: Pathophysiology and prevention. Clin Symp 1987;39:2.
5. Chrischilles EA, Butler CD, Davis CS, et al. A model of lifetime osteoporosis impact. Arch Intern Med 1991;151:2026.
6. Donald CL, Hulley SB, Vogel JM, et al. Effect of prolonged bed rest on bone mineral. Metabolism 1970; 9:1071.
7. Panin N, Gorday WJ, Paul BJ. Osteoporosis in hemiplegia. Stroke 1971;2:41.
8. Hamdy RC, Krishnaswamy G, Cancellaro V, et al. Changes in bone mineral content and density after stroke. Am J Phys Med Rehabil 1993;72:188.
9. Chiu KY, Pun WK, Luk KD, Chow SP. A prospective study on hip fractures in patients with previous cerebrovascular accidents. Injury 1992;23:297.
10. Ragnarsson KT, Sell GH. Lower extremity fractures after spinal cord injury: A retrospective study. Arch Phys Med Rehabil 1981;62:418.
11. Lewinnek GE, Kelsey J, White AA, et al. The significance and a comparative analysis of the epidemiology of hip fractures. Clin Orthop 1980;152:35.
12. Gallagher JC, Melton LJ, Riggs BL, et al. Epidemiology of fractures of the proximal femur in Rochester, Minnesota. Clin Orthop 1980;150:163.
13. Cummings SR, Rubin SM, Black D. The future of hip fractures in the United States. Numbers, costs and potential effects of postmenopausal estrogen. Clin Orthop 1990;252:163.
14. Kaplan PE, Roden W, Gilbert E, et al. Reduction of hypercalciuria in tetraplegia after weight-bearing and strengthening exercises. Paraplegia 1981;19:289.
15. Parfitt AM. Bone Remodeling: Relationship to the Amount and Structure of Bone, and the Pathogenesis and Prevention of Fractures. In BL Riggs, LJ Melton III (eds), Osteoporosis: Etiology, Diagnosis, and Management. New York: Raven, 1988;45.
16. Garn SM. The Phenomenon of Bone Formation and Bone Loss. In HF DeLuca, HM Frost, WSS Jee, et al. (eds), Osteoporosis. Recent Advances in Pathogenesis and Treatment. Baltimore: University Park Press, 1981;3.
17. Gong JK, Arnold JS, Cohn SH. Composition of trabecular and cortical bone. Anat Rec 1964;149:325.
18. Rockoff SD, Sweet E, Bleustein J. The relative contribution of trabecular and cortical bone to the strength of human lumbar vertebrae. Calcif Tissue 1969;3:163.
19. Riggs BL, Wahner HW, Dunn WL, et al. Differential changes in bone mineral density of the appendicular and axial skeleton with aging: Relationship to spinal osteoporosis. J Clin Invest 1981;67:328.
20. Mazess RB. On aging bone loss. Clin Orthop 1982;165:239.
21. Dempster DW, Shane E, Horbert W, et al. A simple method for correlative light and scanning electron mi-

croscopy of human iliac crest bone biopsies: Qualitative observations in normal and osteoporotic subjects. J Bone Mineral Res 1986;1:15.

22. Nordin BEC, Need AG, Chatterton BE, et al. The relative contributions of age and years since menopause to postmenopausal bone loss. J Clin Endocrinol Metab 1990;70:83.

23. Nordin BEC, Chatterton BE, Steurer TA, et al. Forearm bone mineral content does not decline with age in premenopausal women. Clin Orthop Rel Res 1986;211:252.

24. Brown JP, Delmas PD, Arlot M, et al. Active bone turnover of the cortico-endosteal envelope in postmenopausal osteoporosis. J Clin Endocrinol Metab 1987;64:954.

25. Frost HM. Bone "mass" and the "mechanostat": A proposal. Anat Rec 1987;219:1.

26. Riggs BL, Wahner HW, Seeman E, et al. Changes in bone mineral density of the proximal femur and spine with aging: Differences between the postmenopausal and senile osteoporosis syndromes. J Clin Invest 1982;70:716S.

27. Patel U, Skingle S, Campbell GA, et al. Clinical profile of acute vertebral compression fractures in osteoporosis. Br J Rheumatol 1991;30:418.

28. Cohn SH, Abesamis C, Yasumura S, et al. Comparative skeletal mass and radial bone mineral content in black and white women. Metabolism 1977;26:171.

29. Smith DM, Nance WE, Kang KW. Genetic factors in determining bone mass. J Clin Invest 1973;52:2800.

30. Riggs BL, Melton LJ III. Evidence for two distinct syndromes of involutional osteoporosis. Am J Med 1983;75:899.

31. Daniell HW. Postmenopausal tooth loss: Contributions to edentulism by osteoporosis and cigarette smoking. Arch Intern Med 1983;143:1678.

32. Deitrick JE, Whedon GD, Shorr E. Effects of immobilization upon various metabolic and physiologic functions of normal men. Am J Med 1948;4:3.

33. Morey ER, Baylink DJ. Inhibition of bone formation during space flight. Science 1978;201:1138.

34. Wronski TJ, Morey ER. Effect of spaceflight on periosteal bone formation in rats. Am J Physiol 1983;244:R305.

35. Simmons DJ, Russell JE, Winter F, et al. Effect of spaceflight on the non–weight-bearing bones of rat skeleton. Am J Physiol 1983;244:R319.

36. Jee WSS, Wronski TJ, Morey ER, et al. Effects of spaceflight on trabecular bones in rats. Am J Physiol 1983;244:R310.

37. Whedon GD. Disuse osteoporosis: Physiological aspects. Calcif Tissue Int 1984;36:S146.

38. Griffiths HJ, Bushueff B, Zimmerman RE. Investigation of the loss of bone mineral in patients with spinal cord injury. Paraplegia 1976;14:207.

39. Garland DE, Steward CA, Adkins RH, et al. Osteoporosis after spinal cord injury. J Orthop Res 1992;10:371.

40. Garland DE, Faulkes GD, Adkins RH, et al. Regional osteoporosis following incomplete spinal cord injury. Contemp Orthoped 1994;28:134.

41. Coman AE, Hutchinson RH, Bors E. Extremity fractures of patients with spinal cord injuries. Am J Surg 1962;103:732.

42. Claus-Walker J, Halstead LS. Metabolic and endocrine changes in spinal cord injury: IV. Compounded neurologic dysfunctions. Arch Phys Med 1982;63:632.

43. Naftchi NE, Viau AT, Sell GH, et al. Mineral metabolism in spinal cord injury. Arch Phys Med Rehabil 1980;61:139.

44. Ohry BA, Shemesh Y, Zac R, et al. Zinc and osteoporosis in patients with spinal cord injury. Paraplegia 1980;18:174.

45. Pilonchery G, Minaire P, Milan JJ, et al. Urinary elimination of glycosaminoglycans during the immobilization osteoporosis of spinal cord injury patients. Clin Orthop 1983;174:230.

46. Aloia JF, Cohn SH, Ostuni JA, et al. Prevention of involutional bone loss by exercise. Ann Intern Med 1978;89:356.

47. Sinaki M, Mikkelsen BA. Postmenopausal spinal osteoporosis: Flexion versus extension exercises. Arch Phys Med Rehabil 1984;65:593.

48. Brighton CT, Tadduni GT, Pollack SR. Treatment of sciatic denervation disuse osteoporosis in the rat tibia with capacitively coupled electrical stimulation. J Bone Joint Surg [Am] 1985;67:1022.

49. Leeds EM, Klose KJ, Ganz W, et al. Bone mineral density after bicycle ergometry training. Arch Phys Med Rehabil 1990;71:207.

50. Frost HM. The pathomechanics of osteoporosis. Clin Orthop 1985;200:198.

51. Parfitt AM. The cellular basis of bone remodeling: The quantum concept reexamined in light of recent advances in the cell biology of bone. Calcif Tissue Int 1984;36:S37.

52. Eriksen EF. Normal and pathological remodeling of human trabecular bone: Three dimensional reconstruction of the remodeling sequence in normals and in metabolic bone disease. Endocr Rev 1986;7:379.

53. Raisz LG. Local systemic factors in the pathogenesis of osteoporosis. N Engl J Med 1988;318:818.

54. Baron R, Neff L, Tran Van P, et al. Kinetic and cytochemical identification of osteoclast precursors and their differentiation into multinucleated osteoclasts. Am J Pathol 1986;122:363.

55. Parfitt AM. Trabecular bone architecture in the pathogenesis and prevention of fracture. Am J Med 1987;82:68.

56. Baron R, Neff L, Louvard D, et al. Cell-mediated extracellular acidification and bone resorption: Evidence for a low pH in resorbing lacunae and localization of a 100-kD lysosomal membrane protein at the osteoclast ruffled border. J Cell Biol 1985;101:2210.

57. Parfitt AM. Age-related structural changes in trabecular and cortical bone: Cellular mechanisms and biomechanical consequences. Calcif Tissue Int 1984;36:S123.

58. Peck WA, Woods WL. The Cells of Bone. In BL Riggs, LJ Melton III (eds), Osteoporosis: Etiology, Diagnosis, and Management. New York: Raven, 1988;1.

59. Kleerekoper M, Villanueva AR, Stanciu J, et al. The role of three-dimensional trabecular microstructure in the pathogenesis of vertebral compression fractures. Calcif Tissue Int 1985;37:594.

60. Parfitt AM, Matthews CHE, Villanueva AR, et al. Relationships between surface, volume, and thickness of iliac trabecular bone in aging and in osteoporosis. J Clin Invest 1983;72:1396.

61. Melton LJ III, Riggs BL. Clinical spectrum. In BL Riggs, LJ Melton III (eds), Osteoporosis: Etiology, Diagnosis, and Management. New York: Raven, 1988;155.

62. Bell NH, Greene A, Epstein S, et al. Evidence for alteration of the vitamin D-endocrine system in blacks. J Clin Invest 1985;76:470.

63. Davies M, Mawer EB, Hann JT, et al. Seasonal changes in the biochemical indices of vitamin D deficiency in the elderly: a comparison of people in residential homes, long-stay wards and attending a day hospital. Age Ageing 1986;15:77.

64. Lamberg-Allardt C. Vitamin D intake, sunlight exposure, and 25-hydroxyvitamin D levels in the elderly during one year. Ann Nutr Metab 1984;28:144.

65. Gardsell P, Lindberg H, Obrant KJ. Osteoporosis and heredity. Clin Orthop 1989;240:164.

66. Seeman E, Hopper JL, Bach, LA. Reduced bone mass in daughters of women with osteoporosis. N Engl J Med 1989;320:554.

67. Armamento-Villareal R, Villareal DT, Avioli LV, et al. Estrogen status and heredity are major determinants of premenopausal bone mass. J Clin Invest 1992;90:2464.

68. Davis ME, Strandjord NM, Lanzl LH. Estrogens and the aging process: The detection, prevention and retardation of osteoporosis. JAMA 1966;196:129.

69. Meema HE, Bunker ML, Meema S. Loss of compact bone due to menopause. Obstet Gynecol 1965;26:333.

70. Melton LJ III, Wahner HW, Richelson LS, et al. Osteoporosis and the risk of hip fracture. Am J Epidemiol 1986;124:254.

71. Raisz LG. Osteoporosis. J Am Geriatr Soc 1982;30:127.

72. Richelson LS, Wahner HW, Melton LJ, et al. Relative contributions of aging and estrogen deficiency to postmenopausal bone loss. N Engl J Med 1984;311:1273.

73. Johnston CC Jr, Hui SL, Witt RM. Early menopausal changes in bone mass and sex steroids. J Clin Endocrinol Metab 1985;61:905.

74. Marcus R, Cann C, Madvig P, et al. Menstrual function and bone mass in elite women distance runners. Ann Intern Med 1985;102:158.

75. Lloyd T, Buchanan JR, Bitzer S, et al. Interrelationships of diet, athletic menstrual status, and bone density in collegiate women. Am J Clin Nutr 1987;46:682.

76. Lindsay R, Hart DM, Forrest C, et al. Prevention of spinal osteoporosis in oophorectomised women. Lancet 1980;2:1151.

77. Foresta C, Ruzza G, Mioni R, et al. Osteoporosis and decline of gonadal functions in the elderly male. Horm Res 1984;19:18.

78. Kelepouris N, Harper KD, Gannon F, et al. Severe osteoporosis in men. Ann Intern Med 1995;123:452.

79. Lukert BP. Glucocorticoid-induced osteoporosis. South Med J 1992;85:2S-48.

80. Chyun YS, Kream BE, Raisz LG. Cortisol decreases bone formation inhibiting periosteal cell proliferation. Endocrinology 1984;114:477.

81. Auwerx J, Bouillon R. Mineral and bone metabolism in thyroid disease: A review. Q J Med 1986;60:737.

82. Baran DT. Editorial: Detrimental skeletal effects of thyrotropin suppressive doses of thyroxine: Fact or fantasy? J Clin Endocrinol Metab 1994;78:816.

83. Sotaniemi EA, Hakkarainen HK, Puranen JA, et al. Radiologic bone changes and hypocalcemia with anticonvulsant therapy in epilepsy. Ann Intern Med 1972;77:389.

84. McCrea ES, Rao K, Diaconis JN. Roentgenographic changes during long-term diphenylhydantoin therapy. South Med J 1980;73:312.

85. Stoffer SS, Rahman Z-U, Meier DA, et al. Prompt resolution of osteomalacia by switching from phenytoin to phenobarbital. Arch Intern Med 1980;140:852.

86. Jubiz W, Haussler MR, McCain TA, et al. Plasma 1,25-dihydroxyvitamin D levels in patients receiving anticonvulsant drugs. J Clin Endocrinol Metab 1977;44:617.

87. Sackler JP, Liu L. Heparin-induced osteoporosis. Br J Radiol 1973;46:548.

88. Wise PH, Hall AJ. Heparin-induced osteopenia in pregnancy. Br Med J 1980;281:110.

89. Avioli LV. Heparin-induced osteopenia: An appraisal. Adv Exp Med Biol 1975;52:375.

90. Slemenda CW, Christian JC, Reed T, et al. Long-term bone loss in men: Effects of genetic and environmental factors. Ann Intern Med 1992;117:286.

91. Diamond T, Stiel D, Lunzer, M. Ethanol reduces bone formation and may cause osteoporosis. Am J Med 1989;86:282.

92. Seeman E, Melton LJ III, O'Fallon WM, et al. Risk factors for spinal osteoporosis in men. Am J Med 1983;75:977.

93. Baran DT, Teitelbaum SL, Bergfeld MA, et al. Effect of alcohol ingestion on bone and mineral metabolism in rats. Am J Physiol 1980;238:E507.

94. Farley JR, Fitzsimmons R, Taylor AK, et al. Direct effects of ethanol on bone resorption and formation in vitro. Arch Biochem Biophys 1985;238:305.

95. Krawitt EL. Effect of ethanol ingestion on duodenal calcium transport. J Lab Clin Med 1975;85:665.

96. Hernandez-Avila M, Colditz GA, Stampfer MJ, et al. Caffeine, moderate alcohol intake, and risk of fractures of the hip and forearm in middle-aged women. Am J Clin Nutr 1991;54:157.

97. Daniell HW. Osteoporosis of the slender smoker: Vertebral compression fractures and loss of metacarpal cortex in relation to postmenopausal cigarette smoking and lack of obesity. Arch Intern Med 1976;136:298.

98. Byrjalsen I, Haarbo J, Christiansen C. Role of cigarette smoking on the postmenopausal endometrium during sequential estrogen and progestogen therapy. Obstet Gynecol 1993;81:1016.

99. Smith EL Jr, Smith PE, Ensign CJ, et al. Bone involution decrease in exercising middle-aged women. Calcif Tissue Int 1984;36:S129.

100. Cummings SR. Are patients with hip fractures more osteoporotic? Am J Med 1985;78:487.

101. Johnston CC Jr, Norton J, Kernek KD, et al. Heterogeneity of fracture syndromes in postmenopausal women. J Clin Endocrinol Metab 1985;61:551.

102. Aitken JM. Relevance of osteoporosis in women with fracture of the femoral neck. Br Med J 1984;288:596.

103. Riggs BL, Wahner HW, Melton LJ III, et al. Dietary calcium intake and rates of bone loss in women. J Clin Invest 1987;80:979.

104. Dawson-Hughes B, Jacques P, Shipp C. Dietary calcium intake and bone loss from the spine in healthy postmenopausal women. Am J Clin Nutr 1987;46:685.

105. Riis B, Thomsen K, Christiansen C. Does calcium supplementation prevent postmenopausal bone loss? N Engl J Med 1987;316:173.

106. Tsai K-S, Heath H III, Kumar R, et al. Impaired vitamin D metabolism with aging in women: Possible role in pathogenesis of senile osteoporosis. J Clin Invest 1984;73:1668.

107. Slovik DM, Adams JS, Neer RM, et al. Deficient production of 1,25-dihydroxyvitamin D in elderly osteoporotic patients. N Engl J Med 1981;305:372.

108. Vigorita VJ, Lane JM, Suda MK, et al. Differences between lactase deficient and non-lactase deficient women with spinal osteoporosis. Clin Orthop 1987;215:248.

109. Margen S, Chu J-Y, Kaufmann NA, et al. Studies in calcium metabolism: I. The calciuretic effect of dietary protein. Am J Clin Nutr 1974;27:584.

110. Barrett-Connor E, Chang JC, Edelstein SL. Coffee-associated osteoporosis offset by daily milk consumption. The Rancho Bernardo Study. JAMA 1994;271:280.

111. Massey LK, Whiting SJ. Caffeine, urinary calcium, calcium metabolism and bone. J Nutr 1993;123:1611.

112. Rigotti NA, Neer RM, Skates SJ, et al. The clinical course of osteoporosis in anorexia nervosa. A longitudinal study of cortical bone mass. JAMA 1991;265:1133.

113. Maynard FM. Immobilization hypercalcemia following spinal cord injury. Arch Phys Med Rehabil 1986;67:41.

114. Cochran G, Van B. A Primer of Orthopaedic Biomechanics. Edinburgh: Churchill-Livingstone, 1982.

115. Currey JD. The Mechanical Adaptations of Bones. Princeton: Princeton University Press, 1984.

116. Meythaler JM, Tuel SM, Cross LL. Successful treatment of immobilization hypercalcemia using calcitonin and etidronate. Arch Phys Med Rehabil 1993;74:316.

117. Minaire P, Meunier P, Edouard C, et al. Quantitative histological data on disuse osteoporosis. Comparison with biological data. Calcif Tissue Res 1974;17:57.

118. Wronski TJ, Morey ER. Skeletal abnormalities in rats induced by simulated weightlessness. Metab Bone Dis Rel Res 1982;4:69.

119. Forster J, Querusio L, Burchard KW, et al. Hypercalcemia in critically ill surgical patients. Ann Surg 1985;202:512.

120. Somjen D, Binderman I, Berger E, et al. Bone remodeling induced by physical stress is prostaglandin E2 mediated. Biochim Biophys Acta 1980;627:91.

121. Urist MR, DeLange RJ, Finerman GAM. Bone cell differentiation and growth factors. Science 1983;220:680.

122. Syftestad GT, Urist MR. Bone aging. Clin Orthop 1982;162:288.

123. Bertolini DR, Nedwin GE, Bringman TS, et al. Stimulation of bone resorption and inhibition of bone formation in vitro by human tumor necrosis factors. Nature 1986;319:516.

124. Canalis E. Interleukin-1 has independent effects on deoxyribonucleic acid and collagen synthesis in cultures of rat calvariae. Endocrinology 1986;118:74.

125. Smith DD, Gowen M, Mundy GR. Effects of interferon-γ and other cytokines on collagen synthesis in fetal rat bone cultures. Endocrinology 1987;120:2494.

126. Raisz LR, Kream BE. Regulation of bone formation: I. N Engl J Med 1983;309:29.

127. Raisz LG, Kream BE. Regulation of bone formation: II. N Engl J Med 1983;309:83.

128. Thompson DD, Rodan GA. Immobilization produces increased bone resorption and decreased formation in rats. [Abstract.] J Bone Mineral Res 1986;1(Suppl 1):S23.

129. Stracke H, Schulz A, Moeller D, et al. Effect of growth hormone on osteoblasts and demonstration of somatomedin-C/IGF I in bone organ culture. Acta Endocr 1984;107:16.

130. Gray TK, Mohan S, Linkhart TA, et al. Estradiol stimulates in vitro the secretion of insulin-like growth factors by the clonal osteoblastic cell line, UMR106. Biochem Biophys Res Com 1989;158:407.

131. Finkelman RD, Bell NH, Strong D, et al. Ovariectomy selectively reduces the concentration of transforming growth factor b in rat bone: Implications for estrogen deficiency-associated bone loss. Proc Natl Acad Sci USA 1992;89:12190.

132. Oursler MJ, Cortese C, Keeting P, et al. Modulation of transforming growth factor-b production in normal human osteoblast-like cells by 17b-estradiol and parathyroid hormone. Endocrinology 1991;129:3313.

133. Marie PJ, Hott M, Launay JM, et al. In vitro production of cytokines by bone surface-derived osteoblastic

cells in normal and osteoporotic postmenopausal women: Relationship with cell proliferation. J Clin Endocrinol Metab 1993;77:824.

134. Price PA, Baukol SA. 1,25-dihydroxyvitamin D_3 increases synthesis of the vitamin K-dependent bone protein by osteosarcoma cells. J Biol Chem 1980;25:11660.

135. Pun KK, Lau P, Wong FGW, et al. 25-Hydroxycholecalciferol and insulin-like growth factor I are determinants of serum concentration of osteocalcin in elderly subjects with and without spinal fractures. Bone 1990;11:397.

136. Ljunghall S, Johansson AG, Burman P, et al. Low plasma levels of insulin-like growth factor 1 (IGF-1) in male patients with idiopathic osteoporosis. J Intern Med 1992;232:59.

137. Wuster C, Blum WF, Schlemilch S, et al. Decreased serum levels of insulin-like growth factors and IGF binding protein 3 in osteoporosis. J Intern Med 1993;234:249.

138. Mundy GR. Editorial: An OAF by any other name. Endocrinology 1996;137:1149.

139. Margolis RN, Canalis E, Partridge NC. Invited review of a workshop: anabolic hormones in bone: basic research and therapeutic potential. J Clin Endocrinol Metab 1996;81:872.

140. Marcus R. Clinical review 72. The nature of osteoporosis. J Clin Endocrinol Metab 1996;81:1.

141. Wishart JM, Horowitz M, Bochner M, et al. Relationships between metacarpal morphometry, forearm and vertebral bone density and fractures in postmenopausal women. Br J Radiol 1993;66:435.

142. Genant HK, Faulkner KG, Gluer C-C. Measurement of bone mineral density: Current status. Am J Med 1991;9l:5B-49S.

143. Chestnut CH III. Noninvasive techniques for measuring bone mass: A comparative review. Clin Obstet Gynecol 1987;30:812.

144. Geusens P, Dequeker J, Verstraeten A, et al. Age-, sex-, and menopause-related changes of vertebral and peripheral bone: Population study using dual- and single-photon absorptiometry and radiogrammetry. J Nucl Med 1986;27:1540.

145. Cummings SR, Black DM, Nevitt MC, et al. Bone density at various sites for prediction of hip fractures. Lancet 1993;341:72.

146. Wahner HW, Dunn WL, Brown ML, et al. Comparison of dual-energy x-ray absorptiometry and dual photon absorptiometry for bone mineral measurements of the lumbar spine. Mayo Clin Proc 1988;63:1075.

147. Bellantoni MF, Blackman MR. Osteoporosis: Diagnostic screening and its place in current care. Geriatrics 1988;43:63.

148. Hall FM, Davis MA, Baran DT. Bone mineral screening for osteoporosis. N Engl J Med 1987;316:212.

149. Tosteson ANA, Rosenthal DI, Melton LJ III, et al. Cost effectiveness of screening perimenopausal white women for osteoporosis: Bone densitometry and hormone replacement therapy. Ann Intern Med 1990;113:594.

150. Riggs BL, Wahner HW. Bone densitometry and clinical decision-making in osteoporosis. Ann Intern Med 1988;108:293.

151. Heaney RP, Avioli LV, Chestnut CH III, et al. Ultrasound velocity through bone predicts incident vertebral deformity. J Bone Mineral Res 1995;10:341.

152. Schott AM, Weill-Engerer S, Hans D, et al. Ultrasound discriminates patients with hip fractures equally well as dual energy x-ray absorptiometry and independently of bone mineral density. J Bone Mineral Res 1995;10:243.

153. Delmas PD. Biochemical markers of bone turnover: Methodology and clinical use in osteoporosis. Am J Med 1991;91:5B.

154. Eyre DR, Koob TJ, Van Ness KP. Quantitation of hydroxypyridinium crosslinks in collagen by high-performance liquid chromatography. Anal Biochem 1984;137:380.

155. Christiansen C, Riis BJ, Rodbro P. Prediction of rapid bone loss in postmenopausal women. Lancet 1987;1:1105.

156. Hansen MA, Overgaard K, Riis BJ, et al. Role of peak bone mass and bone loss in postmenopausal osteoporosis: 12 year study. Br Med J 1991;303:961.

157. Frisch B, Eventov I. Hematopoiesis in osteoporosis—Preliminary report comparing biopsies of the femoral neck and iliac crest. Isr J Med Sci 1986;22:380.

158. Riggs BL. Practical Management of the Patient with Osteoporosis. In BL Riggs, LJ Melton III (eds), Osteoporosis: Etiology, Diagnosis, and Management. New York: Raven, 1988;481.

159. Buchanan JR, Myers CA, Greer RB. Determinants of atraumatic vertebral fracture rates in menopausal women: Biologic v mechanical factors. Metabolism 1988;37:400.

160. Peck WA, Riggs BL, Bell NH, et al. Research directions in osteoporosis. Am J Med 1988;4:275.

161. Weaver CM, Martin BR, Plawecki KL, et al. Differences in calcium metabolism between adolescent and adult females. Am J Clin Nutr 1995;61:577.

162. Matkovic V, Kostial K, Simonovic I, et al. Bone status and fracture rate in two regions of Yugoslavia. Am J Clin Nutr 1979;32:540.

163. Horowitz M, Need AG, Philcox JC, et al. Effect of calcium supplementation on urinary hydroxyproline in osteoporotic postmenopausal women. Am J Clin Nutr 1984;39:857.

164. Horowitz M, Need AG, Philcox JD, et al. The effect of calcium supplements on plasma alkaline phosphatase and urinary hydroxyproline in postmenopausal women. Horm Metab Res 1985;17:311.

165. Horsman A, Gallagher JC, Simpson M, et al. Prospective trial of estrogen and calcium in postmenopausal women. Br Med J 1977;2:789:92.

166. Ettinger B, Genant HK, Cann CE. Postmenopausal bone loss is prevented by treatment with low-dosage estrogen with calcium. Ann Intern Med 1987;106:40.

167. Dawson-Hughes B, Dallal, GE, Krall EA, et al. A controlled trial of the effect of calcium supplementation on bone density in postmenopausal women. N Engl J Med 1990;323:878.

168. Recker RR. Calcium absorption and achlorhydria. N Engl J Med 1985;313:70.

169. Chapuy MC, Arlot ME, Duboeuf F, et al. Vitamin D_3 and calcium to prevent hip fractures in elderly women. N Engl J Med 1992;327:1637.

170. Heaney RP. Effect of calcium on skeletal development, bone loss, and risk of fractures. Am J Med 1991;91:5B-23S.

171. Lloyd T, Andon MB, Rollings N, et al. Calcium supplementation and bone mineral density in adolescent girls. JAMA 1993;270:841.

172. Johnston CC Jr, Miller JZ, Slemenda CW, et al. Calcium supplementation and increases in bone mineral density in children. N Engl J Med 1992;327:82.

173. Heaney J. Bone mass, nutrition and other lifestyle factors. Am J Med 1993;95(Suppl 5A):295.

174. Elders PJM, Netelenbos JC, Lips P, et al. Calcium supplementation reduces vertebral bone loss in perimenopausal women: A controlled trial in 248 women between 46 and 55 years of age. J Clin Endocrinol Metab 1991;73:533.

175. Reid IR, Ames RW, Evans MC, et al. Effect of calcium supplementation on bone loss in postmenopausal women. N Engl J Med 1993;328:460.

176. Abramowicz MA. Prevention and treatment of postmenopausal osteoporosis. Med Lett 1987;29:75.

177. Weiss NS, Ure CL, Ballard JH, et al. Decreased risk of fractures of the hip and lower forearm with postmenopausal use of estrogen. N Engl J Med 1980;303:1195.

178. Riggs BL, Seeman E, Hodgson SF, et al. Effect of the fluoride/calcium regimen on vertebral fracture occurrence in postmenopausal osteoporosis: Comparison with conventional therapy. N Engl J Med 1982;306:446.

179. Felson DT, Zhang Y, Hannan MT, et al. The effect of postmenopausal estrogen therapy on bone density in elderly women. N Engl J Med 1993;329:1141.

180. Lindsay R, Tohme JF. Estrogen treatment of patients with established postmenopausal osteoporosis. Obstet Gynecol 1990;76:290.

181. Hillner BE. Estrogen therapy for geriatric osteoporosis: Just one ball in a complex juggling act. South Med J 1992;85:2S-10.

182. Mack TM, Pike MC, Henderson BE, et al. Estrogens and endometrial cancer in a retirement community. N Engl J Med 1976;294:1262.

183. Weiss NS, Szekely DR, English DR, et al. Endometrial cancer in relation to patterns of menopausal estrogen use. JAMA 1979;242:261.

184. Cummings SR. Evaluating the benefits and risks of postmenopausal hormone therapy. Am J Med 1991;91:5B-14S.

185. Cummings SR, Black DM, Rubin SM. Lifetime risks of hip, Colles', or vertebral fracture and coronary heart disease among white postmenopausal women. Arch Intern Med 1989;149:2445.

186. Christianson C, Riis BJ, Nilas L, et al. Uncoupling of bone formation and resorption by combined estrogen and progestagen therapy in postmenopausal osteoporosis. Lancet 1985;12:800.

187. Judd HL, Cleary RE, Creasman WT, et al. Estrogen replacement therapy. Obstet Gynecol 1981;58:267.

188. Weinerman SA, Bockman RS. Medical therapy of osteoporosis. Orthop Clin North Am 1990;21:109.

189. Lufkin EG, Wahner HW, O'Fallon WM, et al. Treatment of postmenopausal osteoporosis with transdermal estrogen. Ann Intern Med 1992;117:1.

190. Ott SM. Estrogen therapy for osteoporosis—Even in the elderly. Ann Intern Med 1992;117:85.

191. Watts NB. Bisphosphonate therapy for postmenopausal osteoporosis. South Med J 1992;85:2S-31.

192. Kanis JA, Gertz BJ, Singer F, et al. Rationale for the use of alendronate in osteoporosis. Osteoporosis Int 1995;5:1.

193. Parfitt AM. Use of bisphosphonates in the prevention of bone loss and fractures. Am J Med 1991;91:5B-42S.

194. Watts NB, Harris ST, Genant HK, et al. Intermittent cyclical etidronate treatment of postmenopausal osteoporosis. N Engl J Med 1990;323:73.

195. Storm T, Thamsborg G, Steiniche T, et al. Effect of intermittent cyclical etidronate therapy on bone mass and fracture rate in women with postmenopausal osteoporosis. N Engl J Med 1990;322:1265.

196. Harris ST, Watts NB, Jackson RD, et al. Four-year study of intermittent cyclic etidronate treatment of postmenopausal osteoporosis: Three years of blinded therapy followed by one year of open therapy. Am J Med 1993;95:557.

197. Marcus R. Cyclic etidronate: has the rose lost its bloom? Am J Med 1993;95:555.

198. Reginster J-Y. Effect of calcitonin on bone mass and fracture rates. Am J Med 1991;91:5B-19S.

199. Avioli LV. Calcitonin therapy in osteoporotic syndromes. South Med J 1992; 85:2S-17.

200. MacIntyre I, Whitehead MI, Banks LM, et al. Calcitonin for prevention of postmenopausal bone loss. Lancet 1988;1:900.

201. American Hospital Formulary Service Drug Information 1994;2076.

202. Overgaard K, Hansen MA, Nielsen V-AH, et al. Discontinuous calcitonin treatment of established osteoporosis—Effects of withdrawal of treatment. Am J Med 1990;89:1.

203. Buclin T, Randin JP, Jacquet AF, et al. The effect of rectal and nasal administration of salmon calcitonin in normal subjects. Calcif Tissue Int 1987;41:252.

204. Nishioka T, Kurayama H, Yasuda T, et al. Nasal administration of salmon calcitonin for prevention of glucocorticoid-induced osteoporosis in children with nephrosis. J Pediatr 1991;118:703.

205. Overgaard K, Riis BJ, Christiansen C, et al. Effect of calcitonin given intranasally on early postmenopausal bone loss. BMJ 1989;299:477.

206. Thiebaud D, Jacquet AF, Burckhardt P. Fast and effective treatment of malignant hypercalcemia. Combination of suppositories of calcitonin and a single infusion of 3-amino 1-hydroxypropylidene-1-bisphosphonate. Arch Intern Med 1990;150:2125.

207. Kleerekoper M, Balena R. Fluorides and osteoporosis. South Med J 1992;85:2S-34.

208. Riggs BL. Treatment of osteoporosis with sodium fluoride or parathyroid hormone. Am J Med 1991;91:5B-37S.

209. Riggs BL, Hodgson SF, O'Fallon WM, et al. Effect of fluoride treatment on the fracture rate in postmenopausal women with osteoporosis. N Engl J Med 1990;322:802.

210. Schnitzler CM, Wing JR, Gear KA, Robson HJ. Bone fragility of the peripheral skeleton during fluoride therapy for osteoporosis. Clin Orthop 1990;261:268.

211. Wing JR, Gear KA, Robson HJ. Bone fragility of the peripheral skeleton during fluoride therapy for osteoporosis. Clin Orthop 1990;261:268.

212. Dambacher MA, Ittner J, Ruegsegger P. Long term fluoride therapy of postmenopausal osteoporosis. Bone 1986;7:199.

213. Pak CYC, Sakhaee K, Piziak V, et al. Slow-release sodium fluoride in the management of postmenopausal osteoporosis. Ann Intern Med 1994;120:625.

214. Heaney RP. Fluoride and osteoporosis. Ann Intern Med 1994;120:689.

215. Lafage M-H, Balena R, Battle MA, et al. Comparison of alendronate and sodium fluoride effects on cancellous and cortical bone in minipigs. J Clin Invest 1995;95:2127.

216. Hodsman AB, Fraher LJ, Ostbye T, et al. An evaluation of several biochemical markers for bone formation and resorption in a protocol utilizing cyclical parathyroid hormone and calcitonin therapy for osteoporosis. J Clin Invest 1993;91:1138.

217. Canalis E, Centrella M, Burch W, et al. Insulin-like growth factor I mediates selective anabolic effects of parathyroid hormone in bone cultures. J Clin Invest 1989;83:60.

218. Reeve J, Meunier PJ, Parsons JA, et al. Anabolic effect of human parathyroid hormone fragment on trabecular bone in involutional osteoporosis: a multicentre trial. BMJ l980;280:1340.

219. Finkelstein JS, Klibanski A, Schaefer EH, et al. Parathyroid hormone for the prevention of bone loss induced by estrogen deficiency. N Engl J Med 1994;331:1618.

220. Shen V, Birchman R, Xu R, et al. Effects of reciprocal treatment with estrogen and estrogen plus parathyroid hormone on bone structure and strength in ovariectomized rats. J Clin Invest 1995;96:2331.

221. Gallagher JC. Vitamin D metabolism and therapy in elderly subjects. South Med J 1992;85:2S.

222. Meunier PJ, Chapuy MC, Arlot ME, et al. Effects of a calcium and vitamin D_3 supplement on non-vertebral fracture rate, femoral bone density and parathyroid function in elderly women. A prospective placebo-controlled study. J Bone Min Res 1991;6(Suppl 1):S135.

223. Tilyard MW. 1,25-Dihydroxyvitamin D_3 vs calcium in the treatment of established postmenopausal osteoporosis. J Bone Min Res 1990;5(Suppl 2):S275.

224. Orimo H, Shiraki M, Hayashi R, et al. Reduced occurrence of vertebral crush fractures in senile osteoporosis treated with 1 α(OH)-vitamin D_3. Bone Mineral 1987;3:47.

225. Ott SM, Chestnut CH III. Calcitriol treatment is not effective in postmenopausal osteoporosis. Ann Intern Med 1989;110:267.

226. Eichenholtz SN. Management of long bone fractures in paraplegic patients. J Bone Joint Surg 1963;45:299.

227. Lukert BP. Osteoporosis: Review and update. Arch Phys Med Rehabil 1982;63:480.

228. Cook DJ, Guyatt GH, Adachi JD, et al. Quality of life issues in women with vertebral fractures due to osteoporosis. Arthritis Rheum 1993;36:750.

229. Sinaki M. Exercise and Physical Therapy. In BL Riggs, LJ Melton III (eds), Osteoporosis: Etiology, Diagnosis, and Management. New York: Raven, 1988;457.

230. Lal S. Usefulness of cross anterior spinal hyperextension orthosis in patients with osteoporotic problems. Arch Phys Med Rehabil 1991;72:773.

231. Kaplan RS, Sinaki M. Posture training support: Preliminary report on a series of patients with diminished symptomatic complications of osteoporosis. Mayo Clin Proc 1993;68:1171.

232. Levin RM. Osteoporosis: Prevention is key to management. Geriatrics 1993;48(Suppl 1):18.

233. Matkovic V, Heaney RP. Calcium balance during human growth: Evidence for threshold behavior. Am J Clin Nutr 1992;55:992.

234. Sentipal JM, Wardlaw GM, Mahan J, et al. Influence of calcium intake and growth indexes on vertebral bone mineral density in young females. Am J Clin Nutr 1991;54:425.

235. Matkovic V, Fontana D, Tominac C, et al. Factors that influence peak bone mass formation: A study of calcium balance and the inheritance of bone mass in adolescent females. Am J Clin Nutr 1990;52:878.

236. Baran D, Sorensen A, Grimes J, et al. Dietary modification with dairy products for preventing vertebral bone loss in premenopausal women: A three-year prospective study. J Clin Endocrinol Metab 1989;70:264.

237. Saltman PD, Strause LG. The role of trace minerals in osteoporosis. J Am Coll Nutr 1993;12:384.

238. Herzberg M, Foldes J, Steinberg R, et al. Zinc excretion in osteoporotic women. J Bone Mineral Res 1990;5:251.

239. Angus RM, Sambrook PN, Pocock NA, et al. Dietary intake and bone mineral density. Bone Mineral 1988;4:265.

240. Kiel DP. New strategies to prevent hip fractures. Hospital Practice February 15, 1994;47.

241. Ensrud KE, Nevitt MC, Yunis C, et al. Postural hypotension and postural dizziness in elderly women. Arch Intern Med 1992;152:1058.

242. Tinetti ME, Baker DI, Garrett PA, et al. Yale FICSIT: Risk factor abatement strategy for fall prevention. Am Geriatr Soc 1993;41:315.

243. Krall EA, Dawson-Hughes B. Walking is related to bone density and rates of bone loss. Am J Med 1994;96:20.

244. Dalsky GP, Stocke KS, Ehsani AA, et al. Weight-bearing exercise training and lumbar bone mineral content in postmenopausal women. Ann Intern Med 1988;108:824.

245. Limburg PJ, Sinaki M, Rogers JW, et al. A useful technique for measurement of back strength in osteoporotic and elderly patients. Mayo Clin Proc 1991;66:39.

246. Itoi E, Sinaki M. Effect of back-strengthening exercise on posture in healthy women 49 to 65 years of age. Mayo Clin Proc 1994;69:1054.

247. Sinaki M, Wahner HW, Offord KP, et al. Efficacy of nonloading exercises in prevention of vertebral bone loss in postmenopausal women: A controlled trial. Mayo Clin Proc 1989;64:762.

248. Bloomfield SA, Williams NI, Lamb DR, et al. Non weightbearing exercise may increase lumbar spine bone mineral density in healthy postmenopausal women. Am J Phys Med Rehabil 1993;72:204.

249. Tremollieres FA, Pouilles J-M, Ribot C. Vertebral postmenopausal bone loss is reduced in overweight women: A longitudinal study in 155 early postmenopausal women. J Clin Endocrinol Metab 1993;77:683.

250. Pi-Sunyer FX. Medical hazards of obesity. Ann Intern Med 1993;119(7 pt 2):655.

251. Young N, Formica C, Szmukler G, et al. Bone density at weight-bearing and nonweight-bearing sites in ballet dancers: The effects of exercise, hypogonadism, and body weight. J Clin Endocrinol Metab 1994;78:449.

252. Draper J, Roland M. Perimenopausal women's views on taking hormone replacement therapy to prevent osteoporosis. Br Med J 1990;300:786.

253. Rubin SM, Cummings SR. Results of bone densitometry affect women's decisions about taking measures to prevent fractures. Ann Intern Med 1992;116(12 pt 1):990.

254. Finkelstein JS, Klibanski A, Neer RM, et al. Increases in bone density during treatment of men with idiopathic hypogonadotropic hypogonadism. J Clin Endocrinol Metab 1989;69:776.

255. Cosman F, Shen V, Xie F, et al. Estrogen protection against bone resorbing effects of parathyroid hormone infusion. Ann Intern Med 1993;118:337.

Chapter 5
Heterotopic Ossification

Santosh Lal

Historically, persons with disabilities due to congenital disorders, trauma, and neurologic insults did not survive to face the effects of chronicity and disability. The increase in chronic disabilities and their consequences is multifactorial; increased life span is reflected by improved health care, prevention, and therapeutic and supportive care. Technological advances have resulted in the survival and maintenance of persons who otherwise would have died. Persons with recent disabilities are going to be the chronic disabled patients of the future. Postpolio syndrome is on the increase because of these factors.

Factors responsible for increasing disability and functional impairment should be monitored, controlled, and reduced to maintain the highest level of function for as long as possible. Adverse complications affecting the disability need to be prevented or appropriately treated with interventions using current knowledge. More research is needed to develop new modalities and technology for future applications.

Most of the disabling complications of prolonged immobilization are related to the neuromusculoskeletal system. Heterotopic ossification is a frequent complication seen in many clinical conditions and hinders rehabilitation. Heterotopic ossification is defined as the formation of mature lamellar bone in the soft tissues [1].

Heterotopic ossification is a biological process of new bone formation in nonosseous tissues where bone is not normally found [2–11]. It has been described in the literature by many names. Most nomenclatures describe its location or its pathophysiology (Table 5-1).

This new bone is not mere calcification in the soft tissues but is true bone radiologically and histologically. Heterotopic ossification varies greatly in its incidence and severity. Its effect on disability depends on its severity and location. Various researchers have made efforts to understand the natural history of this complication, but to date, the etiology remains obscure. The etiology, pathophysiology, and management of heterotopic ossification continue to be controversial. No definite criteria are available to identify high-risk persons in all diagnostic categories. Heterotopic ossification is seen in many conditions, both common and uncommon (Table 5-2). These include spinal cord injury [12], traumatic brain injury [13], total hip replacement [12, 14], stroke [15–17], burns [18], amputations [19], and even drug abuse. At least one-third of these patients have significant heterotopic ossification, causing functional difficulties owing to restriction in joint motion or ankylosis (Figure 5-1). Free joint motion is especially important to achieve independence via rehabilitation for transfer activities, sitting, lower extremity dressing, perineal care, and elimination functions. Heterotopic ossification can also affect orthotic or prosthetic fittings.

Natural History

Heterotopic ossification occurs in neuromuscular injury with prolonged immobilization. It is found in the regions of neurologic deficits, most often in hips, knees, shoulders, and elbows. Involvement

Table 5-1. Genesis of Nomenclature of Heterotopic Ossification

Nomenclature	Genesis	Year	Author
Traumatic ossifying myositis		1914	Fay [2]
Paraosteoarthropathy	New bone formation in tissues where bone normally is not formed	1918	Dejerine and Ceillier [8]
Soft-tissue calcification	New bone formation in tissues where bone normally is not formed	1949	Abramson and Kamberg [3]
Soft tissue ossification	New bone formation in tissues where bone normally is not formed	1958	Ackerman [4]
Pseudomalignant osteoma	New bone formation in tissues where bone normally is not formed	1958	Ackerman [4]
Heterotopic ossification	New bone formation in tissues where bone normally is not formed	1961	Damanski [9]
Neurogenic osteoma	New bone formation in tissues where bone normally is not formed	1971	Benassy and Chambelles [5]
Calcifying hematoma	New bone formation in tissues where bone normally is not formed	1966	Benassy [6]
Para-articular ossification	New bone formation in tissues where bone normally is not formed	1966	Freehafter et al. [10]
Ectopic bone	New bone formation in tissues where bone normally is not formed		
Neurogenic ossifying myopathy	Disease of the muscle	1945	Soule [7]
Myositis ossificans in paraplegia	Inflammatory disease of the muscles	1949	Miller and O'Neil [11]
Funny bone	Abnormal bone		

Table 5-2. Incidence of Heterotopic Ossification in Various Conditions

Common [Reference]	Uncommon
Spinal cord injury (16–53%) [12]	Multiple sclerosis
Traumatic brain injury (11–76%) [13]	Arachnoiditis
Total hip replacement (8–53%) [12, 14, 15]	Tetanus
Burns (11.2%) [18, 19]	Spinal cord tumors (meningioma)
Amputations*	Poliomyelitis
Cerebrovascular accidents (10%) [15–17]	Encephalitis

*Amputations secondary to burns have a higher incidence of heterotopic ossification development (82%) [19].

distal to the elbow and knee has been virtually unknown. A recent report described the presence of heterotopic bone formation involving wrists and fingers in three patients in prolonged comas [20]. It is associated with skeletal atrophy in the paralyzed extremity. The severity of the heterotopic ossification depends on the severity of the neurologic insult. The exact time of onset is variable; it usually occurs within 4–10 weeks, but it may be observed as early as 19 days [21, 22] or as late as several months [8–10, 21] after spinal cord injury. The highest risk period for the occurrence of heterotopic ossification after spinal cord injury is 5 months, and after total hip replacement it is 3 months; heterotopic ossification is unlikely to develop after these periods [14, 23–26]. Its growth may cease spontaneously or continue to progress for 6–14 months. Heterotopic ossification may be unilateral or bilateral and can affect more than one site. It can be asymptomatic, but clinical features such as soft tissue swelling can be the first indication of its development. The clinical picture depends on the stage

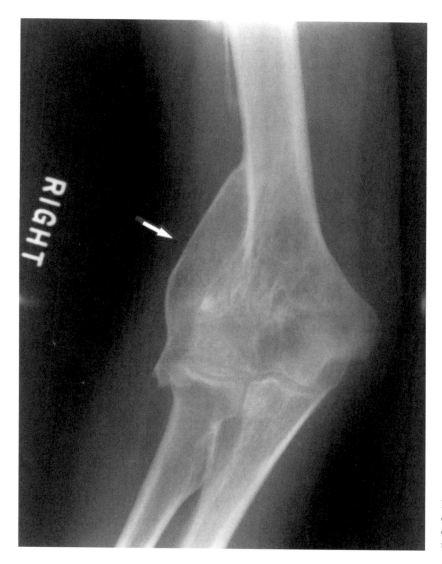

Figure 5-1. Ankylosis of the elbow (arrow) caused by heterotopic ossification in a patient with acute brain injury.

of the disorder. Clinically, four stages have been described: acute, subacute, chronic immature, and chronic mature (Table 5-3). Using serial bone scans, heterotopic ossification is seen to progress through five stages [27]. The time period for progression from one stage to another varies, ranging from months to years. The maturity of the bone is important when considering surgical treatment and prevention of recurrence.

The incidence of heterotopic ossification seems to be higher in adult men. The disorder has not been reported in children, and there is no relationship to racial group [28]. The incidence of heterotopic ossification is reported to be lower in spinal cord injury resulting from stab injuries [28]. In traumatic brain injury heterotopic ossification seems to be related to the severity of the injury and spasticity. Four risk factors, including age (older than 30 years), completeness of injury, presence of spasticity, and coexistence of pressure ulcers, have been identified in spinal cord injury [29]. The risk factors seem to be additive. The greater the number of risk factors, the higher the incidence of the disorder (Table 5-4). Risk factors for the occurrence of the

Table 5-3. Stages of Heterotopic Ossification

Stage	Duration	Clinical Signs	Alkaline Phosphatase	Sedimentation Rate	Radiologic	Bone Scan
I Acute	2 wks	Inflammation	↑	↑	Negative	± Activity
II Subacute	2–8 wks	↓ Inflammation ↓ Range of motion Hard welling	↑	↑	Grade I activity	Increasing
III Chronic active immature	6–8 mons	↓ Range of motion Irregular palpable bony masses	↑	↑	Grade II	Decreasing activity
IV Chronic mature	8–18 mons	↓ Range of motion Ankylosis Hard bony masses	↓ Normal	Normal	Grade III	Active to normal scan

↑ = increased; ↓ = decreased.

Table 5-4. Risk Factors for Heterotopic Ossification

Spinal Cord Injury	Traumatic Brain Injury	Total Hip Replacement
Males older than age 30 years Complete lesion + Pressure ulcers + Spasticity	Males Severity of injury + Pressure ulcers + Spasticity	Males Bilateral condition Associated arthritis Previous total hip replacement with heterotopic ossification Infection after total hip replacement

+ = present.

disorder in total hip replacement have also been identified. These factors include the presence of osteophytes, pre-existing heterotopic bone formation due to previous surgery, history of infection, traumatic osteoarthritis, ankylosing spondylitis, and idiopathic skeletal hyperostosis [30]. No associated risk factors have been reported in the infection group. Incidence of severe disability involving heterotopic ossification is reported in 0.5–3.0% of the total hip arthroplasty cases [31].

Classification

Like everything else related to heterotopic ossification, confusion exists regarding its classification. Publications prior to 1960 do not reflect any differentiation between heterotopic ossification after local trauma and after neuromuscular insults. Some authors have claimed no difference in the two forms. At present, the condition can be best classified as congenital and acquired forms with their subdivisions (Table 5-5).

Clinical Features

Congenital Heterotopic Ossification

Myositis Ossificans Progressiva

Myositis ossificans progressiva is a congenital form of heterotopic ossification that is believed to be an inheritable and sometimes familial disorder (also reported in monozygotic twins). Recently, a family with five affected persons in three generations has

Table 5-5. Classification of Heterotopic Ossification

Congenital
    Myositis ossificans progressiva or fibrodysplasia ossificans
Acquired
    Traumatic myositis ossificans or myositis ossificans circumscripta
Neuromuscular
    Neurologic insult: traumatic brain injury, spinal cord injury, cerebrovascular accident
    Musculoskeletal insult: total hip replacement, amputations, burns
    Infections: tetanus, arachnoiditis, encephalitis
Idiopathic

been described, providing further evidence of autosomal dominant inheritance. A wide range of phenotypic severity was apparent. Disabling ectopic bone formation led to premature death in an asymptomatic adult with characteristic big toe abnormalities [32]. It is associated with other congenital skeletal anomalies: commonly bilateral hallux valgus, microdactyly of the toes, and ankylosis of interphalangeal and metatarsophalangeal joints. It is more common in female patients, with the disease being evident by 6 years of age. The progression of congenital heterotopic ossification is not random, rather it proceeds with a characteristic anatomic pattern—i.e., axial to appendicular, cranial to caudal, and proximal to distal [33].

Although diagnosis may be made later, the disease is progressive, with loss of movement. The muscle ligaments and tendons are involved. The disease advances by a series of exacerbations. The victim gradually freezes, and terms such as *petrified man* have been used to describe the effect on the patient.

Death occurs from pneumonia as a result of restrictive pulmonary disease [34, 35]. A male patient with myositis ossificans progressiva is shown in Figures 5-2 and 5-3, with heterotopic ossification present in the shoulders, elbows, knees, and back. The radiologic appearance of heterotopic ossification is shown in Figures 5-4 and 5-5.

Case Report 1. A 20-year-old man was admitted to a spinal cord injury unit in 1981 with traumatic incomplete C6 cervical myelopathy as a result of a motor vehicle collision. The patient had pre-existing diffuse myositis ossificans progressiva (fibrodysplasia ossificans progressiva) from an early age. Het-

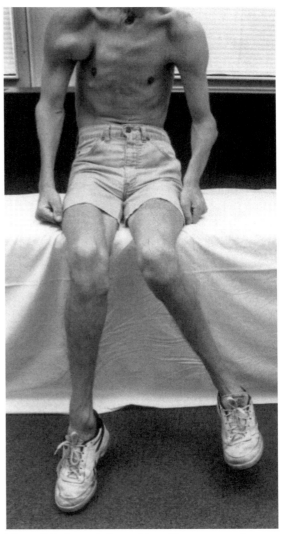

Figure 5-2. Congenital myositis ossificans progressiva (shoulders, elbows, and knees).

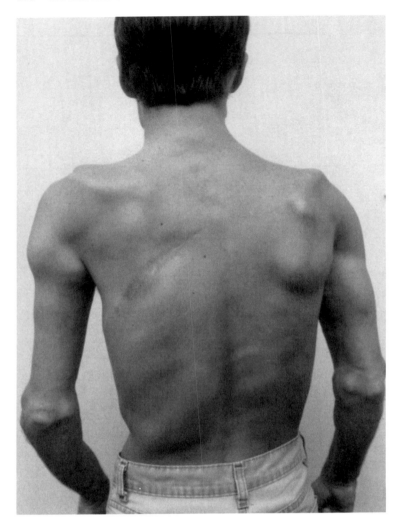

Figure 5-3. Myositis ossificans progressiva of the back, elbows, and shoulders, with healed incision where heterotopic ossification has been removed.

erotopic bone was present at all of the sites described in the literature (see Figures 5-2 through 5-5), with the exception of the spine. The patient underwent spine stabilization surgery for a C6 vertebral fracture. HLA-DR typing revealed HLA-DR5 and another unidentified locus. The patient was last seen in the outpatient department in 1993 at the age of 35 years. He continued to experience quadriparesis, multiple contractures, limitation of movement with multiple bony masses, pulmonary restrictive diseases, and neurogenic bladder and bowel. In 1990, the patient had undergone surgery for partial excision of bony masses from the back and right upper arm. He continued to maintain independence in physical activities and ambulated with assistive devices. He also was a volunteer at a hospital. This patient is an interesting and determined individual with complex congenital and acquired neuromusculoskeletal problems.

Acquired Heterotopic Ossification

Traumatic Ossificans or Myositis Ossificans Circumscripta

The lesion is usually solitary and associated with trauma.

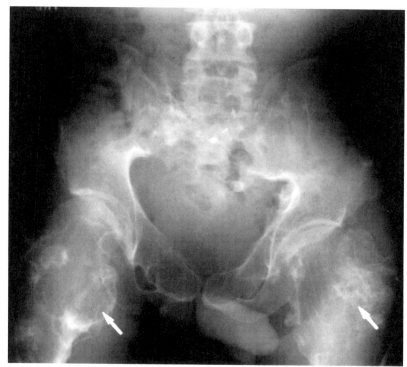

Figure 5-4. Radiologic appearance of myositis ossificans progressiva around the hips (arrows).

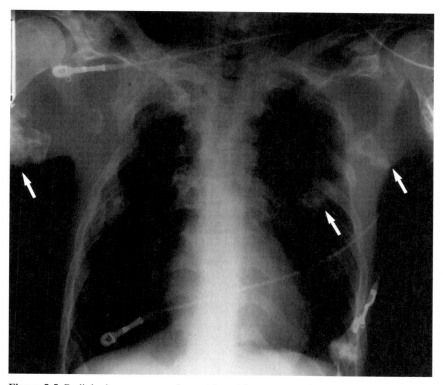

Figure 5-5. Radiologic appearance of myositis ossificans progressiva around the shoulders and chest (arrows).

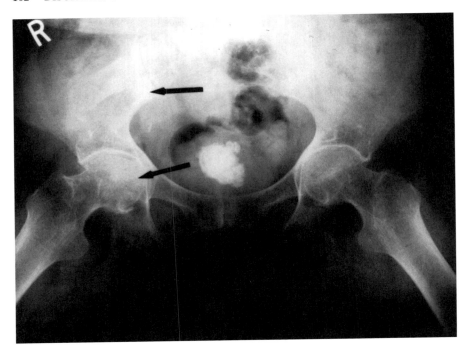

Figure 5-6. Heterotopic ossification at the hip (arrows) with osteoporosis in a normal individual with osteoporosis of the spine (see Case Report 2 in text).

Neuromuscular Heterotopic Ossification

Heterotopic ossification can be caused by neuromuscular insult. The etiology continues to be unknown. There are three different subcategories:

1. Neurologic: spinal cord injury, traumatic brain injury, and stroke [36].
2. Musculoskeletal: amputations, burns, total hip replacement, and arthralgia.
3. Infections: poliomyelitis, Guillain-Barré syndrome, tetanus, encephalitis, and arachnoiditis.

Idiopathic Heterotopic Ossification

Heterotopic ossification has been reported in otherwise healthy persons [37].

Case Report 2. An 82-year-old woman was initially seen for back pain resulting from vertebral compression fractures at T9, T10, T11, and T12 in October 1990. She responded well to spinal bracing, pharmacologic intervention, and a well-planned exercise program. The patient was taking disodium etidronate (Didronel) and calcium carbonate for osteoporosis. She continued to progress nicely, and in April 1991 was gradually weaned off of the spinal orthosis, which was being used for prolonged upright position, standing, and ambulation.

In March 1994, the patient, then 85 years old, reported some pain and stiffness in the hips as well as balance problems, but she had not experienced any falls. A physical examination revealed no swelling, but there was decreased range of motion in both hips in abduction and external rotation. The patient was able to walk without any assistive device, displaying not only flexion at the hips and knees, but also internally rotated hips.

Osteoarthritis of the hips was suspected and roentgenograms were taken. Soft tissue calcification adjacent to the medial aspect of both femoral necks was observed due to early heterotopic ossification and hypertrophic degenerative arthritis (Figure 5-6). This case demonstrates the development of heterotopic ossification with no risk factors while the patient was taking Didronel, a heterotopic ossification and osteoporosis prophylactic agent that lacked efficacy in this case.

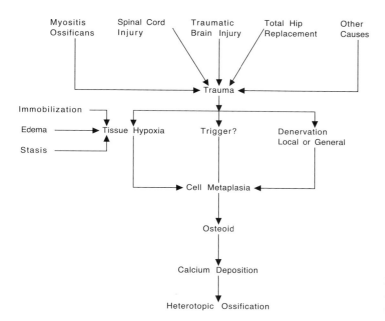

Figure 5-7. Schematic representation of the pathogenesis of heterotopic ossification.

Pathogenesis

The exact cause and mechanism of heterotopic ossification remain unknown. There is evidence that heterotopic ossification is the result of rapid metaplastic osteogenesis and some chondrogenesis, resulting in the formation of lamellar corticospongiosal bone [22]. Two major questions about the pathogenesis of heterotopic ossification remain unanswered:

1. Where do the osteoblasts come from?
2. What triggers the osteoblastic activity?

A review of the literature suggests five contenders as precursors of osteoblasts [38]:

1. The primitive mesenchymal cells.
2. Undifferentiated fibroblasts.
3. Cartilage cells (normally present in many muscle tendons).
4. Capillary endothelial cells.
5. Periosteal cells within the connective tissue. "Periosteal rests" hypothetically form periosteum of neighboring bones.

What triggers the cellular metaplasia and why it does not materialize in all cases with similar conditions remain unanswered. Devitalized and dead tissues act as inducers of bone formation [39]. Common theories proposed to explain the triggering pathogenetic mechanism are tissue hypoxia, neurogenic factors, genetic factors, autoimmunity, and hypersensitivity.

No positive correlation exists between heterotopic ossification and autoimmune responses [40–46]. Tissue hypoxia due to immobilization, local edema resulting from circulatory stasis [22, 47], and an unidentified neurogenic factor in denervated tissues may be responsible for tissue metaplasia resulting in heterotopic ossification. This mechanism could explain the pathogenesis of traumatic myositis ossificans. Tissue damage and necrosis resulting from trauma and inflammatory reactions precipitate cellular metaplasia and bone formation. A combination of immobilization and forcible mobilization experimentally has led to the development of heterotopic ossification in rabbits [48, 49]. The role of passive exercises and spasticity in heterotopic ossification continues to be controversial [49–51]. The common features in all the conditions in which heterotopic ossification is seen are immobilization due to trauma, surgery, or forced therapeutic rest, followed by mobilization with exercise or spasticity (Figure 5-7). The prevalence of

Table 5-6. Symptoms and Signs of
Heterotopic Ossification

General
    Elevated temperature
    Malaise
    Increased spasticity
Local
    Local swelling with brawny induration
    Increase in local temperature and redness
    Joint effusion
    Decreased range of motion
    Ankylosis
    Skin breakdown may or may not be present
    Unilateral or bilateral
    Common sites: hips, medial side of thigh, knees,
       femoral condyles, shoulder, and elbows

and relationship of pressure ulcers to heterotopic ossification is also controversial [9, 52, 53].

The incidence of heterotopic ossification is greater in osteoarthritic men than women following total hip replacement [54]. Surgical trauma in total hip replacement causes undifferentiated fibroblasts to produce osteoid matrix instead of connective tissue. Little or no osteoclastic activity is seen.

Diagnosis

Often heterotopic ossification is diagnosed accidentally when radiographs are obtained for some other reason. The most important point for early diagnosis is a high index of suspicion for its presence in high-risk patient populations.

Clinical Picture

Systematic evaluation should include a clinical examination, radiographs, bone scan, and determination of serum alkaline phosphatase levels. Symptoms similar to those in trauma, inflammation, or tumor occur in the early stages and include swelling, erythema, redness, and increased temperature, followed by limitation in range of motion in either the hips, knees, or inner side of the thigh in the adductor or iliopsoas muscles. Pain may or may not be present, depending on whether sensation is intact. In 2–4% of

cases, patients report pain at any stage. Spasticity may be enhanced. Bilateral knee effusion has been reported to occur early [24]. Fever and malaise may also be present (Table 5-6).

Laboratory Tests

Routine blood chemistry values, including elevated levels of serum calcium, inorganic phosphorus, and alkaline phosphatase, have limited diagnostic value. However, persistent elevation of both serum alkaline phosphatase and phosphorus concentrations are more likely to be associated with the development of heterotopic ossification [55]. The interpretation of an increased serum alkaline phosphatase level and increased urinary hydroxyproline level is controversial, but these abnormalities often parallel the evolution of heterotopic ossification [22, 24, 25, 53]. The serum alkaline phosphatase value is usually elevated during active bone formation. It becomes normal when bone is mature but may remain normal throughout. Serial determinations of the serum alkaline phosphatase value are valuable in determining the progress of heterotopic ossification.

The sedimentation rate is elevated in both acute and subacute stages. An elevated creatine phosphokinase value indicates involvement of muscle by heterotopic ossification [22].

Radiologic Evaluation

Radiologically, heterotopic ossification has been described to have four grades (Table 5-7). Roentgenograms may either appear normal or show soft tissue swelling in the initial stages (grade 0) (Figure 5-8). After 2–3 weeks, soft irregular flocculated deposits, described as "dotted veil or hazy shell," are seen adjacent to bone (Figure 5-9). Heterotopic ossification is separate from the periosteum of the bone (grade I). At 8–10 weeks, a dense lacy pattern of bone with peripheral flocculation may be seen (Figure 5-10). Maturation with a trabeculated pattern and a decrease in the fluffy appearance occurs at 6–8 months or longer (grade II). The bone matures in 12–18 months [57] and is more homogeneous and well defined (grade III) (Figure 5-11). Most observers

Table 5-7. Histologic and Radiographic Grading of Heterotopic Ossification

Grade	Radiologic Appearance	Histologic Picture
0	Soft-tissue swelling; negative for heterotopic ossification	Profuse proliferation of fibroblasts; appearance of hyaline mass
I	Soft irregular flocculation; "dotted veil or hazy shell" appearance	Cellular metaplasia with osteoid; dilated capillaries; central necrosis
II	Dense, lacy pattern; trabecular pattern; decreased fluffy appearance	Zoning phenomenon: four clearly defined zones (see text)
III	Homogenous, well-defined trabecular pattern; atrophy of adjacent bone	True bone with cortex; tightly latticed spongiosa

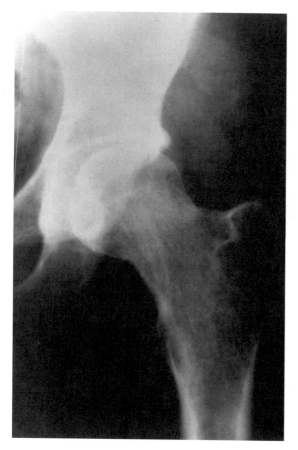

Figure 5-8. Grade 0: no heterotopic ossification.

have noted associated osteoporosis in adjacent bone. Determination of the maturity of heterotopic ossification is of great significance in planning surgical treatment.

Bone Scan

Serial bone scans are an important tool for diagnosing heterotopic ossification early, studying its evolution, and evaluating the effectiveness of treatment. Single random bone scans are of little assistance [22, 26, 27]. Evaluation studies for heterotopic ossification have been done with strontium 85 [27], technetium 99m three-phase scanning, and gallium-67 scanning [26]. Increasing radionuclide activity indicates growing immature bone, whereas decreased uptake suggests slowing of the disease process.

Angiography

Angiography has been used to study the natural history of heterotopic ossification [22] but is not applied currently in the diagnosis of the disorder. Angiography is not a useful tool in determining the maturity of heterotopic ossification. Doppler combined with ultrasound have proven to be useful tools in ruling out deep vein thrombosis and accurately detecting musculoskeletal abnormalities within hours of clinical manifestations. Ultrasound can also help determine the exclusion or inclusion of the formation of heterotopic ossification in spinal cord injured patients [58].

Histopathology

Tissue diagnosis by biopsy is not done because of the risk of exacerbating the disorder by resec-

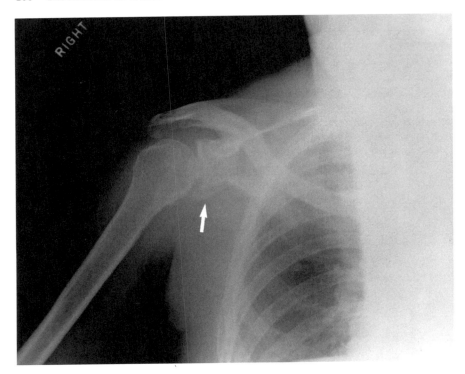

Figure 5-9. Grade I: heterotopic ossification is separate from bone periosteum (arrow).

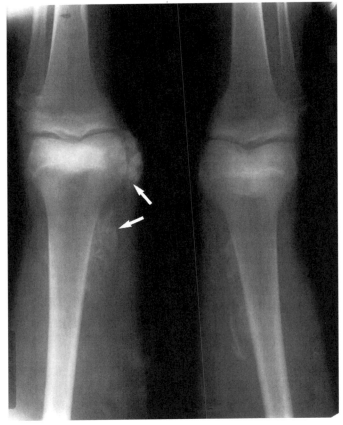

Figure 5-10. Immature heterotopic ossification: grade II (bottom arrow) and grade III (top arrow).

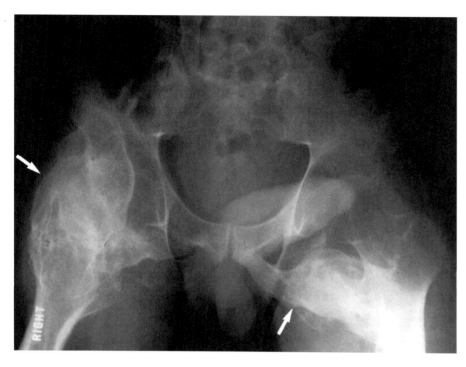

Figure 5-11. Immature grade II heterotopic ossification (top arrow) and mature grade III heterotopic ossification (bottom arrow).

tion of an immature lesion. However, the histologic structure has been studied extensively from surgical samples, using light and electron microscopy [22, 38]. Heterotopic bone is true bone but instead of a true periosteum it has a fibrous covering [59]. The histologic appearance in the different phases is described in the following sections and in Table 5-7.

Early Acute Phase

The early acute phase of heterotopic ossification resembles the sequelae of muscle trauma—i.e., profuse proliferation of fibroblasts, with degeneration of muscle cells into a hyaline mass. Soft tissue swelling is evident. Roentgenograms appear normal at this stage, which lasts for 2–3 weeks.

Early Subacute Phase

In the early subacute phase there is a hypervascular periphery with a relatively avascular center, cellular metaplasia, and dilated capillaries with hyaline matrix (osteoid) formation. Roentgenograms may

or may not be revealing. The duration of this phase is approximately 4 weeks.

Subacute Phase

A zoning phenomenon is seen in the subacute phase. Four zones can be identified that merge with each other from center to periphery: (1) a central zone with undifferentiated highly cellular areas and mitotic figures, (2) a zone of cellular osteoid with loose cellular stroma, (3) a zone showing osteoblastic and fibroblastic activity of new bone formation undergoing trabecular organization, and (4) the outermost zone of well-defined bone encapsulated in fibrous tissue. The subacute phase persists from 4–12 weeks.

Mature Phase

Heterotopic ossification is true bone; it is harder than normal bone and consists of cortex and tightly latticed spongiosa with less-defined corticospongiosal margins than in normal bone. The haversian system and hematopoiesis are discrete [22]. Bone

Table 5-8. Differential Diagnosis of Heterotopic Ossification

Parameter	Heterotopic Ossification	Thrombophlebitis	Inflammatory Condition	Hematoma	Neoplasm
Pain (depending on sensation)	+	+	+	+	Persistent +
Swelling	Rapid, localized ↑ followed by ↓ in uniform hardness	+ Palpable vessel cord	Uniform soft	+	Progressive ↑ Variable consistency
Alkaline phosphatase	↑ Alkaline phosphatase	−	−	−	↑ Alkaline phosphatase
Radiography	New bone with radiolucent demarcation zone from cortex; no destruction of cortex	−	−	−	Periosteal reaction and destruction of cortex of bone
Bone scan	+	−	−	−	+
Doppler flow studies	−	+	−	−	−
Response to antibiotics	No change	No change	Resolves	No change	No change

− = absent; + = present; ↑ = increase; ↓ = decrease.

continues to mature after 24 weeks, and maturation may continue for 18 months or longer.

Differential Diagnosis

The conditions that simulate heterotopic ossification in its early stages are hematoma, inflammatory conditions (periostitis, osteomyelitis), thrombophlebitis, fractures, and neoplasms. The salient features and diagnostic methods of differentiation are presented in Table 5-8.

Management

Therapeutic intervention after early diagnosis of heterotopic ossification continues to be controversial; to date there is no known method to prevent the formation of this disorder. The following treatment modalities are recommended.

Physical Therapy

The role of physical therapy in the management of heterotopic ossification is controversial to the point that it is also considered an etiologic factor in the development of the lesion [9, 21, 22, 52, 60]; however, this point has recently been disputed [61, 62]. Generally, the accepted role for physical therapy is to maintain range of motion and prevent ankylosis by employing gentle, passive range of motion exercises. Forceful joint manipulation has also been used to gain mobility [60, 61]. Routine or forceful physical therapy treatment may cause pseudoarthritis. However, the benefits may be improved range of motion. Crepitus or cracking sounds may be heard during the exercise program [62].

Pharmacologic Agents

The idea of broad, continuous use of medications to prevent heterotopic ossification is controversial. A brief description of pharmacologic agents recommended for prevention of this disorder follows.

Disodium Etidronate

Disodium etidronate does not prevent heterotopic ossification but reduces its severity [12, 14, 51, 64,

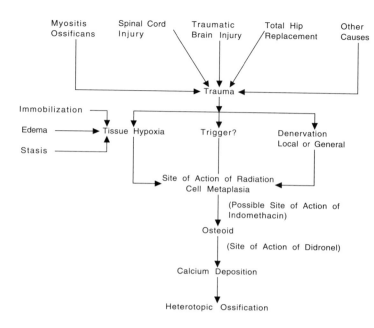

Figure 5-12. Preventive modalities of heterotopic ossification and their site of action.

65]. The drug does not prevent the initial inflammatory process [66] but prevents the ossification [67] (Figure 5-12). Disodium etidronate can be used orally or intravenously. Intravenous administration of 300 mg disodium etidronate can achieve a high concentration at the site of heterotopic bone for 3–5 days. Use of oral disodium etidronate for 6 months subsequently is recommended [68]. The prophylactic use of disodium etidronate is recommended for 3–6 months beginning 3–4 weeks after injury. The customary dosage is 20 mg/kg for 6 months. Disodium etidronate has also been beneficial in preventing recurrence of severe heterotopic ossification after surgery. Therapy with disodium etidronate should start at least 4 weeks before and continue for at least 1 year after surgery. Cost of the drug, gastrointestinal side effects, and its efficacy are controversial issues (see Case Report 2). Prophylaxis with a dose of less than 20 mg/kg needs to be proven.

Indomethacin

The use of indomethacin for retardation and prevention of heterotopic ossification in total hip arthroplasty [69–72] and severe head injury [71] has been recommended. Indomethacin inhibits prostaglandin E_2, thus preventing osteoid formation. Indomethacin

suppresses inflammation, mesenchymal cell proliferation, and woven bone formation. The recommended dose is 25 mg three times per day for 6 weeks in the early stages, but the optimal duration of therapy is still under investigation.

Nonsteroidal Anti-inflammatory Drugs and Aspirin

Nonsteroidal anti-inflammatory drugs and aspirin for the prophylaxis of heterotopic ossification have shown beneficial effects after total hip replacement [73]. Further studies to confirm this report are needed. The use of warfarin (anticoagulant) and verapamil (calcium channel blocker) for heterotopic ossification is suggested, but needs to be investigated [74].

Radiation Therapy for Prophylaxis

The use of postoperative prophylaxis with radiation therapy has been evaluated only after total hip replacement [75–79]. Initially, higher doses (2,000–3,000 rad) were used, but low doses (1,000 rad) have been shown to be equally effective [79]. The rationale behind radiation prophylaxis is prevention of precursor cell differentiation to os-

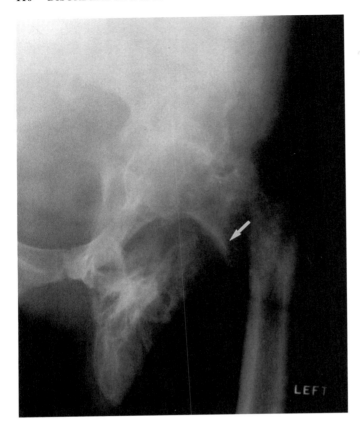

Figure 5-13. Fracture (arrow) as a complication with heterotopic ossification after surgery.

teoblasts. By altering the DNA transcription, osteoid formation is prevented [80]. There is controversy in three areas about the use of radiation: (1) trials have been limited, (2) prophylaxis is incomplete (moderate heterotopic ossification still may develop), and (3) there is a risk of induction of malignancy [81–83]. Low-dose radiation has shown excellent results in providing relief from pain and preventing the recurrence of heterotopic bone in the hip of the arthroplasty patients [31]. Successful use of limited field, single, low-dose radiation—i.e., 600–800 rad administered within 3 postoperative days of total hip arthroplasty to prevent heterotopic ossification—has been reported [80].

Surgical Intervention

Surgery for excision of heterotopic ossification is indicated only in conditions where the lesion interferes with self-care and mobility and prevents reha-bilitation. Surgery should be contemplated when the bone is mature and quiescent and the patient is medically stable (an added risk of hyperreflexia needs to be considered in patients with spinal cord injury). Total excision is usually not possible, and wedge resection is recommended. Appropriate precautions and timing of surgery are very important. The maturity of bone is determined by quiescent clinical condition, an almost normal alkaline phosphatase level, radiologic appearance, and decreased radionuclide activity on the bone scan.

Precautions should be taken to avoid infected skin lesions, urinary tract infection, and poor general condition before and after surgery. Antibiotic and disodium etidronate prophylaxis should be initiated prior to surgery. Range of motion exercises should begin 1 week after the surgery.

Risks of surgery include hemorrhage, infection, fracture (Figure 5-13), and recurrence (Figure 5-14). The effectiveness of surgery is variable depending on the location of the lesion. In patients

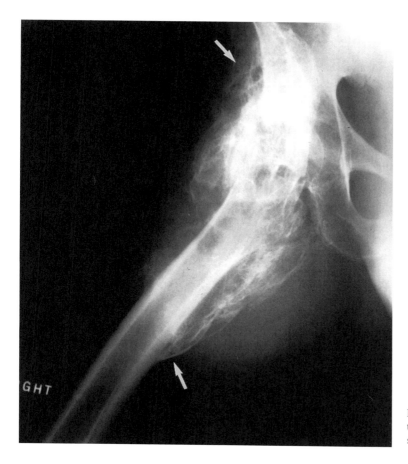

Figure 5-14. Recurrence of heterotopic ossification (arrows) after surgery.

with head trauma, heterotopic ossification involving the elbow has the most favorable outcome [13]. Complications resulting from heterotopic ossification [31, 83] include ankylosis, pressure ulceration, painful arthrosis or pseudoarthrosis, malignant transportation, neurovascular compression, and recurrence.

Conclusion

Prophylactic and corrective treatment of heterotopic ossification continues to be inadequate. Despite vigorous research and interest by specialists from various medical fields, the etiology, pathogenesis, natural history, and medical management of the disorder remain uncertain. Prospective follow-up studies are needed [84] so that better patient care will be forthcoming [85].

References

1. Pittenger DE. Heterotopic ossification. Osteoporosis Review 1991;20(1):33.
2. Fay OJ. Traumatic parosteal bone and callus formation: the so-called traumatic ossifying myositic. Surg Gynecol Obstet 1914;19:174.
3. Abramson DJ, Kamberg S. Spondylitis, pathologic ossification, and calcification associated with spinal cord injury. J Bone Joint Surg [Am] 1949;31:275.
4. Ackerman LV. Extraosseous localized non-neoplastic bone and cartilage formation (so-called myositis ossificans). J Bone Joint Surg [Am] 1958;40:279.
5. Benassy J, Chambelles F. Osteomes tentatives therapeutiques. Ann Med Phys (Paris) 1971;14:467.
6. Benassy J. Ossifications and fracture healing in paraplegia and brain injuries. Proc Annu Clin Spinal Cord Injury Conf 1966;15:55.
7. Soule AB. Neurogenic ossifying fibromyopathies. A preliminary report. Neurosurgery 1945;2:485.

8. Dejerine M, Ceillier A. Para-ostéoarthropathies des paraplégives par lésions medullaires (étude clinique et radiographique). Ann Med 1918;5:497.

9. Damanski M. Heterotopic ossification in paraplegia—A clinical study. J Bone Joint Surg [Br] 1961;43:286.

10. Freehafter AA, Yurik R, Mast WA. Para-articular ossification in spinal cord injury. Med Serv J Can 1966;22:471.

11. Miller LF, O'Neil CJ. Myositis ossificans in paraplegics. J Bone Joint Surg [Am] 1980;62:811.

12. Finerman GAM, Stover SL. Heterotopic ossification following hip replacement or spinal cord injury: Two clinical studies with EHDP. Metab Bone Dis Rel Res 1981;4&5:337.

13. Garland DE, Razza BE, Waters RL. Forceful joint manipulation in head injured adults: Incidence and location. J Bone Joint Surg [Am] 1980;62:1143.

14. Spielman G, Bennarellia TA, Rogers CR. Disodium etridonate: Its role in preventing HO in severe head injury. Arch Phys Med Rehabil 1983;64:539.

15. Nakajo M, Endo H. HO with hemiplegia caused by cerebral apoplexy. Orthop Surg (Tokyo) 1969;20:193.

16. Rosin AJ. Periarticular calcification in a hemiplegic limb. A rare complication of stroke. J Am Geriatr Soc 1970;18:916.

17. Hajek VE. Heterotopic ossification in hemiplegia following stroke. Arch Phys Med Rehabil 1987;68:313.

18. Munster AM, Bruck HM, Johns LA, et al. Heterotopic ossification following burns: a prospective study. J Trauma 1973;12:1071.

19. Helm PA, Walker SC. New bone formation at amputation sites in electrically burn-injured patients. Arch Phys Med Rehabil 1987;68:284.

20. Sazbon L, Groswasser Z. Heterotopic bone formation involving wrist and fingers in brain-injured patients. Brain Injury 1989;3:57.

21. Hardy AG, Dickson JW. Pathological ossification in traumatic paraplegia. J Bone Joint Surg [Br] 1963;45:76.

22. Rossier AB. Current facts of paraosteoarthropathy (POA). Paraplegia 1973;11:36.

23. Urist MR, Strates BS. Bone formation in implants of partially and wholly demineralized bone matrix. Clin Orthop 1970;71:271.

24. Furman R, Nicholas JJ, Jovoff L. Elevation of serum alkaline phosphatase coincident with ectopic bone formation in paraplegic patients. J Bone Joint Surg [Am] 1970;52:1131.

25. Nicholas JT. Bone formation in patients with spinal cord injury. Arch Phys Med Rehabil 1973;54:334.

26. Freed JH, Hahn H, Menter R, Dillon T. The use of the three-phase bone scan in the early diagnosis of heterotopic ossification (HO) and in the evaluation of Didronel therapy. Paraplegia 1982;20:208.

27. Tibon J, Sakimura I, Nickel VL, Hsu E. Heterotopic ossification around the hip in spinal cord injured patients. J Bone Joint Surg [Am] 1978;60:769.

28. Scher AT. The incidence of ectopic bone formation in post-traumatic paraplegic patients of different racial groups. Paraplegia 1976;14:202.

29. Lal S, Heineman A, Hamilton B, Betts HB. Risk factors for heterotopic ossification in spinal cord injury. Arch Phys Med Rehabil 1987;68:653.

30. Finerman GAM, Kregel WF, Lowel JD, et al. Role of diphosphonate (EHDP) in the prevention of heterotopic ossification after total hip arthroplasty: A preliminary report. In Proceedings of the Fifth Open Scientific Meetings of the Hip Society, St. Louis, 1977.

31. Warren S, Brooker A. Excision of heterotopic bone followed by irradiation after total hip arthroplasty. J Bone Joint Surg [Am] 1992;74:201.

32. Connor JM, Skirton H, Lunt PW. A three generation family with fibrodysplasia progressiva. J Med Genet 1993;30:687.

33. Cohen RB, Hahn GV, Tabas JA, et al. The natural history of heterotopic ossification in patients who have fibrodysplasia ossificans progressiva. J Bone Joint Surg [Am] 1993;75:2.

34. Aegerter E, Kirkpatrick JA. Orthopaedic Diseases: Physiology, Pathology, Radiology (3rd ed). Philadelphia: Saunders, 1968.

35. Geho WB, Whiteside JA. Experience with disodium etidronate in disease of ectopic calcification. Research Paper. Cincinnati, OH: Procter & Gamble, 1971.

36. Rosin AJ. Ectopic calcification around joints of paralyzed limb in hemiplegia, diffuse brain damage and other neurological disease. Ann Rheum Dis 1975;34:499.

37. Samuelson K, Coleman SS. Nontraumatic myositis ossificans in healthy individuals. JAMA 1976;235:1132.

38. Bayley SJ. Resident review #14. Funny bones: A review of the problems of heterotopic bone formation. Orthop Rev 1979;8:1.

39. Ostrowicki K, Wlodarski K. Induction of heterotopic bone formation. In GH Bourne (ed), Biochemistry and Physiology of Bone (2nd ed). Vol 3. New York: Academic, 1971.

40. Hunter T, Hidahl CR, Smith NJ, et al. Histocompatibility antigens in paraplegic or quadriplegic patients with sacroiliac joint changes. J Rheumatol 1979;6:1.

41. Hunter T, Dubo HJ, Hidahl CR, et al. Histocompatibility antigens in patient with spinal injury or cerebral damage complicated by HO. Rheum Rehabil 1980;19:97.

42. Weiss S, Grosswassner Z, Ohri A, et al. Histocompatibility (HLA) antigens in heterotopic ossification associated with neurological injury. J Rheumatol 1979;6:88.

43. Minaire P, Betuel H, Girard R, Piloncherry G. Neurologic injuries, paraosteoarthropathis and human leukocyte antigens. Arch Phys Med Rehabil 1980;51:214.

44. Larson JM, Michalski JP, Collacott EA, et al. Increased prevalence of HLA-B27 in patients with ectopic ossification. Rheum Rehabil 1981;20:193.

45. Garland DE, Alday B, Venos KG. Heterotopic ossification and HLA antigens. Arch Phys Med Rehabil 1984;65:531.

46. Ritter MA, Biegel AA, Bray RA, Blintz M. HLA antigens and ectopic ossification following total hip arthroplasty. J Bone Joint Surg [Am] 1984;59:345.

47. Major P, Resnick D, Greenway G. HO in paraplegia: A possible disturbance of the paravertebral sinuses. Radiology 1980;136:797.
48. Michelson JE, Granforth G, Anderson LC, Helsinki F. Myositis ossification following forcible manipulation of the leg. J Bone Joint Surg [Am] 1980;62:811.
49. Izumi K. Study of ectopic bone formation in experimental spinal cord injured rabbits. Paraplegia 1983;21:331.
50. Hassack DW, King A. Neurogenic heterotopic ossification. Med J Aust 1967;1:325.
51. Stover SL, Niemann KMW, Miller JM. Disodium etidronate in the prevention of post-operative recurrence of HO in SCI patients. J Bone Joint Surg [Am] 1976;58:683.
52. Silver JR. HO: A clinical study of its possible relationship to trauma. Int J Paraplegia 1969;7:220.
53. Hassard GH. HO about the hip and unilateral decubitus ulcers in SCI. Arch Phys Med Rehabil 1975;56:355.
54. Ritter MA, Vaughn RB. Ectopic ossification after total hip arthroplasty. J Bone Joint Surg [Am] 1977;59:345.
55. Kim SW, Charter RA, Chal CJ, et al. Serum alkaline phosphatase and inorganic phosphorus values in spinal cord injury patients with heterotopic ossification. Paraplegia 1980;28:441.
56. Bolger JT. Heterotopic bone formation and alkaline phosphatase. Arch Phys Med Rehabil 1975;56:36.
57. Wharton GW. Heterotopic ossification. Clin Orthop 1975;112:142.
58. Bodley R, Jamous A, Short D. Ultra-sound in the early diagnosis of heterotopic ossification in patients with spinal cord injury. Paraplegia 1993;31:500.
59. Wlodarski KH. Normal and heterotopic periosteum. Clin Orthop Res (Sect III Basic Science and Pathology) 1989;241:265.
60. Wharton GW, Morgan TH. Ankylosis in the paralyzed patient. J Bone Joint Surg [Am] 1970;52:105.
61. Garland DE, Razza BE, Waters RL. Forceful joint manipulation in head injured adults with heterotopic ossification. Clin Orthop 1982;169:133.
62. Stover SL, Hataway CJ, Zieger HE. Heterotopic ossification in spinal cord injured patients. Arch Phys Med Rehabil 1975;56:199.
63. Subbarao JV. Pseudoarthrosis in heterotopic ossification in spinal cord-injured patients. Am J Phys Med Rehabil 1990;69:88.
64. Hahn HR. Heterotopic ossification following spinal cord injury: The case for prophylactic therapy. Procter & Gamble (Craig Hospital, Englewood, CO), 1982.
65. Stover SL. Spinal cord injury update. J Am Paraplegia Soc 1983;3:66.
66. Bassett CAL, Bonath A, Macagno F, et al. Diphosphonates in the treatment of myositis ossificans. Lancet 1969;2:7627.
67. Thomas BJ, Amstutz HC. Results of administration of disphosphonate for the prevention of heterotopic ossification after total hip arthroplasty. J Bone Joint Surg [Am] 1985;67:400.
68. Banovac K, Gonzalez F, Wade N, Bowker JJ. Intravenous disodium etidronate therapy in spinal cord injury patients with heterotopic ossification. Paraplegia 1993;31:660.
69. Ritter MA, Gide TJ. The effect of indomethacin on para-articular ectopic ossification following THR. Clin Orthop 1982;167:113.
70. Ritter MA. Indomethacin counters ectopic bone growth. Orthopedics Today 1984;May:13.
71. Ritter MA. Indomethacin: An adjunct to surgical excision of immature heterotopic bone formation in a patient with severe head injury. Orthopedics 1987;10:1379.
72. Schmidt R. Heterotopic ossification in severe head injury: A preventive program. Brain Injury 1988;2:169.
73. Eyb R, Knahr K. The effect of prophylaxis for thrombosis on heterotopic ossification following total hip joint replacement. Arch Orthop Trauma Surg 1983;102:114.
74. Buschbacher R. Heterotopic ossification: A review. Crit Rev Phys Rehabil Med 1992;4:199.
75. Coventry MD, Scranton PW. The use of radiation to discourage ectopic bone. J Bone Joint Surg [Am] 1981;63:201.
76. Parkinson JR, McCollister CE, Hubbard LF. Radiation therapy in the prevention of heterotopic ossification after total hip arthroplasty. In JP Nelson (ed), The Hip: Proceedings of the Tenth Open Scientific Meeting of the Hip Society. St. Louis: Mosby, 1982;211.
77. MacLennan I, Keys HM, Evarts CM, Phillips R. Usefulness of postoperative hip irradiation in the prevention of heterotopic bone formation in a high risk group of patients. Int J Radiat Oncol Biol Phys 1984;10:49.
78. Ayers DC, Evarts CM, Parkinson JR. The prevention of heterotopic ossification in high-risk patients by low-dose radiation therapy after total hip arthroplasty. J Bone Joint Surg [Am] 1986;68:1423.
79. Brunner R, Morscher E, Hunig R. Para-articular ossification in total hip replacement: An indication for irradiation therapy. Arch Orthop Trauma Surg 1987;106:102.
80. Hedley A, Hendren D. The prevention of heterotopic bone formation following total hip arthroplasty using 600 rads in a single dose. J Arthroplasty 1989;4:319.
81. Hutchinson GB. Neoplastic changes following irradiation. Radiology 1972;105:645.
82. Pelligrini V, Konski A, Gastel J, et al. Prevention of heterotopic ossification with irradiation after total hip arthroplasty. J Bone Joint Surg [Am] 1992;74:186.
83. Colachis SC III, Clinchot MD, Venesy DMD. Neurovascular complications of heterotopic ossification following spinal cord injury. Paraplegia 1993;31:51.
84. Roger RC. "Programme idea," heterotopic calcification in severe head injury, a preventive programme. Brain Injury 1988;2:169.
85. Gennarelli T. Heterotopic ossification. Brain Injury 1988;2:175.

Part III
Endocrinology

Chapter 6
Endocrinologic Disorders

Przemyslaw Lastowiecki and Mark E. Molitch

A number of endocrine disorders may be found in patients with long-term disabilities. This chapter focuses on (1) chronic conditions whose treatment may need to be modified because of superimposed illness—e.g., tube feedings in patients with diabetes mellitus; (2) acute endocrine dysfunction related to the trauma, surgery, or other circumstance that may require an admission for rehabilitation—e.g., diabetes insipidus (DI) resulting from head trauma; and (3) endocrine conditions specifically related to the disability state—e.g., hypercalcemia associated with prolonged bed rest. Attempts have been made to provide the pathophysiologic background for these disorders in a brief fashion so as to give the rationale for the various therapeutic choices given.

Anterior and Posterior Pituitary

Hypopituitarism

Many disorders that may lead to chronic disability such as head trauma, brain and pituitary tumors, cerebrovascular accidents, brain metastases, and cranial irradiation can cause disruption of hypothalamic and pituitary function (Table 6-1).

The hypothalamus and pituitary are linked in a tightly coordinated system in which hormones released from hypothalamic neurons traverse the portal vessels of the hypothalamic-pituitary stalk to inhibit or stimulate appropriate pituitary hormones. These, in turn, have stimulatory effects on growth and the hormonal function of several target organs.

Although the neurons producing these hypophysiotropic factors are distributed throughout the hypothalamus, their axons all project toward the mediobasal hypothalamus.

Isolated deficiencies of pituitary hormone secretion may occur, but more often two or more pituitary hormones are affected [1]. The distinction between hypothalamic and pituitary injury may be quite difficult and for most practical purposes is not necessary.

The size of the lesion and the rapidity of growth are the most important factors dictating the extent of dysfunction [2]. The frequency of postoperative hypopituitarism depends on the size of the tumor and the degree of destruction of the adjacent normal tissues [3].

Most patients undergoing radiation therapy to the brain will eventually develop hypopituitarism. Regardless of the mode of the therapy (gamma knife, proton beam, conventional methods, etc.) or the primary objectives (treatment of the brain tumor, pituitary tumor, or head and neck cancer), if a sufficient dose is delivered to the hypothalamic area, complete or partial hypopituitarism may be expected. Hypopituitarism occurs in 50% of patients a mean of 4.2 years following the treatment and is caused mainly by hypothalamic failure [4].

Head trauma is also a frequent cause of hypopituitarism. Clinical manifestations may occur immediately (adrenal crisis) or be delayed for weeks to months or even years following injury. Trauma rarely causes isolated hormonal deficiency [5]. If hypopituitarism develops, 100% of the patients will have growth hormone deficiency, 95% adrenocorti-

Table 6-1. Causes of Hypopituitarism

Pituitary tumor
Parasellar tumor (meningioma)
Suprasellar tumor (craniopharyngioma, meningioma, optic nerve glioma, chordoma)
Irradiation (pituitary, nasopharyngeal, cranial)
Surgery
Pituitary apoplexy (including Sheehan's syndrome)
Infiltrative diseases
Granulomatous diseases
    Sarcoidosis, eosinophilic granuloma, giant cell granuloma, Wegener's granulomatosis, lymphocytic hypophysitis
Infection
    Tuberculosis, fungi
Metastatic tumor
    Breast, colon, prostate, lung
Miscellaneous
    Empty sella, trauma, carotid artery aneurysm, hemochromatosis

---

cotropic hormone (ACTH) and gonadotropin deficiency, and 85% thyroid-stimulating hormone (TSH) deficiency. The hypopituitarism develops because of hypothalamic damage or shearing of the pituitary stalk. Spontaneous recovery from hypopituitarism following head trauma is rare [6].

In the acute setting, symptoms and signs of adrenal crisis (hypotension) with or without DI (polydipsia, polyuria) predominate. Hypothyroidism and hypogonadism take weeks to develop. Manifestations of growth hormone and prolactin deficiency are not well established (see sections on thyroid and adrenal disease for description of clinical manifestations).

Patients suspected of hypopituitarism should have hormone tests to determine which hormones are deficient and then be started on replacement therapy. Glucocorticoid therapy should be started immediately, however, without waiting for test results when panhypopituitarism is strongly suspected. It is sufficient to perform tests of trophic and appropriate target organ hormones—e.g., ACTH and cortisol, TSH and free T4, luteinizing hormone, and testosterone. The diagnosis is clear if a low level of a target organ hormone is associated with a low or inappropriately "normal" level of its pituitary hormone—e.g., low T4 with low or normal TSH in the setting of pituitary adenoma. Often, however, partial hormonal deficiencies are present that may be detected only by dynamic hormonal testing.

Patients with suspected or documented partial hypopituitarism should be assumed to have adrenal insufficiency until proven otherwise. This requires appropriate coverage with steroids (see adrenal section). Replacement doses should be increased to "stress" doses during severe illness (sepsis, myocardial infarction, cerebrovascular accident, etc.) and doubled or tripled with any minor stress. This approach must be continued until further testing determines whether there is a need for lifelong steroid supplementation. Patients with diminished ACTH reserve (baseline cortisol greater than 5 µg/dl but less than 20 µg/dl with stress or after ACTH stimulation test) may require steroid coverage only during periods of stress.

Patients with known central hypothyroidism should be treated with thyroxine. It is of crucial importance to delay thyroxine therapy until after ACTH secretion is determined to be intact or until replacement therapy with steroids is started. A sudden increase in thyroxine concentration in patients with undetected ACTH deficiency can cause a dramatic increase in cortisol metabolism in the liver that cannot be compensated for with increased secretion, and this results in adrenal crisis. The TSH level cannot be used as a tool in adjusting the dose of thyroxine in central hypothyroidism. Thyroxine should be gradually increased at 6- to 8-week intervals until the free T4 or free T4 index is in the normal range.

Hypogonadism caused by hypopituitarism should be treated in all premenopausal women and those postmenopausal women who would otherwise benefit from estrogen replacement therapy. For that purpose, combinations of estrogen and progestogen should be used.

The need for testosterone replacement therapy in the chronically disabled man should be determined on an individual basis. Benefits of the therapy— e.g., increased energy, increased libido, disappearance of hot flashes, and improved bone density—should be weighed against potential adverse effects of the therapy, which include the conflict of increased libido in a patient with a chronic physical disability that may preclude sexual intercourse. Testosterone is given in intramuscular injections as cypionate or enanthate in a dose of 200–300 mg every 3–4 weeks. The initial dose should be much lower—e.g., 50–100 mg every month, particularly in a patient with long-standing hypogonadism.

Disorders of Vasopressin Secretion

Abnormal regulation of water balance and its principal determinant, plasma sodium (P_{Na}), is commonly encountered in chronically disabled patients. Plasma osmolality (P_{Osm}) and P_{Na} are normally maintained within very narrow ranges (P_{Osm}, 285–295 mOsm/kg; P_{Na}, 135–145 mEq/liter). This consistency is accomplished by fine-tuned mechanisms regulating arginine vasopressin (AVP; also called antidiuretic hormone [ADH]) secretion and water intake. Osmoreceptors for AVP secretion and thirst perception are localized in the hypothalamus. AVP is produced in the supraoptic and paraventricular nuclei of the hypothalamus and then transported through the neurons to the posterior pituitary where it is released to the circulation [7]. Secretion of AVP is under control of a variety of osmotic, and to a lesser degree, nonosmotic stimuli. When P_{Osm} decreases below 280 mOsm/kg (corresponding to P_{Na} of 135 mEq/liter) AVP secretion is shut off. As a result, urine becomes maximally dilute (U_{Osm} <100 mOsm/kg), urine flow increases, and a water diuresis ensues. With an increase of P_{Osm}, the plasma vasopressin concentration increases maximally and causes an antidiuresis, with U_{Osm} increasing above 800 mOsm/kg [8].

AVP secretion is also regulated by changes in blood pressure and blood volume, mediated

through atrial and aortic baroreceptors. Hypotension and hypovolemia lower the "set point" for osmoreceptor-dependent AVP release. Hypertension and hypervolemia have the opposite effect. These mechanisms contribute to the hyponatremia associated with the states of decreased "effective" plasma volume—e.g., congestive heart failure. Other nonosmotic stimuli such as nausea, hypoxemia, hypercapnia, and mechanical ventilation can occasionally also come into play and cause inappropriate AVP secretion [8].

Intake of water is regulated by the thirst mechanism, which remains under control of the same factors as AVP secretion. An increase of osmolality above a certain threshold for thirst will increase water intake sufficiently to compensate even for the highest rate of water loss, if access to water is secured. If the thirst osmoreceptors are damaged and the thirst mechanism is not controlled, then inappropriately excessive water intake or lack of sufficient water intake will result in hyponatremia or hypernatremia, respectively.

Hyponatremia

Hyponatremia (P_{Na} <135 mEq/liter) occurs commonly in chronically disabled, hospitalized patients in whom injudicious use of intravenous fluids is often superimposed on an abnormal thirst mechanism or inappropriate AVP secretion. (See also Chapter 1.)

Manifestations of hyponatremia include symptoms of central nervous system dysfunction such as confusion, agitation, lethargy, and headache, as well as nausea and bloating. The severity of the symptoms depends not only on the degree of hyponatremia but also on the rate at which the disorder developed. Coma and seizures can be manifestations of severe or rapidly developing hyponatremia.

The first step in the evaluation of the patient with hyponatremia is to rule out a spurious decrease in P_{Na} concentration (pseudohyponatremia) that might result from hypertriglyceridemia, hyperglycemia, or hyperproteinemia. A good clue to pseudohyponatremia is a normal level of P_{Osm} in the face of hyponatremia.

The next step is to assess the patient's volume status. Volume depletion is characterized by orthostatic or frank hypotension, tachycardia, de-

Table 6-2. Medications Causing Hyponatremia

Hydrochlorothiazide
Chlorpropamide
Clofibrate
Vincristine

creased skin turgor, dry mucous membranes, flat jugular veins, and low urinary sodium level (U_{Na} <20 mEq/liter). Water is retained despite hypo-osmolality because nonosmotic stimuli override hypo-osmotic AVP suppression. A level of U_{Na} greater than 40 mEq/liter, despite obvious volume depletion, indicates that the kidneys are the source of volume loss (e.g., diuretic use, salt-losing nephropathies, Addison's disease, or osmotic diuresis).

Volume expansion is suggested by jugular venous distension, bibasilar rales, edema, and ascites. Hyponatremia develops as the effective arterial blood volume is paradoxically decreased, despite total body volume overload, and again overrides osmotically mediated AVP suppression. This mechanism operates in congestive heart failure, nephrotic syndrome, and cirrhosis. U_{Na} is usually less than 20 mEq/liter, which indicates a normal Na-conserving mechanism in hypoperfused kidneys.

*Syndrome of Inappropriate
Antidiuretic Hormone Secretion*

Most patients with hyponatremia do not have evidence of volume contraction or overload. U_{Na} is usually high (greater than 40 mEq/liter) and urine omolality is higher than plasma osmolality, thus being "inappropriate." (See also Chapter 1.) There are several conditions associated with such a clinical picture. Hypothyroidism and adrenal insufficiency cause decreased free water clearance and hyponatremia. They should always be sought and ruled out. There are numerous medications that can cause water retention and euvolemic hyponatremia (Table 6-2).

Once hypothyroidism, adrenal insufficiency, and drug effect have been ruled out, the only diagnostic possibility is the syndrome of inappropriate

ADH secretion (SIADH). Vasopressin can be produced ectopically, usually by a variety of cancers or inflammatory tissues, and such production is not subjected to normal regulatory mechanisms. More commonly, vasopressin is directly released from the posterior pituitary gland as a result of a direct stimulus (tumor, inflammatory process) or because of a "reset osmostat." The list of disorders causing SIADH is long and, in addition to malignancies, includes a variety of pulmonary diseases, central nervous system disorders, trauma, and surgery. Every patient with the diagnosis of SIADH should be evaluated for possible malignancy unless the cause is obvious—e.g., head trauma or neurosurgery involving the hypothalamus. In such cases, SIADH usually develops 3–5 days after the initial insult [8].

Treatment. Acute hyponatremia occurring within 24 hours with a decrease of P_{Na} to less than 120 mEq/liter is a true medical emergency. It may cause severe symptoms and carries a mortality up to 30–50% in adults. Recent weight gain and low serum blood urea nitrogen and uric acid support the diagnosis. U_{Na} is usually greater than 40 mEq/liter.

Severe symptomatic hyponatremia (P_{Na} <120 mEq/liter) puts the patient at risk for seizures, coma, and respiratory arrest and warrants aggressive therapy. Correction of hyponatremia is accomplished with infusion of 3% saline. The rule of thumb is that the P_{Na} level should not increase faster than 1 mEq/liter per hour in cases of acute (less than 48 hours) and not faster than 0.5 mEq/liter per hour in cases of chronic hyponatremia. The immediate goal of therapy is to elevate P_{Na} concentration to approximately 120 mEq/liter during the first 24 hours of therapy. Under no circumstances should the P_{Na} level be allowed to increase above 130 mEq/liter in the first day of the treatment. Too rapid correction may cause central pontine (and extrapontine) myelinolysis, a demyelinating condition clinically presenting with quadriplegia, aphasia, and urinary incontinence. Central pontine myelinolysis usually occurs in malnourished patients (alcohol abusers) who have undergone too rapid a correction of hyponatremia, but it has also been reported in patients without this risk factor.

The amount of Na needed to increase the P_{Na} concentration to a given level can be calculated from the following formula; total body water is 60% of the actual body weight:

$$\text{Na needed (in mEq)} = \text{total body water (TBW)} \times (\text{desired } P_{Na} - \text{measured } P_{Na})$$

A 3% NaCl solution contains 513 mEq of Na per liter. The calculated amount of Na is given over 24–30 hours to effect a P_{Na} increase of 0.5–1.0 mEq/liter per hour. The usual rate of administration is 0.1 ml/min per kilogram. Because hypertonic saline causes a significant fluid shift to the vascular compartment, the concomitant use of loop diuretics may be necessary, particularly in the elderly. After P_{Na} is brought to 120–130 mEq/liter, further therapy can be limited to fluid restriction. Most cases of SIADH are reversible within 1–2 weeks and therefore even suboptimal fluid restriction often seems effective because the disease simply remits.

Mild to moderate ($P_{Na} > 120$ mEq/liter) asymptomatic hyponatremia that evolves over more than 48 hours is best managed conservatively with water restriction and occasionally increased NaCl intake. The goal of the therapy is to create a negative water balance; therefore, the total water intake must be restricted to less than renal and insensible losses. As there is between 800 and 1,000 ml of water in the ordinary diet, the discretionary water intake often must be restricted to 250–500 ml per 24 hours. If intravenous solutions are needed, the patient should be given 0.9% NaCl. Dextrose 5% in water and 0.45% NaCl are inappropriate in this setting.

Noncompliance with fluid restriction is a common problem in a patient whose SIADH does not remit within 1–2 weeks. Chronic SIADH can be managed with demeclocycline, a tetracycline that interferes with the renal action of AVP and causes reversible nephrogenic DI. The effective dose of demeclocycline is 900–1,200 mg/day given in two divided doses. Demeclocycline causes a urinary concentration defect within 1–2 weeks from the start of the therapy and therefore is not suitable for treatment of acute SIADH. The induced nephrogenic DI also resolves slowly, usually within 1–2 weeks after the discontinuation of the medication.

Diabetes Insipidus

DI is a condition characterized by an excretion of large volumes of hypotonic urine. It needs to be distinguished from polyuria caused by solute diuresis (glucosuria, mannitol, myoglobinuria, postobstruction diuresis, etc.). The diagnosis is suspected when a 24-hour urine sample has a volume of more than 2–3 liters and an osmolality of less than 300 mOsm/liter. Careful documentation of polyuria also helps to rule out urinary frequency.

Hypotonic polyuria may result from three different defects. (1) Hypothalamic DI (also known as central or neurogenic) occurs because of the absence of vasopressin (AVP). (2) Nephrogenic DI is characterized by the lack of renal response to AVP. (3) Primary polydipsia occurs when AVP secretion is inhibited by excessive water intake. AVP secretion is directly correlated with plasma osmolality. Therefore, in the patient with hypotonic polyuria unexplained by solute diuresis, the distinction between central and nephrogenic DI can be made by measurement of plasma vasopressin. Because the vasopressin assay is technically difficult and often not available, the diagnosis is made on the basis of indirect tests of AVP secretion and action plasma and urine osmolality during controlled dehydration. A water deprivation test will distinguish these two forms of DI if there is a complete lack of AVP secretion or action.

Etiology

Central DI is rarely a familial disorder of autosomal dominant pattern. Neurosurgery, head trauma, and tumors are the most common causes of central DI. Infiltrative disorders, such as histiocytosis X and sarcoidosis, can lead to hypothalamic or posterior pituitary destruction.

Pathophysiology

The primary defect in central DI is the inability to secrete AVP sufficiently to produce adequate antidiuresis and maintain appropriate water balance. Urine flow increases exponentially with decreased AVP secretion and causes loss of total body water with an increase in plasma osmolality. Even a 1% increase in plasma osmolality will stimulate thirst and cause incremental water intake. Therefore, with an intact thirst mechanism, plasma osmolality remains normal or only slightly elevated no matter how severe the polyuria [9]. Hyperosmolality in a patient with central DI and unrestricted water intake suggests a concurrent defect in thirst. It occurs more commonly in the elderly or patients after extensive neurosurgical procedures involving the hypothalamus [10].

In primary polydipsia, abnormal water intake suppresses plasma osmolality and expands total volume. The decrease of AVP concentration leads to polyuria. Polyuria is maintained as long as inappropriate water intake is continued. Plasma osmolality stabilizes slightly below the normal range. Significant reduction of plasma osmolality suggests a concurrent defect in AVP suppression.

Clinical Features and Therapy

Patients with DI usually remain asymptomatic until urinary output reaches 3–4 liter/day and nocturia develops. As noted previously, patients do not present with significant hypernatremia unless a thirst defect is present or free access to water is denied. This may happen if fluid restriction is recommended in a hospitalized polyuric patient. Previously optimal management of DI may not be adequate if there is an impairment of mental status precluding appropriate water intake and compliance with a prescribed medical regimen. In such cases management should be changed to parenteral 1-deamino-(8-D-arginine)-vasopressin (DDAVP; subcutaneously or intravenously) and hypotonic fluid infused to match obligatory losses.

There are some distinct patterns of DI in neurosurgical patients. Polyuria developing within 24 hours after a neurosurgical procedure, particularly involving the pituitary stalk, median eminence, or hypothalamus, might represent DI but more often is caused by osmotic or water diuresis. The mere measurement of urine flow is insufficient to make the diagnosis. An osmotic diuresis should be sought, because steroids might cause hyperglycemia and mannitol is frequently prescribed for the treatment of cerebral edema. A water diuresis usually ensues as patients excrete excessive amounts of fluids given during the procedure. In such cases, the intravenous fluid replacement given in the ratio of 1 to 1 to the urine output will only support polyuria. DDAVP or vasopressin (Pitressin) should never be given empirically because it may result in severe hyponatremia. The proper management includes the initial reduction of the intravenous fluid rate to below urinary losses and monitoring hourly urine rate and P_{Na} levels. If urine concentration does not occur, plasma osmolality increases above 300 mOsm/liter (in the absence of mannitol therapy), and P_{Na} increases above 145 mEq/liter, a diagnosis of central DI is established. The patient can then be given 1–2 μg of DDAVP parenterally.

Polyuria with onset at 12–24 hours following surgery or head trauma often signifies major hypothalamic injury and severe DI. DI after transsphenoidal hypophysectomy usually resolves within 2–5 days [11]. Less commonly it is prolonged or even permanent. Postoperative DI may occur as part of the so-called "triple response." Initial impairment of AVP secretion is caused by neural shock. Polyuria resolves within 2–5 days and is followed by 2–14 days of antidiuresis caused by excessive release of stored AVP. There is a great propensity for hyponatremia if DDAVP is continued at this period. This is followed by the third phase of impaired AVP secretion and polyuria that might be either transient or permanent. As the course of DI following surgery or head trauma is unpredictable, it is prudent to hold each dose of DDAVP and allow some hypotonic diuresis for 2–4 hours, thereby avoiding unnecessary continuation of therapy when the DI was only transient.

Patients with DI resulting from neurosurgery or trauma should be assumed to have anterior pituitary insufficiency and treated with stress doses of steroids intravenously until further evaluation of their hypothalamic-pituitary-adrenal axis can be undertaken.

The general goal of therapy is to reduce polyuria to tolerable levels, preferably without or with only minimal nocturia. Control of polyuria will be followed by normalization of polydipsia, assuming that there is no concurrent thirst mechanism abnormality. Desmopressin (dDAVP) is a long-acting analogue of AVP. It has a half-life of 4–6 hours and a duration of action that varies from patient to patient, usually 12–24 hours. It is delivered parenterally, either subcutaneously or intravenously; both routes are equally effective. Stable patients are treated with intranasal dDAVP. The typical parenteral dose ranges between 1–2 μg every 8–24 hours. As the bioavailability of the intranasal preparation is about 10% of the parenteral dose, the typical outpatient dose of dDAVP is 5–20 μg every 8–24 hours. Milder forms of central DI are sometimes managed with chlorpropamide, clofibrate, or carbamazepine. Hydrochlorothiazide will also reduce polyuria but is more effective in the nephrogenic form of DI.

Thyroid

Thyroid Function Studies

For most clinical situations the best initial test of thyroid hormone action is the measurement of TSH using an ultrasensitive assay. Other TSH assays cannot be recommended as an initial test for all clinical situations because they lack sensitivity in differentiating low normal from suppressed TSH values [12]. The concentration of thyroxine (T4) depends on its binding proteins (thyroxine-binding globulin, albumin, prealbumin). For most clinical questions, the free T4 is estimated rather than measured directly. Estimates of free T4 (free thyroxine index) can be inappropriately elevated in some cases of euthyroid hyperthyroxinemia associated with distorted binding of T4 to albumin and prealbumin. Use of TSH as a primary screening test avoids any confusion associated with binding protein abnormality [12, 13].

Up to 10% of all hyperthyroid patients have an elevated level of triiodothyronine (T3) but a normal T4 concentration, a condition known as T3 toxicosis.

Radioiodine uptake measures the percentage of radioactive tracer accumulated in the thyroid gland 4 and 24 hours after delivery of the isotope. Indications for the use of radioiodine uptake are now quite limited. It is used primarily to distinguish hyperthyroidism of atypical Graves' disease (no goiter or ophthalmopathy) from the thyrotoxicosis of thyroiditis in which an inflammatory process causes a leakage of preformed thyroid hormone, along with a low radioiodine uptake.

Hypothyroidism

Hypothyroidism is called primary (the overwhelming majority of cases) when it is caused by the failure of the thyroid gland. Central (secondary or tertiary) hypothyroidism results from a failure of the pituitary or hypothalamus. In primary hypothyroidism TSH levels are elevated, and levels of free

Table 6-3. Manifestations of Hypothyroidism

Weakness, fatigue
Dry, coarse skin
Edema of the extremities
Cold intolerance
Coarsening of the voice
Weight gain
Decreased memory
Arthralgias, paresthesias
Constipation
Muscle cramps

T4 or free T4 index are low. An elevated TSH level in the face of a normal free T4 level represents a preclinical stage of hypothyroidism.

The typical symptoms and signs of hypothyroidism are given in Table 6-3. Hypothyroidism may cause diastolic hypertension that resolves with appropriate hormonal therapy. Sleep apnea is common; it is either caused by pharyngeal obstruction or central hypoventilation [14]. In some patients cardiomegaly (usually due to a pericardial effusion) associated with an elevated creatine phosphokinase level (MM band) with nonspecific electrocardiographic changes can be mistaken for cardiac disease.

Causes of Hypothyroidism

The most common cause of hypothyroidism is Hashimoto's thyroiditis, which is an autoimmune disease with lymphocytic infiltration and destruction of the thyroid [15]. Patients usually have a goiter that may vary in consistency, from rubbery to hard. A thyroid scan will show inhomogeneous uptake. Ninety-five percent of patients have high titers of antimicrosomal (antiperoxidase) antibodies. Although it has been thought that Hashimoto's thyroiditis leads to permanent destruction of the gland and irreversible hypothyroidism, recent data from Japan indicate that up to 25% of patients may actually have a reversible form of thyroid disease [16].

Hypothalamic or pituitary disease may lead to a decrease in the secretion of biologically active TSH, resulting in central (secondary or tertiary) hypothyroidism. The defect in TSH synthesis may be isolated but more often is combined with other pituitary hormonal deficiencies. TSH levels may be low, normal, or even rarely elevated, but in the last circumstance the circulating hormone is immunoreactive but less bioactive. The diagnosis is suspected when, in the appropriate clinical setting, a low T4 level is associated with low or low normal TSH level.

Therapy

The only recommended form of thyroid hormone replacement therapy is levothyroxine. Other preparations, such as desiccated thyroid, triiodothyronine, and combinations of T4 and T3, should be avoided because they cause a disproportionate increase in serum T3 levels. There are differences in bioavailability of different brands of levothyroxine and it is best to continue the same brand. Eighty percent of the oral dose of thyroxine is absorbed [17]. Absorption is diminished in malabsorption syndromes such as sprue, chronic pancreatitis, or Crohn's disease. Many medications interfere with L-thyroxine absorption, including cholestyramine, aluminum hydroxide, sucralefate, and ferrous sulfate. Dosing of these medications should be separated from thyroxine by at least 4–6 hours.

Before initiating thyroxine therapy, it is important to evaluate the patient for potential adrenal insufficiency and underlying coronary artery disease. Thyroxine increases cortisol metabolism and may precipitate adrenal crisis in patients with diminished adrenal reserve. This is particularly true in central hypothyroidism, which is rarely an isolated abnormality and is often associated with secondary adrenal insufficiency. In such cases thyroxine therapy must not be started without glucocorticoid coverage. Elderly patients and those with several risk factors for coronary artery disease should be started on very low doses of thyroxine, such as 12.5–25.0 µg/day with frequent follow-up [17–19]. Doses are increased by 12.5–25.0 µg every 4–6 weeks, as tolerated, until the TSH level returns to normal. Therapy of patients with unstable angina may have to be delayed until definitive therapy of coronary artery disease is accomplished.

The average replacement dose of thyroxine is 1.6 µg/kg per day [17]. Younger patients may be started on a dose slightly lower than the estimated replacement requirement [19]. Thyroxine therapy in central hypothyroidism is not adjusted on the basis of TSH level; here, the goal of the therapy is to return the patient to a clinically euthyroid state, with T4 levels in the normal range.

Hyperthyroidism

Hyperthyroidism is a clinical and biochemical state triggered by excessive amounts of thyroid hormone. Thyrotoxicosis may develop from endogenous disease or when thyroxine is supplied as a medication or surreptitiously taken. In thyroiditis normal synthetic function of the thyroid gland may be accompanied by increased release of preformed hormone.

The most common cause of hyperthyroidism is Graves' disease. Women have a much higher incidence than men. The underlying abnormality is a production of abnormal immunoglobulins acting as thyroid gland stimulators and known as thyroid-stimulating immunoglobulins [20, 21]. The thyroid is typically enlarged and highly vascular; however, a small gland does not rule out Graves' disease. The most common manifestations of thyrotoxicosis are given in Table 6-4. The unique features of Graves' disease are infiltrative ophthalmopathy and dermopathy. Lid lag, "stare," and lid retraction are common in hyperthyroidism, regardless of the cause. The course of ophthalmopathy does not correlate well with the degree of hyperthyroidism, nor its therapy. In the absence of goiter or ophthalmopathy further studies may need to be undertaken to establish the diagnosis, such as demonstration of thyroid-stimulating immunoglobulins or a high radioiodine uptake (Table 6-5). Thyroid scan usually shows a homogeneous image. A hot nodule on the scan, with suppression of the rest of the gland, supports the diagnosis of toxic adenoma or toxic multinodular goiter.

Treatment

Treatment options for Graves' disease include radioiodine, antithyroid medications, and surgery. Radioactive iodine is the most common treatment for Graves' disease, toxic adenoma, and multinodular goiter. Radioiodine may result in transient exacerbation of thyrotoxicosis associated with radiation thyroiditis, which usually occurs within the first week following therapy [22]. The risk is minimal if prior to the time of iodine-131 therapy, the patient has been made euthyroid with antithyroid drugs. Therefore, all patients above the age of 40 years and with large goiters and any significant comorbid factors should be carefully prepared for radioiodine therapy with antithyroid

Table 6-4. Manifestations of Thyrotoxicosis

General
   Heat intolerance
   Diaphoresis
   Goiter
Skin
   Velvety appearance
   Palmar erythema
   Smooth elbows and knees
   Vitiligo
Hair
   Fine and friable
Eyes
   Lid lag
   Ophthalmopathy (see text)
Heart
   Tachycardia
   Atrial fibrillation
   Systolic murmur
   Coronary heart failure
Lungs
   Dyspnea
Gastrointestinal
   Increased appetite
   Hyperdefecation
   Malabsorption
Central nervous system
   Irritability
   Insomnia
   Fatigue
   Tremor
Muscles
   Proximal weakness
   Myasthenia gravis picture
   Hypokalemic periodic paralysis
Skeleton
   Clubbing
   Osteoporosis
Renal
   Polyuria
Blood
   Increased red blood cell mass
   Pernicious anemia
Reproductive
   Oligomenorrhea, amenorrhea
   Decreased fertility

Table 6-5. Etiology of Thyrotoxicosis

Radioiodine Uptake	
High	**Low**
Graves' disease	Subacute thyroiditis
Toxic adenoma	Silent thyroiditis
Multinodular goiter	Factitious thyrotoxicosis
Pituitary adenoma	Struma ovarii
Partial thyroid hormone resistance	Post–radioiodine-131 therapy
	Iodine induced
Trophoblastic disease	
Iodine induced	
Follicular carcinoma	

therapy depends on the dose and is about 10–20%. In later years the rate of development of hypothyroidism is a steady 2–5% a year, regardless of the dose [22].

Thionamide medications interfere with several steps of thyroid hormone synthesis. Recommended initial doses of methimazole are 30–40 mg/day in one to two doses and propylthiouracil, 300–450 mg, in three to four doses. Most patients respond within 6–8 weeks, and after the state of euthyroidism is achieved, the dose may be gradually tapered under close follow-up and regular thyroid hormone studies. Remission may be achieved in 30% [12]. Unfortunately, the relapse rate is high and most patients require retreatment with antithyroid medication or radioiodine therapy. The most serious side effect of thionamide drugs is agranulocytosis. It occurs in less than 1% of treated patients [23]. Agranulocytosis is an idiosyncratic reaction, and frequent monitoring of the blood count is usually not helpful in preventing this complication. Patients should be warned about possible manifestations of agranulocytosis and instructed to stop the medication if they develop fever or sore throat. Because Graves' disease per se may be associated with a mild neutropenia, a white blood cell count with differential should be obtained prior to starting therapy, in case a later comparison is needed. Other side effects include rash and hepatitis.

Thyroidectomy is no longer performed for hyperthyroidism but should be considered in children and pregnant women in whom there is poor re-

medications. Younger individuals without large goiters may be prepared for the radioiodine with only propranolol. There is no evidence that iodine-131 causes any complications from radiation injury except for hypothyroidism. The incidence of hypothyroidism in the first year following the sponse to antithyroid medications. Patients with large goiters and compressive symptoms or suspicious nodules also benefit from surgery.

Hyperthyroidism in the Elderly

The prevalence of overt hyperthyroidism in patients above the age of 65 is estimated to be 0.1%. The diagnosis is easy to miss, because the characteristic manifestations of thyrotoxicosis are often not found (apathetic hyperthyroidism). Weight loss and atrial fibrillation are the most common findings. The treatment options are similar to those for general population.

Subclinical Hyperthyroidism

A patient with a suppressed TSH level associated with a normal free T4 level is said to have subclinical hyperthyroidism. Although such patients are usually asymptomatic, the nocturnal heart rate may be increased and the systolic time interval shortened. Other biochemical abnormalities may include elevated liver function test results, creatine phosphokinase levels, and sex hormone–binding globulin concentrations. Significant bone loss has been reported in patients whose TSH level was suppressed by thyroxine therapy [24]. It is still unclear whether decreased bone density translates into morbidity in this population. Patients with suppressed TSH levels are also at risk of atrial fibrillation.

Asymptomatic patients should be observed with thyroid function studies every 6–12 months to detect progression to overt hyperthyroidism. Patients who have symptoms and signs attributable to hyperthyroidism as well as those at significant risk of osteoporosis or atrial fibrillation should be treated.

Thyroid Storm

The most severe, life-threatening form of hyperthyroidism is called thyroid storm. It usually occurs in the setting of unrecognized hyperthyroidism, with a superimposed precipitating event such as surgery, trauma, infection, exposure to iodine (even in the form of a medication or radiocontrast agent), or even vigorous thyroid gland palpation during physical examination. Thyroid storm may be also triggered by radioiodine therapy of hyperthyroidism. The diagnosis is established on clinical grounds only because there is no characteristic laboratory

feature, although the free T4 levels correlate best with severity. Patients usually present with hyperthermia, mental status changes, and severe tachycardia. The condition is life threatening and should be treated promptly. High doses of antithyroid drugs are given, if necessary through a nasogastric tube. Propylthiouracil is preferred because of its inhibition of T4 to T3 conversion. Inorganic iodine (SSKI, Lugol's solution) is usually given shortly after the first dose of antithyroid medications. Dexamethasone also interferes with peripheral conversion of thyroid hormones. Propranolol is given intravenously as needed to control tachyarrythmias. Precipitating events should be sought and treated when possible (e.g., infections).

Adrenals

Adrenal Insufficiency

Adrenal insufficiency is a potentially life-threatening disorder that results from deficient adrenocortical function owing to either destruction of both adrenal glands (primary adrenal insufficiency) or abnormal pituitary (ACTH) or hypothalamic (corticotropin-releasing hormone) function (secondary adrenal insufficiency). Diminished function of the adrenal cortex is not clinically evident until more than 90% of both glands are destroyed. In the case of primary adrenal failure, all three distinct histologic layers of the gland are affected, which results in diminished secretion of glucocorticoids, aldosterone, and adrenal androgens. Secondary adrenal insufficiency does not affect aldosterone secretion, because more than 90% of its production is under control of the renin-angiotensin system and the plasma potassium concentration.

Etiology

By far the most common cause of adrenal insufficiency is iatrogenic glucocorticoid therapy with subsequent suppression of the hypothalamic-pituitary-adrenal axis [25]. The incidence of other causes of adrenal insufficiency (except for AIDS) is low and estimated at 40–60 per million per year [26] (Table 6-6). The exact incidence of adrenal insufficiency in the course of AIDS is not known but is certainly increasing. Its etiology is complex

Table 6-6. Causes of Adrenal Insufficiency

Primary
   Idiopathic (autoimmune) (65%)
   Tuberculosis (20%)
   Other (15%)
     Fungi
     Adrenal hemorrhage
     Sarcoidosis
     Amyloidosis
     Adrenoleukodystrophy
     AIDS
     Congenital adrenal hyperplasia
     Medications (ketoconazole, metyrapone,
       mitotane)
Secondary
   Hypothalamic suppression by exogenous: glucocorticoids,
     adrenocorticotropic hormone
   Lesions of the hypothalamus and pituitary
     Pituitary adenoma
     Craniopharyngioma and other tumors
     Infection
     Sarcoidosis
     Head trauma
   Isolated adrenocorticotropic hormone deficiency

and includes cytomegalovirus adrenalitis, *Mycobacterium avium intracellulare* infection, cryptococcal infection, and ketoconazole therapy [27]. In the hospital setting other causes become important, such as hemorrhage into both adrenal glands during cardiovascular surgery and anticoagulant use.

Diagnosis

The symptoms and signs of adrenal insufficiency are nonspecific and include weakness, nausea, abdominal pain, weight loss, hypotension, and hyponatremia. Hyperkalemia is a feature of primary adrenal insufficiency but not secondary, because in these disorders aldosterone secretion is intact.

The diagnosis of adrenal insufficiency requires a high index of suspicion. Random cortisol levels are of minimal value unless obtained during significant stress such as severe hypotension, mechanical ventilation, or organ failure. Low cortisol levels in such circumstances may suggest adrenal insufficiency. A morning cortisol level below 3 µg/dl is always diagnostic of adrenal insufficiency [28]. A morning cortisol level above 14 µg/dl always predicts normal hypothalamic-pituitary-adrenal function [28]. The rapid synthetic ACTH stimulation test (cosyntropin; Synacthen) is commonly used in the evaluation of patients suspected of adrenal insufficiency. After a baseline cortisol level is obtained, cosyntropin, 0.25 mg, is injected intravenously and a second cortisol level determination is done at 60 minutes. In ill patients this test can be performed at any time. Obviously, glucocorticoid therapy should be held until after the test but in certain circumstances even a 1- to 2-hour delay may be detrimental—e.g., the hypotensive patient suspected of having bilateral adrenal hemorrhage. In such cases dexamethasone in stress doses should be started immediately, before the ACTH stimulation test because dexamethasone will not interfere with the assay for cortisol. Patients with normal adrenal reserve have cortisol levels above 20 µg/dl after ACTH at 30 or 60 minutes or the cortisol will increase 8 µg/dl or more above the baseline [28, 29]. A rapid ACTH stimulation test is also done in the patients suspected of secondary adrenal insufficiency on the assumption that the prolonged absence of "trophic" ACTH action diminishes adrenal reserve and the subsequent response to injection of synthetic hormone. This is true for some but not for all patients with secondary adrenal insufficiency. Patients with acute onset of ACTH deficiency—e.g., pituitary apoplexy or head trauma—have low or undetectable baseline with normal poststimulatory cortisol levels, and, of course, the clinical picture of acute adrenal failure. These patients require full glucocorticoid coverage, with further hypothalamic and pituitary testing done at a later date.

Acute adrenal insufficiency is a medical emergency and, if not recognized and treated properly, leads to death. The treatment should be started empirically before results of confirmatory biochemical studies are available. Patients are usually hypotensive and resistant to volume expansion and vasopressors. The risk of adrenal insufficiency increases if the patient has AIDS, sepsis, major abdominal trauma, tuberculosis, disseminated intravascular coagulation, or is anticoagulated. Normal adrenal glands are capable of secreting 300 mg cortisol for 24 hours during maximal stress [30]. This corresponds to 300 mg hydrocortisone, 60 mg prednisolone, and 8–12 mg dexamethasone. The glucocorticoid should be administered intravenously in three to four divided doses. Higher doses of glucocorticoids have no advantage and should not be used in the treatment of adrenal crises. When severe stress lessens, the dose of steroid may be tapered rapidly to maintenance replacement doses. At this point patients with a clinical picture suggesting secondary adrenal insufficiency can be further studied. Tests include stimulation with insulin-induced hypoglycemia and the metyrapone test.

The treatment of chronic adrenal insufficiency is a challenging task. Even slightly higher than needed doses of steroid will result in the clinical picture of iatrogenic Cushing's syndrome over a period of months to years. On the other hand, any additional illness as well as physical stress will increase the need for steroids. Shorter acting steroids (hydrocortisone) are preferred over longer acting (dexamethasone) because of difficulties in adequate titration. Hydrocortisone (20 mg) or prednisone (5 mg) should be given in the morning after awakening. Often a second dose (hydrocortisone, 5–10 mg; prednisone, 2.5 mg) is needed in early afternoon to control symptoms in the late evening. In patients with primary adrenal insufficiency, a small dose of mineralocorticoid (fludrocortisone, 50–100 μg) is usually needed to control hyperkalemia or othostatic hypotension [31].

Pheochromocytoma

Pheochromocytoma is a catecholamine-producing tumor arising from the chromaffin cells of the adrenal medulla or, rarely, sympathetic ganglia. The prevalence of pheochromocytoma is estimated at 0.01–0.50% of the hypertensive population [32]. It mainly affects people in the third through fifth decade of life, without sex preference. Paragangliomas (pheochromocytomas derived from sympathetic ganglia) localize along the para-aortic sympathetic chain and may be found in the abdomen, chest, or neck. The "rule of ten" helps to understand the natural behavior of pheochromocytomas [33]: 10% extra-adrenal, 10% bilateral, 10% familial, 10% malignant, 10% extra-abdominal, and 10% without hypertension.

Symptoms of pheochromocytoma are caused by the effects of excess circulating catecholamines. Suspicion of pheochromocytoma is usually raised in

a hypertensive patient with episodic symptoms of headache, perspiration, and palpitations. Approximately 50% of all patients have episodic "spells" of variable presentation. They can be precipitated by exercise, stress, or even physical examination. Hypertension may also be severe and nonremitting. Less than 10% of patients are normotensive or have profound orthostatic hypotension. The absence of headaches, perspiration, and palpitations in a hypertensive individual virtually rules out the diagnosis of pheochromocytoma. Other symptoms may include pallor (but not flushing), tremor, weight loss, postural dizziness, nausea, and vomiting.

Physical examination of a patient with pheochromocytoma may reveal orthostatic hypotension, hypertensive retinopathy, mild tremor, and tachycardia. Café au lait spots suggest neurofibromatosis, which is associated with pheochromocytoma in about 1% of cases [33]. Other familial syndromes with pheochromocytoma include multiple endocrine neoplasia IIA, multiple endocrine neoplasia IIB, and von Hippel-Lindau disease.

Vanillylmandelic acid is the most commonly used test but is also the least specific, with 10–15% false-positive results. Measurement of 24-hour urinary metanephrines provides the most useful initial information (98% sensitivity). When clinical suspicion is high, tests for urinary metanephrines, catecholamines, and vanillylmandelic acid should be ordered [34]. Plasma catecholamines and pharmacologic testing are not generally used in the initial evaluation for pheochromocytoma. In the acute setting treatment may need to be started before the diagnostic testing is completed.

The alpha-blocker, phenoxybenzamine, has been used for treatment, beginning with 10 mg twice a day and gradually increasing over several days as necessary. Only after adequate control of blood pressure is established can a beta-blocker be added to control tachycardia. Hypertensive crisis in the course of pheochromocytoma should be treated with phentolamine (Regitine) and nitroprusside intravenously.

Calcium and Parathyroids

Hypercalcemia

With the introduction of automated chemistry profiles, hypercalcemia has been recognized as one of the most common metabolic abnormalities. Hypercalcemia may range from mild and asymptomatic to severe, resulting in dysfunction of several organ systems.

The usual normal concentration of calcium (P_{Ca}) is 8.8–10.4 mg/dl. Approximately 47% of total calcium is present in the unbound, physiologically active ionized form. This portion of calcium usually remains constant despite fluctuations of binding proteins. The simplest formula to correct calcium for a change in albumin concentration is to allow 0.8 mg/dl of calcium more for each gram per deciliter of albumin that is below the normal level of 4 g/dl. Measurement of ionized calcium is rarely necessary, except in the conditions that interfere with calcium-protein binding such as acidosis or alkalosis.

The differential diagnosis of hypercalcemia is quite large, although the two most important conditions, primary hyperparathyroidism and malignancy, are responsible for more than 90% of all cases [35]. Primary hyperparathyroidism is the most common cause of hypercalcemia and is more prevalent among the elderly. Malignancy is implicated in about 30% of all cases and should be sought and ruled out in all hospitalized patients with hypercalcemia [35]. Other causes include immobilization, medications, thyrotoxicosis, multiple myeloma, vitamin D intoxication, and familial hypocalciuric hypercalcemia. Rarely, hypercalcemia accompanies granulomatous disease (sarcoidosis, histiocytosis), lymphoma, Addison's disease, and milk-alkali syndrome.

The duration of hypercalcemia can be a useful clue to the diagnosis because it can often be tracked for years in patients with primary hyperparathyroidism or familial hypocalciuric hypercalcemia. Hypercalcemia of malignancy usually has a rapid course, because it occurs late when the disease process is advanced. It may be the presenting sign of malignancy in 5–10% of cases [36]. Most commonly, hypercalcemia of malignancy is caused by lung cancer (squamous carcinoma, almost never small cell carcinoma), breast cancer, head and neck cancer, and renal cell cancer. Rarely, it may precede the final diagnosis for months or even years when it is caused by slow growing cancers such as islet cell carcinoma, cholangiocarcinoma, or medullary thyroid carcinoma. The hypercalcemia of malignancy is usually the result of osteolysis from bone metastasis or the production of parathyroid hormone–related protein (PTH-RP) by the cancer [36].

Symptoms of hypercalcemia usually appear when the corrected P_{Ca} level exceeds 11.5–12.0 mg/dl. Nausea, anorexia, abdominal discomfort, constipation, vomiting, polyuria, and polydypsia may occur. Central nervous system symptoms include lethargy, weakness, hyporeflexia, and ultimately coma when P_{Ca} concentrations exceed 16–18 mg/dl.

The hypercalcemia of primary hyperparathyroidism is usually mild to moderate (P_{Ca} 11.0–12.5 mg/dl) with few symptoms and often is diagnosed incidentally. It later tends to be associated with nephrolithiasis, metabolic bone disease, and possibly peptic ulcer disease.

The most valuable step in the further evaluation of hypercalcemia is measurement of intact PTH (iPTH), which in most instances will clearly separate primary hyperparathyroidism from other causes of hypercalcemia [35]. The patient with elevated iPTH may also have familial hypocalciuric hypercalcemia or thiazide- or lithium-induced hypercalcemia but these conditions are easy to rule out by history and measurement of a 24-hour urinary calcium level. In the group of patients with suppressed iPTH, further evaluation should include a careful search for malignancy with chest radiography, barium swallow, mammography, and bone scanning [35, 36]. Additional studies such as serum and urine protein electrophoresis and a 25-OH-D_3 level may be needed as dictated by the clinical picture. Ultimately if there is still a question of potential malignancy induced hypercalcemia and other studies are negative, PTH-RP can be measured [37].

Therapy for Hypercalcemia

The only effective therapy for primary hyperparathyroidism is parathyroidectomy. However, as many patients are now diagnosed in a preclinical stage, the question of whether the surgery is always necessary arises. Some patients will have stable P_{Ca} levels of 11.0–11.5 mg/dl with minimal or no symptoms for years. Whether individuals without contraindications should have surgery is controversial. The presence of metabolic bone disease or nephrolithiasis even in the face of a near normal calcium level would favor surgery [35]. Chronically disabled patients with several comorbid factors might have unacceptably high surgical risk factors and limited life expectancy and therefore would not benefit from surgery. In these cases, after adequate hydration is ensured, calcium level stabilization can be accomplished with intravenous fluids. Pamidronate given at 1- to 4-week intervals and estrogen replacement therapy in postmenopausal women will also lower the P_{Ca} level by an average of 0.5–0.8 mg/dl.

Treatment of symptomatic hypercalcemia should begin with hydration. Hypercalcemia causes a form of nephrogenic diabetes insipidus, which is often superimposed on gastrointestinal symptoms (nausea and vomiting) and therefore can lead to severe dehydration. A vicious cycle ensues, as volume contraction worsens the problem further by decreasing renal perfusion and urinary calcium excretion. Loop diuretics (furosemide, bumetanide [Bumex]) have a calciuric effect but diuresis should not be started until volume status is fully restored. In milder or reversible causes of hypercalcemia, rehydration usually suffices. Severe and chronic hypercalcemia, particularly the hypercalcemia of malignancy, warrants further therapy. Most of the pharmacologic agents inhibit osteoclastic bone resorption. First-line therapy includes pamidronate, which is effective in moderate to severe hypercalcemia. Pamidronate is available only in the intravenous form and should be given in doses of 30–90 mg over 4–24 hours. The infusion can be repeated at daily or weekly intervals as needed. The total dose of pamidronate should not exceed 200–300 mg. The maximal calcium lowering effect occurs within 2–5 days and lasts for up to 2–3 weeks [38]. Other factors such as chemotherapy for malignancy will modify the response to pamidronate. Pamidronate is not approved in the United States for use in other conditions causing hypercalcemia except malignancy; however, it has proved effective in hypercalcemia of immobilization and some cases of primary hyperparathyroidism.

Calcitonin is effective in mild to moderate hypercalcemia. Its calcium-lowering effect occurs within 6–12 hours and therefore it can be a suitable bridge between hydration and pamidronate in the treatment of severe and chronic hypercalcemia. The starting dose is usually 200 IU subcutaneously three times a day and can be decreased later to a lower maintenance dose if an adequate response is accomplished. Some patients do not tolerate calcitonin because of its unpleasant side effects (nausea, hypotension, allergy). In some patients tachyphylaxis may develop [38].

Phosphate given orally not only inhibits bone resorption but also significantly decreases Ca absorp-

tion. Phosphate is used with modest effect in the medical treatment of primary hyperparathyroidism; however, diarrhea limits its use.

Estrogen decreases total and ionized calcium in postmenopausal women with or without primary hyperparathyroidism. Severe hypercalcemia cannot be controlled with the use of estrogen alone. In mild cases, however (P_{Ca}, 11.0–11.5 mg/dl, with no evidence of target organ damage), the addition of estrogen may lower the calcium level and obviate surgery. Estrogen therapy is strongly recommended for all postmenopausal women with primary hyperparathyroidism.

Diabetes Mellitus

Management of the Diabetic Patient Requiring Nutritional Support

It is difficult to predict an individual diabetic patient's glucose response to nutritional support. Glycemic control often deteriorates due to the high carbohydrate load and the catabolic response to infection, surgery, trauma, or organ failure [39].

There are significant differences between non–insulin-dependent diabetes mellitus (NIDDM) and insulin-dependent diabetes mellitus (IDDM) patients in terms of treatment adjustment during nutritional support. The required alteration of the therapy is also determined by the specific type of nutritional support (enteral versus parenteral) [40].

About half of the patients with NIDDM started on enteral nutrition will need insulin therapy. In one study of 40 diabetic patients, 38% of the patients did not require a change in the therapy and remained on a diet or a diet plus oral medications alone. Fifteen percent of the NIDDM patients required only an increase in the dose of oral hypoglycemic agent [40].

Patients with NIDDM treated with diet or diet and oral medications when started on parenteral nutrition will require insulin therapy in 77% of cases. The mean insulin dose of this patient population is 100 units (U) per 24 hours [40].

Most patients with IDDM will need significant alterations of their insulin regimens once started on enteral or parenteral nutrition. Insulin requirements may increase by 50% or more during parenteral nutrition (see Chapter 7).

Severity of the underlying illness has a great impact on insulin requirements. The dose of insulin usually has to be increased by more than 50% in septic patients, regardless of the mode of nutritional support [40, 41]. The likelihood that there will be a need for a major change in the diabetic therapy depends on the severity of illness, type of the feeding, and type of diabetes (IDDM versus NIDDM). It is not dependent on the age of the patient or preadmission therapy. The specific type of enteral nutrition (continuous versus cyclic) does not have any impact on the need for a therapy adjustment.

Diabetic patients should be meticulously followed with regular capillary blood glucose monitoring during nutritional support. We recommend at least four blood glucose measurements (6 A.M., 12 noon, 6 P.M., and 12 midnight) or before main meals. On the introduction of nutritional support the patient should be maintained on the usual prefeeding regimen unless there is marked, persistent hyperglycemia. The exception is the NIDDM patient started on parenteral nutrition. As noted previously, because the vast majority of these patients will require insulin, there is a good reason to switch the therapy at the beginning of the total parenteral nutrition. It is usually safer to err on the side of undertreatment than to risk recurrent hypoglycemia. The goal of the therapy should be to maintain glycemia in the range of 140–250 mg/dl.

In NIDDM patients treated with oral hypoglycemic agents and started on enteral nutrition, it is reasonable to continue this therapy because up to 40% of patients will not require insulin. The dose of oral medication should be increased up to maximal recommended doses (e.g., glyburide, 20 mg/day) as needed to control glycemia in the optimal range. With constant hyperglycemia (blood glucose greater than 250 mg/dl) insulin therapy is warranted. General principles of switching to insulin therapy apply, but there are some important differences. The initial dose of insulin can be somewhat higher than in other circumstances because patients have a significant carbohydrate load with nutritional support and they will be closely monitored. In the patient on continuous enteral nutrition it is reasonable to start intermediate-acting insulin (neutral protamine Hagedorn [NPH] or Lente) in a dose of 20–25 U in the morning. In most cases NPH will not act for the whole 24-hour period and a second evening or night injection of insulin may be needed to control morning hyperglycemia. Regular insulin may also be needed. Fur-

ther adjustments should be made every 2–3 days. The ultimate algorithm is quite variable, with some patients having higher insulin requirements in the night or early morning hours. This rule pertains particularly to patients on cyclic enteral nutrition overnight. An average dose of insulin for the NIDDM patient treated with parenteral nutrition and switched from an oral hypoglycemic is approximately 100 U/day. The initial dose should be much lower, approximately 20–30 U of regular insulin, put into the total parenteral nutrition bag. Additional coverage can be provided with regular insulin subcutaneously up to four times a day to achieve a goal of blood glucose at 140–250 mg/dl. The total insulin requirement can be used as a guide to gradually increase the amount of insulin given directly intravenously with nutritional support. If the anticipated use of insulin is temporary, it is important to use human insulin rather than pork or beef insulin to reduce antigenicity and prevent an anamnestic response should insulin have to be given again subsequently.

Patients with IDDM should be managed in a similar way. The preadmission dose of insulin is a useful starting point and then the dose is gradually adjusted during nutritional support.

If longer acting insulin solutions such as NPH or Lente are not given, then regular insulin should be given at least four times a day. Small doses of 1–2 U can be given for blood glucose levels below 100 mg/dl. In addition, this regimen will provide coverage for the period when long acting insulin has not yet started to work and will avoid a "brittle" course of glycemia when additional short-acting insulin is given only for very high blood sugars. Continued attention to blood glucose will minimize the potential for acute metabolic complications of decompensated diabetes. Urine and plasma ketones should be ordered when hyperglycemia greater than 300 mg/dl persists or an additional illness or event (sepsis, surgery, etc.) complicates the course of the therapy.

References

1. Arafah BM. Reversible hypopituitarism in patients with large nonfunctioning pituitary adenomas. J Clin Endocrinol Metab 1986;62:1173.
2. Vance ML. Hypopituitarism. N Engl J Med 1994; 330:1651.
3. Nelson PB, Goodman ML, Flickenger JC, et al. Endocrine function in patients with large pituitary tumors

treated with operative decompression and radiation therapy. Neurosurgery 1989;24:398.

4. Constine LS, Woolf PD, Cann D, et al. Hypothalamic-pituitary dysfunction after radiation for brain tumors. N Engl J Med 1993;328:87.

5. Edwards OM, Clark JDA. Post traumatic hypopituitarism: Six cases and a review of the literature. Medicine (Baltimore) 1986;65:281.

6. Eiholzer U, Zachmann M, Gnehm HE, Prader A. Recovery from post-traumatic anterior pituitary insufficiency. Eur J Pediatr 1986;145:128.

7. Robinson AG. The neurohypophysis: Recent developments. J Lab Clin Med 1987;109:336.

8. Robertson GL. Posterior pituitary. In P Felig, JD Baxter, AE Broadus, LA Frohman (eds), Endocrinology and Metabolism (2nd ed). New York: McGraw-Hill, 1987;338.

9. Goldman MB, Luchins DJ, Robertson GL. Mechanisms of altered water metabolism in polydipsic, hyponatremic, psychotic patients. N Engl J Med 1988;318:397.

10. Robertson GL. Dipsogenic diabetes insipidus: A newly recognized syndrome caused by a selective defect in the osmoregulation of thirst. Transactions of the Association of American Physicians 1987;100:241.

11. Bononi PL, Robinson AG. Central diabetes insipidus: Management in the postoperative period. Endocrinologist 1991;2:180.

12. Hay ID, Bayer MF, Mariash CN, et al. Assessment of current free thyroid hormone and thyrotropin measurements and guidelines for future clinical assays. Clin Chem 1991;37:2007.

13. Bayer MF. Effective laboratory evaluation of the thyroid status. Med Clin North Am 1991;75:1.

14. Grunstein RR, Sullivan CE. Sleep apnea and hypothyroidism: Mechanisms and management. Am J Med 1985;85:775.

15. Dussault JH, Rosseau F. Immunologically mediated hypothyroidism. Endocrinol Metab Clin North Am 1987;16:417.

16. Takasu N, Yamada T, Takasu M, et al. Disappearance of thyrotropin-blocking antibodies and spontaneous recovery from hypothyroidism in autoimmune thyroiditis. N Engl J Med 1992;326:513.

17. Fish LH, Schwartz HL, Cavanaugh J, et al. Replacement dose, metabolism and bioavailability of levothyroxine in the treatment of hypothyroidism. N Engl J Med 1987;316:764.

18. Helfand M, Crapo LM. Monitoring therapy in patients taking levothyroxine. Ann Intern Med 1990;113:450.

19. Kaplan M. Thyroid hormone therapy. Postgrad Med 1993;93:249.

20. Spaulding SW, Lippes H. Hyperthyroidism. Clinical features and diagnosis. Med Clin North Am 1985;69:937.

21. Farid NR. Immunogenetics of autoimmune thyroid disease. Endocrinol Metab Clin North Am 1987;16:229.

22. Graham GD, Burman KD. Radioiodine treatment of Graves' disease: An assessment of its potential risks. Ann Intern Med 1986;105:900.

23. Cooper DS. Antithyroid drugs. N Engl J Med 1984;311:1353.

24. Ross DS. Subclinical hyperthyroidism: Possible danger of overzealous thyroxine replacement therapy. Mayo Clin Proc 1988;63:1223.

25. Speigel RJ, Vigersky RA, Oliff AJ. Adrenal suppression after short term corticosteroid therapy. Lancet 1979;1:630.

26. Sin SC, Kitzman DW, Sheddy PF, Northart RC. Adrenal insufficiency from bilateral adrenal hemorrhage. Mayo Clin Proc 1990;65:664.

27. Dobs AS, Dempsey MA, Ladenson PW, Polk BF. Endocrine disorders in men infected with human immunodeficiency virus. Am J Med 1988;84:611.

28. Grinspoon SK, Biller BMK. Laboratory assessment of adrenal insufficiency. J Clin Endocrinol Metab 1994;79:923.

29. Kehlet H, Lindholm J, Bjerre P. Value of the 30 minute ACTH test in assessing hypothalamic-pituitary-adrenocortical function after pituitary surgery in Cushing's disease. Clin Endocrinol 1984;20:349.

30. Chin R. Adrenal crisis. Crit Care Clin 1991;7:23.

31. Loriaux DL, Cutler GB Jr. Diseases of the adrenal gland. In PO Kohler (ed), Clinical Endocrinology. New York: Wiley, 1986;167.

32. Bravo EL, Gifford RW. Pheochromocytoma: Diagnosis, localization and treatment. N Engl J Med 1984;311:1298.

33. Kalff V, Shapiro MB, Lloyd R, et al. The spectrum of pheochromocytoma in hypertensive patients with neurofibromatosis. Arch Intern Med 1982;142:2092.

34. Sheps SG, Jiang N-S, Klee GG. Diagnostic evaluation of pheochromocytoma. Endocrinol Metab Clin North Am 1988;17:397.

35. Bilezikian A. Management of acute hypercalcemia. N Engl J Med 1992;326:1196.

36. Mundy GR. Hypercalcemia of malignancy revisited. J Clin Invest 1988;82:1.

37. Ratcliff WA, Hutchesson ACJ, Bundred NJ, et al: Role of assays for parathyroid-hormone-related protein in investigation of hypercalcemia. Lancet 1992;339:164.

38. Attie MF. Treatment of hypercalcemia. Endocrinol Metab Clin North Am 1989;18:807.

39. Knapke CM, Owens JP, Mirtallo JM. Management of glucose abnormalities in patients receiving total parenteral nutrition. Clin Pharmacol 1989;8:136.

40. Park RM, Hansell DT, Davidson LE. Management of diabetic patients requiring nutritional support. Nutrition 1992;8:316.

41. Overett TK, Bistrian BR, Lewry SF, et al. Total parenteral nutrition in patients with insulin dependent diabetes mellitus. J Am Coll Nutr 1986;5:79.

Part IV

Gastroenterology

Chapter 7

Weight Loss and Malnutrition

Robert M. Craig

Depending on the clinical problem, weight loss and loss of muscle mass are variably present in the disabled patient. Some have an obligate loss of muscle from disuse atrophy. Others have nutritional deficits secondary to failure to aliment, as in neurogenic dysphagia. Still others have deficits of nutrient stores secondary to underlying diseases rather than diminished supplies of nutrients.

Regardless of the process, it is clear that rehabilitation has to include nutrient supply and replenishment of nutritional deficits. This chapter discusses the pathophysiology, nutritional assessment, complications, and management of nutrient deficits in the disabled patient.

Pathophysiology

If malnutrition is defined as a deficient nutrient store, correctable by replacement of the nutrient, then malnutrition can ensue in the disabled through many routes (Table 7-1). The purest example of malnutrition results from an inadequate gastrointestinal tract, which could occur from trauma—e.g., a motor vehicle collision that traumatized the duodenum or necessitated surgical exploration. During this acute phase, not only are there enormous obligate losses secondary to the hypercatabolic rate from the trauma, but the gastrointestinal tract is unusable for replenishing these losses. If the gastrointestinal tract remains impaired for more than a week, intravenous hyperalimentation (IVH) should be considered (see the section on Management).

There are other, more chronic situations in which the gastrointestinal tract is inadequate. An obvious example is the stroke victim who has problems with deglutition (see Chapter 8 for a full discussion of these motility problems). These patients frequently have bronchopulmonary aspiration complicating their swallowing problems. If severe, the problem may necessitate nasogastric or gastrostomy feeding.

The recumbent position that is often necessitated in the disabled patient predisposes to other problems of gastrointestinal inadequacy. Gastroesophageal reflux with resultant stricture occurs more commonly in those who require bed rest for prolonged periods. Until the stricture is treated, special nutritional problems may ensue. In addition, the superior mesenteric artery syndrome, in which the transverse duodenum becomes obstructed by the superior mesenteric arterial mesentery and the lumbar spine, occurs more frequently in the disabled. Thin individuals, with little paraspinal fat, who have to be on their backs for prolonged periods are particularly susceptible to this problem. Therapy includes restitution of body mass by intense nutritional support, with resultant increased paraspinal fat and less duodenal compression. Enteral or parenteral nutrition may be required to promote this restitution. If the compression does not resolve, a surgical duodenojejunostomy may be required.

Disabled patients may also suffer from a host of gastrointestinal problems that the nondisabled patient may have. Patients with diabetes mellitus require special mention because they have an increased incidence of physical disability—e.g.,

Table 7-1. Pathophysiology of Nutrient Deficits in the Disabled

Inadequate gastrointestinal tract
   Acute abdominal trauma with adynamic ileus
   Problems with deglutition
   Motility problems of stomach, small bowel, and colon
   Esophageal stricture
   Superior mesenteric artery syndrome
Other problems, unrelated to underlying disability (intestinal obstruction, fistulae, pancreatitis, etc.)
Nutrient deficits, unrelated to supply of nutrients
   Related to sick organism
   Not correctable by supply of nutrients
Obligate loss of muscle mass
   Neurogenic disuse atrophy
Depression

strokes or leg amputations. Other gastrointestinal problems that occur in the diabetic patient are the dysmotility syndromes that can be particularly vexing to treat (see Chapter 8 for a more complete discussion). If gastroparesis diabeticorum becomes severe, it can interfere with sufficient nutrient intake, making both diabetic control and nutritional restitution difficult.

Besides these situations in which a nutrient deficit is due to an inadequate gastrointestinal tract, there are situations in which there are diminished nutrient stores secondary to an underlying host deficit from other disease processes. For example, a sick individual often will have diminished protein synthesis with hypoalbuminemia, unrelated to nutrient supplies, but caused by the disease process itself. Unless the disease is corrected, the nutrient deficit will not be rectified. If an infected decubitus ulcer is not treated with antibiotics, debridement, skin grafting, etc., the attendant hypoalbuminemia will not resolve in spite of intense nutritional support. This is not to say that nutritional support is of no value; rather it is to stress that nutritional support by itself will be insufficient to promote restitution of these deficits.

There are some circumstances in which there is an obligate loss of some nutrients that is part of the disabled process. For example, a quadriplegic will necessarily lose muscle mass and be in negative nitrogen balance until the muscle mass is lost. No matter how intensely nutritional support is provided, it cannot prevent this disuse muscle loss.

Finally, diminished nutrient intake can ensue from mental depression that often exists in the disabled. Any good rehabilitation program must include the assessment and management of mental depression. Usually intense nutritional support is unnecessary in this process, but rarely enteral nutrition has to be instituted.

Nutritional Assessment

The first aspect of a nutritional assessment, and perhaps the most important, is the overall medical evaluation. To interpret whether deficits are due to diminished nutrient supplies, it is imperative that one is aware of the patient's medical problems. For example, if someone is dying of metastatic carcinoma and is disabled from the spread to the spine, it would be unreasonable to assert that a low serum albumin is due to a lack of nutrients. Rather, this deficit is a manifestation of the sick host and will not be rectified by forcing intense nutritional support on the system. This initial assessment, then, will attempt to separate the effects of malnutrition (nutrient supply) from underlying disease processes. In addition, the assessment should include an evaluation of the individual's emotional state and how it relates to the illness.

Inherent in the previously mentioned process is an analysis of the adequacy of the gastrointestinal tract. Frequently, malnutrition ensues when the gastrointestinal tract is insufficient, and the resolution of the nutritional problem often requires treatment of the gastrointestinal tract. For example, an esophageal stricture would have to be dilated, and it should be prevented in the future by diminishing gastric acid production.

In this analysis, a nutritional or prognostic judgment can be made on a patient that is as precise as a formal nutritional assessment. However, we often perform a nutritional assessment that includes measurements that can be followed as a patient improves (Table 7-2). The first of these measurements may be protein-calorie counts if it is unclear whether or not nutritional support will be required. A nitrogen balance test is performed with these counts to see if a negative nitrogen balance is present. This is calculated by the following formulation:

$$\text{Nitrogen in} - \text{nitrogen out} = \text{Balance}$$
$$\text{Protein in (by count)}/6.25 \text{ g protein per g nitrogen} - 24\text{-hour urinary urea nitrogen} - 3 \text{ g} = \text{Balance}$$

Table 7-2. Nutritional Assessment

Evaluation of disease processes
    Are deficits due to supply of nutrients or underlying
      disease?
    Is the gastrointestinal tract adequate?
Overall nutritional, prognostic index
Measurement of body composition
    Fat, triceps skin fold
    Muscle, midarm muscle circumference
    Impedance plethysmography
    Whole body potassium measurements
    Creatinin height index
    Body weight and recent weight loss
Visceral protein measurements
    Serum protein, albumin, transferrin
    Skin test reactivity to recall antigens
Measurement of specific nutrients
    Serum electrolytes: Na, K, Cl, Ca, P, Mg
    Micronutrients: Cr, Cu, Se, I, Mn, Zn
    Vitamins: Prothrombin time, vitamin B_{12}, folic acid,
      vitamin D
Nitrogen balance

Specific measurements of fat stores with a triceps skin fold and of muscle stores with a midarm muscle circumference are also performed, and there are published charts relating these to standards. In addition, serum proteins, including total protein, albumin, transferrin, and others, have been used to assess stores of visceral protein. The short half-life proteins, such as retinal-binding protein, may more accurately reflect acute changes in protein stores. Skin test reactivity to the recall antigens, mumps, *Candida*, and trichophyton has also been used as an assessment of visceral protein stores. Finally, total body muscle protein can be approximated by measuring urinary creatinine excretion and relating it to height. The reliability and availability of these methods of estimating protein stores are outlined in Table 7-3.

Overall, these measurements provide important prognostic information, regardless of whether they are a reflection of host disease or lack of nutrient supply. Some have expressed these measurements in terms of a polynomial equation that can be used in following nutritional restitution.

Management

It is not clear in every circumstance when intense nutritional support should be provided, but a reasonable guideline is 1–2 weeks without satisfactory nutrient intake. If the weight loss and decreased intake are due to metastatic cancer or another uncorrectable medical illness, intense nutritional support should rarely be used. In the initial assessment, the effects of the underlying illness must be separated from those of decreased nutrient supply, and the adequacy of the gastrointestinal tract should be assessed. Although there are no controlled studies of nutritional support in the disabled, it is reasonable to ensure sufficient nutrient supplies to optimize rehabilitation.

Adequate Gastrointestinal Tract

If possible the gastrointestinal tract should be used instead of parenteral hyperalimentation. There are theoretical problems with providing IVH that include atrophy of the gastrointestinal tract and, in experimental animals, diminished immune surveillance with translocation of bacteria from the gastrointestinal tract into adjacent lymph nodes and eventually into the vascular system. This gastrointestinal atro-

Table 7-3. Methods for Assessing Total Body Protein Stores

Method	Reliability	Feasibility
Nitrogen balance	Fair	All hospital laboratories
Creatinine height index	Fair	All hospital laboratories
Total body potassium	Good	Only in research centers
Impedance plethysmography	Good	Many medical centers
Serum chemistries	Fair	All hospital laboratories
Anergy to skin test antigens	Fair	All hospitals

phy may be minimized if small amounts of oral feeding are administered even when IVH is provided. Additionally, the use of the gastrointestinal tract is safer and less costly than total parenteral nutrition.

If the patient is able to swallow, oral feedings are preferred over tube feedings. Sometimes the evaluation of swallowing by speech pathology is useful. Often the patient with a stroke or some other central nervous system disability is able to swallow textured foods but unable to swallow liquids or solids. In addition certain positional manipulations may promote improved swallowing. Further nutritional supplements either in a pudding or liquid form can sometimes augment the supply of nutrients. Almost all of the nutritional supplements are lactose free so lactose does not become a cause of diarrhea. Some of these nutritional supplements cause gastrointestinal intolerance including abdominal cramping and diarrhea, but most are quite well tolerated.

If a patient is unable to swallow but has an open gastrointestinal tract, some type of tube feeding is generally recommended. One can administer tube feeding by a nasogastric tube, nasoenteric tube, gastrostomy tube, or jejunostomy tube. The gastrostomy tubes are preferred over the jejunostomy tubes. The latter are reserved for circumstances such as repeated gastric aspiration and aspiration pneumonitis. The types of tube feedings and their indications and common complications are outlined in Tables 7-4, 7-5, and 7-7. Included in the decision about what type of tube feeding to administer are considerations such as long-term feeding, interference with rehabilitation, the type of nursing care that is required, and potential complications.

Nasogastric Feeding

Nasogastric feedings are generally provided during an individual's acute illness. The major advantage of nasogastric feeding is the ability to measure gastric residuals. A reasonable guideline for gastric residuals is 75 ml. If the residual volume is greater than that, continuous feeding should be stopped. In addition, bolus feedings should be discontinued if the gastric residual is greater than 75 ml just before the next feeding. The nasogastric tube should be placed in the distal antrum, between the second and third mark of the nasogastric tube at the naris. Feedings should be started with an isotonic solution at a slow, continuous rate. An isotonic solution is preferred, because hypotonic or hypertonic solutions in the duodenum delay gastric emptying. Generally, if the nasogastric feeding has to be used longer than 2 or 3 weeks, the patient should be considered a candidate for a percutaneous gastrostomy.

Nasoenteric Feeding Tube

A number of small flexible nasoenteric tubes have become available. These are generally coated with a hydromer that becomes lubricated with water. They are easily passed through the nose into the stomach and then into the duodenum. Some studies have demonstrated that if the tube is in the proximal duodenum, the incidence of aspiration and pneumonitis is not decreased below that from gastrostomy feedings. Therefore, the tip of the nasoenteric tube should be placed at least into the third or fourth portion of the duodenum. These catheters have an internal stylet that stiffens the catheter for easy placement through the nose and into the stomach. The stylet increases the risk of perforation of the esophagus or lung, with eventual pneumothorax. Following passage into the stomach, the stylet should be removed and the tip of the nasoenteric tube should be allowed to pass distally into the duodenum. Sometimes the passage of the tube out of the stomach and into the duodenum is facilitated by the use of motility agents such as metoclopramide. The assistance of a radiologist is sometimes useful. Rarely, it becomes necessary for the tube to be placed into the duodenum endoscopically, but this is difficult because the endoscope often drags the tube out as the endoscope is removed.

Nasoenteric tubes should receive only continuous feeding. One of their disadvantages is the inability to measure gastric residuals. The usual polymeric feedings are satisfactory for nasoenteric feeding, preferably with an isotonic solution. Once the tube is in the optimal location, it should be secured so that it does not ride up into the esophagus, with attendant aspiration of feedings.

Gastrostomy

Surgical gastrostomies were first used in the nineteenth century. One of the revolutions in gastroenterology was the introduction of the percutaneous gastrostomy. Since the percutaneous gastrostomy was introduced, surgically placed gastrostomies have been performed rarely. Critical analysis of the literature, however, does not show a clear medical advantage of percutaneous gastrostomy over surgically placed gastrostomy. However, the percutaneous approach is perhaps simpler, quicker, and less costly than the surgically placed gastrostomy. The gastrostomy tube is a satisfactory method for long-term feeding in patients who have functional dysphagia or other problems with swallowing.

Usually placement of a gastrostomy is reserved for patients who will need nutritional supplementation longer than 2 or 3 weeks. A percutaneous gastrostomy can be placed at the bedside with endoscopic guidance. Other percutaneous options include a push technique with radiologic guidance and a laparoscopic technique with direct visualization of the gastric wall. Most medical centers, however, use the endoscopically guided percutaneous gastrostomy. This technique is safe and successful more than 95% of the time, and feedings can be instituted within 24 hours of placement. Unless the patient is on antibiotics, prophylactic use of cefazolin will decrease the incidence of wound infection. Feedings should be started with a continuous infusion of full-strength isotonic solution at 50 ml/hour and gradually increased to the required feeding rate. Once a continuous feeding is well tolerated, it can be switched to bolus. Gastric residuals should be checked frequently. If the gastric residuals are greater than 75 ml, the feeding should be temporarily stopped. Occasionally gastroparesis ensues, which can be assisted by the use of metoclopramide.

Major complications of percutaneous gastrostomy occur 5% of the time. These include a fracture of the gastric wall, with perforation secondary to pulling the gastrostomy tube through the stomach, bleeding at the site of the percutaneous gastrostomy, and necrotizing fasciitis. The latter condition is a devastating illness, with aerobic and anaerobic organisms, necessitating wide debridement of the infection. Minor wound infections and leakage around the tube are found relatively commonly but are generally not troublesome.

If the percutaneous gastrostomy tube is removed inadvertently, it can be replaced with another gastrostomy tube so long as it is performed relatively soon. The gastrostomy tract closes quickly and often will be completely sealed in 3 hours or so. Sometimes the tract can be dilated with gastroenterologic dilators.

In general, these gastrostomy tubes are sturdy and can remain in place for 6 months or even longer. There are replacement gastrostomy tubes that are commercially available. Most of the percutaneous gastrostomy tubes can be pulled through the tract because the internal bumper is collapsible. However, there are some percutaneous gastrostomy tubes that require removal by a gastroscope, with snaring of the tip of the tube. Long-term gastrostomy tubes that lie flush to the skin, called gastrostomy buttons, can also be used. These have the advantage of having no external tube except during feeding times.

If possible, only liquid medicines should be administered through gastrostomy tubes, because tablets can clog the tube even if they are crushed finely. If there are no liquid preparations for the drug, then crushed tablets can be used, so long as the tube is flushed vigorously with 20 ml of water. In addition, the tube should be flushed with 50 ml of water after each bolus tube feeding to decrease clogging.

Jejunostomy

Jejunostomy tubes are used much less frequently than gastrostomy tubes. They are generally used in circumstances in which the patient has repeated gastric aspiration and pneumonitis. Jejunostomy tubes are usually placed surgically, either the needle jejunostomy type or a larger tube. Sometimes jejunostomy tubes are placed surgically when it is anticipated that there would be prolonged adynamic ileus. Continuous feeding should be used in jejunostomy tubes rather than bolus feeding, and polymeric isotonic solutions are preferred. Residual volumes cannot be checked. Although some crushed tablets can be used with the larger jejunostomy tubes with liberal irrigation, they should only be introduced when no liquid substitution is available.

Particularly in the postoperative period, the jejunostomy has an advantage over the gastrostomy tube, because it can be used immediately rather than after resolution of adynamic ileus. Generally the small intestine does not take part in adynamic ileus, which is a problem primarily of the stomach and colon. The major disadvantages of the jejunostomy tube are frequent clogging of the tube, the inability to give bolus feeding, and more diarrhea. Although elemental tube feedings have been advocated by some, this is rarely necessary, because polymeric feedings are well tolerated and do not produce more tube obstruction than the elemental diets.

Specialized Tube Feeding Formulations

Although it is possible to process food in a blender and provide this as tube feeding, this rarely is exercised currently because the canned formulations are isotonic, have a satisfactory mix of lipid and carbohydrate calories, and provide 1 calorie per milliliter of feeding. The amount of free water contained in the currently available commercial products is also satisfactory. These products are often called polymeric formulations because the carbohydrate is in a polymeric form and the protein is comprised of long peptides rather than small peptides or individual amino acids. Occasionally a patient will not be able to tolerate a polymeric diet and an elemental diet has to be provided. The elemental diets have amino acids or dipeptides or tripeptides instead of the longer peptide chains, and the carbohydrate is provided as monosaccharide or disaccharides. Consequently, the osmolality is greater with these tube feedings, which may produce diarrhea.

There are many specialty formulations that have become available in the past few years. A formulation providing increased branch chain amino acids has been advocated for portosystemic encephalopathy and trauma. However, controlled studies have failed to show a distinct advantage of this solution over standard polymeric diets. In addition, there may be a theoretical advantage with tube feedings supplemented with glutamine, but experimental data in humans supporting this recommendation are lacking.

Major Problems with Tube Feedings

Aspiration

One of the problems in looking at data on aspiration is to determine what material has been aspirated. Some series do not make it clear whether or not someone has aspirated the normal salivary contents, which can produce pneumonia, or whether there is truly aspiration of the tube feeding. If a nasoenteric or jejunostomy tube is placed in the third or fourth portion of the duodenum or more distally into the small intestine, the risk of tube feeding aspiration is decreased. This is the major indication for using this type of tube feeding. However, if the tube is in the proximal duodenum, there is really no advantage of this type of feeding over nasogastric or gastrostomy feedings.

Nasogastric or nasoenteric tube feeding also traverses the two sphincteric zones in the upper and lower esophageal areas, which can predispose to aspiration or gastroesophageal reflux. A feeding jejunostomy or gastrostomy should eliminate these risks.

The feedings should be delivered under close observation if the patient has diminished mentation so that the tube feeding can be stopped immediately if the patient vomits or regurgitates. In addition, the head should be elevated in bolus tube feedings to reduce this risk. Sometimes vomiting or gastric aspiration can be decreased with the use of some motility agents such as metoclopramide. Hypertonic or hypotonic solutions should be avoided in the stomach because they may inhibit gastric emptying.

Diarrhea

Diarrhea is the most common problem seen with tube feeding. Often the diarrhea is due to something other than the tube feeding such as antibiotic-induced diarrhea due to *Clostridium difficile* or some other change in bacterial flora. None of the currently available tube feedings contain lactose. However, foods blended using milk can sometimes produce a lactose-induced diarrhea. Hypertonic solutions may produce more diarrhea than isotonic or hypotonic solutions, particularly if they are administered into the jejunum. Some other drugs such as oral phosphate or magnesium can induce diarrhea. Magnesium and phosphate deficiencies should not be corrected orally. Finally, diarrhea can sometimes be secondary to a colonic obstruction with overflow through the obstructed area. An endoscopic and radiologic evaluation is sometimes required. Generally, antimotility agents such as deodorized tincture of opium, loperamide, diphenoxylate, or codeine can be used.

Table 7-4. Peripheral Vein Intravenous Nutrition

Substance	Amount
3.5% Amino acid	500 ml
5% Dextrose	500 ml
Multivitamin	1 vial per day
NaCl	20 mEq/liter
KCl	20 mEq/liter
Other additives as needed	
Rate	125 ml/hr, providing 3 liters daily
Intralipid, 20%	21 ml/hr, providing 1,000 kcal/day

Table 7-5. Possible Indications for Intravenous Hyperalimentation

Scleroderma of small intestine
Intestinal obstruction
Postoperative adynamic ileus (if anticipated 2 weeks)
Prolonged acute pancreatitis, pancreatic pseudocyst, pancreatic ascites
Inflammatory bowel disease: acute, chronic, fistulous disease, obstruction
Short gut syndrome
Irradiation enteritis
Small intestinal fistula
Esophageal obstruction until obstruction relieved
AIDS enteropathy
Premature infants
Thermal injury

Metabolic Complications

Metabolic complications of tube feeding are not as severe as those seen with intravenous hyperalimentation. Hyperglycemia and, rarely, hyperosmolarity can ensue. The latter is unusual with the current isotonic polymeric feedings. If a patient has diabetes mellitus, the hyperglycemia can be managed easily by administering appropriate amounts of insulin or by adjusting the tube feeding rate. Potassium, magnesium, or phosphate abnormalities can sometimes be seen with tube feedings. If someone is hypophosphatemic or hypomagnesemic, it is generally unwise to correct these deficiencies by the gastrointestinal tract because either oral or tube fed phosphate or magnesium will induce a severe secretory diarrhea. Liver abnormalities occur rarely with enteral feeding. If someone has liver test abnormalities with total parenteral nutrition, the abnormalities usually resolve when enteral alimentation is introduced. Problems with carbon dioxide retention induced by high carbohydrate feeding in patients with chronic obstructive pulmonary disease can occur, although infrequently. Usually a standard polymeric formula has sufficient carbohydrate and lipid to give a balanced caloric mix so that a patient with chronic obstructive pulmonary disease does not run into problems with excessive carbon dioxide production.

Inadequate Gastrointestinal Tract

There may be circumstances in which the gastrointestinal tract is inadequate. A patient may have an intestinal obstruction, adynamic ileus, gastroparesis, intestinal fistulae, or inflammatory disease of the gastrointestinal tract. Under these circumstances total parenteral nutrition may be advisable. Rarely, a peripheral amino acid and carbohydrate solution supplemented with intravenous fat can be provided. This solution usually has insufficient calories, but it can supplement nutrients in a patient partially maintaining oral intake. Hypertonic solutions will damage peripheral veins, which are often precious commodities in sick patients. A sample of a peripheral intravenous mixture is shown in Table 7-4.

IVH should be considered in patients who are nutritionally depleted, or who are expected to become depleted, whose gastrointestinal tracts cannot be used. Examples of its indications are given in Table 7-5. Timing is important, because most patients with a temporary loss of gastrointestinal function do not require IVH. A reasonable rule of thumb for postoperative patients is to provide IVH when the gastrointestinal tract is dysfunctional for 2 weeks (or it is anticipated that it will be dysfunctional for 2 weeks). IVH may have to be employed preoperatively if the patient is depleted prior to surgery. Controlled studies for postoperative patients support these recommendations; however,

Table 7-6. Modification of Intravenous Hyperalimentation Solutions Based on Medical Problems

Medical Problem	Modifications
Respiratory failure	Fewer carbohydrates and calories when weaning off ventilator
Acute or chronic renal failure	Restriction of phosphate, magnesium, and potassium
	Fluid restriction
	Occasionally more NaCl to facilitate dialysis
	Preferential use of essential amino acids?
Hepatic failure	Fluid and sodium restriction
	Branch chain amino acid solution with encephalopathy
Congestive heart failure	Sodium and water restriction
Syndrome of inappropriate secretion of antidiuretic hormone	Increased NaCl concentration with diuretics
	Demethyltetracycline

guidelines for other acute abnormalities of the gastrointestinal tract are not as clear. Nevertheless, 2 weeks without feeding is a reasonable standard for most conditions. Considerable clinical judgment is necessary in other conditions in predicting the value of IVH. The closer the patients are to having what resembles short gut syndrome, the more likely they will benefit from IVH.

Contraindications to IVH include an uncooperative patient, such that a central line cannot be safely introduced or maintained; hopeless circumstances in which long-term survival is not expected; coagulopathy precluding central line placement; metastatic or far advanced cancer (relative contraindication); and situations in which the gastrointestinal tract is functional (relative contraindication). Some of these patients will have a dysfunctional gastrointestinal tract and may benefit from IVH, in spite of their having metastatic carcinoma. In addition, a functional gastrointestinal tract does not absolutely contraindicate IVH. In some circumstances, it may be used for patient convenience.

IVH should be provided through a designated line, with as few interruptions as possible (blood drawing, infusions of blood products, administration of drugs). However, exceptions are sometimes necessary when venous access is difficult, and when the patient's problems are complex—e.g., following bone marrow transplantation.

IVH is monitored best by a team of people, usually composed of physicians, dieticians, pharmacists, and nurses. One pharmacist, one dietician, and one physician are usually sufficient; however, most hospitals require more than one nurse. In smaller institutions that do not have a nutritional support service, IVH is preferably performed in an intensive care unit under the direction of an attending physician aware of the indications and methods employed. When IVH is considered, consultative advice is often provided to the managing service regarding the advisability and type of intense nutritional support. The type of solution given and data regarding the patient's clinical status and laboratory findings are monitored and recorded daily.

Standard order forms are employed to minimize errors in writing IVH orders. One form is used for nursing orders for the general care of the patient receiving IVH. These are individualized among hospitals, but include orders on laboratory studies, whom to call for various problems, glucose monitoring, vital sign monitoring, and confirmation by chest radiography on the central location of the venous catheter before initiation of IVH. A second form is the usual IVH solution that is provided for patients with no special medical problem. A third form is for nonstandard solutions for patients with special medical problems, in which the electrolytes are not specified, but are left blank in the chart to be filled in by the managing service.

Modifications are required for special medical problems (Table 7-6). The volume can be restricted by concentrating the dextrose to 30% or 35% in final concentration and infusing the solution more slowly. Likewise, the amino acid concentration can be concentrated to 5% or 7.5% in final concentration, and the more concentrated fat emulsion, 20%, can be used. Electrolyte changes can be made easily, based on serial serum chemistries. Special amino acid so-

Table 7-7. Complications of Intravenous Hyperalimentation and Prevention or Therapy

Complication	Therapy or Prevention
Mechanical	Experience of inserting physician
Pneumothorax	
Hemothorax	
Thoracic duct injury	
Brachial plexus injury	
Air embolism	Care in the institution of the infusion
	Breath holding when lines are opened
	Use of clamps when the lines are opened
Catheter clotting	1,000 U heparin per liter IVH
Electrolyte disturbance	Watch for increased potassium and phosphate requirements early
	Careful monitoring of potassium, magnesium, phosphate for renal disease
	Low sodium, look for SIADH
Hyperglycemia, hypoglycemia	Careful glucose monitoring, especially early
	Gradually increase rate
	Put regular insulin in IVH bottle
	Avoid long-acting insulin
Hepatic: cholestasis, fatty liver	Avoid overfeeding
	Mixed carbohydrate, lipid
	Possibly benefited by cyclic alimentation
Catheter sepsis	Designated line for IVH; avoid other uses
	If no other source for fever, remove line
	Careful aseptic technique with insertion

IVH = intravenous hyperalimentation; SIADH = syndrome of inappropriate secretion of antidiuretic hormone.

lutions for acute renal failure (essential amino acids) and portosystemic encephalopathy (branch-chain enriched) are of equivocal value, because controlled studies do not show clear-cut advantages.

Overfeeding, especially with high dextrose infusions, will increase CO_2 production and may be disadvantageous when a patient is being weaned off a ventilator. The amount of calories required can be estimated by the Harris Benedict equation, which relates age, height, weight, and metabolic activity to estimated energy expenditure. Overfeeding the patient with respiratory insufficiency may aggravate CO_2 retention, because the laying down of fat from carbohydrates produces excessive CO_2 (the respiratory quotient, or the amount of CO_2 produced per O_2 consumed, is high). Carbohydrates are metabolized with more CO_2 production than lipids, making a higher lipid infusion more suitable for patients with respiratory insufficiency. A reasonable carbohydrate to lipid calorie ratio for most patients is 2 to 1, shifting to 1 to 1 in some patients with ventilatory insufficiency. These modifications can be implemented by de-creasing or increasing the concentrations of intravenous fat or glucose and their rates of infusion.

Complications of Intravenous Hyperalimentation

The complications of IVH can be divided into mechanical, related to the catheter insertion and maintenance, and medical. The major morbidity from IVH is related to catheter insertion. Surveys of IVH indicate that the misadventure rate correlates inversely with the experience of the physician, suggesting that the procedure should be performed by a few designated individuals. The complications and their treatment and prevention are outlined in Table 7-7.

Many of the metabolic complications occur early in the course of IVH. With refeeding there may be a large requirement for phosphate, which lessens with each day of infusion. The rate of infusion should not be increased until the metabolic derangements are corrected. Special attention to magnesium, phosphate, and potassium is necessary in renal insufficiency, because elevated levels can occur quickly if the usual quantities are infused. The most common metabolic disturbances are with glucose. Hyperglycemia may occur in the absence of diabetes mellitus and is easily treated by the acute use of subcutaneous regular insulin, with the gradual increase of regular insulin in the IVH infusion. Long-acting insulin should be avoided. Although some insulin may bind to the infusion lines or to heparin, the amount bound is approximately the same from infusate to infusate. Because glucose and insulin are given concurrently, the risks of hypoglycemia or hyperglycemia are minimized.

Slight elevations of the liver enzymes, alkaline phosphatase, and amino transferases are commonly seen during IVH, and the pathophysiology remains obscure. Liver biopsy specimens generally show only excessive fat and cholestasis, but sometimes fibrosis and cirrhosis occur, especially when the IVH is given for an extended time. It is difficult to separate out the effects of the underlying diseases from IVH, because similar hepatic derangements are seen with inflammatory bowel disease and the short gut syndrome. It is not certain how to manage the problem, but excessive calories, particularly glucose, may be disadvantageous. The hepatic abnormalities are benign in the short-term and are not a reason to terminate therapy.

Clotting of the central catheter can be devastating, because it may limit access sites, which are the lifeline for some patients with chronic bowel insufficiency. Sometimes the clot can be lysed with fibrinolytic infusions, but often the line has to be sacrificed. The use of heparin in the infusate lessens this complication. Patients prone to this complication may require long-term full anticoagulant treatment with heparin or warfarin.

The careful evaluation of fever should precede the removal of a central line catheter. Urinary, pulmonary, and gastrointestinal sources should be investigated and treated. Peripheral blood and central line blood cultures should be obtained. The central catheter should then be removed and the tip cultured if no other reason for the fever can be identified.

Conclusion

The disabled patient should receive a nutritional evaluation to determine if sufficient nutrients are being delivered. Nutritional support in terms of nutritional supplements, various types of tube feedings, and, sometimes, intravenous feedings should be considered to promote improved rehabilitation.

Case Management Studies

Case 1

A 60-year-old man with a spinal cord injury and chronic obstructive pulmonary disease is placed on a ventilator. His pulmonary disease is bad enough that he needs positive pressure breathing. Because of the positive pressure breathing he develops subcutaneous emphysema. In addition, a muscle relaxant is used. Should we proceed with enteral feedings in this individual? What type of enteral feedings would you choose?

1. The patient improves but continues to have problems with dysphagia, perhaps related to the fact that he has a nasotracheal tube. Tube feeding is introduced into his stomach. Citrotein, which is 95% carbohydrate, is used. A nitrogen balance is performed that shows that he has 5 g nitrogen positive per day. He produces a large quantity of carbon dioxide when this is analyzed on a metabolic cart. Is there something that can be done to help improve this situation?
2. The patient is switched to Magnacal full strength, which provides 2 kcal/ml to the patient. Then he begins vomiting. What do you think might cause this?

Case 2

A 70-year-old woman has neurogenic dysphagia and requires a percutaneous, endoscopically guided gastrostomy.

1. The gastrostomy tube falls out and a Foley catheter is replaced. Shortly afterward the patient vomits, and there is leakage around the tube. What do you think the cause of this might be?
2. On the day following placement of a percutaneous gastrostomy, the gastroenterologist generally loosens the external bumper. What is the purpose of this?

3. When should a gastrostomy tube be changed?
4. What types of gastrostomy tubes are there? What is a PEG button, for example?

Case 3

A 26-year-old quadriplegic man, secondary to closed head trauma, has functional dysphagia. A small polyethylene feeding tube is placed and he has no residuals, but he continues to have considerable vomiting. What is the cause of this problem?

1. A standard nasogastric tube is placed in his stomach. He continues to have vomiting and his gastric residuals are in excess of 100 ml. What medication might you try to improve this situation?
2. The patient is infused with 3,000 kcal and 100 g protein per day but remains in negative nitrogen balance. Why do you think the patient may still be in negative nitrogen balance?

Case 4

A 65-year-old woman with a stroke and chronic renal failure requiring dialysis is started on a nasogastric tube feeding with the hopes that her dysphagia is temporary and that she will not require a long-term percutaneous gastrostomy tube. What tube feeding would be reasonable to consider for her? What ions require special attention? What is a refeeding syndrome?

Case 5

Do you believe that it is ethical to place a percutaneous gastrostomy in a patient who has a vegetative existence, is unable to communicate, and has problems with swallowing to continue that person's existence indefinitely?

True or False Questions

1. A patient who becomes quadriplegic as a result of a motor vehicle collision requires enteral nutrition. Keeping in mind the obligate muscle

mass that ensues from disuse atrophy, the urinary nitrogen loss accurately reflects the goal of nitrogen intake that should be provided.
2. IVH is the preferred method of intense nutritional support over enteral alimentation, since the number of calories and grams of nitrogen can be administered with greater precision.
3. A percutaneous gastrostomy can be performed at the bedside with the assistance of endoscopic guidance, and it has a low incidence of side effects.

Answers to Case Management Questions

Answers for Case 1

One can proceed with tube feeding in this individual; however, the safest approach would be the placement of a larger bore tube in the stomach so that gastric aspirates can be checked for residual volume. The individual's production of carbon dioxide following the use of the high carbohydrate feeding was due to both overfeeding and the carbohydrate preference. Decreasing the feeding rate so that his nitrogen balance was closer to zero and switching the feedings to a more balanced solution between lipid and carbohydrate should have decreased his carbon dioxide production. Magnacal does have a reasonable carbohydrate and lipid balance and can be used in circumstances in which volume is a problem. However, the osmolality is very high and this preparation was probably the cause of his vomiting. Hyperosmolar or hypo-osmolar solutions in the stomach delay gastric emptying by osmoreceptors in the duodenum.

Answers for Case 2

The Foley catheter balloon probably is obstructing the pylorus or the duodenum. The patient can continue to receive feeding but the other contents of the stomach will not empty out of the stomach and will leak around the tube or produce vomiting. The external bumper of a gastrostomy tube is loosened following the placement of a percutaneous gastrostomy so that purulent material does not accumulate in the abdominal wall along the gastrostomy track. A gastrostomy tube does not need to be changed at any special interval, and the tubes can generally last for 6 months or more. There are various types of gastrostomy tubes. Most of them are similar to a Foley catheter, with some modifications. A PEG button, however, is a special modification such that it can be flush to the abdominal wall. An adapter is introduced through the PEG button for feeding.

Answers for Case 3

The polyethylene catheter is not large enough to give reliable gastric residual determinations. The patient probably has considerable gastric retention, perhaps related to central gastroparesis. Metoclopramide can be used to correct gastroparesis, although it is not always effective. The patient remains in negative nitrogen balance in spite of receiving a large amount of calories and protein because patients with central or spinal cord injuries often have an obligate negative nitrogen balance due to disuse atrophy of the muscles. No matter how hard you push the system, there will have to be a negative nitrogen balance owing to the loss of muscle.

Answers for Case 4

There are some special tube feedings that are low in potassium, magnesium, and phosphate that are reasonable in patients with chronic renal failure, and that would be appropriate for this individual. However, she may still need more phosphate than is generally required for patients with renal insufficiency because refeeding requires increased intracellular ions such as phosphate, magnesium, and potassium. All of these ions have to be watched closely with restitution of her problem.

Answers for Case 5

The decision to use intense nutritional support in this individual is difficult and the assistance of the family and other loved ones in the decision is often useful. One need not prolong the existence of an individual who is vegetative and has no hope of improvement.

Answers to True or False Questions

1. False.
2. False.
3. True.

Suggested Reading

Nutritional Assessment

Baker JP, Detsky AS, et al. Nutritional assessment: A comparison of clinical judgment and objective measurements. N Engl J Med 1982;306:969.

Buzby GP, Mullen SL, et al. Prognostic nutritional index in gastrointestinal surgery. Am J Surg 1980;139:160.

Fleck A. Acute phase response: Implications for nutrition and recovery. Nutrition 1988;4:109.

Windsor JA. Nutritional assessment: A pending renaissance. Nutrition 1991;7:377.

Enteral Feeding

Barbul A. Arginine and immune function. Nutrition 1990;6:53.

Caltaldi-Betcher EL, Seltzer MH, et al. Complications occurring during enteral nutrition support: A prospective study. J Parenter Enteral Nutr 1984;7:56.

Kelly TWJ, Patrick MR, Hillman KM. Study of diarrhea in critically ill patients. Crit Care Med 1983;11:7.

Keohane PP, Attrill H, et al. Limitations and drawbacks of "fine bore" nasogastric feeding tubes. Clin Nutr 1986;2:85.

Kirby DF, Craig RM, et al. Percutaneous endoscopic gastrostomies: A prospective evaluation and review of the literature. J Parenter Enteral Nutr 1986;10:155.

Olivares L, Segovia A, Revuelta R. Tube feeding and lethal aspiration in neurosurgical patients: A review of 720 autopsy cases. Stroke 1974;5:654.

Silk DBA. Diet formulation and choice of enteral diet. Gut 1986;27:S1.

Troyman DL, Young AB, et al. High protein enteral feedings: A means of achieving positive nitrogen balance in head injured patients. J Parenter Enteral Nutr 1985;9:679.

Yeung CK, Young GA, et al. Fine needle catheter jejunostomy: An assessment of new method of nutritional support after major gastrointestinal surgery. Br J Surg 1979;66:727.

Rocchi E, Casanelli M, et al. Standard or branched chain amino acid infusion as short term nutrition support in liver cirrhosis? J Parenter Enteral Nutr 1985;9:447.

Williams WW. Infection control during parenteral nutrition therapy. J Parenter Enteral Nutr 1985;9:735.

Wilson DO, Rogers RM, Hoffman RM. Nutrition and chronic lung disease. Am Rev Respir Dis 1985;132:1347.

Parenteral Hyperalimentation

Benotti PN, Bistrian BR. Practical aspects and complications of total parenteral nutrition. Crit Care Clin 1987;3:115.

Feinstein EI. Total parenteral nutritional support of patients with acute renal failure. Nutr Clin Pract 1988;3:9.

Hammarqvist F, Wernermen J, et al. Addition of glutamine to total parenteral nutrition after elective abdominal surgery spares free glutamine in muscle, counteracts the fall in muscle protein synthesis, and improves nitrogen balance. Ann Surg 1989;209:455.

Hiyama DT, Fischer JE. Nutritional support in hepatic failure. Nutr Clin Pract 1988;3:96.

McMahon M, Manji N, et al. Parenteral nutrition in patients with diabetes mellitus: Theoretical and practical considerations. J Parenter Enteral Nutr 1989;13:545.

Perdum PP, Kirby DF. Short-bowel syndrome: A review of the role of nutrition support. J Parenter Enteral Nutr 1991;15:93.

Sax HC, Bower RH. Hepatic complications of total parenteral nutrition. J Parenter Enteral Nutr 1988;12:615.

Solomon SM, Kirby DF. The refeeding syndrome: A review. J Parenter Enteral Nutr 1990;14:90.

Ziegler TR, Young LS, et al. Clinical and metabolic efficacy of glutamine-supplemented parenteral nutrition after bone-marrow transplantation. Ann Intern Med 1992;116:821.

Chapter 8
Disorders of Alimentation and Bowel Motility

Gene Z. Chiao and Peter J. Kahrilas

Gastrointestinal motility is frequently a focus of one's sense of well-being. Even in a nondisabled, relatively young population, disorders of swallowing, gastroesophageal acid reflux, altered gastric emptying, constipation, diarrhea, or abdominal pain prompt numerous physician visits. In the case of the disabled population, the individual's ability to cope with these difficulties is limited, and thus problems can be more profound.

As a generalized description, the gastrointestinal tract is a long, smooth muscle tube with striated muscle control points at the esophagopharyngeal area above and the external anal sphincter below. Thus, in discussing motor function of the gut, an immediate distinction must be made between structures under central nervous system (CNS) control (striated muscle structures) and those under autonomic nervous system control (smooth muscle structures). Fortunately, the portion of the gut under autonomic control functions reasonably well, even when freed of CNS control. After experimental destruction of the spinal cord at the T2 to T3 level, gastric emptying is transiently impaired but the small intestine functions relatively normally. During a recovery period of about 2 weeks, gastric emptying returns to normal coincident with the return of motilin secretory function [1, 2]. Thus, the function of the smooth muscle structures of the gastrointestinal tract, namely the esophagus, stomach, gallbladder, small bowel, and colon, are relatively preserved when freed of CNS control. However, the situation is quite different in the striated muscle structures under direct CNS control, namely the

oropharynx and the external anal sphincter. These structures do not regain normal function after injury to the relevant CNS control mechanisms and as a result represent a focus of continued disability. For this reason, a large part of this chapter focuses on two relatively small areas of the gastrointestinal tract: the oropharynx and the external anal sphincter, control points to the entry to and exit from the gastrointestinal tract.

Oropharynx

Swallowing is so fundamental to our existence that we rarely take note of it. Just how important it is becomes apparent when swallowing difficulty develops. However, before attempting to understand the scope of the problem of dysphagia, the details of the normal swallow response must first be considered. Similarly, illustrative cases are used to exemplify mechanisms of dysfunction, but no attempt is made to be encyclopedic regarding etiologies of oropharyngeal dysphagia.

Central Nervous System Control of Swallowing

Swallowing is composed of an initial oral phase, a pharyngeal phase, and an esophageal phase. The oral phase of swallowing is largely voluntary and highly variable depending on taste, environment, hunger, motivation, etc. The pharyngeal phase is the complex motor event referred to as the swallow re-

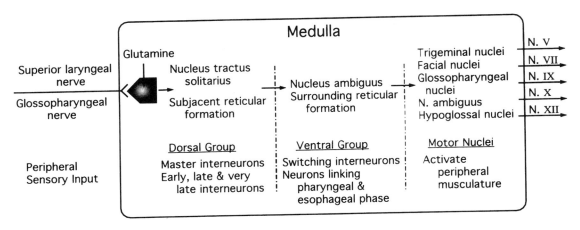

Figure 8-1. Model of the medullary swallowing center. Sensory input enters the medulla at and below the nucleus of the tractus solitarius, and motor output exits via five cranial nerves. The presumed function of each group of neurons is itemized beneath each anatomic grouping.

sponse. Afferent sensory fibers from the larynx capable of initiating swallowing travel centrally through the internal branch of the superior laryngeal nerve and afferents from the pharyngeal plexus travel centrally through the glossopharyngeal nerve [3]. Sensory fibers crucial to the initiation of swallowing converge in the spinal trigeminal system and fasciculus solitarius before terminating in the medullary swallow center. The location and architecture of the medullary swallowing center has been extensively investigated [4]. The evolving model is summarized in Figure 8-1. The "master neurons" that establish the timing of sequential excitation of specific cranial motor nuclei are believed to be among the dorsal group in Figure 8-1, located in and around the nucleus tractus solitarius [5]. Once activated, the master neurons can establish the entire motor sequence of the swallow without further sensory input. However, even if not necessary, afferent feedback does facilitate the discharge of swallow interneurons, emphasizing the potential for modifying the swallow in response to bolus characteristics [6]. Also among the dorsal group shown in Figure 8-1 are interneurons activated at specific times within the swallow pattern, corresponding to the activity of specific groups of pharyngeal and esophageal muscles. These neurons exhibit either a phasic discharge or a modification of spontaneous

activity with swallowing [6]. Depending on the temporal relationship of neuronal activity with the onset of deglutition, Jean has classified these medullary neurons as early, late, or very late neurons. The second group of interneurons, consisting of the medullary swallow center, are the ventral group in Figure 8-1, located in and around the nucleus ambiguus. These interneurons probably function as switching neurons to relay the swallowing orders from the dorsal pattern generators to the various motoneuron pools involved in enacting the muscular response [7]. Electrical stimulation of the ventral group of interneurons will not elicit a pharyngeal swallow but will evoke the esophageal phase, suggesting that these cells may serve to link the pharyngeal and esophageal phases [4]. Although swallowing can be elicited or facilitated by electrical stimulation of higher brain centers [8, 9], these areas are not necessary for the response to occur. Rather, the higher structures probably function to modify the oral phase of swallowing and to integrate feeding with visceral and somatic reflexes. The significance of this neuronal architecture is that swallowing is relatively protected from disturbance by diseases affecting brain centers higher than the medulla. However, medullary motoneuron diseases such as bulbar polio or amyotrophic lateral sclerosis can lead to severe dysfunction.

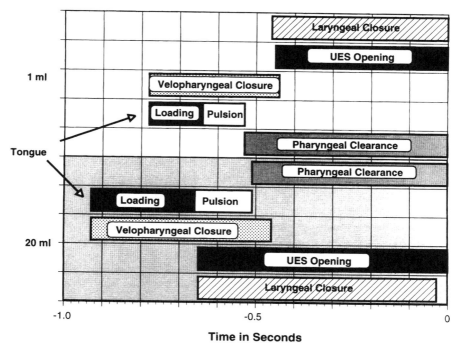

Figure 8-2. Time lines of 1- and 20-ml swallows. The upper, unshaded area depicts time relationships among swallow events during 1-ml swallows, whereas the lower, shaded area depicts the same events during 20-ml swallows. In both instances, time 0 is the end of the swallow, determined by the timing of upper esophageal sphincter (UES) closure, and all other events are given negative timing values. When so viewed, it is clear that the apparent prolongation of the 20-ml swallow is associated with an earlier mechanical reconfiguration of the pharynx from a respiratory to a swallowing pathway. The earlier reconfiguration is associated with a prolonged tongue-loading period. Propulsive events, however, occur within a similar time frame, resulting in more vigorous expulsion of the larger bolus. The mechanics and timing of the pharyngeal contraction, important in the process of pharyngeal clearance and in UES closure, are remarkably constant among swallow volumes. (Reprinted with permission from PJ Kahrilas, JA Logemann. Volume accommodation during swallowing. Dysphagia 1993;8:259.)

Mechanics of Swallow

Although physiologically described in neurophysiologic and electromyographic patterns, swallowing is clinically evaluated in biomechanical terms. Unlike neuromuscular or manometric studies, biomechanical studies focus on how the swallowed bolus is manipulated by actions of oropharyngeal structures. The biomechanical analysis by videofluoroscopic or cineradiographic swallowing techniques is the foundation for the clinical evaluation of oropharyngeal dysphagia.

The pharyngeal swallow results in a transient rearrangement of pharyngeal structures and is normally completed within 1 second. The swallow encompasses several closely coordinated actions: (1) elevation and retraction of the soft palate with closure of the nasopharynx, (2) upper esophageal sphincter (UES) opening, (3) laryngeal vestibule closure, (4) tongue loading (ramping), (5) tongue pulsion, and (6) pharyngeal clearance. Initial attempts at defining the relationship among these swallow elements focused on timing them relative to each other. However, that timing is affected by the volume of the swallowed bolus, making it difficult to establish a temporal reference among events (Figure 8-2). Having examined these timing relationships from a number of perspectives, the most glaring constancy of the swallow response is the duration and propagation of pharyngeal constrictor contraction associated with pharyngeal clearance [10]. Thus, in order to construct a time line of the biomechanical events within the swallow and still preserve the constancy of the most stereotyped aspect of the swallow, events must be timed from the end rather than the beginning as illustrated in Figure 8-2, in which the completion of pharyngeal clearance occurs at time 0 and all earlier events occur before time 0 [11].

The events charted in Figure 8-2 can be divided into two groups: (1) those resulting in the reconfiguration of the oropharynx from a respiratory to a swallow pathway (velopharyngeal closure, UES opening, laryngeal vestibule closure, and tongue loading), and (2) those associated with moving the bolus into the esophagus (tongue pulsion and pharyngeal clearance). When so divided, the fundamental distinction between small and large volume swallows is that with large volume swallows, the anatomic reconfiguration is achieved earlier and persists longer than observed with small volume swallows; tongue loading with associated velopharyngeal closure starts earlier and takes longer, and UES opening with associated closure of the laryngeal vestibule commences sooner and persists longer. Events associated with moving the bolus into the esophagus, however, occur within a similar time period regardless of swallow volume, resulting in more vigorous expulsion of larger volumes. Because large and small volumes must be transferred from the oropharynx to the proximal esophagus in the same time increment, it follows that the rate of transfer is greater for the larger volume bolus [11].

The most obvious anatomic reconfiguration required to transform the oropharynx from a respiratory to a swallow pathway is to open the inlet to the esophagus and seal the inlet to the larynx. As suggested in Figure 8-2, these events occur in close synchrony. The mechanical determinants of UES opening are laryngeal elevation and anterior traction on the hyoid [12, 13]. The mechanical determinants of laryngeal vestibule closure, which is almost exactly synchronized with UES opening, are laryngeal elevation and anterior tilting of the arytenoid cartilages against the base of the epiglottis [14]. Thus, examining the efficacy of either of these events should focus on laryngeal elevation. Figure 8-3 illustrates the pattern of laryngeal elevation for 2-, 5-, and 20-ml swallows [15]. Note that the degree of elevation achieved and its persistence is greater for larger volume swallows. Note also that UES relaxation occurs at roughly the same degree of elevation regardless of swallow volume. What changes with volume is the persistence of laryngeal elevation above this critical value. On the closure side of Figure 8-3, the onset of the hypopharyngeal contraction (indicative of the pharyngeal clearance wave) always occurs in a fixed relationship to UES contraction, whereas the larynx is still elevated.

Once the larynx is elevated, UES opening results from traction on the anterior sphincter wall caused by contraction of the suprahyoid and infrahyoid musculature that also results in a characteristic pattern of hyoid displacement [12, 13]. Both the diameter and duration of sphincter opening increase with increased bolus volumes. The increased duration of UES opening is related to subtle modifications in the persistence of the hyoid excursion (Figure 8-4), whereas changes in the diameter of opening are related to increased intrabolus pressure with larger volume swallows. The electrophysiologic correlate of this observation is that the period of neuronal and subsequent suprahyoid and infrahyoid musculature activation is modified by bolus-specific input. Presumably, the sensory cue for this differential activation is related to the degree of tongue deformation and consequent proprioceptive activation associated with larger volume swallows. Sphincter closure coincides with the arrival of the propagated pharyngeal contraction [10, 13].

Larger volume swallows are associated with more vigorous bolus expulsion from the oropharynx; 1-ml swallows may have a maximal expulsion velocity of 15 cm per second, whereas larger volume swallows may have a velocity of 50 cm per second [16]. The two main determinants of bolus transport out of the oropharynx are the action of the tongue and pharyngeal constrictors. In the case of the pharyngeal constrictors, the propagated pharyngeal contraction has similar propagation and vigor regardless of bolus volume [10, 17]. However, the propagated pharyngeal contraction is more involved with the process of clearance than of bolus propulsion; it strips the final bolus residue from the pharyngeal walls, minimizing the chance that aspiration will occur with the resumption of respiration. This is graphically evident in Figure 8-5, showing the relationship between bolus movement and contraction of the pharyngeal constrictors. Tongue motion, however, varies substantially with bolus volume,

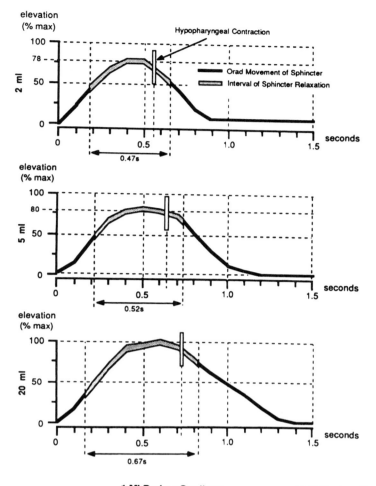

Figure 8-3. The relative timing of events within the pharyngeal swallow during 2-, 5-, and 20-ml swallows. Values of laryngeal elevation were normalized for each subject so that 100% was the maximal elevation occurring during 20-ml swallows. Note that as the interval of manometric relaxation increased, the period of laryngeal elevation was prolonged, the upper esophageal sphincter relaxed earlier, and the interval between the onset of laryngeal elevation and hypopharyngeal contraction increased. (Reprinted with permission from PJ Kahrilas, WJ Dodds, J Dent, et al. Upper esophageal sphincter function during deglutition. Gastroenterology 1988;95:52.)

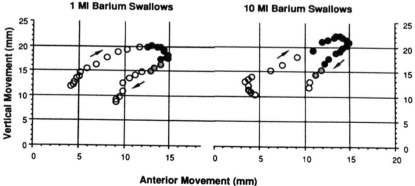

Figure 8-4. Movement patterns of the hyoid during 1- and 10-ml swallows. Each circle represents the hyoid position during a single video frame of the recorded fluoroscopic sequence (1/30th-second interval), and the arrows indicate the direction of movement. Open circles denote frames during which the sphincter was closed, filled circles denote frames during which the sphincter was open, and gray circles denote frames during which the sphincter was variably open, depending on the subject. Note that sphincter opening and closing occurred at nearly identical hyoid coordinates among subjects and among volumes. The larger volume swallows were associated with persistence of the hyoid superior to and anterior to the opening coordinates. (Reprinted with permission from P Jacob, PJ Kahrilas, JA Logemann, et al. Upper esophageal sphincter opening and modulation during swallowing. Gastroenterology 1989;97:1469.)

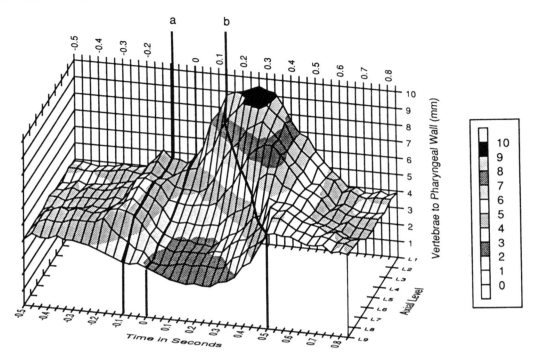

Figure 8-5. Posterior pharyngeal wall movement during 5-ml barium swallows. The axial level of measurement (L1 to L9) is shown on the *y*-axis such that lines 4 and 9 are at the levels of the valleculae and the uppermost margin of the upper esophageal sphincter. The remainder of the lines are evenly spaced. Time is on the *x*-axis, with time 0 indicating upper esophageal sphincter opening, time a indicating bolus head contact with the sensor at the level of L2, and time b indicating the time of luminal closure at each axial level. Distance from the pharyngeal wall to the anterior surface of the vertebral bodies at each level is shown on the *z*-axis, with the key on the right applying to the shading of the surface graph. Because upper esophageal sphincter opening corresponds with the arrival of the bolus head at the sphincter, the interval a-0 (0.1 second) approximates the period during which the bolus head traverses the pharynx. The bolus tail traverses the pharynx much more slowly (0.37 second). Note that the period of bolus head passage precedes any significant contractile activity of the pharyngeal constrictors but that the pharyngeal constrictor contraction is intimately associated with passage of the bolus tail through the pharynx. (Reprinted with permission from PJ Kahrilas, JA Logemann, S Lin, GA Ergun. Pharyngeal clearance during swallowing: A combined manometric and videofluoroscopic study. Gastroenterology 1992;103:128.)

suggesting that it has a cardinal role in determining differences in bolus propulsion among swallow volumes [18–20].

In the course of the swallow, each tongue region exhibits either centrifugal motion (front and center of tongue) or centripetal motion followed by centrifugal motion (posterior oral tongue and tongue base). The resultant pattern of tongue motion forms a bolus chamber between the tongue surface and the pharyngeal walls. The volume of the pharyngeal chamber is related to the depth of the central groove that is greater for larger volume swallows. However, the bolus chamber is typically 10–15 ml greater in volume than the bolus [20]. A corollary to this is that substantial aerophagia must be a normal consequence of swallowing. This can be demonstrated by cine computed tomographic imaging of the pharyngeal chamber during swallow (Figure 8-6). Volume calculations using this technique concluded that approximately 15 ml of air were typically ingested with each swallowed bolus under the conditions of that experiment [21].

Oropharyngeal Dysphagia

Oropharyngeal dysphagia can result from structural or propulsive abnormalities of the orophar-

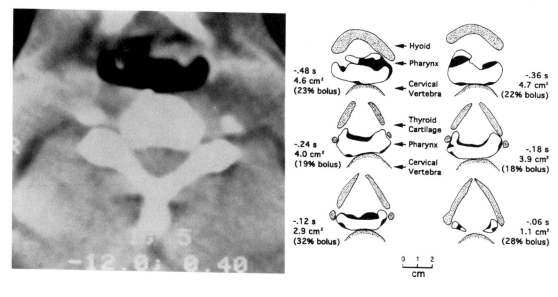

Time: -.48 s

○ Air   ● Bolus   ◎ Bone or Cartilage

Figure 8-6. Cine computed tomographic (CT) image and tracings at the level of the valleculae during swallowing. The actual image on the left was obtained 0.48 second before luminal closure, whereas the tracings on the right illustrate the dynamic changes of the bolus cavity through the course of the swallow, terminating with luminal closure at time 0. Although the hyoid elevates out of the CT plane between –0.36 and –0.24 second, anterior hyoid movement is readily evident between –0.48 and –0.36 second. Note the absence of posterior wall motion (pharyngeal constrictors) until –0.06 second, supporting the notion that this action is a clearance event rather than an element of bolus propulsion. Also note that the epiglottis and valleculae effectively occlude the medial part of the bolus chamber, splitting the bolus, before closure. Finally, the bolus is seemingly randomly distributed around the perimeter and mixed with a substantial quantity of air. (Reprinted with permission from GA Ergun, PJ Kahrilas, S Lin, et al. Shape, volume, and content of the deglutitive pharyngeal chamber imaged by ultrafast computerized tomography. Gastroenterology 1993;105:1396.)

ynx or proximal esophagus. Structural abnormalities of these areas may result from trauma, surgery, tumors, caustic injury, congenital conditions, or acquired deformities. Propulsive abnormalities can result from dysfunction of either intrinsic musculature, peripheral nerves, or CNS control mechanisms. Thus, whereas esophageal dysphagia usually results from esophageal diseases, most cases of oropharyngeal dysphagia are the result of neurologic or muscular diseases, with oropharyngeal dysfunction being just one pathologic manifestation.

The patient history is crucial in the evaluation of oropharyngeal dysphagia. Major objectives of the history are to differentiate oropharyngeal dysphagia from globus, esophageal dysphagia, or xerostomia. Unlike dysphagia, which occurs only during swallowing, globus sensation is most prominent between swallows. Unlike esophageal dysphagia, in which patients mistakenly identify the neck as the locus of bolus hang-up approximately 30% of the time, patients almost invariably accurately recognize the locus and consequence of oropharyngeal dysphagia. Therefore, identification of associated symptoms such as aspiration, nasopharyngeal regurgitation, esophagopharyngeal regurgitation, drooling, chest pain, or intermittent esophageal obstruction can be of great value in distinguishing esophageal from oropharyngeal dysphagia. Finally, patients with xerostomia may complain of dysphagia but the associated history of dry mouth, dry eyes, rheumatoid arthritis, radiation therapy, or use of anticholinergic medications should lead the clinician to suspect xerostomia.

Structural Causes of Oropharyngeal Dysphagia

Implicit in the mechanical description of swallowing summarized previously is that normal swallowing is associated with minimal outflow resistance from the oropharynx. A postcricoid web causes dysphagia as a result of outflow resistance at this level. Similarly, because the posterior wall of the pharynx is so closely opposed to the anterior aspect of the cervical vertebrae, cervical osteophytes result in an anterior bulging into the hypopharynx that can make passage of a normal-sized bolus difficult. An analogous situation can arise as a result of edema after the surgical stabilization of the vertebral column, implantation of metal stabilization devices, or after cervical laminectomy.

The most common structural cause of oropharyngeal dysphagia is a hypopharyngeal diverticulum. Acquired hypopharyngeal diverticula occur most commonly in men after the sixth decade of life. Although there is a tendency to refer to all hypopharyngeal diverticula as Zenker's diverticula, the location of pouches varies and it is probably better to classify the diverticula according to their site of origin. The most frequent site of herniation is an area between the oblique fibers of the inferior pharyngeal constrictor and the cricopharyngeus muscle in the midline posteriorly [22]. However, the unifying theme of all locations for false diverticula is that they occur through sites of potential weakness of the muscular lining of the hypopharynx. Hypopharyngeal diverticula are generally asymptomatic until they enlarge sufficiently to accommodate and store a significant amount of food or liquid. In most instances, symptoms are of postswallow regurgitation or even aspiration of material from the pharyngeal pouch.

The pathogenesis of hypopharyngeal diverticula has been the subject of much speculation and debate [23]. Diverticula have been hypothesized to result from delayed UES relaxation, failure of relaxation, and premature contraction. However, few credible data exist to support any of these hypotheses and other manometric investigations have not demonstrated any abnormalities. A more recent and plausible pathophysiologic explanation for the development of diverticula is that they form as a result of a restrictive myopathy associated with diminished compliance of the cricopharyngeus muscle. Surgical specimens of cricopharyngeus muscle strips from 14 patients with hypopharyngeal

diverticula demonstrated structural changes that would decrease UES compliance and opening [24]. The cricopharyngeus samples from these patients had "fibro-adipose tissue replacement and fiber degeneration." The process that led to the histologic changes is unclear, but whatever the case may be, these findings support the hypothesis that fibrosis of the cricopharyngeus impairs UES opening by decreasing sphincter compliance. Thus, although the muscle relaxes normally during a swallow, it cannot distend normally, resulting in the appearance of a cricopharyngeal bar during a barium swallow (Figure 8-7). Diminished sphincter compliance is associated with increased hypopharyngeal intrabolus pressure in order to maintain transsphincteric flow through the smaller UES opening. Whereas normal individuals have extremely compliant sphincters such that the range of upstream intrabolus pressure only varies from 6–18 mm Hg as the swallow volume is increased from 2–30 ml, patients with cricopharyngeal bars showed upstream pressures ranging from 13–68 mm Hg for the same range of bolus volumes [25]. The same phenomena have been demonstrated in patients with Zenker's diverticula, suggesting that diverticula formation is an eventual consequence of the increased stress on the hypopharynx resulting from the increased intrabolus pressure [26]. Presumably, the increased intrabolus pressure is also the cause of perceived dysphagia.

Propulsive Causes of Oropharyngeal Dysphagia

Primary neurologic or muscular diseases involving the oropharynx can be associated with dysphagia. Although the specifics of the diseases vary, the net effect on swallowing can be analyzed according to the mechanical description of the swallow described previously. A nasal voice and instances of nasopharyngeal regurgitation reflect on either weakness or paresis of the soft palate elevators. Poor control of the bolus within the mouth can result from tongue weakness. Postswallow residua in the valleculae or hypopharynx reflect on an ineffective, presumably weakened pharyngeal contraction. Aspiration suggests either weakened laryngeal elevators with a resultant impairment of laryngeal closure during swallowing or a defective swallow that results in significant postswallow residua, which is then aspirated after the swallow sequence

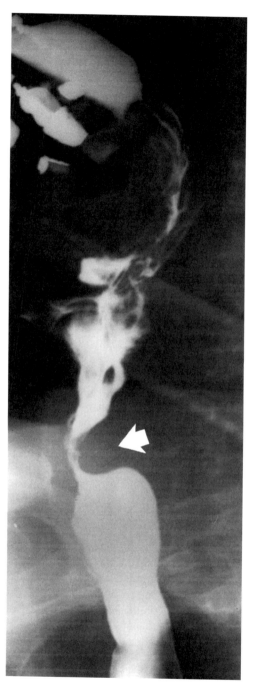

Figure 8-7. A roentgenogram showing a cricopharyngeal bar (arrow) with diminished upper esophageal sphincter opening during a swallow of barium contrast. (Courtesy of Richard Gore, M.D.)

is completed. All of these potential mechanisms can be evaluated with a thorough history and a videofluoroscopic swallowing study. The videofluoroscopic swallowing study can be analyzed in accordance with the mechanical elements of the swallow described previously. Table 8-1 summarizes the mechanical elements of the swallow along with the manifestation and consequence of dysfunction and potential for therapy. Dysfunction of the swallow does not necessarily obligate an individual to non-oral feeding. Depending on the severity of the impairment, level of motivation, and neurologic intactness, defective elements of the swallow can be selectively compensated. Impaired laryngeal closure can be compensated for by tucking the chin during swallow and use of the "supraglottic swallow" (hold breath during swallow and cough to clear residue before inhaling after swallow). Impaired nasopharyngeal closure can be compensated for by using palatal elevators and by avoiding thin liquid foods. Impaired UES opening can be improved by using Mendelsohn's maneuver, a biofeedback technique that purposefully prolongs the anterosuperior laryngeal traction at mid-swallow [27, 28]. Finally, impaired pharyngeal clearance can be compensated for by turning the head toward the paretic side in the case of unilateral dysfunction [29] or by postswallow cough to clear residue in the case of bilateral paresis.

A final note is on the utility of cricopharyngeal myotomy. Cricopharyngeal myotomy can be an effective mode of therapy for patients with cricopharyngeal bars or hypopharyngeal diverticula. In general, the criteria for performing a myotomy should be (1) the presence of significant dysphagia leading to local discomfort, weight loss, or aspiration; (2) confirmation of UES dysfunction by videoradiography, preferably with intraluminal manometry; and (3) absence of clinically significant gastroesophageal reflux or gastroesophageal regurgitation. These criteria are often met in the case of hypopharyngeal diverticula but probably not in many other clinical situations. Performing myotomies in questionable cases is not advisable because, although it is a relatively safe procedure, it can further impair diminished pharyngeal constrictor function, and sudden death from aspiration is a reported complication, emphasizing the need to assess lower esophageal competence preoperatively.

Table 8-1. Functional Elements of a Swallow

Swallow Element	Biomechanical Mechanism	Evidence of Dysfunction (Typical Diseases)	Therapeutic Techniques
Airway protection	Laryngeal elevation, arytenoid tilt, cord closure	Aspiration during bolus transit (amyotrophic lateral sclerosis)	Chin down, biofeedback (supraglottic swallow)
Nasopharyngeal closure	Soft palate elevation	Nasopharyngeal regurgitation (myasthenia gravis)	Avoid thin liquids (cholinomimetics for myasthenia)
Upper esophageal sphincter opening	Upper esophageal sphincter relaxation, laryngeal elevation, anterior hyoid traction	Dysphagia, postswallow residue/aspiration, diverticulum formation (cricopharyngeal bar, cerebrovascular accident, Parkinson's)	Biofeedback (Mendelsohn's maneuver), myotomy
Bolus propulsion	Tongue contour, sensation, motor control	Sluggish, misdirected bolus (Parkinson's, surgical defects, cerebral palsy)	Avoid thin liquids
Pharyngeal clearance	Pharyngeal shortening, propagated pharyngeal contraction, epiglottic flip	Postswallow residue/aspiration (polio, postpolio, muscular dystrophy, cerebrovascular accident)	Head turning (unilateral weakness), postswallow cough

Esophagus

Esophageal peristalsis is initiated shortly after the bolus traverses the upper esophageal sphincter. The peristaltic contraction moves from the striated muscle of the upper third of the esophageal body to the smooth muscle of the distal two-thirds of the esophagus at a speed between 2 and 4 cm per second. Esophageal peristalsis initiated by a swallow is referred to as primary peristalsis; secondary peristalsis can be initiated at any level of the esophagus in response to local luminal distention. The peristaltic contraction produced by swallowing is under CNS control and is abolished by bilateral cervical vagotomy [30]. The striated muscle of the esophagus receives only somatic excitatory innervation, and the peristaltic contraction of this segment results from the sequential activation of motor units in a craniocaudal sequence. Physiologic evidence of this arrangement was provided by studies in which the central end of the proximally severed vagus nerve was reimplanted in the sternocleidomastoid muscle. Sequential activation of the reinervated musculature could then be demonstrated directly in response to swallowing [30]. The smooth muscle esophagus behaves somewhat differently than the striated muscle portion in that although the peristaltic contraction is triggered by vagal activation, the progressive nature of the peristaltic contraction results from some programming mechanism in the esophagus itself. Support for this conclusion is based on the observation that secondary peristalsis (initiated by local esophageal distention) persists after vagotomy [31] as well as the observation that even simultaneous stimulation of the entire vagal trunk results in peristaltic rather than simultaneous contraction of the smooth muscle segment [32].

The lower esophageal sphincter (LES) is a segment of tonically contracted smooth muscle at the distal end of the esophagus that is approximately 2 cm in length. The resting tone of the LES varies between 10 and 30 mm Hg among individuals. LES pressure is lowest in the postprandial period and highest at night. Intra-abdominal pressure, gastric distention, peptides, hormones, various foods, and many drugs affect the LES pressure. The mechanism of its tonic contraction is not fully understood but seems to be a property of the muscle itself rather than of a unique population of nerves affecting the sphincter [33]. Basal LES tone is inhibited with swallowing concurrently with the inhibitory front that traverses the smooth muscle esophagus. LES relaxation is vagally mediated by preganglionic cholinergic nerves and postganglionic noncholinergic, nonadrenergic nerves. Recent evidence strongly suggests that the neurotransmitter is nitric oxide [34–36]. The vagal fibers affecting LES relaxation enter the esophagus relatively proximally in the body as the physiologic response is unaffected by high abdominal truncal vagotomy [37, 38].

Esophageal Dysphagia

Dysphagia can result from esophageal disorders. Unlike pharyngeal dysphagia in which patients accurately localize the site of dysfunction, with esophageal dysphagia a patient's identification of the locus of bolus hang-up is of limited accuracy. The actual level of bolus hang-up or obstruction occurs at or above the level of hang-up identified by the patient. Thus, the sensation of dysphagia from a distal esophageal obstruction caused by a ring or an esophageal motor disorder will often be referred to the level of the neck. Therefore, identification of associated symptoms such as aspiration, nasopharyngeal regurgitation, esophagopharyngeal regurgitation, weight loss, drooling, chest pain, or intermittent esophageal obstruction can be of great value in further localizing the problem. The physiologic correlate of esophageal dysphagia is of impaired bolus transit through the esophageal body into the stomach. This may be the result of a failed propulsive mechanism or a structural problem impairing the bolus flow. Structural abnormalities may partly or completely compromise the esophageal lumen. Failure of the propulsive mechanism may be intermittent or constant. However, it is important to note that not all instances of impaired esophageal aperistalsis are symptomatic. Certainly it has been shown that a significant number of elderly individuals have asymptomatic peristaltic failure, sometimes referred to as presbyesophagus [39]. The proportion of individuals with peristaltic dysfunction who experience dysphagia is not known.

Esophageal strictures, rings, or webs result in a situation in which the limited opening aperture of the esophagus can impair bolus transit. This problem only occurs with solids and is frequently intermittent. It is a frequent fluoroscopic observation that impaired bolus transit of a solid bolus, such as a marshmallow, coincides temporally with the subjective experience of dysphagia. Obstructive esophageal lesions can be congenital (Schatzki's ring, webs), malignant, or the result of benign processes, most commonly the result of reflux esophagitis. Rings formed at the gastroesophageal junction, described by Schatzki, are generally symptomatic only when the internal diameter of the ring is less than 13 mm (approximately 41 French) and hence dilation is generally recommended when this circumstance is detected [40].

Dysphagia can also result from external structures impinging on the esophagus or limiting the distensibility of the esophagus. Dysphagia lusoria is caused by compression of the esophagus by an anomalous right subclavian artery arising from the descending aorta and passing behind the esophagus. Vertebral osteophytes, especially on the cervical vertebral bodies, can similarly transiently obstruct the intraluminal flow through the esophagus and result in dysphagia.

If there is a physiologic correlate of dysphagia, unrelated to a luminal narrowing from within or without, it relates to a peristaltic defect. This may relate to a major motor disorder of the esophagus such as achalasia or diffuse esophageal spasm [41] in which bolus transport is obviously impaired, or it may result from more subtle abnormalities of peristalsis. Recent evidence suggests that although normal peristaltic amplitude is considerably in excess of what is necessary for bolus transport, hypotensive peristalsis is associated with impaired volume clearance of the esophagus [42]. Failed peristalsis is associated with grossly impaired esophageal volume clearance. Nonpropagated, or simultaneous, esophageal contractions are also associated with impaired esophageal bolus transit and dysphagia. This can be the case regardless of the amplitude of the contractions. Overall, the critical esophageal peristaltic amplitude necessary to accomplish complete clearance of liquid barium from the esophagus is dependent on the esophageal region in question but does not exceed 40 mm Hg regardless of the region [42]. Although no data exist on the subject, one might predict that the successful transport of solid boluses would require somewhat greater peristaltic amplitudes.

A potential cause of peristaltic failure in the disabled population is vagotomy, which occurs either as the result of surgical intervention or of a neurologic disorder interfering with the motor nuclei of the vagus nerve. In instances of bilateral vagotomy at or above the cervical level, aperistalsis of the esophageal body results [37]. The effects of unilateral vagotomy are variable, sometimes resulting in aperistalsis or a diminished amplitude of peristalsis. Bilateral vagotomy also results in a diminution of the resting LES pressure.

Gastroesophageal Reflux Disease

Gastroesophageal reflux disease (GERD) is the most common esophageal disorder [43]. It is characterized by excessive reflux of gastric contents, including acid and pepsin, into the esophagus. Prolonged exposure of the esophageal epithelium to these noxious substances can lead to mucosal inflammation and injury (esophagitis). Gastroesophageal reflux is subjectively experienced as heartburn, or pyrosis (retrosternal burning sensation), acid regurgitation, chest pain, dysphagia, or water brash (excess salivation). Other potential consequences of gastroesophageal acid reflux are laryngitis, bronchospasm, and persistent aspiration pneumonia. Evidence suggests that a relatively minor quantity of refluxed acid can be extremely injurious to the respiratory tree [44]. An increasing body of literature suggests that reflux disease may be responsible for a significant proportion of intrinsic asthma and even some instances of anoxic encephalopathy in the pediatric population [45–47]. Experimentally, the occurrence of reflux-related aspiration laryngitis or pneumonitis has proved difficult to quantify. Technetium radionuclide scanning has been used wherein the patient ingests technetium sulfacolloid and after a 24-hour period the lung fields are scanned for evidence of aspiration. This test lacks sensitivity and is also hampered by the normal process of gastric emptying.

The presence of reflux symptoms does not necessarily imply the presence of esophagitis. Esophagitis is a histologic or endoscopic diagnosis. Mild esophagitis is seen histologically as a thickening of the basal cell layer and a heightening of the vascular papillae in the squamous epithelium of the esophagus [48]. These changes are induced by accelerated shedding of the surface cells. As the esophagitis gets more severe there is erythema, exudate, ulceration, and finally stricture formation in the distal esophagus. With severe esophagitis, epithelial metaplasia (Barrett's esophagus) can occur in which case the normal squamous epithelium is replaced by a specialized columnar epithelium. Dysplastic Barrett's epithelium is a premalignant condition.

Symptomatic GERD results when the balance between aggressive forces (acid reflux, potency of refluxate) and defensive forces (esophageal acid clearance, mucosal resistance) tilt in favor of the aggressive forces. The intermittent nature of symptoms in some individuals with GERD suggests that the aggressive and defensive forces are part of a rather delicately balanced system. Significant aberration in any one of these pathophysiologic influences can result in tipping the balance of forces acting on the esophageal mucosa from a compensated condition to a decompensated condition (heartburn, esophagitis).

Individual gastroesophageal reflux events occur by three mechanisms: (1) transient LES relaxations, (2) abdominal straining, and (3) free reflux across a patulous LES [49, 50]. Transient LES relaxations occur in both normal individuals and in GERD patients and are the only potential mechanism of reflux during periods in which the LES pressure is normal. These relaxations are part of the reflex that normally allows for gas escape from the stomach, better known as belching, and can be triggered by fundic distention with gas [51, 52]. Stress reflux events, on the other hand, occur during periods of abdominal straining when the increased intra-abdominal pressure drives the gastric content retrograde across a hypotensive LES [53]. What then determines pathologic gastroesophageal junction incompetence? Current thinking is that this depends on both the LES and the diaphragmatic sphincter [54]. Patients with hiatal hernia have progressive disruption of the diaphragmatic sphincter, depending on the extent of axial herniation. Therefore, although neither condition in and of itself (hiatal hernia or hypotensive LES) results in severe gastroesophageal junction incompetence, the two conditions interact with each other in more than an additive fashion. A recent paper modeling the susceptibility of the gastroesophageal junction to stress reflux events suggested the relationship illustrated in Figure 8-8 between instantaneous LES pressure and the size of hiatal hernia in determining gastroesophageal junction incompetence [55].

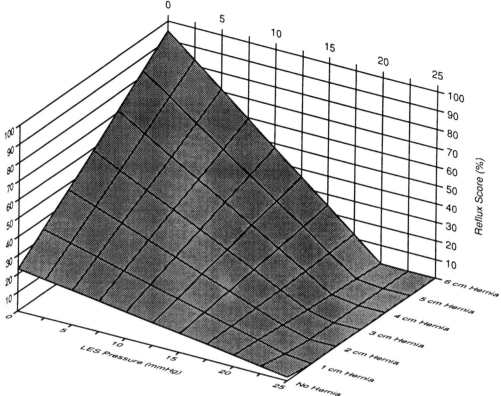

Figure 8-8. Model of the relationship between lower esophageal sphincter (LES) pressure, size of hernia, and the susceptibility to gastroesophageal reflux induced by provocative maneuvers as reflected by the reflux score. The overall equation of the model is Reflux score = 22.64 + 12.05 (Hernia size) − 0.83 (LES pressure) − 0.65 (LES pressure × Hernia size). The hernia size is in centimeters and the LES pressure is in mm Hg. The multiple correlation coefficient of this equation for the 50-subject data set was 0.86 ($R^2 = 0.75$). (Reprinted with permission from S Sloan, AW Rademaker, PJ Kahrilas. Determinants of gastroesophageal junction incompetence: Hiatus hernia, lower esophageal sphincter, or both? Ann Intern Med 1992;117:977.)

Once a reflux event has occurred, the defensive forces acting to prevent the development of esophagitis are (1) effective esophageal emptying to clear refluxed material from the esophagus, (2) neutralization of refluxed acid by salivary bicarbonate, and (3) an intact mucosal diffusion barrier [53]. The most common aberration encountered in GERD patients is of a prolonged acid clearance time, which is seen in an estimated half of esophagitis patients [56]. An elegant demonstration of the normal mechanism of acid clearance simultaneously assessed volume clearance (elimination of detectable fluid volume from the esophagus) and acid clearance (restoration of esophageal mucosal pH to a value of 4) using 0.1N HCl radiolabeled with technetium sulfur colloid [57]. Esophageal volume clearance almost immediately follows acid instillation but volume clearance does not equate with acid clearance. Rather, the restoration of esophageal pH is achieved in increments with each subsequent swallow. Thus, the normal process of esophageal acid clearance is a two-step process; virtually all acid volume is cleared by esophageal peristalsis, leaving a minimal residue that sustains an acidic pH in the esophageal mucosa until it is neutralized by swallowed saliva.

It follows from the previous discussion that impaired volume clearance in reflux disease results in a prolonged acid clearance time. Two mechanisms of impaired volume clearance have been identified: peristaltic dysfunction [58] and "re-reflux" associated with some hiatal hernias [59, 60]. Peristaltic dysfunction is defined as either failed peristalsis or peristaltic sequences with contractions in the distal esophagus sufficiently feeble to impair esophageal emptying. Aside from prolonging the process of acid clearance, peristaltic dysfunction is also correlated with dysphagia [61]. The prevalence of peristaltic dysfunction increases dramatically with increasing severity of esophagitis, rising from 25% in individuals with mild esophagitis to 50% in patients with severe esophagitis. Hiatal hernias impair esophageal emptying by re-reflux from the hernia sac during swallowing. This is particularly problematic in patients with nonreducing hernias, and these patients have the greatest impairment of both esophageal volume clearance and acid clearance.

Therapy of reflux esophagitis is aimed at improving esophageal acid clearance, decreasing the acidity of refluxed material, and increasing gastroesophageal junction competence [62]. Postural maneuvers (elevating the head of the bed 6–8 inches and remaining in an upright posture after meals) employ gravity to aid in esophageal clearance. Chewing gum or using oral lozenges increase both saliva production and swallowing frequency, thereby speeding esophageal acid clearance. Antacids reduce the acidity of refluxed material, bathe the esophagus in neutralizing solution, and promote salivation. H2 blockers, or more recently, omeprazole, diminish the causticity of the refluxate. Cisapride speeds gastric emptying so that there is less material to reflux. Bethanechol increases salivation. Helpful dietary measures are to avoid specific substances (fats, chocolate, alcohol, cigarettes, peppermint, and caffeine) that are known to decrease LES pressure and to refrain from eating just before going to bed. In most cases, diet (including weight loss), postural maneuvers, and antacids are adequate therapy. However, as detailed in the following section, it is unlikely that severe disease will respond to nonpharmacologic therapy.

A constant feature of the recent pharmacologic trials of therapy for peptic esophagitis is the propensity for endoscopic recurrence of mucosal lesions after the discontinuation of antisecretory therapy [63]. This is particularly true if the initial severity of mucosal disease was endoscopically grade 2 or worse, and the rationale for treating grade 2 or worse disease differently than mild disease is because of its tendency to recur. Data from Hetzel et al. demonstrated that with the complete discontinuation of antisecretory therapy, 80% recurrence of mucosal disease can be anticipated within 180 days. This finding has led to wide experimentation with various schemes of maintenance therapy [64–68].

Analyzing the data from these pharmacologic trials inevitably leads to the conclusion that if the maintenance of mucosal healing is the object of therapy, the level of antisecretory therapy required for maintenance must equal that used for healing. Use of a lesser regimen results in a significantly higher relapse rate. What is not immediately evident on first inspection of the data is that each trial selected patients of a given disease severity because they were healed by a particular antisecretory regimen. If patients were not healed by that regimen, they were not entered into the maintenance phase of the trial. Thus, the patients in the trial by Stein et al. healed by famotidine are not equivalent to those in the Koop trial healed by 40 mg/day omeprazole, and one would not anticipate good maintenance results if the Koop patients were maintained on famotidine.

Another maintenance treatment option available for the patient with severe esophagitis is antireflux surgery. The surgical solution has the appeal of being a potentially permanent solution, freeing the patient of all disease-related limitations. Clearly, this laudable goal is achieved by some surgeons with some patients. However, there are few data in the form of an objective quantitative assessment of surgical efficacy. To quote the eminent British surgeon, Bancewicz, regarding efficacy data on antireflux surgery, "Unfortunately, reading the surgical literature and talking to disillusioned gastroenterologists does not inspire confidence. It is clear that the methods of assessment and definitions of success vary widely and it is tempting to suggest that some publications are designed more to bolster the confidence of the surgeon than to find out how the patient is feeling" [69]. These reservations aside, the best controlled data on antireflux surgery are those recently published by Spechler et al. [70]. In that study, limited medical therapy (devised in the pre-omeprazole era) was compared with surgery in a well-controlled blinded design. Fundoplication surgery was done by a limited number of qualified, experienced surgeons who met at the outset of the study and agreed to the particulars of the operation to be employed. All three therapies worked acceptably well in terms of symptom reduction, resolution of esophagitis, and patient satisfaction. The surgical group did marginally better than the medical groups and they accomplished this without any antisecretory therapy. Hence, one must conclude that surgery can work quite nicely in patients with severe esophagitis. It is, however, unlikely that the surgical group would have done any better than the medical group had omeprazole been used as the continuous medical therapy. Nonetheless, a strong argument for surgery can be made in the following circumstances: (1) failed medical therapy with demonstrable, persistent, symptomatic esophagitis (the ubiquitous 10%); (2) medical "success" but at too high a cost in a young, relatively healthy patient; or (3) problematic symptoms from regurgitation (laryngitis, asthma). On the other hand, a strong argument can be made against surgery in other circumstances: (1) elderly patients with substantial concomitant disease; (2) patients with poor or absent peristaltic function who might incur problematic dysphagia; (3) patients with highly functional symptoms likely to be made worse or blamed on surgical intervention; and (4) lack of available necessary antireflux surgery expertise.

Stomach

Physiologically, the stomach serves as a reservoir for ingested food and as a grinder, sieve, and pump to deliver food into the duodenum. Consider each function in turn. With filling, the gastric fundus relaxes to accommodate the increased volume, a process called receptive relaxation, which is mediated by a vagovagal reflex and allows ingested food to be stored in the fundus. For efficient enzymatic digestion and small bowel absorption of nutrients, the ingested food must be reduced to less than 1-mm particles and introduced slowly into the small bowel. The gastric antrum and pylorus accomplish this function. Repetitive concentric peristaltic contractions originate in the proximal gastric body and propel the chyme toward the pyloric aperture in the distal stomach. The larger particles settle out and are recirculated, whereas the smaller ones traverse the pylorus. The mechanical shearing force in the fluid reduces the larger particles so that they may pass into the duodenum during later contractions. Thus, under vagal influence, the dynamic antrum and pylorus serve as a pump, grinder, and sieve to feed the duodenum.

Outflow from the stomach is closely regulated by feedback inhibition from chemoreceptors and osmoreceptors in the duodenum so that the caloric and osmotic content of food entering the intestine is controlled. Fat, glucose, and hypertonic fluids markedly inhibit gastric emptying and stimulate pyloric contraction. Neural reflexes and possibly gastrointestinal hormones mediate gastric emptying by determining fundic tone, antral contractility, pyloric diameter, duodenal segmentation, and gastroduodenal coordination [71]. Gastric emptying can be assessed by a radionuclide scan of labeled solid and liquid meals. In normal subjects, the time required to empty half of a solid meal is less than 120 minutes, whereas a liquid meal requires less than 60 minutes.

The food particles that cannot be mechanically reduced into 1 mm or less are retained in the stomach until the fasting state. About 2 hours after the meal, the motility of the stomach converts from the fed state, as described previously, to a fasting state. Under the influence of motilin, a gastrointestinal hormone, a series of contractile waves, known as the migrating motor complex, originates from the proximal gastric body every 60–90 minutes and propagates distally, sweeping any remaining large food particles into the duodenum. This gastric "housekeeping" activity that occurs after each meal prevents the accumulation of mechanically unreducible material in the stomach.

Diabetic Gastroparesis

Delayed gastric emptying can be caused by anatomic or functional abnormalities. Autonomic neuropathy due to diabetes is the most commonly encountered cause of delayed gastric emptying accompanied by symptoms of nausea, vomiting, bloating, weight loss, or early satiety. Other signs of peripheral or autonomic neuropathies are a "stocking-glove" paresthesia or orthostatic hypotension. Because gastric emptying of solids is dependent on the grinding action of the antral contraction, solid food emptying is affected initially in gastroparesis whereas liquid emptying remains normal. In severe cases of diabetic gastroparesis, both liquid and solid emptying can be affected. The migrating motor complex or gastric "housekeeper" is also often reduced or absent, causing larger mechanically unreducible food particles to accumulate in the stomach and form bezoars. Because episodes of hyperglycemia can aggravate the gastric dysmotility, treatment begins with improving glucose control. A variety of prokinetic medicines are available: cholinergic agonists (i.e., metoclopramide [72], domperidone [73], and cisapride [74]) and a motilin receptor agonist (i.e., erythromycin [75]). Paradoxically, symptomatic improvement in gastroparesis often does not correlate with objective evidence of improved gastric emptying. Especially in the case of metoclopramide, the agent can suppress the nausea by a CNS mechanism without having an impact on gastric emptying. Patients with severe, refractory gastroparesis have been managed surgically by pyloroplasty or partial gastrectomy. Nutritional support is discussed in Chapter 6.

Postsurgical Gastric Emptying Disorders

Historically, selective vagotomy or truncal vagotomy was an integral part of the surgical treatment of peptic ulcer disease. The desired effect of vagotomy is to reduce gastric acid secretion; however, denervation impairs contractile activity of the stomach and duodenum as well. Truncal vagotomy denervates the entire stomach and pylorus. Selective gastric vagotomy is limited to the acid-secreting portions of the stomach (fundus and corpus). The motor effect of a selective vagotomy is to impair receptive relaxation of the fundus and corpus, thereby hindering gastric accommodation to an ingested meal. Consequently, the liquid portion of a meal that is normally stored in the proximal stomach is rapidly emptied. The motor effect of truncal vagotomy is disruption of the antral pumping and grinding, resulting in delayed gastric emptying of solid food and mandating that a concomitant gastric drainage procedure (pyloroplasty or antrectomy) be done concurrently [76]. On the other hand, a selective gastric vagotomy typically does not require a concomitant drainage procedure, which can result in premature and rapid emptying of gastric contents, exacerbating rather than alleviating the effects of vagotomy in some patients.

Approximately 5–10% of patients undergoing truncal vagotomy and pyloroplasty (or antrectomy) will have chronic abdominal cramping and diarrhea related to rapid gastric emptying [77]. These symptoms may be associated with systemic symptoms resulting from hypovolemia (flushing, palpitations, hypotension), often referred to as "early dumping syndrome." Other symptoms related to the aftereffects of an oversecretion of insulin in the immediate postprandial period (hypoglycemia, palpitations, sweating) are referred to as "late dumping syndrome."

Patients with disabling symptoms due to a dumping syndrome are instructed on dietary measures that delay the delivery of hyperosmolar loads to the small intestine. General measures include frequent, small meals with a high protein to carbohydrate ratio and refraining from the simultaneous consumption of liquids and solids. Although many ingenious surgical procedures have been devised to correct dumping syndrome, none have gained wide acceptance, and in general, they should be avoided.

Small Bowel

In the broadest sense, the postprandial function of small intestinal motor function is to mix food with digestive enzymes, bile, and fluids, and then to disperse the mixture across the absorptive mucosal surface. In the interdigestive period, on the other hand, the motor activity functions to sweep clean the small intestinal lumen of indigestible debris. Thus, like the stomach, the small intestine also has two distinct motility patterns: the fed pattern and the fasting pattern. Both motility patterns are orchestrated by the enteric nervous system, the meshwork of autonomic neurons situated between the muscular layers of the intestine. Switching between the patterns of small intestinal contractility is probably accomplished by the action of enteric peptides. Serum motilin levels characteristically increase with the initiation of the migration motor complex, probably functioning to coordinate the LES and stomach with the fasting intestinal contractile activity. The entry of nutrients into the small intestine causes a rapid reversion to the fed contractile pattern, characterized by segmentation; the unorganized, non-propagated local contractions of individual intestinal segments causing the mixing and to-and-fro movement of luminal contents. The fasting pattern of small intestinal motility is characterized by a migrating motor complex that completes a cycle approximately every 90 minutes and is characterized by a propagated contractile front going from duodenum to ileum. This sweeping activity serves to empty the indigestible residua from the small intestinal lumen [78]. The migrating motor complex is also thought to prevent the development of small bowel overgrowth by colonic bacteria.

Superior Mesenteric Artery Syndrome

In any instance of apparent intestinal obstruction that is characterized by postprandial vomiting and pain, mechanical obstruction of the gut needs to be considered. In the disabled population, as in any population, adhesions from previous surgery, malignancies, and incarcerated hernias represent some of the most common causes of intestinal obstruction. An additional consideration in chronically disabled or bedridden individuals is the superior mesenteric artery syndrome. The superior mesenteric artery, traveling with the mesentery, traverses the small bowel at, and actually defines the division between, the third and fourth portion of the duodenum. In individuals who have incurred significant weight loss, thereby decreasing their mesenteric fat, the superior mesenteric artery stretches like a bowstring across the duodenum and can be obstructive. The obstruction is complete when the individual is supine and can be relieved by an upright posture. Superior mesenteric artery syndrome is demonstrable radiographically by the characteristic cutoff between the third and fourth portions of the duodenum, eliminated by altering posture. Figure 8-9 illustrates the radiographic findings in a case of superior mesenteric artery syndrome.

Small Bowel Motility Disorders: Idiopathic Intestinal Pseudo-obstruction

Intestinal motility disorders associated with stasis comprise two broad categories: neuropathic and myopathic. Chronic idiopathic intestinal pseudo-obstruction is an example of a neurologic disorder affecting the intrinsic nervous system. A common symptom of an intestinal motility disorder is of frequent, intermittent episodes of abdominal disten-

tion. A radiographic film of the abdomen discloses air and fluid levels suggestive of a mechanical obstruction. Conservative medical management includes nasogastric suction fasting, correction of dehydration or electrolyte depletion, and nutritional support. In the initial evaluation, mechanical obstruction must be excluded and an underlying condition must be sought. Common causes of pseudo-obstruction include drugs (narcotics, tricyclic antidepressants, alpha-adrenergic agonists, and calcium channel blockers); infection (gram-negative bacterial sepsis); heavy metal poisoning (lead); paraneoplastic syndrome (small cell carcinoma of the lung); and endocrine (hypothyroidism), metabolic (hypercalcemia), and collagen vascular diseases (scleroderma). Exploratory laparotomy may sometimes be necessary to exclude mechanical obstruction. In instances in which no mechanical obstruction or metabolic derangement exists, the apparent obstruction may result from poorly understood small intestinal motor defects. Unfortunately, the rare diagnosis of intestinal motility disorder is usually considered only after multiple laparotomies have been performed, making it even more difficult to distinguish between mechanical obstruction from adhesions and a primary motor disorder.

Small bowel manometry can assist in the differentiation of neuropathic (e.g., chronic intestinal pseudo-obstruction) and myopathic (e.g., hollow visceral myopathy) processes that result in dysmotility. Manometric recordings show normal amplitude, but uncoordinated contraction in the case of extrinsic or intrinsic neuropathic disorders; in contrast, low amplitude but normally coordinated intestinal phasic pressure activity is characteristic of myopathic disorders [79]. Ultimately, however, the diagnosis of chronic intestinal pseudo-obstruction can only be made by silver staining full-thickness biopsy specimens of the gut and demonstrating abnormalities of the myenteric plexus. In the cases of visceral myopathies, abnormal intestinal smooth muscle is seen on small bowel biopsy specimens [80].

The differentiation of neuropathic and myopathic processes can help to formulate the management strategy. In myopathic disorders, treatment includes antibiotics for bacterial overgrowth and consideration of surgical decompression or surgical resection of segmental disease. In contrast, prokinetic drugs are the mainstay of treatment for neuropathic disorders. Pharmacologic agents aimed at

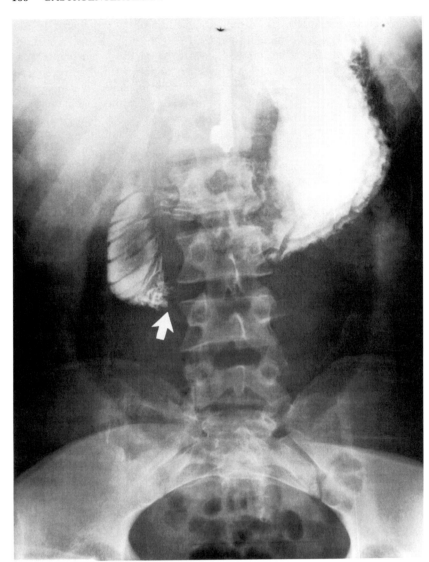

Figure 8-9. Radiographic appearance of superior mesenteric artery syndrome. The stomach and first parts of the duodenum are distended with barium, but there is a sharp cutoff at the junction (arrow) between the third and fourth portions of the duodenum, corresponding to the crossing of the superior mesenteric artery. (Courtesy of Richard Gore, M.D.)

restoring normal intestinal propulsion include cisapride, erythromycin, and octreotide. Cisapride [81] and octreotide [82] can be effective in restoring small intestinal transit time, inducing migrating motor complex, and improving symptoms. Nutritional support is paramount and is tailored to the severity of the motility disorders. An enteral diet of low-lactose, low-fiber polypeptide is usually successful in those with mild-to-moderate symptoms. Patients with severe motility disorder require home parenteral nutrition when dietary and medical treat-

ments are ineffective and surgery is not indicated. Parental nutrition continues to be the mainstay of treatment for patients with myopathic pseudo-obstruction, in whom prokinetic agents are unlikely to be beneficial.

Colon and Anorectum

Constipation and fecal incontinence are common gastrointestinal complaints in disabled patients. To

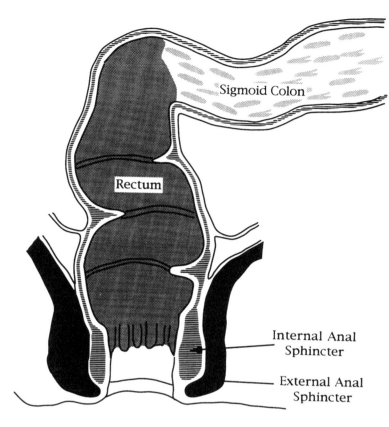

Figure 8-10. Anal sphincters. The internal anal sphincter is contiguous with the distal end of the circular smooth muscle layer of the colon. Tonic contraction of the internal anal sphincter generates the majority of the resting anal tone. Rectal distention produces a transient relaxation of the internal sphincter mediated by the enteric nervous system: myenteric and Auerbach's plexus. The external anal sphincter is a group of concentric striated muscle fiber that is part of the pelvic floor. This muscle surrounds the anal canal and overlaps with the internal anal sphincter, contributing to the anal tone at rest. During periods of stress where the intra-abdominal pressure is increased, the external anal sphincter contracts to augment the anal tone and prevent fecal incontinence.

understand the pathophysiology of these conditions, some appreciation of the normal physiology is necessary. The lower gastrointestinal tract is best described as two functional units: (1) the right colon reabsorbs water and electrolytes; and (2) the left colon (descending and sigmoid colon) together with the anorectum serve as the storage compartment, allowing the desiccated feces to be eliminated in a socially appropriate manner.

Approximately 1,000 ml of effluent is normally delivered through the ileocecal valve to the cecum and the right colon each day. Efficient reabsorption of water and electrolyte must occur in order to reduce the fecal stream to the normal volume of less than 200 ml per day. The uncoordinated, brief contractions of the circular colonic smooth muscles produce local contractions called segmentation. This action causes a to-and-fro mixing motion of the stool to facilitate water and electrolyte absorption by the colonic mucosa. The aboral movement of the fecal matter is achieved through coordinated contractions of the circular and longitudinal smooth muscles called giant migrating contractions. Such contractions cause mass movement that propels fecal matter from one colonic segment to another and can occur just before defecation [83]. However, the movement of feces into the distal colon does not always trigger defecation. As the feces enter the rectum, a combination of reflexive continence mechanisms and voluntary control can suppress the defecatory urge, storing the stool for later elimination.

The mechanical barrier of the anorectal continence mechanism consists of (1) the internal anal sphincter, which is contiguous with the distal end of the tubular colon, (2) the striated muscle of the external sphincter (Figure 8-10), and (3) the puborectalis muscle. The tonic activity of the smooth muscle internal sphincter maintains a resting high

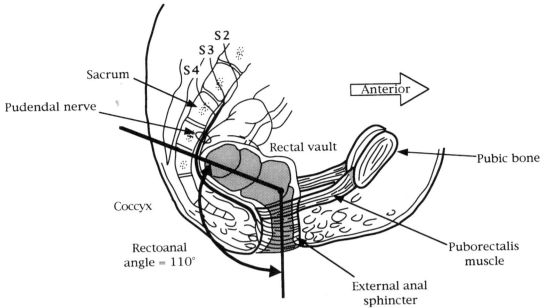

Figure 8-11. Mechanism of continence. The high compliance of the rectum permits the rectal vault to accommodate increasing volumes with minimal increases in compartmental pressure and effectively store the fecal material. The puborectalis forms a sling around the anal canal. The rectoanal angle formed by the tonic contraction of the puborectalis impairs the passage of stool from the rectal vault into the anal canal. The tonic contraction of the external and internal anal sphincters produces the resting tone in the anal canal. The rectoanal reflex coordinates the interaction of these continence mechanisms. When stool enters the rectum, the stretch stimuli produces a relaxation of the internal anal sphincter mediated by the local enteric nervous system. The stool is allowed to enter the proximal anal canal. Sensory nerve endings in the anal canal sense the fecal threat. The afferent signal is carried by the pudendal nerve to S2 to S4 and triggers the "rectoanal reflex." This spinal reflex sends an efferent response back down the pudendal nerve and augments the external anal sphincter, increasing the anal tone. Simultaneously, the consciousness is alerted to the presence of the stored feces.

pressure zone in the anal canal, preventing the passage of stool. The puborectalis muscle (Figure 8-11) forms a sling around the anal canal and under tonic activity pulls the anal canal to an acute angle of typically less than 100 degrees, sealing the anal canal from the rectum and providing mechanical resistance against distal propulsion of feces [84, 85]. At rest, the activity of the internal sphincter and the puborectalis sling afford the majority of continence; however, certain physical activities such as coughing or lifting can increase intra-abdominal pressure and stress the mechanism, leading to incontinence. Additional reflexes are called into play. The pelvic diaphragm together with the external sphincter and puborectalis contract, augmenting the sphincter pressure and decreasing the already sharp angle of the anal canal [85]. Through these measures, the

anorectum maintains continence at rest and during conditions of stress.

The storage function of the anorectum is equally important in controlling defecation. As stool enters the rectum and distends the rectal vault, smooth muscle of the internal sphincter relaxes reflexively [86], allowing the stool to descend into the proximal anal canal. The anal canal is densely innervated by sensory receptors that trigger a reflexive contraction of the external anal sphincter, preventing the stool from descending further into the anal canal [87]. This rectoanal inhibitory reflex is a locally mediated spinal response where the sensory input is carried by the pudendal nerve to spinal cord segments (L4 to S1) and the efferent response also returns via the pudendal nerve to the external anal sphincter. The highly compliant rectum stretches to accommodate the added stool volume and maintains a relatively low pressure as compared with the higher pressure in the anal canal. As the rectum distends, a sensory message is conveyed centrally, alerting the individual to the presence of stool. If the conditions are socially acceptable, the person may defecate or alternatively suppress the urge.

Defecation is aided by assuming a squatting position, during which hip flexion straightens the acute angle of the anal canal made by the puborectalis sling. The puborectalis and the external sphincter are then relaxed. Valsalva's maneuver increases intra-abdominal pressure and forces the stool down the anal canal. A giant migrating contraction may be initiated at the mid or distal colon to evacuate feces from the sigmoid colon and higher up [88, 89]. Thus, the anorectal continence mechanism depends on a complex interplay of sphincters, rectal compliance, and crucial anatomy that is mediated by a local spinal reflex and is controlled by the consciousness. A defect in any of the factors of the continence mechanism can lead to constipation or fecal incontinence.

Fecal Incontinence

Fecal incontinence can be a severe, psychologically disabling condition leading to social isolation. As discussed previously, fecal continence is maintained by a host of cognitive and physiologic factors. Hence, a variety of conditions can compromise the continence mechanisms. An important element of the history is whether the stool is solid or liquid. Severe diarrheal disease of any cause can produce a sufficiently large volume of liquid stool to overwhelm even a normal continence mechanism. Mild defects in the continence mechanism may result in fecal incontinence only during conditions of stress such as laughing, coughing, sneezing, or lifting. The common effect of these activities is to increase intra-abdominal pressure, overwhelming the continence mechanism and leading to stress incontinence. Liquid stool incontinence is also a consequence of fecal impaction. Fecal incontinence occurs as liquid stool flows around the impacted stool. Diminished awareness associated with Alzheimer's disease, drug sedation, dementia, or immobility may also lead to fecal impaction. Functional immobility can prevent one from reaching an appropriate setting to defecate. Spinal cord lesions (traumatic or mass lesions) can impair the sensory awareness of rectal filling and cause incontinence. Careful neurologic examination will usually reveal cord signs in the lower extremities.

Anorectal surgery can result in fecal incontinence. A variety of common procedures including rectal tears during vaginal delivery, hemorrhoidectomy, or fistulectomy can disrupt the internal and external anal sphincter and impair the continence mechanism. The most common scenario of incontinence occurs in elderly multiparous women. Studies have suggested that their prior multiple "uneventful" vaginal deliveries may have caused mechanical trauma to the anal sphincter and repetitive stretch injury to the pudendal nerve as the fetus traversed the pelvic diaphragm during its passage through the birth canal [90]. The resultant pudendal neuropathy impairs the afferent and efferent signals responsible for rectal sensation and anal sphincter tone. Similar peripheral neuropathy of the pudendal nerve is believed to be the cause of fecal incontinence in the diabetic patient.

Anorectal manometry is useful in assessing rectal sensation, basal anal sphincter tone, and the ability to volitionally augment the anal sphincter. An individual is normally able to sense a rectal volume of less than 30 ml. The threshold for rectal sensation is tested through graded inflation of a rectal balloon that also assesses the afferent, efferent, and spinal components of the rectoanal inhibitory reflex [91, 92]. The finding of decreased resting anal sphincter tone and a poor voluntary "squeeze" anal pressure (decreased voluntary augmentation of the sphincter tone) in a multiparous woman with incontinence is consistent with anal sphincter trauma during vaginal births [90]. Similarly the manometric findings of decreased rectal sensation and poor voluntary augmentation of the anal sphincter pressure in a diabetic patient with incontinence suggest diabetic neuropathy. Anorectal manometry can be useful in confirming the clinical impression.

Treatment of fecal incontinence is most frustrating in patients with a neuropathic cause (e.g., diabetic neuropathy or pudendal stretch injury from obstetric trauma) because the damage is irreparable. Biofeedback sessions that train the subjects to increase their sensory awareness of rectal distention during balloon inflation and to voluntarily respond by maximally contracting their external anal sphincter may be of some benefit. Through progressively

Table 8-2. Causes of Constipation in the Elderly

Misperception
  Misinterpretation
  Psychogenic
Dietary causes
  Low fiber intake
  Poor fluid intake
  Reduced caloric intake
Functional causes
  Depression
  Confusion, weakness
  Inadequate toilet arrangements
  Immobility
Secondary causes
  Neuromuscular disorders: scleroderma, hollow visceral
    myopathy
  Chronic intestinal pseudo-obstruction
  Endocrine disorders: hypothyroidism, hyperthyroidism
  Colonic obstruction: tumors, diverticulitis, radiation
    strictures, ischemia, volvulus
Medications
  Aluminum-containing antacids
  Narcotic analgesics
  Anticholinergic agents, antidepressants
  Iron, bismuth, diuretics

smaller rectal distention volumes, sensory awareness of stool in the rectum is enhanced. In the process, the subjects also strengthen their external anal sphincter. Centers experienced with this technique report complete continence or substantial reduction of spontaneous incontinence in about 70% of the patients who can be trained [93]. Appropriate patient selection is important. Good candidates for anal biofeedback training should be able to follow instructions, have some degree of rectal sensation, be motivated to follow the training program, and have the ability to voluntarily contract their external anal sphincter.

Modifying stool consistency can also be used as a treatment of incontinence. Because the continence mechanism handles solid stool more effectively than liquid stool, subjects with mild incontinence may respond by simply converting their stool from a liquid to a solid consistency. This can be achieved by dietary fiber supplements or antidiarrheal agents such as loperamide.

Surgical management of incontinence should be considered in patients who fail medical therapy or who have altered anorectal anatomy such as rectal prolapse. Sphincteroplasty, which involves resection of scarred sphincteric muscle and reapproximation of viable sphincter to recreate an intact ring of muscle, appears to be the best choice for incontinence due to obstetric, traumatic, and iatrogenic disruption of the external anal sphincter [94]. In general, sphincteroplasty along with other surgical procedures have unpredictable results and have been associated with a variable outcome. Patients with coexisting neurologic defects tend to do worse. Unfortunately no prospective randomized studies have analyzed this group to determine other preoperative characteristics that may influence the surgical outcome.

Constipation: Symptoms, Causes, and Treatment

The symptom of constipation must be carefully interpreted because it can mean infrequent defecation, excessive straining, a sense of incomplete evacuation, too small stools, or too hard stools. Most commonly, however, constipation refers to infrequent defecation. Special attention should be given to elderly patients who experience a recent change in their bowel habits. This symptom can represent partial obstruction by a colonic malignancy and warrants stool hemoccult test, a colonoscopy, or a barium enema study. Those patients with life-long symptoms of constipation may have a more benign course such that extensive evaluation is not necessary. Other causes of constipation include dietary factors, functional factors, systemic diseases, and medications (Table 8-2).

Serious concerns should be given to patients with constipation associated with findings of abdominal distention or tenderness. A digital rectal examination may reveal fecal impaction as the cause of obstruction. In the elderly, who may be poorly communicative, rectal examination may reveal inflamed hemorrhoids, tender anal fissures, or a perirectal abscess that may cause rectal pain and a reluctance to defecate. A plain abdominal roentgenogram is sometimes helpful, showing either fecal matter filling the left colon in the case of fecal impaction, or the "bird's beak" taper of a sigmoid volvulus (Figures 8-12 and 8-13). The roentgenogram can also indicate colonic distention that can result in colonic perforation (Figure 8-14). Perforation risk increases

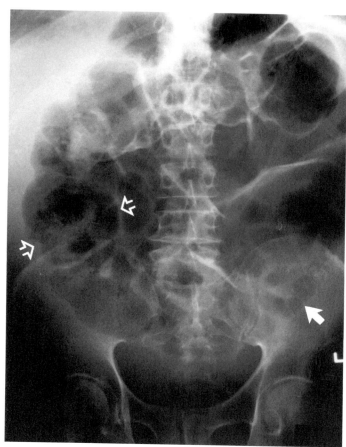

Figure 8-12. Colonic obstruction. This abdominal roentgenogram of an elderly man with constipation and abdominal distention shows dilated colonic segments (between open arrows) filled with air and feces. Loops of air-filled small bowel can be seen over the left iliac crest (closed arrow). These radiographic features can be seen in any causes of obstruction: fecal impaction, obstructing carcinoma, sigmoid volvulus, etc. Fecal impaction usually shows large amount of fecal material filling the rectum and left colon; such a finding is absent in this roentgenogram. (Courtesy of Scott Wu, M.D.)

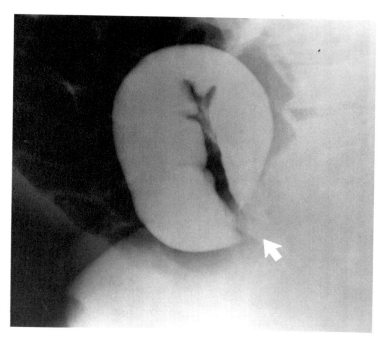

Figure 8-13. Sigmoid volvulus. In this roentgenogram, liquid barium contrast has been instilled rectally and can be seen filling the closed loop of the sigmoid segment. The mobile sigmoid colon has torsed on itself, forming a closed loop obstruction, a sigmoid volvulus. Both ends of the loop taper to a point (arrow) and represent the axial twisting on the rectum and the proximal sigmoid. An open loop obstruction occurs above the torsion point of the sigmoid colon. This patient was treated with immediate endoscopic decompression and untwisting of the sigmoid loop. The diagnosis of sigmoid volvulus can be made without rectal barium instillation when a similar air-filled sigmoid loop is recognized in the left lower quadrant of an abdominal roentgenogram. (Courtesy of Scott Wu, M.D.)

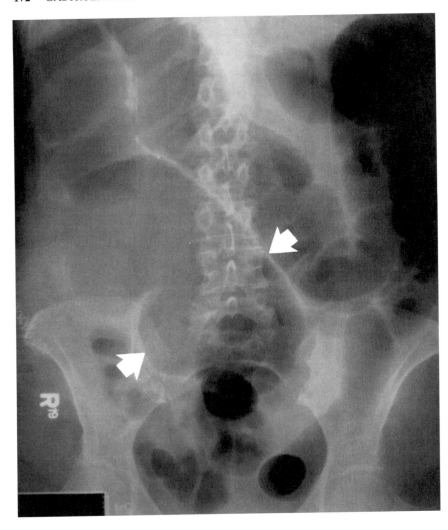

Figure 8-14. Colonic ileus with massive dilation. This postoperative patient has a paralytic colonic ileus from excessive narcotic use. The abdominal roentgenogram demonstrates massively dilated colon and cecum. The cecum, measuring approximately 12 cm (between arrows), is at risk for perforation. The patient was treated with endoscopic decompression of colonic air and stool. Subsequent narcotic use was minimized and electrolyte abnormalities were corrected. The diagnosis of postoperative paralytic ileus is made on clinical grounds. In some cases, the clinical picture and abdominal roentgenogram can be identical to colonic obstruction and obstructive etiologies must be excluded (by endoscopy or barium contrast studies). (Courtesy of Gary G. Ghahremani, M.D.)

when the diameter of the colon or the cecum exceeds 8 or 10 cm, respectively. Fecal impaction is treated with digital disimpaction, laxatives, or enemas. One recommended therapy for fecal impaction is the 3 to 2 to 1 regimen with a stool softener (docusate sodium, 100 mg orally 3 times a day), colonic stimulant (senna tablets, 2 orally each day 8 hours before bowel routine), and rapidly acting rectal stimulant (bisacodyl enema, 1 each day after a meal) to trigger the routine [95]. Sigmoid volvulus can be successfully resolved with an endoscope. Whatever the cause of the distention may be, the underlying condition should be treat promptly to prevent further colonic dilation and potential perforation.

Most patients with constipation can be treated with dietary modification and correction of the underlying condition (i.e., hypothyroidism or discontinuing the offending medication). The patients who are more difficult to treat should be considered for further evaluation with flexible endoscopy, colonic transit, evacuation proctography (defecography), and anorectal manometry.

Colonic transit is measured by tracking ingested radiopaque markers through the colon with sequential abdominal radiographs over several days. Most normal subjects pass the markers within approximately 70 hours [96, 97]. Persistence of markers in the distal colon or the rectum suggests a distal colonic or anorectal dysfunction [98, 99]. Transit studies are also useful to assess subjects who misperceive or misrepresent their symptoms [99, 100]. Defecography is a technique to assess the anorectal dynamics. The evacuation of a thick barium paste is studied under videofluoroscopy. The efficacy of rectal emptying and rectal diameter and any abnormalities may be seen only during straining. These include intussusceptions, rectoceles, excessive perineal descent, and insufficient puborectalis relaxation. Anorectal manometry can identify rare cases of adult Hirschsprung's disease when the internal anal sphincter fails to relax during rectoanal inhibitory reflex testing. Inappropriate contraction of the puborectalis muscle during voluntary straining is indicative of pelvic floor dyssynergy.

Management of Constipation

Studies of institutionalized elderly have shown that the addition of supplemental fiber and fluids improves constipation [101, 102]. There is no evidence that constipated subjects have a lower dietary fiber intake, but it is commonly believed that their symptoms are related to poor toilet habits and dietary deficiencies. In normal subjects, the addition of fiber supplements increases stool weight, shortens transit time, and increases frequency of defecation. Laxatives represent the next level of therapy. There are several classes of laxatives: stimulants, lubricants, osmotic agents, and stool softeners. Each class of laxative has a different mode of action. Osmotic laxatives such as sorbitol and lactulose are nonabsorbable agents that produce an osmotic diarrhea. Stimulant laxatives (senna, phenolphthalein, bisacodyl) produce propagating propulsive waves when applied topically. Long-term use of these agents can cause degeneration of the myenteric plexus or fluid electrolyte disturbances. Mineral oil works as a lubricant but can cause malabsorption of fat-soluble vitamins. Rectal enemas of tap water or sodium phosphate and biphosphate may be necessary to treat fecal impaction.

Diarrhea: Symptoms, Causes, and Treatment

Similar to constipation, diarrhea represents a constellation of symptoms ranging from an abnormal increase in stool volume (normally <200 ml/day), an

Table 8-3. Categories of Diarrhea

Infectious diarrhea
  Viral
  Bacterial: Enterotoxic *Escherichia coli, Campylobacter*
  Protozoan: *Giardia*, amoebae
Osmotic diarrhea
  Lactase deficiency
  Magnesium-containing agents
  Malabsorbed sugars: lactulose, sorbitol
Secretory diarrhea
  Bile acid malabsorption
  Bacterial overgrowth causing bile acid deficiency
  Pancreatic exocrine insufficiency with steatorrhea
Inflammatory diarrhea
  Acute/chronic radiation enteritis
  Inflammatory bowel disease: Crohn's disease and
    ulcerative colitis
Laxative-induced diarrhea
  Colonic stimulants
Rapid transit diarrhea
  Short bowel syndrome
  Chronic radiation enteritis
  Enterocolonic fistula
Obstructive diarrhea
  Fecal impaction
  Colonic tumor
  Strictures

abnormal increase in stool liquidity, or an abnormal increase in stool frequency often accompanied by urgency, perineal discomfort, or incontinence. Technically, diarrhea is defined on the basis of stool volume whereas abnormalities of bowel pattern or consistency are indicative of functional bowel difficulties. The causes of diarrhea are numerous (Table 8-3) and this discussion is focused on those common in disabled patients. Of the various causes of acute diarrhea, most are self-limited, resolving within 24–48 hours. No pathogens are usually identified even after extensive evaluation. Furthermore, even if an organism is isolated on stool culture, antibiotic therapy is not warranted for such self-limited infections. Therefore, the most cost-effective strategy is observation and supportive measures. If, however, the patient is severely ill, immunocompromised, or appears toxic, stool cultures can be obtained and empiric antibiotics (trimethoprim-sulfamethoxazole or ciprofloxacin) started. In controlled studies, antibiotic therapy use in immunocompetent ambulatory subjects does not shorten the symptom duration. The effect on the frequency of bacteremia and mortality in chronically disabled subjects is unclear. Widespread antibiotic use can lead to the emergence of resistant bacterial strains or, in the case of *Salmonella*, development of carrier status.

Clostridium Difficile–*Related Diarrhea*

A common clinical scenario is of diarrhea in an institutionalized subject who may have received antibiotic therapy. A common cause in this setting is *Clostridium difficile* colitis. A recent bacteriologic study of 115 rehabilitation hospital inpatients with diarrhea identified *C. difficile* as the cause in 25% [103]. Other pathogens were rare; no evidence of *Salmonella*, *Shigella*, *Campylobacter*, or *Yersinia* infection was found. Giardiasis was detected in one patient. In the majority of cases, no pathologic organisms could be isolated. This suggests that *C. difficile* is an important cause of diarrhea among rehabilitation hospital inpatients. Stool cultures for *Salmonella*, *Shigella*, *Campylobacter*, *Yersinia*, or *Giardia*, on the other hand, have a very low yield. The investigators suggest that eliminating routine testing for these pathogens would reduce costs without compromising care.

Enzyme immunoassay of stool specimens for *C. difficile* toxin is the most common method for detecting *C. difficile* infection with good sensitivity (69–87%) and specificity (99–100%) [104, 105]. Tissue culture cytotoxin assay for *C. difficile* toxin has a higher sensitivity (94–100%) but the test is expensive and requires overnight incubation of samples. Therapy of *C. difficile* colitis requires discontinuing the offending antibiotic (almost all antibiotics have been implicated) and institution of either oral metronidazole or the more costly vancomycin. Alternatively, mild diarrhea may abate on discontinuing the antibiotics alone and require no further specific therapy. A parenteral alternative is intravenous metronidazole. Relapse of *C. difficile*–related diarrhea is common, recurring in up to 30% of patients after successful initial therapy. A repeat course of metronidazole or vancomycin is usually successful. Many of the institutionalized or hospitalized patients are asymptomatically colonized with *C. difficile*. A study of 428 inpatients showed that 21% became colonized with *C. difficile* organism during their hospital stay [106]. The mode of transmission is presumed to be through health care workers. There is no indication for repeat stool study to document eradication of *C. difficile* because most will remain colonized. Treatment of asymptomatic carriers to control *C. difficile* nosocomial outbreaks is not recommended because treatment is only temporarily effective and recolonization is common after therapy [107]. Prevention is through judicious use of antibiotics, especially clindamycin and other broad-spectrum agents.

Medication-Induced Diarrhea

Medication-induced diarrhea is another common scenario. As part of the initial evaluation, the medication list should also be reviewed. Some of the main culprits are sorbitol in theophylline elixir preparations and laxatives. In addition, diarrhea can be a side effect of antibiotic use, unrelated to *C. difficile* infection. The onset of antibiotic-related diarrhea closely coincides with the use of antibiotics and abates when the antibiotic is discontinued. *C. difficile* infection is rarely associated with diarrhea that begins within 7 days of antibiotic use.

Diet-Related Diarrhea

Dietary factors can also produce diarrhea. Malabsorption due to acquired disaccharidase deficiency, especially lactase deficiency, is common. In the majority of the individuals, the enzyme activity at the brush border of the enterocytes slowly decreases throughout life. Most individuals will begin having mild-to-moderate lactose intolerance later in life [108]. The diagnosis of lactose malabsorption can be made on the results of a lactose hydrogen breath test. This test detects increased hydrogen production from colonic bacterial fermentation of malabsorbed lactose test dose. However, such a test is usually not necessary; improvement of symptoms on a trial of lactose-free diet is sufficient for a presumptive diagnosis.

Individuals on tube feedings of hypertonic commercial enteral formulas, especially those with a jejunostomy feeding tube receiving bolus feeding, can experience an osmotic diarrhea. The uncontrolled delivery of the nutrient directly into the small bowel is presumed to overwhelm the absorptive capacity of the small bowel. In addition to bypassing the controlled delivery system of the stomach, the diarrhea in these individuals may also be related to the relative decrease in the disaccharidase level or abnormal enterocyte transport function that occurs during an acute illness or malnutrition. Bolus feeding into a jejunostomy tube should be changed to a continuous drip feeding program. A trial of an isotonic or half-strength enteral formula may be attempted in the appropriate patients or when an extensive evaluation is unrevealing.

Conclusion

A variety of alimentary disorders are commonly associated with the chronically disabled. Many disabled individuals are elderly; hence, they are susceptible to age-related alimentary disorders. Furthermore, chronic disability, deconditioning, and aging leave these individuals with little functional reserve and increased susceptibility to decompensation during acute illnesses. Homeostasis may be restored when the acute illness is treated. Similar principles hold for the alimentary tract. In many cases, the motility disorder of the alimentary tract (dysphagia, constipation, etc.) is only one sign of a more general illness. Colonic ileus during gram-negative bacterial infection and sepsis presenting as constipation and abdominal distention are classic examples. In other cases, the relation may be more subtle, such as constipation as the presenting symptom of hypercalcemia related to hyperparathyroidism. In both cases, constipation resolves with the treatment of the underlying condition. In these days of polypharmacy, the number of prescribed medications parallels the severity of the patient's illness. With greater pharmacologic exposure, the risk of a medication-related gastrointestinal side effect increases. A common compound in elixir medications is sorbitol, a malabsorbed sugar, that can produce an osmotic diarrhea. So, before embarking on an extensive and often expensive evaluation of a gastrointestinal symptom, a review of medications may reveal the culprit. When confronted with a symptom that suggests a disorder of the alimentary tract, rather than just treating the symptom, iatrogenic causes and underlying conditions should be considered.

References

1. Telford GL, Go VLW, Szurszewski JH. Effect of central sympathectomy on gastric and small intestinal myoelectric activity and plasma motilin concentrations in the dog. Gastroenterology 1985;89:989.
2. Fealey RD, Szurszewski JH, Merritt JL, DiMagno EP. Effect of traumatic spinal cord transection on human upper gastrointestinal motility and gastric emptying. Gastroenterology 1984;87:69.
3. Sinclair WJ. Role of the pharyngeal plexus in initiation of swallowing. Am J Physiol 1971;221:1260.
4. Miller AJ. The search for the central swallowing pathway: The quest for clarity. Dysphagia 1993;8:185.
5. Jean A. Brainstem control of swallowing: Localization and organization of the central pattern generator for swallowing. In A Taylor (ed), Neurophysiology of the Jaws and Teeth. London: Macmillan, 1990.
6. Jean A. Localisation et activité des neurons déglutiteurs bulbaires. J Physiol Paris 1972;64:227.
7. Jean A. Control of the central swallowing program by inputs from the peripheral receptors. A review. J Auton Nerv Syst 1983;7:87.
8. Miller AJ. Deglutition. Physiol Rev 1982;62:129.
9. Martin RE, Sessle BJ. The role of the cerebral cortex in swallowing. Dysphagia 1993;8:195.
10. Kahrilas PJ, Logemann JA, Lin S, Ergun GA. Pharyngeal clearance during swallowing: A combined manometric and videofluoroscopic study. Gastroenterology 1992;103:128.
11. Kahrilas PJ, Logemann JA. Volume accommodation during swallowing. Dysphagia 1993;8:259.
12. Cook IJ, Dodds WJ, Dantas RO, et al. Opening mechanism of the human upper esophageal sphincter. Am J Physiol 1989;257:G748.
13. Jacob P, Kahrilas PJ, Logemann JA, et al. Upper esophageal sphincter opening and modulation during swallowing. Gastroenterology 1989;97:1469.
14. Logemann JA, Kahrilas PJ, Cheng J, et al. Closure mechanisms of the laryngeal vestibule during swallow. Am J Physiol 1992;262:G338.
15. Kahrilas PJ, Dodds WJ, Dent J, et al. Upper esophageal sphincter function during deglutition. Gastroenterology 1988;95:52.
16. Fisher M, Hendrix T, Hurst J, Murrills A. Relation between volume swallowed and velocity of the bolus ejected from the pharynx into the esophagus. Gastroenterology 1978;74:1238.
17. Ekberg O, Olsson R, Sundgren-Borgstrom P. Relation of bolus size and pharyngeal swallow. Dysphagia 1988;3:69.
18. Kier WM, Smith KK. Tongues, tentacles and trunks: The biomechanics of movement in muscular-hydrostats. Zoological Journal of the Linnean Society 1985;83:307.
19. Wein B, Böckler R, Klajman S. Temporal reconstruction of sonographic imaging of disturbed tongue movements. Dysphagia 1991;6:135.

20. Kahrilas PJ, Lin S, Logemann JA, et al. Deglutitive tongue action: Volume accommodation and bolus propulsion. Gastroenterology 1993;104:152.

21. Ergun GA, Kahrilas PJ, Lin S, et al. Shape, volume, and content of the deglutitive pharyngeal chamber imaged by ultrafast computerized tomography. Gastroenterology 1993;105:1396.

22. Wilson CP. Diverticula of the pharynx. J R Coll Surg Edinb 1959;4:236.

23. Goyal RK. Disorders of the cricopharyngeus muscle. Otolaryngol Clin North Am 1984;17:115.

24. Cook IJ, Blumberos P, Cash K, et al. Structural abnormalities of the cricopharyngeus muscle in patients with pharyngeal (Zenker's) diverticulum. J Gastroenterol Hepatol 1992;7:556.

25. Dantas RO, Cook IJ, Dodds WJ, et al. Biomechanics of cricopharyngeal bars. Gastroenterology 1990;99:1269.

26. Cook IJ, Gabb M, Panagopoulos V, et al. Pharyngeal (Zenker's) diverticulum is a disorder of upper esophageal sphincter opening. Gastroenterology 1992;103:1229.

27. Logemann JA, Kahrilas PJ. Relearning to swallow post stroke—Application of maneuvers and indirect biofeedback: A case study. Neurology 1990;40:1136.

28. Kahrilas PJ, Logemann JA, Krugler C, Flanagan E. Volitional augmentation of upper esophageal sphincter opening during swallowing. Am J Physiol 1991;260:G450.

29. Logemann JA, Kahrilas PJ, Kobara M, Vakil NB. The benefit of head rotation on pharyngoesophageal dysphagia. Arch Phys Med Rehabil 1989;70:767.

30. Roman C. Nervous control of peristalsis in the esophagus. J Physiol Paris 1966;58:479.

31. Kravitz JJ, Snape WJ, Cohen S. Effect of thoracic vagotomy and vagal stimulation on esophageal function. Am J Physiol 1966;238:233.

32. Dodds WJ, Christensen J, Dent J, et al. Esophageal contraction induced by vagal stimulation in the opossum. Am J Physiol 1978;235:E392.

33. Goyal RK, Ratan S. Genesis of basal sphincter pressure: Effect of tetrodotoxin on lower esophageal sphincter pressure in opossum in vivo. Gastroenterology 1976;71:62.

34. Conklin JL, Du C, Murray JA, Bates JN. Characterization and mediation of inhibitory junction potentials from opossum lower esophageal sphincter. Gastroenterology 1993;104:1439.

35. Tøttrup A, Svane D, Forman A. Nitric oxide mediating NANC inhibition in opossum lower esophageal sphincter. Am J Physiol 1991;260:G385.

36. Yamato S, Spechler SJ, Goyal RK. Role of nitric oxide in esophageal peristalsis in the opossum. Gastroenterology 1992;103:197.

37. Gonella J, Niel JP, Roman C. Vagal control of lower esophageal motility in the cat. J Physiol (Lond) 1977;273:647.

38. Rattan S, Goyal RK. Neural control of the lower esophageal sphincter: Influence of the vagus nerves. J Clin Invest 1974;54:899.

39. Soergel KH, Zboralske F, Amberg JR. Presbyesophagus: Esophageal motility in nonagenarians. J Clin Invest 1964;43:1472.

40. Schatzki R, Gary JE. Dysphagia due to a diaphragm-like localized narrowing in the lower esophagus (lower esophageal ring). AJR Am J Roentgenol 1953;70:911.

41. Kahrilas PJ, Clouse RE, Hogan WJ. American Gastroenterological Association technical review on clinical use of esophageal manometry. Gastroenterology 1995;109:2053.

42. Kahrilas PJ, Dodds WJ, Hogan WJ. The effect of peristaltic dysfunction on esophageal volume clearance. Gastroenterology 1988;94:73.

43. Kahrilas PJ, Hogan WJ. Gastroesophageal reflux disease. In MH Sleisenger, JS Fordtran (eds), Gastrointestinal Disease: Pathophysiology, Diagnosis, Management (5th ed). Philadelphia: Saunders, 1993;378.

44. Little FB, Kohut RI, Koufman JA, Marshall RB. Effect of gastric acid on the pathogenesis of subglottic stenosis. Ann Otol Rhinol Laryngol 1985;94:516.

45. Malfroot A, Vandenplas Y, Verlinden M, et al. Gastroesophageal acid reflux and unexplained chronic respiratory disease in infants and children. Pediatr Pulmonol 1987;3:208.

46. Harper PC, Bergner A, Kaye MD. Antireflux treatment for asthma: Improvement in patients with associated gastroesophageal acid reflux. Arch Intern Med 1987;147:56.

47. Mays EE, Dubois JJ, Hamilton GB. Pulmonary fibrosis associated with tracheobronchial aspiration. Chest 1976;69:512.

48. Ismail-Beigi F, Horton PF, Pope CE II. Histological consequences of gastroesophageal reflux in man. Gastroenterology 1970;58:163.

49. Dent J, Dodds WJ, Friedman RH, et al. Mechanism of gastroesophageal reflux in recumbent asymptomatic human subjects. J Clin Invest 1980;65:256.

50. Dodds WJ, Dent J, Hogan WJ, et al. Mechanisms of gastroesophageal reflux in patients with reflux esophagitis. N Engl J Med 1982;307:1547.

51. Kahrilas PJ, Dodds WJ, Dent J, et al. Upper esophageal sphincter function during belching. Gastroenterology 1986;91:133.

52. Wyman JB, Dent J, Heddle R, et al. Control of belching by the lower esophageal sphincter. Gut 1990;31:639.

53. Kahrilas PJ. Esophageal motor activity and acid clearance. Gastroenterol Clin North Am 1990;19:537.

54. Mittal RK, Rochester DF, McCallum RW. Sphincteric action of the diaphragm during a relaxed lower esophageal sphincter in humans. Am J Physiol 1989;256:G139.

55. Sloan S, Rademaker AW, Kahrilas PJ. Determinants of gastroesophageal junction incompetence: Hiatus hernia, lower esophageal sphincter, or both? Ann Intern Med 1992;117:977.

56. Johnson LF. 24-Hour pH monitoring in the study of gastroesophageal reflux. J Clin Gastroenterol 1980;2:387.

57. Helm JF, Dodds WJ, Pelc LR, et al. Effect of esophageal emptying and saliva on clearance of acid from the esophagus. N Engl J Med 1984;310:284.

58. Kahrilas PJ, Dodds WJ, Hogan WJ, et al. Esophageal peristaltic dysfunction in peptic esophagitis. Gastroenterology 1986;91:897.

59. Mittal RK, Lange RC, McCallum RW. Identification and mechanism of delayed esophageal acid clearance in subjects with hiatus hernia. Gastroenterology 1987;92:130.

60. Sloan S, Kahrilas PJ. Impairment of esophageal emptying with hiatal hernia. Gastroenterology 1991;100:596.

61. Jacob P, Kahrilas PJ, Vanagunas A. Peristaltic dysfunction associated with nonobstructive dysphagia in reflux disease. Dig Dis Sci 1990;35:932.

62. Sontag SJ. The medical management of reflux esophagitis. Role of antacids and acid inhibition. Gastroenterol Clin North Am 1990;19:683.

63. Hetzel DJ, Dent J, Reed WD, et al. Healing and relapse of severe peptic esophagitis after treatment with omeprazole. Gastroenterology 1988;95:903.

64. Dent J. Australian clinical trials of omeprazole in the management of reflux oesophagitis. Digestion 1990;47:69.

65. Marciano-D'Amore DA, Paterson WG, Da Costa LR, Beck IT. Omeprazole in H2 receptor antagonist-resistant reflux esophagitis. J Clin Gastroenterol 1990;12:616.

66. Lundell L. Prevention of relapse of reflux oesophagitis after endoscopic healing: The efficacy and safety of omeprazole compared with ranitidine. Digestion 1990;47:72.

67. Stein DT, Simon TJ, Berlin RG, et al. Controlling 24 hour esophageal acid exposure in patients with healed erosive esophagitis (EE) prevents recurrence and symptomatic deterioration: Results of a 6 month randomized, double-blind, US, placebo controlled trial comparing famotidine (F) 20 mg bid and 40 mg bid. Gastroenterology 1991:100:A167.

68. Koop H, Arnold R. Long-term maintenance treatment of reflux esophagitis with omeprazole. Prospective study in patients with H2-blocker-resistant esophagitis. Dig Dis Sci 1991;36:552.

69. Banciewicz J. What is the place of surgery in the therapy of reflux esophagitis? Gullet 1993;3(Suppl):85.

70. Spechler SJ, Department of Veterans Affairs Gastroesophageal Reflux Disease Study Group. Comparison of medical and surgical therapy for complicated gastroesophageal reflux disease in veterans. N Engl J Med 1992;326:786.

71. Meyer JH. Motility of the stomach and gastroduodenal junction. In LR Johnson, J Christensen, ED Jacobsen, SG Schultz (eds), Physiology of the Digestive Tract. New York: Raven, 1987;613.

72. Malagelada JR, Rees WDW, Mazzotta LJ, Go VLW. Gastric motor abnormalities in diabetic and postvagotomy gastroparesis: Effect of metoclopramide and bethanechol. Gastroenterology 1980;78:286.

73. Horowitz M, Harding PE, Chatterton BE, et al. Acute and chronic effects of domperidone on gastric emptying in diabetic autonomic neuropathy. Dig Dis Sci 1985;30:1.

74. Horowitz M, Maddox A, Harding PE, et al. Effect of cisapride on gastric and esophageal emptying in insulin-dependent diabetes mellitus. Gastroenterology 1987;92:1899.

75. Janssens J, Peeters TL, Vantrappen G, et al. Improvement of gastric emptying in diabetic gastroparesis by erythromycin. N Engl J Med 1990;322:1028.

76. Binswanger RO, Aeberhard P, Walther M, Vock P. Effect of pyloroplasty on gastric emptying: Long term results as obtained with a labeled test meal 14–43 months after operation. Br J Surg 1978;65:27.

77. Stadaas JO. Gastric motility one year after proximal gastric vagotomy. Scand J Gastroenterol 1980;15:799.

78. Hara Y, Kubota M, Szurszewski JH. Electrophysiology of smooth muscle of the small intestine of some mammals. J Physiol (Lond) 1986;372:501.

79. Colemont LJ, Camilleri M. Chronic intestinal pseudo-obstruction: Diagnosis and treatment. Mayo Clin Proc 1989;64:60.

80. Krishnamurthy S, Schuffler MD. Pathology of neuromuscular disorders of the small intestine and colon. Gastroenterology 1987;93:610.

81. Camilleri M, Brown ML, Malagelada J-R. Impaired transit of chyme in chronic intestinal pseudo-obstruction: Correction by cisapride. Gastroenterology 1986;91:619.

82. Soudah HC, Hasler WL, Owyang C. Effect of octreotide on intestinal motility and bacterial overgrowth in scleroderma. N Engl J Med 1991;325:1461.

83. Hardcastle JK, Mann CV. Study of large bowel peristalsis. Gut 1968;9:412.

84. Hill JR, Kelley ML, Schlangel JF, Code CF. Pressure profile of the rectum and anus of healthy persons. Dis Colon Rectum 1960;3:203.

85. Schuster MM. The riddle of the sphincters. Gastroenterology 1975;69:249.

86. Bouvier M, Gonella J. Nervous control of the internal anal sphincter of the cat. J Physiol (Lond) 1981;310:457.

87. Read NW, Bortolo DCC, Read MG. Differences in anal function in patients with incontinence to solid and in patients with incontinence to liquids. Br J Surg 1984;71:39.

88. Karaus M, Sarna SK. Giant migrating contractions during defecation in the dog colon. Gastroenterology 1987;92:925.

89. Garcia D, Hita G, Mompean B, et al. Colonic motility: Electric and manometric description of mass movement. Dis Colon Rectum 1991;34:577.

90. Sultan AH, Kamm KA, Hudson CN, et al. Anal-sphincter disruption during vaginal delivery. N Engl J Med 1993;329:1905.

91. Parks AG, Porter NH, Melzak J. Experimental study of the reflex mechanism controlling the muscles of the pelvic floor. Dis Colon Rectum 1962;5:407.

92. Lane RH. Clinical application of anorectal physiology. Proc R Soc Med 1975;68:28.

93. Macleod JH. Management of anal incontinence by biofeedback. Gastroenterology 1987;93:291.

94. Wexner SD, Marchetti F, Jagelman DG. The role of sphincteroplasty for fecal incontinence reevaluated: A prospective physiologic and functional review. Dis Colon Rectum 1991;34:22.

95. Staas WE Jr, Cioschi HS. Neurogenic bowel dysfunction. Crit Rev Phys Rehabil Med 1989;1:11.

96. Metcalf AM, Phillips SF, Zinsmeister AR, et al. Simplified assessment of segmental colon transit. Gastroenterology 1987;92:40.

97. Chaussade S, Roche H, Khyardi A, et al. A new method for measuring colonic transit time. Description and validation. Gastroenterol Clin Biol 1986;10:385.

98. Whitehead WE, Drinkwater D, Cheskin LJ, et al. Constipation in the elderly living at home: Definition, prevalence and relationship to life style and health status. J Am Geriatric Soc 1989;37:423.

99. Eastwood HGH. Bowel transit studies in the elderly: Radiopaque markers in the investigation of constipation. Gerontol Clin 1972:14:154.

100. Wald A, Hinds JP, Caruana BJ. Psychological and physiological characteristics of patients with severe idiopathic constipation. Gastroenterology 1983;97:932.

101. Hope AK, Down EC. Dietary fiber and fluid in the control of constipation in a nursing home population. Med J Aust 1986;144:306.

102. Hull C, Greco RS, Brooks DC. Alleviation of constipation in the elderly by dietary fiber supplementation. J Am Geriatric Soc 1980;28:410.

103. Yahlon SA, Krotenherg R, Fruhmann K. *Clostridium difficile*-related disease: Evaluation and prevalence among inpatients with diarrhea in two freestanding rehabilitation hospitals. Arch Phys Med Rehabil 1993;74:9.

104. DeGirolami PC, Hanff PA, Eichelberger K, et al. Multicenter evaluation of a new enzyme immunoassay for detection of *Clostridium difficile* enterotoxin A. J Clin Microbiol 1992;30:1085.

105. Doern GV, Coughlin RT, Wu L. Laboratory diagnosis of *Clostridium difficile*-associated gastrointestinal disease: Comparison of a monoclonal antibody enzyme immunoassay for toxin A only and two cytotoxicity assays. J Clin Microbiol 1992;30:2042.

106. McFarland LV, Mulligan ME, Kwok RYY, Stamm WE. Nosocomial acquisition of *Clostridium difficile* infection. N Engl J Med 1989;320:204.

107. Johnson S, Homann SR, Bettin KM, et al. Treatment of asymptomatic *Clostridium difficile* carriers (fecal excretors) with vancomycin or metronidazole. A randomized placebo-controlled trial. Ann Intern Med 1992;117:297.

108. Buller HA, Grand RJ. Lactose intolerance. Annu Rev Med 1990;41:141.

Part V
Genitourinary Disorders

Chapter 9

Urinary Tract Dysfunction and Complications

Yeongchi Wu and John B. Nanninga

Urinary tract dysfunction is a long-standing problem in chronically disabled patients after severe neuro-musculoskeletal disease. It is also a problem that cuts across virtually all fields of medical practice. When urinary problems are associated with disabling disease, they often accentuate the inability of the patient to cope with his or her handicap. Urinary incontinence contributes to embarrassment and social isolation and thwarts attempts at rehabilitation. Also, the inability to empty the bladder may contribute to renal infection, calculi, and nephron failure. Thus, the diagnosis and management of urinary tract disorders in the disabled is an important component of total rehabilitation. A wide variety of diseases involving the nervous system can alter normal urinary bladder function. These diseases include stroke, dementia, trauma, tumor, multiple sclerosis, spinal cord injury, spina bifida, and diabetes. Also, disabilities that limit a patient's mobility, such as arthritis or amputation, make urinary control relatively difficult because of the impaired ability to reach a toilet.

Pathophysiology

The nervous system is involved at several levels in the control of urinary storage and expulsion [1, 2]. The brain has the function of sensing when the urinary bladder is full and then informing the conscious mind to prepare for or postpone urination. When ready, the person then initiates voiding. There are several areas of the brain involved in these functions (Figure 9-1). The net effect of disease of the cortex and higher centers in the brain is to lose inhibition so that the patient has difficulty maintaining normal bladder capacity. This leads to the unexpected loss of urine.

The pontine-medullary region contains areas that bring about a bladder contraction and simultaneous relaxation of the urethral sphincter [3]. The impulses from this region are carried down the spinal cord via the reticulospinal tracts. Interruption of this system tends to produce a sphincter that does not relax and is, in fact, relatively obstructive, even though the bladder can contract via a local sacral cord reflex. Sensation of bladder filling may be intact with lesions of the brain stem, but the ability to void on command is lost. The sensation of bladder filling is carried in the dorsolateral column of the spinal cord, and the motor impulses to the sacral cord are carried by the reticulospinal system to the sacral detrusor motor cells in the intermediolateral cell group at S2 to S4. Interruption of the cord by whatever disease process causes failure of the striated urethral sphincter to relax normally during urination, a condition often referred to as sphincter dyssynergia.

The peripheral nerves to the bladder are located at the sacral levels S2 to S4 and form the pelvic nerve containing both sensory and motor fibers. The nerve travels to the bladder where it synapses with a parasympathetic ganglion. From the ganglia, short postganglionic nerves go to the smooth muscle cells of the bladder. Damage to the peripheral nerves leaves the patient with motor and at least some degree of sensory loss. The previously mentioned anatomy is shown in Figure 9-2.

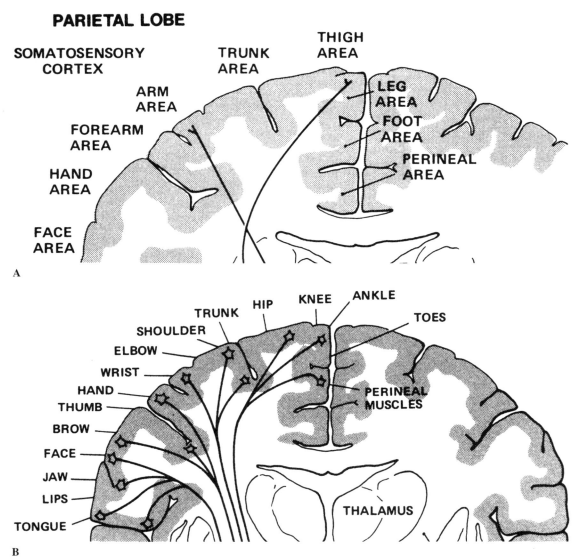

Figure 9-1. A. The region of sensation from the perineal area that produces sensation of bladder and urethral fullness and pain. B. The motor cortex with the representation of the perineal (sphincter) muscles. (Adapted with permission from S Gilman, S Winans. Manter and Gatz's Essentials of Clinical Neuroanatomy and Neurophysiology [7th ed]. Philadelphia: Davis, 1987;49. Copyright by F.A. Davis Company.)

Neurotransmitters involved in bladder function are those that provide storage function and expulsive activity. The storage function seems to depend at least in part on sympathetic (norepinephrine) activity and the presence of leucine enkephalin [1, 4, 5]. The contraction of the bladder is brought about by the release of acetyl-choline from the nerve endings in the bladder. There are undoubtedly other neurotransmitters involved in bladder function, and future investigative efforts should define these agents and their role in bladder function.

In chronically ill persons there may be problems in either retaining urine or expelling it. The

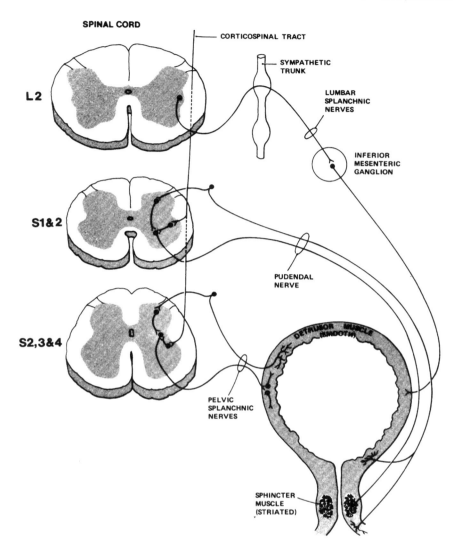

Figure 9-2. The segments of the lumbosacral spinal cord that regulate bladder and sphincter function. The lumbar cord (sympathetic cord) provides nerves that aid in the storage of urine; the postganglionic nerves to the bladder neck aid in maintaining continence and, in men, prevent retrograde ejaculation. The sacral cord gives off parasympathetic fibers that are sensory and motor to the bladder muscle. The anterior horn of the sacral cord gives off the pudendal nerve that provides sensation in the urethra and closure of the striated sphincter. (Adapted with permission from S Gilman, S Winans. Manter and Gatz's Essentials of Clinical Neuroanatomy and Neurophysiology [7th ed]. Philadelphia: Davis, 1987; 31. Copyright 1987 by F.A. Davis Company.)

inability to retain urine, owing to an unexpected or uninhibited bladder contraction or impaired mobility, may result in loss of urine. This can be managed by a collecting device, frequent voiding, or the use of medication. On the other hand, the inability to expel urine results in urinary retention because of structural or functional obstruction, such as from sphincter dyssynergia in spinal cord disease, and this requires intermittent or indwelling catheter drainage, antispasticity medication, or surgical correction of the obstruction, depending on the exact cause.

Diagnosis

History and Physical Examination

The patient's history will reveal whether the patient can urinate and whether there is some degree of control of urination. At times, a diary is helpful in documenting the frequency of urination and the circumstances during which incontinence occurs. The neurologic examination will point to disease that may be affecting bladder function. In performing a rectal examination, it is important for the examiner to check for voluntary control of the anal sphincter as well as the anal wink or bulbocavernosus reflex. The presence of voluntary activity indicates functioning motor tracts, whereas the anal reflex indicates only that the sacral reflex arc is intact. This is the same as checking for the voluntary versus spastic movement of the limb to determine functionality. Voluntary activity of the toes and ankles also indicates that the urethral sphincter is functioning. In our experience, in patients with central cord syndrome or Brown-Séquard syndrome, the ability to contract the anal sphincter on command is a favorable prognostic sign for the recovery of bladder and sphincter function.

Finally, an attempt should be made to observe the urinary stream. A weak, intermittent stream suggests sphincter dyssynergia or at least some form of obstruction, although one cannot tell for sure if the bladder (detrusor) muscle itself is weak. More sophisticated flow studies can be performed with electronic flow devices that give a precise measurement of the degree of impairment. Also, it is worth noting during urination whether the lower extremities exhibit spasticity. This often indicates sphincter spasticity as well, which will produce some degree of obstruction to the outflow of urine.

Urodynamic Studies

Urodynamic studies of the urinary bladder and its sphincter use electrodiagnostic recording devices. The various studies are of value in defining the impairment of urinary bladder storage or the process of elimination [6]. The cystometrogram documents the functional bladder capacity by measuring or revealing the sensation of bladder filling and the bladder contractile activity. The bladder is filled with sterile fluid, preferably warmed to body temperature, and the bladder pressure is monitored during filling. Notation is made when the patient first senses filling and then when the urge to void occurs. The pressure can be measured by a water column or electronic pressure transducer and recording machine for a permanent record. The measurement of the abdominal pressure component to the total bladder pressure can be measured by inserting a rectal catheter for pressure measurement along with bladder measurement and subtracting the rectal component from the bladder pressure. Normal bladder capacity is 250–500

ml. Pressure during a bladder contraction should increase to at least 30 cm H_2O over several seconds.

The function of the striated sphincter can be studied by electromyography with a needle electrode placed in the sphincter fibers (Figure 9-3). The monitoring of the electromyographic signal is best observed on an oscilloscope so as to identify artifact and to observe typical skeletal muscle activity. Recording is more accurate with needle electrodes, although surface electrodes are sometimes used because of the patient's apprehension at having a needle inserted in the perineal area. For needle electromyography in women, the electrode is inserted perianally or periurethrally to a depth of 10–15 mm; in men, a needle electrode of 50–75 mm is needed to reach the striated sphincter fiber located distal to the prostate.

In patients with spasticity of the lower extremities, the sphincter usually demonstrates dyssynergia; that is, the muscle is overactive when the bladder is contracting. The testing is performed along with a cystometrogram and recorded on a recording machine. If radiography is readily available, the bladder and sphincter activity can also be seen on fluoroscopy to confirm bladder and sphincter activity.

Cystography and Videourodynamics

In cystography, contrast medium is instilled into the bladder and the patient attempts to void. If a small catheter is used (6–8 French) voiding can be observed and an obstructing area in the urethra demonstrated. Modern equipment allows the simultaneous visualization of bladder pressure, sphincter electromyography, and bladder and urethral imaging as voiding occurs. The study demonstrates whether the bladder neck opens and whether the striate sphincter relaxes (Figure 9-4). Reflux of contrast media into the ureters may also be shown by this method. Care should be taken not to overfill the bladder. The volume is usually limited to 750–800 ml. Ideally, the urine should be sterile before testing to reduce the possibility of urosepsis.

Ultrasound, Intravenous Pyelography, and Isotope Renography

One of the most common long-term problems in the chronically disabled population is urinary

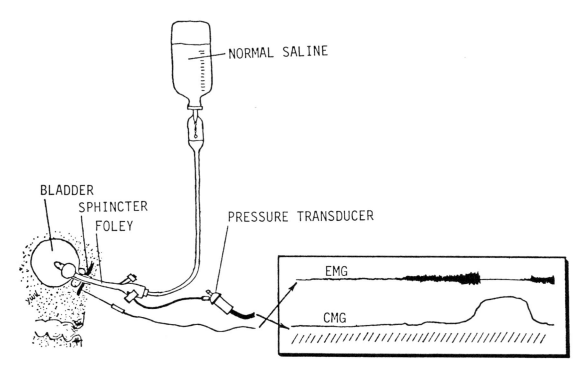

Figure 9-3. Basic setup for performing a cystometrogram (CMG) and sphincter electromyogram (EMG) study. The fluid is seen passing from the sterile fluid container into the bladder through an indwelling urethral catheter (8–14 French). The pressure transducer is attached to the catheter; the transducer is placed at the level of the pubic symphysis in practice. The needle (bipolar here) is shown having been inserted perineally up to the striated sphincter fibers. Activity is monitored on an oscilloscope and recorded on a machine, along with the bladder pressure. The study may be performed with contrast medium in the bladder and the bladder and urethra visualized during an attempt at voiding (see Figure 9-4). (Reprinted with permission from YC Wu. Total bladder care for the spinal cord injured patient. Ann Acad Med Singapore 1983;12:396. Copyright 1983 by Academy of Medicine, Singapore.)

tract complications: calculi, hydronephrosis, and pyelonephritis. Patients at risk for poor bladder emptying with elevated intravesical pressure should be followed for possible upper tract dilatation. Ultrasound and intravenous pyelography will reveal abnormal changes; the intravenous pyelogram gives some estimate of function as well. The isotope renal studies are more sensitive in revealing subtle changes in function and are helpful in determining function in an already compromised kidney. For simply screening patients, the ultrasound has been, in our opinion, safe and effective in detecting abnormalities. The other studies may then be ordered as needed to define the exact problem.

Laboratory Tests

Laboratory tests for the management of impaired bladder function include routine blood chemistry including electrolytes, blood urea nitrogen, creatinine, hemoglobin, and leukocyte count; urinalysis; and urine culture and sensitivity testing. Periodic urine cultures are done to monitor bacteria and identify emerging resistant organisms or to document the exact organism in a febrile patient whose findings on urinalysis point to a urinary tract infection. A simple means of monitoring urinary tract infection in an asymptomatic patient is the dip-slide method. These kits are available from several manufacturers and are an easy and inexpensive means of docu-

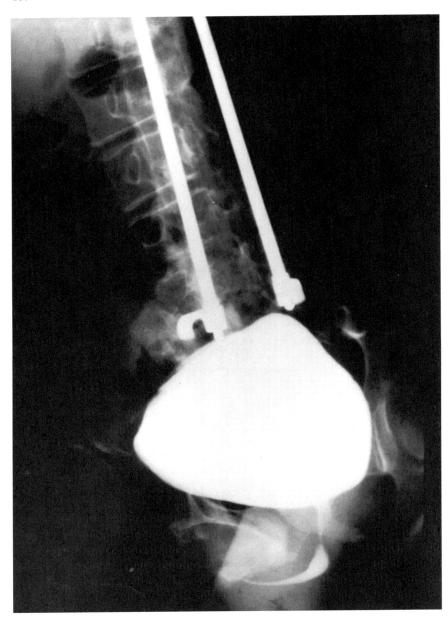

Figure 9-4. A voiding cystourethrogram in a male patient with T11 spinal cord injury shows inadequate opening of the bladder neck and proximal urethra. Despite attempts to urinate, the patient had 200 ml of residual urine. He subsequently was maintained on clean intermittent catheterization.

menting the presence of infection. Selected patients can be taught to use such a technique at home.

Localizing the Site of Urinary Tract Infection

The high frequency of infection, reinfection, and relapse infection and the emergence of antibiotic-resistant organisms led to the difficulty of deciding whether to treat urinary tract infections in patients with permanent neurogenic bladder dysfunction. Finding the site of infection is important because of the possibility of unnecessary overtreatment for bladder infection or insufficient therapy for renal parenchymal infection, which may lead to renal damage.

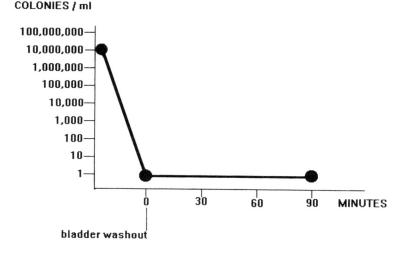

COLONIES / ml

Figure 9-5. In the modified bladder washout procedure, the bladder is irrigated with 50 ml of normal saline 20 times, with or without initial instillation of diluted povidone-iodine solution. Three urine specimens, preirrigation, postirrigation, and 90 minutes postirrigation, were collected for bacterial counting using the semiquantitative dip-slide method. If the bacterial concentration remains low or zero, bacteriuria is probably limited to the bladder.

To date, two techniques, the Fairley bladder washout and the antibody-coated bacteria test, have been reported to be useful in localizing the site of urinary tract infection in patients with non-neurogenic bladders [7–17]. The complexity and expense of the Fairley bladder washout test has limited the applicability in a clinical setting. The antibody-coated bacteria technique, on the other hand, has not been found to be accurate for patients with neurogenic bladder dysfunction.

Attempts were made at the Rehabilitation Institute of Chicago to simplify the Fairley procedure for clinical application for spinal cord injured patients. In the modified bladder washout test, the bladder is first emptied and instilled with 30 ml of half-strength povidone-iodine solution for 1–2 minutes. For patients with significant spasticity, normal saline solution alone is used. The solution is briskly pushed back and forth through the catheter to induce a turbulence in the bladder. This is followed by repetitive irrigation with normal saline solution using 50-ml aliquots for each rinse until a total of 1,000 ml is used.

Three urine specimens (preirrigation, postirrigation, and 90 minutes postirrigation) are collected for counting the bacterial concentration, and the final urine volume is measured for calculating the final total bacterial population. Comparing the change of *bacterial populations*, in addition to the *bacterial concentrations* between postirrigation and final urine specimens (90 minutes postirrigation), provides additional information for localizing the site of urinary tract infection [17]. This simplified procedure appears to have both diagnostic and therapeutic value in managing patients with frequent infection. This simplified procedure can be used as a screening method in patients with urinary tract infection before considering other more involved procedures such as cystoscopy and ureteral catheterization (Figures 9-5 and 9-6).

Infection Versus Colonization

Increased frequency of urinary tract infection in the chronically disabled is due in part to the breakdown of the natural defense mechanism of the bladder against infection. The presence of bacteriuria can be either symptomatic or asymptomatic. Bacteriuria with tissue invasion and resultant tissue response with signs or symptoms has been defined as urinary tract infection [18] (see Chapter 12). Bacteriuria without symptoms or signs may be considered colonization. In patients with spinal cord injury who have no sensation over the kidneys or bladder, it is difficult to decide if antibiotic treatment is needed because of a lack of symptoms. Thus, there is a need for differentiating urinary tract infection from simple colonization of the bladder.

Considering the bladder as a reservoir, there is a constant change of bacterial concentration because of

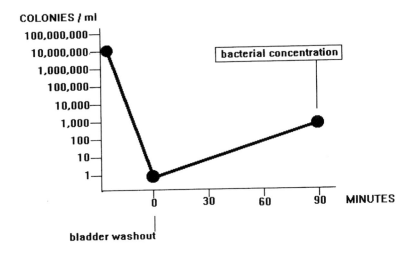

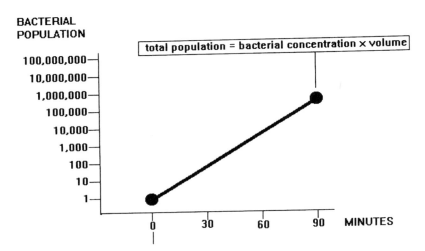

Figure 9-6. In a patient with suspected upper tract infection, the bacterial *concentration* increased 1,000 times (top), whereas the bacterial *population* increased 200,000 times (bottom) as a result of concentration multiplied by the urine volume (200 ml). Such a great change of bacterial population during the lag phase of growth curve (90 minutes after bladder irrigation) is highly suggestive of bacteriuria originating in the upper tract.

the multiplication of bacteria on one hand and the dilution of bacterial concentration from urine excretion on the other. Previous investigators have used mathematical models to explain this dynamic system [19, 20]. After voiding there is always at least a slight residual urine in the bladder. As the urine is drained from the kidneys into the bladder at a linear rate, the remaining bacteria that may be present in the bladder increase at an exponential rate. This results in an initial dilution of the bacterial concentration, which then returns to and exceeds the original concentration. The time from the previous emptying to the time when the bacterial concentration returns to the original level is

defined as a *safe emptying interval* (SEI) (Figure 9-7). When the bladder is emptied within this SEI, the bacterial concentration will decrease until the bacteria are eventually eliminated. Prolongation of emptying beyond the SEI will result in bacterial accumulation to a significant level (Figure 9-8).

Because the bacterial concentration is related to three variables (residual urine, bladder volume, and bacterial doubling time), the SEI will vary from patient to patient and from time period to time period. A decrease or increase of bacterial concentration in the urine will depend on whether the bladder is emptied within or after the SEI (Figure 9-9). The SEI can be

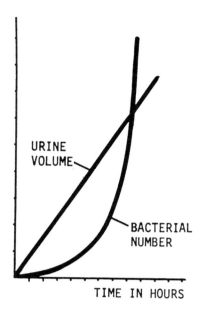
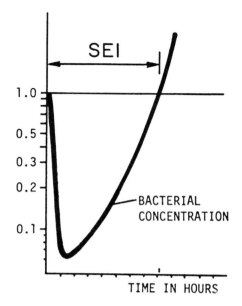

Figure 9-7. As the urine is drained from the kidneys into the bladder at a linear rate, the remaining bacteria increase at an exponential rate. This results in an initial dilution, then a return to the original bacterial concentration. The time interval from the previous emptying to the time when the bacterial concentration returns to the original level is defined as a safe emptying interval (SEI). (Reprinted with permission from YC Wu. Total bladder care for the spinal cord injured patient. Ann Acad Med Singapore 1983;12:388. Copyright 1983 by Academy of Medicine, Singapore.)

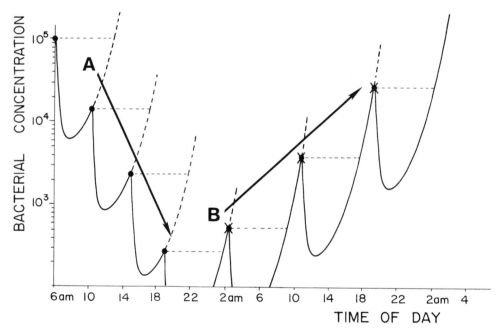

Figure 9-8. A. When the bladder is emptied within the safe emptying interval (filled circle), the bacterial concentration will be lowered gradually until the bacteria are eliminated. B. On the other hand, if the bladder is emptied after the safe emptying interval (filled circle with superimposed x) each time, significant bacteriuria will be inevitable. (Reprinted with permission from YC Wu. Total bladder care for the spinal cord injured patient. Ann Acad Med Singapore 1983;12:389. Copyright 1983 by Academy of Medicine, Singapore.)

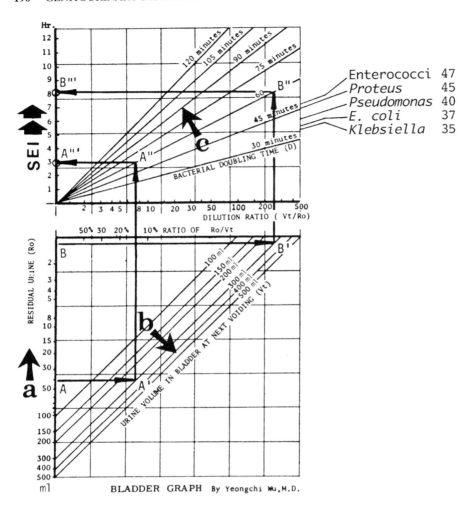

Enterococci 47
Proteus 45
Pseudomonas 40
E. coli 37
Klebsiella 35

BLADDER GRAPH By Yeongchi Wu,M.D.

Figure 9-9. The *bladder graph* is used to determine the safe emptying interval (SEI). By applying residual urine volume (a), bladder urine volume (b), and bacterial doubling time (c), the SEI can be obtained. Reducing the residual urine, increasing the bladder capacity, or prolonging the doubling time will extend the SEI. (Reprinted with permission from YC Wu. Total bladder care for the spinal cord injured patient. Ann Acad Med Singapore 1983;12:389. Copyright 1983 by Academy of Medicine, Singapore.)

easily obtained by tracing on the *bladder graph* from the residual urine amount (R_0), to the estimated urine volume (V_t), to the bacterial doubling time (D), finally yielding the SEI in hours. For example, if a patient (A) has a residual urine of 50 ml, a bladder capacity of 300 ml, and an infection with bacterial doubling time of 60 minutes, the SEI will be about 2.5 hours. The bladder graph represents a mathematical model reported previously by other investigators [19, 20]:

$$C_t \times V_t = C_0 \times R_0 \times 2^{\frac{T}{D}}$$

where C_t = bacterial concentration at time t, C_0 = bacterial concentration at time 0, T = time interval (minutes) between time 0 and time t, D = bacterial doubling time (minutes) or time required for the number of organism to double, R_0 = residual urine (ml) in bladder at time 0, and V_t = urine volume (ml) in bladder at time t.

Theoretically, to maintain sterile urine or eliminate infection, the patient should void more frequently and/or the residual urine should be reduced so that bladder emptying will be within the SEI. Antibacterial agents prolong the doubling time, thus prolonging the SEI. Of interest is the fact that infrequent voiding (every 6–10 hours) has been attributed as a cause for recurrent urinary tract infection [21, 22].

Management

Understanding the dynamics of urinary bladder storage and elimination is the first step toward developing a long-term management program for bladder dysfunction in chronically disabled persons. From the earlier discussion in this chapter, it is important to recognize that both bladder and sphincter dysfunction may occur in disabled patients. In fact, in some neurologically disabled patients, the term *neurogenic sphincter* might be more appropriate than *neurogenic bladder*.

No matter what the etiology of bladder and sphincter dysfunction, there are three phases in the process of urination: (1) sensory feedback informs the person whether the bladder is full; (2) when the bladder is full and voiding is desired, the detrusor muscle contracts; and (3) simultaneously the external (striated) urethral sphincter relaxes; at this moment, the urine in the bladder is expelled through the relaxed outlet.

Impairment of Urinary Drainage in the Elderly

Poor urinary drainage because of structural obstruction in elderly male patients often is related to benign prostatic hyperplasia, which is manifested by slow urinary stream, hesitancy in initiating urination and straining to void, increase in frequency of urination, and a sense of residual urine in the bladder. At times, detrusor hypercontractility will accompany the prostate enlargement, and this will accentuate the urinary frequency. On the other hand, a poorly contracting bladder will also produce incomplete emptying and slow stream. In some instances, a chronically overdistended bladder will have evolved from obstruction. In the elderly population a variety of forms of bladder dysfunction will contribute to incontinence [23].

Classification of Bladder Dysfunction

At this point some attempt should be made to organize the various forms of bladder dysfunction in the elderly beyond what was discussed previously. Problems in the geriatric population will also fit into this discussion. In patients who have suffered from stroke or spinal cord disease, the process of urination may occur too fast for the patient to be prepared. In particular, patients with spinal cord disease lack sensory feedback and have lost the reflex for relaxing the striated sphincter in varying degrees. This leads to the high bladder pressure, elevated residual urine, and risk of bacteriuria related to the high residual urine [24]. In the past bladder dysfunction was classified as being simply upper or lower motoneuron, with varying degree of completeness or incompleteness. Other terms have been used to describe bladder dysfunction such as spastic, cord, paralytic, or autonomous.

Considering that the problem in many disabled patients is both bladder and sphincter dysfunction, we have simply classified patients based on the remaining nervous control of urethral sphincter and the ability of the patient to handle methods of urinary drainage. The classification has evolved into four groups: C, S, P, and Q (Figure 9-10).

Patients in group C have voluntary corticospinal function to some degree: voluntary sphincter function is present, and voluntary bladder function is present at least to some degree. This would include stroke patients and patients with brain injury or incomplete spinal cord injury, including some with Brown-Séquard syndrome or central cord syndrome. These patients demonstrate some impairment in storing urine and have what has been termed a hyperreflexic bladder. The sphincter electromyogram or cystourethrogram will show an open sphincter during voiding.

Group S represents a small group of patients with near-complete loss of voluntary control over the bladder and sphincter, but the bladder contracts and the sphincter relaxes reflexively to allow the unobstructed passage of urine. Such patients require some type of external collection device, although an occasional patient may be able to time or stimulate the bladder to void at a suitable time.

Group Q includes quadriplegic patients with extensive cord disease in whom there is loss of cortical control and sphincter relaxation during voiding. Also the patient has no hand function by which he or she might perform self-catheterization. In these patients, the combination of bladder hyperreflexia and sphincter dyssynergia leads to renal damage if the problem is left untreated.

Group P includes complete or near-complete paraplegic patients, with loss of voluntary control of urethral sphincter and with detrusor–sphincter dyssynergia (if above the sacral cord). These patients

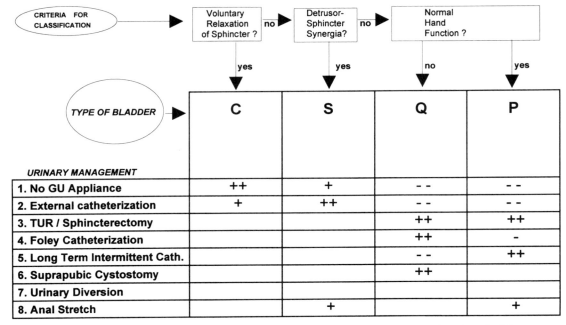

Figure 9-10. In spinal cord injury, the neurogenic bladder can be classified, based on the methods of achieving urethral sphincter opening, into four types of dysfunction: C, S, Q, and P. These bladder dysfunctions are matched with available care methods as shown in the bladder care algorithm. Abbreviations: GU, genitourinary; TUR, trans- urethral resection. +, ++ = preferred method for management; −, -- = nonpreferred method for management. (Reprinted with permission from YC Wu. Total bladder care for the spinal cord injured patient. Ann Acad Med Singapore 1983;12:392. Copyright 1983 by Academy of Medicine, Singapore.)

have hand function, which allows them to perform intermittent self-catheterization. If the bladder does not contract, which would be the case if the sacral cord is damaged, the patient can perform catheterization indefinitely; if a bladder reflex and sphincter dyssynergia are present, the patient will require some means, usually pharmacologic, to provide for low-pressure storage between catheterizations.

Pharmacologic Treatment

The first line of treatment in patients with decreased capacity from hyperreflexia is to give pharmacologic agents that will decrease the frequency of bladder contractions. These are usually anticholinergic drugs such as oxybutynin or propantheline. These drugs are not without side effects, such as dry mouth, constipation, and blurred vision.

In patients who have sphincter dyssynergia, the antispasticity drug baclofen offers some reduction in the amount of spasticity. The drug is not always successful, however, and other means may have to be used to reduce obstruction from the sphincter.

In patients in whom the bladder does not contract very effectively and when there is no detrusor-sphincter dyssynergia, bethanechol chloride is used to promote improved bladder contractility. There is controversy as to how effective this drug really is over a long period. If a bladder does not recover function, the patient is usually placed on intermittent catheterization.

The alpha-adrenergic receptor blocking agents have been used to relax the urethral closure mechanism. A drug such as terazosin is worth trying in patients who have some degree of obstruction at the bladder outlet.

The overall indications for these groups of drugs are discussed in more detail elsewhere, and the reader is encouraged to consult such texts [2].

Intermittent Catheterization

When the patient is not able to void normally because of loss of bladder function or when sphincter obstruction produces bladder retention, the drainage of the bladder *every 4–6 hours or whenever the bladder is full* is recommended. This is often done under sterile conditions in a hospital setting so that organisms from the immediate environment do not colonize the urinary tract. However, such a method is costly and it has been shown that by using a simple, clean technique the urinary tract can be drained with little risk of clinical infection [25–29]. For catheterization, a self-contained catheter encapsulated in a sheath (touchless catheter) can be used. With this system, there is no direct touch of the catheter because it is within a tube. The tube becomes the urinary reservoir. If using the clean system, the urine can be deposited into the toilet as it comes from the end of the catheter. We do not use prophylactic antibiotics as a rule, but occasional patients benefit from a low-dose antibiotic such as nitrofurantoin or sulfa. Probably, the reduced risk of infection with catheterization every 4–6 hours relates to the SEI concept mentioned earlier in the chapter.

Indwelling Urethral Catheterization

Although indwelling catheterization is not the optimal method for bladder care because of bacteriuria, as long as there is a free flow of urine in many patients the asymptomatic bacteriuria may exist but not cause any significant threat. When an indwelling catheter is in place, the drainage tube should be placed so it will not kink. The bag should be below the patient's bladder when in bed or traveling. Cleansing around the catheter–meatus junction aids in reducing ascending infection along the urethra. In male patients the catheter should be taped to the abdominal wall so as to reduce pressure on the urethra and reduce the possibility of penoscrotal fistula. If the catheter tends to plug with debris, irrigation may be done as necessary using a solution such as 0.25% acetic acid or urologic irrigation solution.

Surgical Management

Surgical techniques involve two general goals. One is to facilitate elimination of urine. If obstruction is demonstrated and other means have not been successful in managing the problem, then a procedure such as transurethral resection of the prostate, if that is the obstructing entity, is indicated. At times the sphincter is incised or resected, if this is the obstructing structure and the patient wishes to wear an external collector and not perform catheterization [30]. Another procedure to provide drainage is the placement of a suprapubic catheter. This is done if the patient has not adapted well to other means of bladder management.

The other goal of surgical treatment is to provide a better means of storage. Surgical treatment can be used to expand the capacity of the bladder by augmenting the capacity with a segment of bowel. If the bladder becomes small and contracted, a total bladder substitution may be elected. There are a variety of techniques for this and individual surgeons have their preferences. The various techniques and possible complications are well described [31]. Another means of allowing for bladder expansion is to denervate the bladder and thus eliminate the hyperreflexia. In our experience, patients are reluctant to have nerves destroyed by surgical or chemical means. Furthermore, such procedures do not always produce the desired result of a noncontractile bladder that stores urine at a low pressure.

Occasionally in the chronically disabled population, loss of potency is a problem that adds to the morbidity of the illness. If the patient has a reasonable life expectancy, a penile prosthesis may be considered. Such a prosthesis is also used to facilitate the placement of an external collecting system (usually a condom catheter). In patients with adequate penile blood supply but who have impotence caused by loss of innervation, potency can be achieved with the direct injection of papaverine or prostaglandin into the penis. The dosage varies from patient to patient, and priapism (sustained erection) is always a risk if too large a dose is used.

Anal Stretch

In patients who demonstrate varying degrees of sphincter dyssynergy during the course of their disease, such as multiple sclerosis or paraplegia, the dilation of the anal sphincter will inhibit the sphincter and allow the passage of urine. The patient inserts two fingers in the anal canal and forcefully dilates the sphincter. Pressure may have to be exerted over the bladder to supply pressure to pass the urine [32, 33]. Although this technique is not well suited for use day in and day out, it does have applicability in the small spectrum of patients described previously [34].

References

1. De Groat W, Nadelhaft I, Miline R, Booth A, et al. Organization of the sacral parasympathetic reflex pathways to the urinary bladder and large intestine. J Auton Nerv Syst 1981;3:135.
2. Wein AJ, Levin R, Barrett D. Voiding dysfunction: Relevant anatomy, physiology, and pharmacology. In J Gillenwater, J Grayhack, S Howards, J Duckett (eds), Adult and Pediatric Urology (ed 2). St. Louis: Mosby–Year Book, 1991;933.
3. Holstege G, Griffiths D, De Wall H, Dalm E. Anatomical and physiological observations on supraspinal control of bladder and urethral sphincter muscles in the cat. J Comp Neurol 1986;250:449.
4. De Groat W, Saum W. Sympathetic inhibition of the urinary bladder and the pelvic ganglionic transmission in the cat. J Physiol 1972;220:297.
5. De Groat W, Kawatani M, Hisamitsu T, Lowe I, et al. The role of neuropeptides in the sacral autonomic pathways of the cat. J Auton Nerv Syst 1983;7:339.
6. Abrams P, Blaivas J, Stanton S, Anderson J. Standardization of terminology of lower urinary tract function. Neurourol Urodyn 1988;7:404.
7. Fairley K, Bond A, Brown R, Habersberger P. Simple test to determine the site of urinary tract infection. Lancet 1967;2:427.
8. Giroux J, Perkash I. Limited value of the Fairley test in urologic infections in patients with neurogenic bladders. J Am Paraplegic Soc 1985;8:10.
9. Hawthome N, Kurtz S, Anhalt J. Accuracy of antibody-coated bacteria test in recurrent urinary tract infections. Mayo Clin Proc 1978;53:651.
10. Hellerstein S, Duggan E, Welchert E, et al. Localization of the site of urinary tract infections with bladder washout test. J Pediatr 1981;98:201.
11. Hulter H, Borchardt K, Mahood J, et al. Localization of catheter-induced urinary tract infections: Interpretation of bladder washout and antibody-coated bacteria tests. Nephron 1984;38:48.
12. Jones S. Antibody-coated bacteria in use. N Engl J Med 1976;29:1380.
13. Kuhlemeier K, Lloyd K, Stover S. Failure of antibody-coated bacteria and bladder washout tests to localize infection in spinal cord injury patients. J Urol 1983;130:729.
14. Merritt J, Keyes T. Limitation of the antibody-coated bacteria test in patients with neurogenic bladders. JAMA 1982;247:1723.
15. Naso F, Ditunno J. The Fairley test: An aid in the diagnosis of pyelonephritis in paraplegia. Arch Phys Med Rehabil 1974;55:279.
16. Thomas V, Shelokov A, Farland M. Antibody-coated bacteria in the urine and the site of urinary infection. N Engl J Med 1974;290:588.
17. Wu Y. Localizing the site of urinary infection in spinal cord injured patients using bladder washout and dip-slide technique. National Institute on Disability and Rehabilitation Research, 1988.
18. Ditunno JF, Formal CS. Review article: Current concept—Chronic spinal cord injury. N Engl J Med 1994;330:550.
19. Boen J, Sylvester D. The mathematical relationship among urinary frequency, residual urine and bacterial growth in bladder infection. Invest Urol 1965;2:468.
20. Hinman F, Cox C. The voiding vesical defense mechanism: The mathematical effect of residual urine, voiding interval and volume on bacteriuria. J Urol 1966;96:491.
21. Adatto K, Doebele K, Galland L, Granowetter L. Behavioral factors and urinary tract infection. JAMA 1979;241:2525.
22. Lapides J, Costello R, Zierdt D, Stone T. Primary cause and treatment of recurrent urinary infection in women. J Urol 1968;100:552.
23. Resnick NM, Yalla SV, Laurino E. The pathophysiology of urinary incontinence among institutionalized elderly persons. N Engl J Med 1989;320:1.
24. Hinman F Jr. Obstruction: Back pressure or residual volume and laminar flow. J Urol 1971;105:702.
25. Anderson RU. Prophylaxis of bacteriuria during intermittent catheterization of the acute neurogenic bladder. J Urol 1980;123:364.
26. Lapides J, Diokno A, Cowe B, Kalish M. Follow up on unsterile, intermittent self-catheterization. J Urol 1974;111:184.
27. Lapides J, Diokno A, Gould F, Lowe B. Further observation on self-catheterization. J Urol 1976;116:169.
28. Wu Y, Hamilton B, Boyink M, Nanninga J. Reusable catheter for long term sterile intermittent catheterization. Arch Phys Med Rehabil 1981;62:39.
29. Wu Y, King R, Hamilton B, Betts HB. RIC-Wu catheter kit: New device for an old problem. Arch Phys Med Rehabil 1980;61:455.
30. Perkash I. Contact laser sphincterotomy: further experience and longer follow-up. Spinal Cord 1996;34:227.
31. Rivas DA, Karasick S, Chancellor MD. Cutaneous ileocystostomy (bladder chimney) for the treatment of severe neurogenic vesical dysfunction. Paraplegia 1995;33:530.

32. Donovan WH, Clowers MD, Marci D. Anal sphincter stretch: A technique to overcome detrusor–sphincter dyssynergia. Arch Phys Med Rehabil 1975;58:320.

33. Gans BM, Zimmerman T, Stover WC. Urinary catheterization in severe sphincter spasticity: Report of two cases. Arch Phys Med Rehabil 1975;56:498.

34. Wu Y, Nanninga J, Hamilton B. Inhibition of the external sphincter and sacral reflex by anal stretch in spinal cord urethral injured patient. Arch Phys Med Rehabil 1986;67:135.

Part VI
Hematologic Disorders

Chapter 10

Venous Thromboembolism

David Green

The term *thromboembolism* encompasses deep vein thrombosis (DVT) of the lower extremities and pulmonary embolism (PE). The deep veins involved may be distal (the soleal and peroneal vessels) or proximal (the popliteal, femoral, and iliac veins); clots in the proximal veins usually embolize to the lungs. Thromboembolism is a major problem; some 200,000 persons die each year in the United States of PEs [1]. The incidence of PE confirmed by autopsy in one hospital over a 25-year period was 15.6% [2]. Leg scan results positive for the diagnosis of DVT have been reported in 60–75% of patients with acute stroke [3, 4] and 78% of those with spinal cord injury [5]; 16% of the latter had clinical evidence of thromboembolism. Fatal PE occurs in 2–4% of these patients. The data clearly document the importance of this problem in the disabled.

Risk Factors

In those with disabilities, the major risk factor is immobilization. However, other conditions such as advanced age, obesity, congestive heart failure, and malignancy are commonly associated with DVT and PE. In addition, persons who have sustained trauma to the pelvis or lower extremities, or who have a history of previous DVT, are at a higher risk. Certain other conditions such as the nephrotic syndrome, the presence of antiphospholipid antibodies (lupus anticoagulant), pregnancy, or the administration of oral contraceptives with high estrogen content are known to predispose to thromboembolism.

In summary, there are multiple factors that increase the risk of thrombosis in this patient population.

Pathophysiology

The exact role of immobilization in triggering the thrombotic process is unknown, but some possible mechanisms are shown in Table 10-1. There is loss of the pumping action of the muscles in emptying the leg veins and increased blood viscosity because of dehydration and dependent edema; edema represents loss of fluid into the extravascular space. Persistent external pressure on the more superficial veins as a result of immobility may lead to vascular injury. The stress associated with the underlying disability may increase the levels of important procoagulants such as factor VIII, von Willebrand factor, and fibrinogen, and the latter further contributes to increasing blood viscosity. In addition, protein catabolism as indicated by hypoalbuminemia is often associated with reductions in antithrombin III, a major circulating anticoagulant. Fibrinolytic activity also declines, owing to increases in the concentration of plasminogen activator inhibitor-1, a stress reactant, and diminished release of plasminogen activator from the endothelium; the release of this activator is normally dependent on muscular contraction and increases with exercise.

Many other hemostatic factors are involved in thrombogenesis. For example, platelets are activated by a variety of stimuli, including cigarette smoking, vascular injury, and epinephrine. In patients with

Table 10-1. Factors Associated with the Hypercoagulability of Immobilization

Rheologic
    Decreased venous emptying because of impaired muscular pumping
    Increased viscosity because of dehydration, transudation of fluid into soft tissues, and raised fibrinogen levels
Vascular
    Trauma to vessel wall caused by extrinsic pressure on immobile limbs
Clotting constituents
    Increased levels of procoagulants (factor VIII, von Willebrand factor, fibrinogen) associated with stress and trauma
    Decrease in antithrombin III accompanying protein wasting
    Reduction in fibrinolytic activity due to lack of muscular contraction and increase in plasminogen activator inhibitor-1

acute spinal cord injury, platelet aggregation is enhanced and levels of factor VIII and von Willebrand factor are increased [6, 7]. Platelet coagulant activities have been shown to progressively increase in patients who develop DVT after hip surgery [8]. Other changes, such as decreases in the concentration of antithrombin III and blood fibrinolytic activity, have been used to predict the risk of DVT in patients undergoing abdominal surgery [9]. These factors have not been systematically assessed in patients with chronic disabilities, nor have there been studies of some of the more recently recognized antithrombotic factors such as heparin cofactor II, protein C, or protein S. Alterations in the concentrations or activity of one or more of these hemostatic agents could substantially increase thrombotic risk.

Venous thrombi probably begin in the pocket of valve cusps. Vascular damage or alterations in flow (stasis, changes in shear, turbidity) influence platelets and neutrophils to leave the margins of the blood column, where they are normally found, and attach to the valve pocket or areas where endothelium has been denuded [10]. This sets the stage for the elaboration of cytokines, which attract more neutrophils and macrophages to the site; these latter cells generate procoagulants that eventuate in the elaboration of thrombin. Thrombin converts fibrinogen to fibrin and activates factor XIII, which cross-links the fibrin strands. Fibrin binds to the extended pseudopodia of activated platelets (Figure 10-1). Erythrocytes become trapped in the expanding thrombus, which propagates proximally from the valve cusp to eventually occlude the lumen of the vein. The binding of the thrombus to the vein wall is believed to be tenuous for the first 5–7 days [11]; it is during this period that PE is most likely to occur. Subsequently, the adherent thrombus either

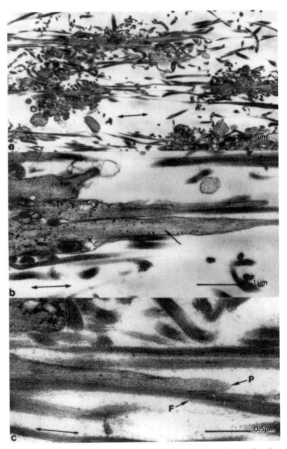

Figure 10-1. a. Platelets and fibrin strands. b. A long platelet pseudopod (arrow). c. Close interaction between platelet pseudopod (P) and fibrin strand (F). (Reprinted with permission from I Cohen, JM Gerrard, JG White. Ultrastructure of clots during isometric contraction. J Cell Biol 1982;93:778. Copyright Rockefeller University Press.)

is lysed, embolizes, or undergoes fibrosis with permanent stricture of the vein.

Most PE arises from the proximal veins of the legs [12]. Small emboli may be clinically silent and physiologically well tolerated. Larger emboli may result in pulmonary infarcts, occasionally accompanied by bronchospasm and cardiac arrhythmias. Massive embolization with occlusion of more than 60% of the pulmonary vasculature is associated with acute right-sided heart failure, circulatory collapse, and death [13]. It should be recognized that thrombi can arise in several vein segments serially or concurrently [14], and therefore there may be waves of PE. In addition to producing multiple lung infarcts, repeated embolization reduces the pulmonary vascular bed and results in pulmonary hypertension and right-sided heart failure.

The important factors that prevent venous thromboembolism are enhanced venous flow and decreased blood viscosity, preservation of the endothelium, maintenance of adequate concentrations of circulating anticoagulants such as antithrombin III and proteins C and S, and a favorable balance of profibrinolytic proteins (tissue plasminogen activator, plasminogen) to inhibitors of fibrinolysis (plasminogen activator inhibitor-1, alpha-2-macroglobulin, antiplasmin). Venous thrombosis probably occurs because these mechanisms are breached.

Diagnosis

Deep Vein Thrombosis

The clinical diagnosis of DVT is often inaccurate; the symptoms and signs usually associated with this disorder (pain, swelling, tenderness, warmth, discoloration, and prominent veins) commonly occur in a variety of other disorders. For example, in a hemiplegic patient leg pain may be neurogenic and leg swelling may be secondary to the paralysis. Paraplegic subjects develop heterotopic bone (see Chapter 5), which presents as pain, warmth, and swelling of the limb. Infections such as cellulitis are common in the chronically disabled and may be accompanied by fever, pain, swelling, warmth, and erythema. Hirsh and Hull [1] have estimated the specificity of clinical diagnosis to be as a low as 30%. Even such a time-honored test as Homans's

sign (calf pain with dorsiflexion of the foot) was observed in fewer than 33% of their patients with documented DVT and, even worse, was noted in 50% of symptomatic patients without DVT.

Of greater concern is the absence of clinical signs in patients found to have DVT by the objective tests described in the following discussion. Seventy-five percent of PEs occur in patients with silent DVT. In patients with spinal cord injury, we and others [15] have observed fever as the only manifestation of thromboembolism. Therefore, clinical suspicion for DVT must be strong, and immobilized patients must be treated as though they will develop DVT. The use of objective tests for monitoring and diagnosis is essential.

In the last few years, there have been major technological improvements in testing, and in most institutions the color-flow ultrasound technique has supplanted the older methods of Doppler flow and impedance plethysmography (IPG). Nevertheless, these latter techniques have advantages in simplicity and low cost and may be used when ultrasound is unavailable. Radioactive fibrinogen scanning has been mainly relegated to use in research settings; the tracer is no longer available commercially. Several studies have examined the sensitivity and specificity of IPG and ultrasound in relationship to each other, and the gold standard, ascending venography. The results of these studies are discussed in the following paragraphs.

IPG measures the rapid decrease in electrical resistance of the limb when an occlusive tourniquet is deflated, taking into account the venous capacitance. Occlusion of the proximal veins significantly reduces the rate of venous outflow and, accordingly, the change in electrical resistance. The method does not indicate whether the occlusion is due to thrombosis or extrinsic compression of the vein, and it is insensitive to DVT below the popliteal vein. False-positive results may occur if venous outflow is impaired because of congestive heart failure or strong muscle contractions or reduced due to arterial disease or use of ergotamine [16]. There is also evidence that venous outflow and capacitance are decreased in patients with spinal cord injury per se [17]. The sensitivity and specificity of IPG were compared with venous ultrasound in patients with symptomatic DVT [18]. The positive predictive value of an abnormal ultrasonogram was 94%, whereas the predictive value of IPG was only 83% ($p = 0.02$).

Ultrasound has two components; the ultrasound beam is reflected from the column of venous blood at a frequency proportional to the flow velocity, the Doppler component. At the same time, the venous flow may be visualized by reconstructing the reflected waves to provide anatomic detail, the scan component. By scanning along the entire length of an accessible vein (such as the superficial femoral or popliteal), a thrombus may be located and its extent recorded. In addition, the operator may look for variations in flow due to respiration, Valsalva's maneuver, or vein compression. The latter manipulation is particularly valuable; noncompressibility is characteristic of obstructed vessels. The limitations of the method are the inability to clearly image such veins as the iliacs, profunda femoris, and soleal sinuses and failure to distinguish external compression on a vein from an occluding thrombus. Also, turbulent blood flow may masquerade as intravascular clot. However, in symptomatic patients with DVT the sensitivity and specificity of color flow ultrasound is greater than 90% [19]. On the other hand, in asymptomatic patients the results have been disappointing. In the study of Davidson et al. [20], the sensitivity of ultrasound was only 38% in patients with venographically confirmed thrombi (a third of whom had proximal vein thrombi). The specificity was much better (92%). Thus, ultrasound is an excellent test in symptomatic patients, but is deficient as a screening tool for DVT.

Venography is the "gold standard" for detecting and localizing DVT. Contrast medium is injected into a dorsal foot vein and radiographs are obtained while the patient is tilted upright. If a large bolus of dye (up to 150 ml) is injected and fluoroscopy is used to monitor the course of the dye, all of the veins of the lower extremity, with the exception of the profunda femoris and internal iliac veins, may be visualized. Thrombi are identified as constant intraluminal filling defects seen in more than one view, cutoffs of the contrast medium at a constant site below a nonfilled segment with reappearance above the site, and persistent nonfilling of the deep venous system above the knee despite adequate dye infusion, especially if abnormal collaterals are seen [21]. False-negative examinations occur when nonobstructing thrombi are present in the common femoral vein, and false-positive studies result from inadequate dye injections and streaming effects in the larger veins [1]. Venography is an invasive procedure; there may be pain at the injection site, phlebitis, and hypersensitivity reactions to the contrast media, but these appear to be less frequent with the nonionic contrast media currently used.

In general, patients in whom DVT is suspected should be initially evaluated with venous ultrasound. If the results are equivocal or negative, but clinical suspicion is high, venography should be performed. Alternatively, the ultrasound may be repeated at 3- to 5-day intervals. Although calf-vein thrombi may go unrecognized, these rarely embolize and only 20% extend to the proximal veins, at which time they should be visualized by ultrasound.

Pulmonary Embolism

The clinical diagnosis of PE is insecure because many of the illnesses that are common in the chronically disabled manifest the same symptoms and signs that are observed in association with PE. Although PE may be accompanied by dyspnea, tachypnea, fever, tachycardia, and chest pain, the same constellation of symptoms characterizes pneumonia or atelectasis. Patients with congestive heart failure have dyspnea, tachycardia, wheezing, and crackles, which initially can be unilateral, simulating a PE. PE occasionally presents as syncope, hypotension, and arrhythmias, which are also signs of septicemia. Adjunctive tests such as arterial blood gas measurements, chest radiographs, and electrocardiograms may help in the differential diagnosis, but there are no patterns of abnormalities that are specific for PE. In the Urokinase/Streptokinase Pulmonary Embolism Study [22], the diagnosis of PE was definitively excluded in as many as 49% of those in whom it was clinically suspected.

Just as in DVT, many PEs are clinically silent. Not only may patients be asymptomatic, but they may have normal blood values, chest films, and electrocardiogram results. In other subjects, fever and tachycardia are the only signs of PE. To establish a diagnosis it is usually necessary to have a high index of suspicion and perform lung scanning and pulmonary angiograms (Figure 10-2).

Ventilation-perfusion ($\dot{V}/\dot{Q}$) lung scans are performed by infusing macroaggregated albumin particles labeled with technetium-99m intravenously to reflect the distribution of lung blood flow, combined with inhalation of xenon-127 gas or tech-

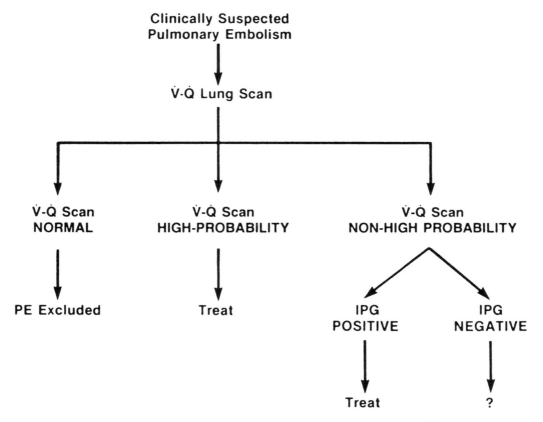

Figure 10-2. Diagnostic approach to a patient with clinically suspected pulmonary embolism. ($\dot{V}/\dot{Q}$ = ventilation-perfusions; IPG = impedance plethysmography; PE = pulmonary embolism). (Reprinted with permission from J Hirsch, RD Hull. Venous Thromboembolism: Natural History, Diagnosis, and Management. Boca Raton, FL: CRC Press, 1987;65. Copyright 1987 CRC Press, Inc.)

netium-99m sulfur colloid aerosol to image the peripheral airways. The scans are interpreted in terms of the probability of PE, which requires concomitant review of the patient's current chest radiograph. They are most informative when the chest roentgenogram is clear, or the $\dot{V}/\dot{Q}$ abnormality is in a noninvolved area of the chest roentgenogram. The sensitivity and specificity of the $\dot{V}/\dot{Q}$ scan were compared with pulmonary angiograms by the PIOPED Investigators [23]. In patients with a high clinical suspicion of PE and high probability scans, or low clinical suspicion of PE and normal scans, accuracy exceeded 90%. On the other hand, if clinical suspicion was high, PE was present in 66% of patients with an intermediate probability scan and 40% of patients with a low probability scan; con-

versely, if clinical suspicion was low, 16% and 4% of patients with PE had intermediate or low probability scans, respectively. The conclusion drawn from these studies is that pulmonary angiography should be performed if clinical suspicion is high, even if the $\dot{V}/\dot{Q}$ scan is read as intermediate or low probability; and that low clinical suspicion does not exclude a PE if the lung scan result is intermediate.

An alternative to pulmonary angiography in a patient with an indeterminate lung scan is an ultrasound study of the lower extremities. This is because 70% of patients with angiographically documented PE have venographic evidence of a DVT, and ultrasound will detect most of these. The diagnosis of DVT will mandate anticoagulant therapy and make further investigations for PE unnecessary. In those patients with negative ultrasound results, either a pulmonary angiogram may be performed or the patient may be followed with serial ultrasound, depending on the clinical circumstances. The rationale of this approach is that the negative ultrasound result makes recurrent emboli unlikely and therefore the patient may be monitored without therapeutic anticoagulation until there is an indication of an active thrombotic process. Of course, such patients would probably be receiving some form of antithrombosis prophylaxis.

Pulmonary angiography is an invasive study involving the injection of radiographic contrast medium into the main pulmonary outflow tract or selected vessels and taking multiple, often magnified views. Pulmonary emboli are visualized as intraluminal filling defects, sharp cutoffs, or absence of filling despite multiple injections. Occasionally, patients experience hypotension, arrhythmias, or exacerbation of respiratory insufficiency during the study. Although it is the definitive test for PEs, the risks, costs, and complications require that it be reserved for those clinical situations in which a diagnosis will initiate important therapeutic interventions. An example would be a patient with evidence of a recent PE despite full anticoagulant therapy for a previously documented DVT. The presence of a new PE indicates failure of the current therapy and the probable need for a vena cava filter.

Screening

From the above discussion, it is clear that recognition of DVT and PE requires strong clinical suspicion. In a patient who is asymptomatic, confirming the diagnosis is problematic because physical examination, venous ultrasound study, and ventilation/perfusion scanning have a low sensitivity for detecting thrombus. A sensitive test for thrombosis is the measurement of circulating d-dimers, which are fragments of fibrin formed during clot dissolution. Using a sensitive method for d-dimer quantitation such as the enzyme-linked immunosorbent assay (ELISA), many investigators have shown that d-dimer testing has a sensitivity for detecting DVT, PE, or both that is greater than 95% [24]. However, the test is nonspecific; positive results are seen in patients with hematomas, renal failure, and liver disease as well as thromboembolism. When a thrombosis is suspected, an ELISA d-dimer test should be performed. If the test result is positive, venous ultrasonography and ventilation/perfusion scanning should be done to confirm the presence and location of thrombi.

Management

Initial Treatment of Acute Thromboembolism

Heparin has been the standard therapy for acute thromboembolism. When given in doses sufficient to prolong the activated partial thromboplastin time (aPTT) to at least 1.5 times the control value, heparin will prevent new thrombus formation and extension of existing thrombus. It will not prevent embolization from existing thrombus, nor induce clot dissolution. An eight-step approach to anticoagulant management is shown in Table 10-2, modified from Raschke et al. [25].

Studies have shown that if an aPTT of at least 1.5 times control is not achieved within 24–72 hours, thromboembolism and recurrence of thrombosis are significantly increased [26]. Although the use of intravenous heparin permits rapid attainment of therapeutic aPTT values, subcutaneous injections of sodium heparin only gradually increase the aPTT. Doyle and colleagues [27] reported that calcium heparin given subcutaneously in an initial dose of 15,000 U and then repeated every 12 hours was as safe and effective as intravenous calcium heparin in preventing new PEs in patients with acute DVT. Although the bioavailability of calcium heparin may be greater than that of sodium heparin, the size of the initial heparin dose was believed to be of greatest importance. In general, however, adequate prolongation of the aPTT with subcutaneous calcium heparin requires more than 24 hours, making the subcutaneous route less attractive for the management of acute thrombosis.

Low molecular weight heparins (LMWH) are prepared by treating standard heparin with depolymerizing agents or enzymes and recovering fragments retaining the ability to bind antithrombin III [28]. These fragments are approximately a third the size of unfractionated heparin (UFH) and have much better bioavailability after subcutaneous injection. Although they have considerably less antithrombin activity than UFH (and produce

Table 10-2. Anticoagulant Management of Acute Thromboembolism

Step 1. Obtain aPTT, PT, and platelet count.
Step 2. Give heparin: intravenous bolus of 80 U/kg, continuous infusion of 18 U/kg per hour
Step 3. Repeat aPTT at 4–6 hours and adjust heparin dose as follows:

aPTT, < 1.5 × control	40 U/kg bolus, then 2 U/kg/hr
aPTT, 1.5–2.3 × control	No change
aPTT, 2.3–3.0 × control	Decrease by 2 U/kg/hr
aPTT, > 3 × control	Hold infusion 1 hr, decrease by 3 U/kg/hr

Step 4. Continue heparin for 5 days, and obtain aPTT daily.
Step 5. Begin warfarin, 10 mg daily, on day 1.
Step 6. Obtain PT on day 2 and daily, and reduce dose of warfarin when international normalized ratio reaches 2.0.
Step 7. International normalized ratio should be at least 2 for 48–72 hours before heparin is discontinued. Target is an international normalized ratio of 2–3.
Step 8. Continue treatment at least 3 months for DVT and 6 months for PE, recurrent DVT, or continued immobility.

aPTT = activated partial thromboplastin time; PT = prothrombin time; DVT = deep vein thrombosis.

much less prolongation of the aPTT), they have potent antifactor Xa activity and are less inactivated by platelets. Furthermore, their predictable dose-response relationship makes laboratory monitoring unnecessary. In clinical trials of patients with acute DVT and PE, daily subcutaneous injections of LMWH were equally as effective and safe as continuous intravenous infusion of UFH [29, 30]. Thus, LMWH would appear to be ideal for the treatment of patients with acute thromboembolism; however, more clinical trials are needed to confirm the promise of these agents, and they are not yet approved by the U.S. Food and Drug Administration (FDA) for this indication.

Follow-Up Management

Warfarin therapy is usually initiated on day 1, after the initial doses of heparin have prolonged the aPTT into the therapeutic range [31]. At least 5 days of overlap therapy of heparin with warfarin is usually necessary to ensure against thrombus extension or embolization. This is because of the rather long half-lives of clotting factors IX and X. Although warfarin administration will result in a rapid decline in the relatively short-lived factor VII, and prolongation of the prothrombin time, depletion of this factor alone does not protect against thrombosis. It is only when the levels of factors IX and X approach 20% of normal that an antithrombotic effect is achieved.

Warfarin therapy is monitored with the prothrombin time, examining the ratio of the patient to the control prothrombin time. Because the various thromboplastin reagents used for the prothrombin time differ in their sensitivity to the effects of warfarin on the coagulant factors, an international normalized ratio (INR) has been developed to assess the intensity of warfarin anticoagulation. By consulting a table, laboratory technicians can compare the sensitivity of their thromboplastin against a well-characterized international reagent and report their results in terms of the INR. The INR has been intensively investigated in patients receiving warfarin, and it has been determined that values of 2.0–3.0 indicate a safe and effective level of anticoagulation in most patients with DVT [32].

Alternative Regimens

Calf-Vein Thrombosis

Some have argued that because calf-vein thrombi rarely embolize, an initial short course of heparin (5–7 days) might be adequate to prevent extension or recurrence of thrombosis. However, Lagerstedt and coworkers [33] observed recurrence within 3 months in 8 of 28 patients who did not receive warfarin therapy after their initial course of heparin. In contrast, none of the warfarin-treated subjects had a recurrence during this time frame. On the other hand, Hull and associates [34] observed a low rate of recurrence in patients receiving low-dose subcutaneous heparin (5,000 U every 12 hours); the rate was similar to those receiving warfarin. However, bleeding complications are much more frequent with warfarin. Therefore, patients with calf-vein DVT should receive initial treatment with either intravenous heparin followed by subcutaneous low doses of heparin or, alternatively, LMWH. Patients can be monitored with serial ultrasound, and if there is evidence of thrombus extension, the dose of subcutaneous heparin or LMWH can be increased, or warfarin therapy initiated.

Maintenance Warfarin Versus Subcutaneous Heparin

Although low-dose subcutaneous heparin was associated with a low rate of complications in *calf-vein* thrombosis, patients with acute *proximal vein* thrombosis receiving low-dose subcutaneous heparin had a 19.3% incidence of recurrent thromboembolism [26]. However, increasing the dose of subcutaneous heparin to prolong the aPTT to 1.5–2.0 times the control value was as effective as warfarin therapy in preventing recurrences and was associated with a lower frequency of bleeding complications [35]. This regimen, or one using LMWH, is particularly attractive for patients likely to have problems with warfarin therapy, such as those with impaired liver function, poor diet, or malignancy.

Pulmonary Embolism

In patients with PE, antithrombin III levels are often low and the doses of heparin required to prolong the aPTT into the therapeutic range may be high. Because recurrent embolization is associated with increased morbidity and mortality, vigorous and prompt anticoagulation is essential. Initial doses of heparin may be two to three times greater than those shown in Table 10-2. Thrombolytic therapy should be considered early in the treatment of massive and submassive embolization.

Contraindications to Anticoagulant Therapy

Some contraindications to anticoagulant therapy are presented in the following list:

1. An intracranial hemorrhage or craniotomy within the preceding 72 hours is considered an absolute contraindication to anticoagulant therapy. Usually a computed tomographic brain scan or magnetic resonance imaging is performed to document the extent and age of the hemorrhage.
2. Serious, ongoing gastrointestinal bleeding.
3. Active bleeding into chest, abdomen, or genitourinary tract.
4. History of heparin-induced thrombocytopenia.

For patients with these serious contraindications to prompt heparin therapy for acute venous thrombosis, as well as for patients who have continued to have major thromboembolism despite adequate anticoagulant therapy, placement of an inferior vena cava filter is recommended [36]. An angiogram is performed to demonstrate the extent of venous thrombosis and to visualize the anatomy of the vena cava. The filter is introduced percutaneously and deployed distal to the renal veins [37]. It should be recognized that although this procedure dramatically reduces the frequency of pulmonary embolization (to 5%), recurrent venous thrombosis occurs and eventually requires long-term warfarin therapy in half the patients as well as elastic hose to control edema.

Complications include misplacement of the filter (occasionally in the renal vein), tilting of the filter permitting pulmonary embolization, and migration of the filter to distant sites. Relative contraindications to anticoagulation, such as recent surgery, hepatic disease, renal failure, or low-grade gastrointestinal bleeding, may be amenable to a lesser intensity of heparin therapy, with aPTTs no longer than 1.5 times control, or the use of LMWH.

Other Antithrombotic Agents

Dextran

This polysaccharide is given by daily intravenous infusions. It impairs platelet function, decreases blood viscosity, and enhances fibrinolysis. Although it has been usually employed in the prophylaxis of venous and arterial thrombosis, it is sometimes used to treat DVT. It has the disadvantages of high cost and risk of inducing allergic (and anaphylactic) reactions and may cause volume overload and oligemic renal failure.

Table 10-3. Thromboembolic Prophylaxis

Mechanical methods
    Early ambulation
    Graduated compression stockings
    Intermittent pneumatic compression leggings
Antithrombotic drugs
    Unfractionated heparin, alone or in combination with
       dihydroergotamine
    Low molecular weight heparin
    Warfarin
    Dextran
Combined approach
    Stockings or leggings plus antithrombotic drug

Thrombolytic Therapy

Streptokinase, urokinase, and tissue plasminogen activator lyse venous thrombi and pulmonary emboli, but their use may be complicated by serious bleeding and a variety of other untoward effects, including the embolization of proximal venous thrombi to the lung. In addition, patients with antibodies to streptococcal proteins may be resistant to therapy or have allergic, usually febrile, reactions to streptokinase. Urokinase and tissue plasminogen activator are considerably more expensive than streptokinase. These agents may be used locally or systemically. The thrombin time may be used to ascertain that an adequate lytic effect is present. The evidence that lysis of proximal vein thrombi reduces the frequency of postphlebitic syndrome is tenuous [1].

Prevention

The importance of prevention with regard to thromboembolism cannot be overemphasized. The particular measure selected for prophylaxis depends on the duration and degree of immobility and becomes especially important if surgical procedures are contemplated. Some of the mechanical agents and antithrombotic drugs in current use for thrombus prevention are listed in Table 10-3; other approaches such as functional electrical stimulation of muscles and newer anticoagulants are under investigation.

Mechanical Agents

Early Ambulation

Early ambulation is clearly desirable, not only to prevent thromboembolism but also to limit osteoporosis (see Chapter 4) and to prevent the development of pressure sores (see Chapter 13); in addition, ambulation improves appetite and a sense of well-being. Miller and coworkers [38] showed that early ambulation of patients with acute myocardial infarction, especially when complicated by congestive failure, significantly reduced the incidence of DVT. If ambulation is not possible, physical therapy with active or passive ranging should be instituted.

Graduated Compression Stockings

Graduated compression stockings apply firm pressure at the foot and ankle and lesser compression more proximally. They may be obtained from commercial sources or can be fabricated by applying several layers of elastic stockinette to the limb. Compression stockings have been shown to provide effective prophylaxis in low-risk postoperative surgical patients (nonorthopedic procedures) and are probably efficacious in nonparalytic medical illnesses. They may also be safely combined with low-dose subcutaneous heparin (5,000 U subcutaneously every 12 hours) to provide prophylaxis in higher risk subjects. Their only drawbacks are that they can be warm, itchy, and tend to slide down the leg.

Intermittent Pneumatic Compression Leggings

Intermittent pneumatic compression leggings are applied to the lower limb to exert rhythmic, sequential compression of the calf and thigh. Investigators have demonstrated that they significantly decrease the incidence of DVT in patients at moderate to high risk of thrombosis, such as those with malignant disease or those having general surgery [39]. The leggings are also useful in neurosurgical patients in whom anticoagulant drugs are contraindicated. Because they require connection to a pump, they restrict patient activities, especially rehabilitation therapies that require the patient to be out of bed. Other problems, such as the constant hum of the pump motor and the sensation of pressure on the limb, are relatively minor annoyances.

Pneumatic leggings have been combined with aspirin to provide effective prophylaxis in patients undergoing knee replacement [40].

Antithrombotic Agents

Subcutaneous Unfractionated Heparin

Recent years have seen a greater flexibility in the use of heparin, with the recognition that the dose should be tailored to the risk of thrombosis. High risk is associated with shortening of the aPTT, primarily due to increases in factor VIII, an acute phase reactant. Normalizing or modestly prolonging the aPTT should decrease the potential for thromboembolism. Thus, a two-tiered approach to the prophylactic use of UFH has been established: low-dose and adjusted dose. Low doses of 5,000 U two to three times daily are used for most medical patients and for patients having general abdominal, urologic, and gynecologic surgery. For those at higher risk (orthopedic procedures on the hip or knee or spinal cord injury), adjusting the dose of heparin to achieve slightly prolonged aPTTs is recommended [41, 42]. Heparin may also be combined with dihydroergotamine; in one study the combination was more effective than heparin alone in preventing DVT in patients undergoing elective abdominal, pelvic, or thoracic surgery [43]. However, this agent should not be used in patients with known or suspected coronary or peripheral arterial disease because of the vasoconstrictive effects of the ergotamine.

Low Molecular Weight Heparin

LMWHs have been used for thromboprophylaxis in general medical and surgical patients, those with stroke and spinal cord injury, and a variety of other settings (recently reviewed in Green et al. [44]). They have usually been given in doses ranging from 3,500–5,000 anti-Xa units subcutaneously either once or twice daily. In most reported studies, the LMWH was either as effective or more effective than UFH, and in many trials its use resulted in less bleeding and fewer injection site hematomas. In the United States, LMWHs have been approved for the prevention of thrombosis in patients undergoing hip replacement surgery or abdominal surgery; other in-

dications are under consideration for approval. A major limitation in the use of LMWH has been cost; the approved preparations are almost ten times more expensive, per dose, than UFH. Therefore, the drug should be prescribed only for those patients who cannot tolerate UFH, or in clinical settings where LMWH has been shown to be superior in preventing major morbidity and mortality from thromboembolic disease (in hip replacement surgery, spinal cord injury, and possibly malignancy).

Warfarin

Warfarin has the advantage of being orally effective, but has the disadvantage of requiring close monitoring of the prothrombin time in order to avoid hemorrhage. This is particularly difficult in the chronically ill, who are frequently receiving other drugs that may potentiate or inhibit the anticoagulant effects of warfarin; and whose nutritional status is poor, which enhances warfarin toxicity. Nevertheless, by using small doses (2.5 mg) and attempting to achieve minimal prolongation of the prothrombin time (4 seconds above control; INR of 1.5–2.0), a prophylactic effect may be achieved. Francis and coworkers [45] used a two-step approach in high-risk patients undergoing total hip or knee replacement; low doses of warfarin were given preoperatively, and full therapeutic doses (to prolong the prothrombin time to 1.5 times control) were given immediately postoperatively. This regimen proved quite effective. In the prevention of recurrent venous thromboembolism, Hull and associates [46] showed that low-dose warfarin (prothrombin time, 4 seconds above control) was as effective and safer than standard warfarin (prothrombin time, 8 seconds above control).

Dextran

Dextran, given as an intravenous infusion in a dose of 10 ml/kg has been an effective antithrombotic agent in patients undergoing surgery [47], but is not as efficacious as low-dose heparin or LMWH in patients having elective hip replacement [39]. Other disadvantages of dextran include high cost, need for intravenous administration, and potential for anaphylactic reactions and oliguric renal failure.

The use of aspirin or other nonsteroidal anti-inflammatory drugs, such as naproxen and ketorolac, should be avoided in patients receiving heparin, LMWH, warfarin, and dextran because these drugs are likely to enhance the risk of serious bleeding.

In Neurology and Neurosurgery

Thrombotic Stroke

Studies using radiolabeled fibrinogen scanning have shown that patients with thrombotic stroke have a high incidence of venous thrombosis; a figure of 75% was reported in one group of elderly subjects [4]. In these patients, low doses of heparin (5,000 U every 8 hours) decreased the number of positive scans to 12.5%. More recently, a low molecular weight heparinoid (ORG 10172) proved to be even more effective than standard heparin for this indication [48]. It is recommended that stroke patients whose computed tomographic or magnetic resonance imaging studies show no evidence of hemorrhage receive either heparin or LMWH until they are ambulatory or at least for the duration of their initial hospitalization. When such patients are readmitted to hospital because of infection, heart failure, or other problems, their anticoagulant prophylaxis should be resumed [49].

Hemorrhagic Stroke and Postcraniotomy

Patients who have had hemorrhagic stroke or a craniotomy are also at high risk for thromboembolism, but there is concern that anticoagulants, even in low doses, may exacerbate hemorrhage. Therefore, compression stockings or boots, which have been shown to be both safe and effective, have been applied in the immediate postoperative period [50]. However, a recent trial demonstrated that LMWH may be safely used in combination with compression hose and continued through the period of rehabilitation [51]. LMWH is recommended rather than standard heparin because in most studies it seems to have a reduced risk of bleeding.

Spinal Cord Injury

The incidence of clinically evident DVT in the spinal cord injured patient is 16.3% and of thrombosis detected by objective tests is 79% [5]. My colleagues and I have shown that external compression leggings can reduce this to 33% and that most of these thrombi will be in the distal rather than proximal veins [7]. In a subsequent study [42], we randomized patients to receive either low-dose heparin (5,000 U every 12 hours) or heparin doses adjusted to prolong the aPTT approximately 1.5 times control (mean dose, 13,200 U every 12 hours). Thromboembolism occurred in 9 of 29 (31%) in the low-dose group and only 2 of 29 (7%) receiving the adjusted dose ($p < 0.05$). However, bleeding necessitated discontinuation of the heparin in 24% of those randomized to the adjusted dose and none on the low dose ($p = 0.02$). It was concluded that patients must be carefully selected and monitored if they are to be treated with adjusted dose heparin. More recently, we compared heparin, 5,000 U every 8 hours, with LMWH, 3,500 U given once daily [52]. After 39 patients had entered the trial, the study was stopped because five of those patients receiving standard heparin had developed either thrombosis or bleeding; no patient on the LMWH had an event ($p = 0.05$). Thereafter, all patients were treated with LMWH; of 68 patients enrolled, only seven have had thrombosis and one has had bleeding [53]. By Kaplan-Meier analysis, the event-free estimate for all patients at 56 weeks is 84.4%, with a standard error of 5.1%. Our studies also suggested that obesity and tetraparesis increased the risk of treatment failure, and that in these higher risk patients, prophylaxis should be continued for more than 8 weeks. Prophylaxis could reasonably be terminated when spasticity has supplanted flaccidity, and patients are capable of actively participating in rehabilitation therapies.

Complications

Pulmonary Embolism

Some PEs have been described as "widow makers" in recognition of their lethality [54]. Death may occur within minutes, preventing application of effective therapy. Therefore, prevention is at the core of patient management, with the more vigorous prophylactic measures used for those at the high-

Table 10-4. Complications of Anticoagulant Therapy

Heparin
1. Bleeding: Dose-related; rare in first 48 hours of therapy; more common in elderly women. Unusual sites of bleeding include gut wall with bowel obstruction, adrenal (may be massive), retroperitoneal, intrapulmonary, compartment syndrome with nerve entrapment
2. Osteoporosis (with long-term therapy)
3. Thrombocytopenia (1–2% incidence; may be associated with thrombosis including stroke, myocardial infarction, or gangrene of an extremity)
4. Alopecia (rare)
5. Transaminase increase

Low molecular weight heparin
1. Bleeding: Appears to be less frequent than with standard heparin. Most often in patients also receiving nonsteroidal anti-inflammatory agents
2. Osteoporosis (may be less common than with standard heparin)
3. Thrombocytopenia (significantly less than with standard heparin, but 90% of patients with heparin-associated thrombocytopenia will also have syndrome with low molecular weight heparin)

Warfarin
1. Bleeding: Dose related; potentiated by various medications, alcohol, starvation, liver disease
2. Teratogenicity in first and possibly second trimester; neonatal bleeding in third trimester
3. Skin and muscle necrosis related to effects on proteins C and S
4. Cholesterol embolization (purple toes syndrome)

est risk. We recently reviewed the histories of spinal cord injured patients who died of acute, massive PE, in comparison with those who had a benign course [55]. The fatal cases were more likely to have higher spinal cord injuries, have less spasticity, and be obese; they also tended to be older and had experienced more adverse medical events such as infection. Recurrent emboli may also lead to pulmonary hypertension and right-sided heart failure.

Postphlebitic Syndrome

The postphlebitic syndrome is characterized by a variety of signs and symptoms, including pain, swelling, induration, pigmentation, and ulceration [56]. The clinical picture depends on which vein has been thrombosed. For example, if the common iliac vein is occluded and fails to recanalize, then the leg may become cyanotic, tense, and subject to venous claudication (pain with exercise). When femoral and popliteal veins are thrombosed, the perforating veins usually become incompetent, leading to pigmentation, swelling, and ulceration around the ankle. In other situations, veins distal to the site of obstruction distend and their valves become incompetent, resulting in persistent edema [1]. The diagnosis is suspected on clinical grounds and confirmed by venous ultrasound studies or venography. It is important to perform these examinations, because the symptoms of the postphlebitic syndrome can mimic those of recurrent DVT, but full-dose anticoagulation is not indicated because no fresh thrombus is present. The patient is spared much discomfort and disability if DVT can be prevented, because postphlebitic syndrome appears unpredictably after DVT. Factors that may be relevant are inadequate initial treatment of the DVT (i.e., an aPTT insufficiently prolonged [57]), and certain distinctive patient characteristics such as obesity or paralysis. We evaluated 50 patients with venographically verified DVT for evidence of vein recanalization [58]. In nonparalyzed subjects, recanalization generally occurred by 33 days after the acute thrombosis, but in paraplegic patients it was delayed by as much as 4 weeks, and several never showed evidence of recanalization.

Complications of Anticoagulant Therapy

Heparin and Low Molecular Weight Heparin

Some of the complications observed with heparin therapy are listed in Table 10-4. Of course, bleeding is the most common and is dose dependent [59]. In addition, bleeding is related to patient characteristics; it is more frequent in the elderly, women, and those with injury or disease of blood vessels. Examples of the latter are patients with peptic ulceration, gastritis, or colitis; these are all relative contraindications to heparin therapy. Bleeding is also more likely in those who have other hemostatic defects, such as deficient or defective platelets or clotting factors. Such defects are observed in patients with hepatic or renal disease, and platelet function is also adversely affected by aspirin, other nonsteroidal anti-inflammatory agents, and alcohol; these should be avoided in patients receiving anticoagulants. The other adverse reactions attributed to heparin are much less common and include osteoporosis (20,000 U daily for more than 6 months [60]), thrombocytopenia (1–2% of those receiving the drug for more than 7–10 days), and an increase in transaminase, which does not appear to be clinically significant. LMWHs appear to cause less bleeding and bone fractures, and infrequently induce thrombocytopenia [61].

Warfarin

The effectiveness and bleeding risk with warfarin are profoundly influenced by patient characteristics and concurrent medications. Bleeding is more likely to occur in subjects whose nutritional status fluctuates unpredictably. During periods of relative starvation, such persons become exquisitely sensitive to the anticoagulant effects of warfarin and are likely to bleed. The situation is aggravated if antibiotics are prescribed during this period. Patients with renal or hepatic disease are also more sensitive to warfarin. In contrast, anticonvulsant agents may confer extreme warfarin resistance, and massive doses may be required to achieve satisfactory levels of anticoagulation. Abrupt cessation of the anticonvulsant may be accompanied by a sudden lengthening of the prothrombin time and bleeding. Alcohol and aspirin have both been implicated as causes of hemorrhage in patients receiving warfarin. The drug is contraindicated in pregnancy because it is teratogenic. An infrequent but devastating complication of warfarin therapy is skin and muscle necrosis due to thrombosis of capillaries and venules. This occurs in patients who either have congenital deficiencies of the vitamin K–dependent anticoagulant proteins C or S or have acquired such deficiencies as a

result of poor vitamin K intake or absorption. The administration of warfarin in doses of 10 mg or more daily to such nutritionally depleted subjects results in a profound decrease in the plasma levels of these anticoagulants with ensuing thrombosis and skin and muscle necrosis. This problem is avoided by giving smaller initial doses of warfarin to such patients, along with full doses of heparin. Purple toes syndrome occurs in patients with ulcerating atheromatous lesions of the abdominal aorta. Administration of warfarin under these circumstances appears to result in loosening of atheromatous debris, principally cholesterol crystals, and distal embolization.

Case Management Studies

Case 1

A 40-year-old man fell at work, sustaining a T12 subluxation with paraplegia. A posterior spinal fusion from T9 to L2 was performed. Two weeks after surgery, the wound was found to be edematous and draining spinal fluid. He was treated conservatively with bed rest and antibiotics, but developed bilateral leg swelling.

1. What diagnostic procedures would be appropriate at this point?
2. Assuming the procedures are positive, how could this complication have been prevented?
3. What treatment would you prescribe?

A vena caval filter was inserted, but migrated to the right renal vein. The patient spiked a temperature of 102°F, and complained of pleuritic chest pain, shortness of breath, and palpitations. Blood gases were 7.4/38/85/94%.

4. What diagnostic procedures are indicated now?
5. If the results are positive, what should be done?

Discussion

Venous thrombosis is the most likely diagnosis and noninvasive venous studies should be done. Seeing a swollen leg in a postoperative patient immediately leads to consideration of DVT. On the other hand, a number of other disorders may simulate venous thrombosis; for example, cellulitis usually presents with a warm, edematous limb. However, the circumscribed area of erythema suggests the correct diagnosis. In young persons with paralysis, heterotopic ossification produces swelling and pain. It is distinguished from venous thrombosis by its characteristic radiographic appearance and positive bone scan result. Leg swelling due to congestive heart failure affects both lower limbs. Swelling of a paralyzed limb may also be due to its being kept in a dependent position, as after prolonged sitting in a wheelchair.

Many patients with postoperative DVT may not have leg swelling. Fever may be the only manifestation of their thrombosis. An unfortunate few will have a pulmonary embolus as the first sign of a previously silent thrombus in the lower extremity. Because the bedside examination for DVT is rarely definitive, it is necessary to establish the diagnosis with objective laboratory tests.

Using IPG, Doppler flow, and duplex ultrasound provides three relatively independent parameters for assessing the presence of venous thrombosis. Occasionally, however, one can be misled; for example, in those patients who have a heterotopic bone formation. The inflammatory mass of bone within the muscle may compress the veins, giving false-positive results in all three tests. In this situation, or to exclude clot in the distal veins of the leg, a venogram is required.

To return to our case, the next question was, assuming the procedure results are positive, how could this complication have been prevented? Table 10-3 shows various methods of prevention of DVT. Of the physical modalities, leg elevation is least effective, and early ambulation most effective in postoperative patients. In those unable to ambulate, compression hose and pneumatic compression boots are widely prescribed. Anticoagulants (warfarin and heparin) are the most efficacious of the pharmacologic agents. The volume expander, dextran, is not only less beneficial but also may be associated with anaphylaxis and acute renal failure. Antiplatelet drugs such as aspirin, although better than placebo, may cause gastritis and bleeding. So, the main ones that are used are external pneumatic compression devices and the anticoagulants.

With regard to the choice of anticoagulant in patients with spinal cord injury, LMWH has been shown to be more efficacious and associated with less bleeding than standard heparin, and is the prophylactic agent of choice. Prophylaxis should be given for at least the first 8 weeks after injury. If the patient is actively involved in physical therapy and

has had an uneventful course, prophylaxis could be safely discontinued at that time.

To return to the case management questions, having now diagnosed a DVT, what therapy is appropriate? Standard heparin by the intravenous route is currently the accepted treatment for acute thrombosis (see Table 10-2). Once the aPTT is within the therapeutic range, warfarin may be started, usually in a dose of 10 mg daily. Heparin may be discontinued when warfarin treatment has resulted in a prolongation of the prothrombin time to greater than 2 times the control value for 48 hours. Some clinicians have been reluctant to begin warfarin treatment concurrently with heparin, but in a randomized, double-blind trial, we found that the early administration of warfarin was as safe and effective as waiting 5 days before starting this agent. The advantages of this approach are that the length of hospital stay is shortened and the patient's exposure to heparin, with its adverse effects on platelets and bleeding, is curtailed.

The patient had a vena cava filter inserted, perhaps because his physicians were reluctant to give full-dose heparin treatment so soon after a major operative procedure. Unfortunately, the filter lodged in the right renal vein, instead of the vena cava. He then developed a temperature of 102°F and pleuritic chest pain, shortness of breath, and palpitations. His blood gases were pH 7.4, pCO_2 38, pO_2 85, and oxygen saturation, 94%. What diagnostic procedures are indicated now?

This presentation is most suggestive of a pulmonary embolus, although pneumonia or pneumothorax could give a similar clinical picture. If there is massive embolus, the patient is breathless, tachycardic, and hypotensive. Smaller emboli may be silent until a lung infarct involves the pleura; then there is pleuritic chest pain, cough, and hemoptysis. In addition to a careful history and physical examination, arterial blood gases should be examined and a $\dot{V}/\dot{Q}$ lung scan performed. Finding hypocapnia and hypoxia support the diagnosis, but a normal examination does not rule it out. A high probability $\dot{V}/\dot{Q}$ scan is over 90% accurate in diagnosing the condition, but an intermediate or low probability scan does not exclude it. In the latter instance, a pulmonary angiogram is required to establish the diagnosis.

The physicians managing this patient were concerned about the possibility of embolization, and tried to prevent this complication by inserting the vena cava filter. Such a filter, seated in the vena cava, has been found to be 90–95% effective in preventing PEs. An unusual occurrence is malpositioning of the filter in the renal vein. To reposition the device requires a major surgical procedure. However, to prevent recurrent PEs, one can simply insert another filter properly positioned in the vena cava, which was done in this case. Other problems with the filter are infrequent and include increased venous pressure in the legs with stasis ulcers and vena caval thrombosis at the site of the filter. It should be noted that eventually 50% of patients with a filter will require anticoagulant therapy because of recurrence of DVT.

Case 2

A 71-year-old woman sustained a left comminuted hip fracture and underwent open reduction and internal fixation. Antithrombotic prophylaxis with warfarin was prescribed, and after 2 weeks on this therapy her prothrombin time was 18 seconds. Over the next 2 weeks she received intensive rehabilitation therapy, but complained of weakness and noted some dark stools. The hemoglobin was 7 g/dl (it had been 11.6 g/dl 2 weeks earlier), and the prothrombin time was 42 seconds.

1. How could this complication have been prevented?
2. What treatment would you recommend?
3. The stools are positive for occult blood. Are additional diagnostic procedures indicated?

Discussion

Patients newly begun on warfarin therapy need careful monitoring with prothrombin times. We are told that after 2 weeks of warfarin treatment, the prothrombin time was 18 seconds, but no further prothrombin times were recorded in the case record. A great many factors influence the response to warfarin. Vitamin K or foods rich in vitamin K, such as raw broccoli, cabbage, and spinach, antagonize warfarin and shorten the prothrombin time. On the other hand, lengthening of the prothrombin time occurs in patients who become anorexic, have diarrhea, or receive antibiotics. In the patient under discussion, the

dose of warfarin prescribed may have been too large, or the intensive rehabilitation program may have kept her in pain, decreasing her food intake. At any rate, failure to monitor the warfarin treatment permitted her prothrombin time to increase to levels associated with bleeding. Warfarin ranks third among all drugs used in the hospital in causing patient injury. Because these agents have a low therapeutic index, they have to be watched closely. Patients should be given a warfarin information sheet, which explains why they need the drug, how it works, why they need to have prothrombin times done, why to take warfarin at a fixed time, why to avoid alcohol (because it may induce gastritis), why to avoid excessive amounts of raw vegetables, why to avoid aspirin, why to inform the doctor about new medications, how to avoid bleeding, and when to contact a physician.

The management of warfarin-induced bleeding is straightforward. If it is minor, holding the warfarin until the prothrombin decreases below 20 seconds will usually result in a cessation of hemorrhage, and the drug can be resumed at a lower dose. If the bleeding is moderate, the administration of fresh frozen plasma, in a dose of 15 ml/kg body weight, will rapidly replenish the clotting factors. If the prothrombin time is prolonged beyond 30 seconds and bleeding is moderate to severe, vitamin K will shorten the prothrombin time within 8–12 hours. The vitamin is usually given subcutaneously in doses ranging from 0.5 mg to 10 mg, repeated daily until the prothrombin time has returned to the therapeutic range.

The stools were positive for occult blood; are additional diagnostic procedures indicated? A recent study showed that if the prothrombin time was over 30 seconds, in the majority of the cases there were no lesions in the gastrointestinal tract. On the other hand, if the prothrombin time was between 10 and 20 seconds, then bleeding was usually due to a specific lesion. Values between 20 and 30 seconds were associated with lesions in about half the cases. In the patient under discussion, the prothrombin time was markedly prolonged, so there would be little point in performing intensive investigation to discover a specific bleeding source.

Case 3

A 26-year-old man suffered a C6 incomplete quadriplegia in a diving accident. Anterior and posterior spinal fusion with an iliac crest bone graft was performed. Three weeks later, while undergoing rehabilitation therapy, he complained of left pleuritic chest pain. His blood pressure was 110/76 mm Hg, pulse was 80, and respirations were 28–30. The pain was reproduced by pressure on the posterior scapular and acromioclavicular areas.

1. What other physical findings might be helpful in clarifying this problem?
2. Are any laboratory studies indicated at this point?

The patient was treated with acetaminophen, but 12 hours later was seen again because of worsening of the chest pain, and "shortness of breath with deep breaths."

3. Should any other therapy be started?
4. What diagnostic studies should be performed?

Discussion

The first consideration in this patient would be musculoskeletal pain. However, one should also listen to the breath sounds and check the temperature to exclude atelectasis or pulmonary infection. In addition, it is important to examine the lower extremities. We recommend measuring the circumference of the legs with a tape measure to detect subtle unilateral edema; this may be a clue to DVT and the origin of PEs.

The main laboratory study indicated at this time is a D-dimer test using ELISA technology. If the test result is negative, PE would be very unlikely. If it is positive, additional studies such as a ventilation/perfusion scan, blood gas measurement, and venous ultrasound examination of the legs would be obtained. These would confirm the presence and location of thrombi. Unfortunately, the ELISA d-dimer test was not available at the time this patient was encountered.

The patient was given analgesics that were temporarily effective, but the pain recurred 12 hours later and he was more short of breath. You might strongly consider giving him heparin at this point and order a $\dot{V}/\dot{Q}$ lung scan. To re-emphasize the point, a high index of suspicion is important in diagnosing thromboembolism; any unexplained fever, tachycardia, dyspnea, or chest pains should prompt investigation. In this patient, a $\dot{V}/\dot{Q}$ scan performed at the time of his first episode of chest pain showed a small defect

at the left apex. The scan was read as low to intermediate probability, and no treatment was given. Three days later, he suddenly experienced marked shortness of breath and became hypotensive; a repeat $\dot{V}/\dot{Q}$ scan showed multiple segmental perfusion defects. A venous flow study, performed at this time, showed thrombus in the proximal veins of the right leg. DVT is often unsuspected in patients who subsequently are shown to have PE. In one study, of 195 patients with autopsy-proven PE, DVT was clinically suspected before death in only 38, but was actually present at autopsy in 162. The other side of the coin is that patients who have DVT will also often have clinically silent PE; 51% of patients in one series had high probability lung scans.

What is the appropriate management for the patient with massive PE? The prompt infusion of a thrombolytic agent will often rapidly clear the emboli and reduce the pulmonary hypertension. There is a whole gamut of thrombolytic agents to choose from, including streptokinase, anisoylated streptokinase, urokinase, single-chain urokinase, and tissue plasminogen activator. Our patient was treated with urokinase because there is a large published literature attesting to its effectiveness in acute PE. He dramatically improved and a repeat $\dot{V}/\dot{Q}$ scan show resolution of the emboli. Intravenous heparin and then warfarin were given and he was transferred back to the rehabilitation institute.

A question often raised is, when is it safe to start mobilizing a patient with a recently diagnosed DVT? Animal studies have suggested that the thrombus is firmly bound to the vein wall within 5 days of its formation. Because thrombus is usually present in most patients for several days before it is recognized, I usually start ambulation or physical therapy 2–3 days after anticoagulant therapy has been instituted. I encourage patients to exercise. Exercise has been shown to increase the fibrinolytic activity of the blood, and may lead to more rapid recanalization of the thrombus. Pulmonary emboli occurring when patients are turned or otherwise manipulated are usually clots that have formed acutely. They are clinically unsuspected because the leg has not had time to become edematous.

References

1. Hirsh J, Hull RD. Venous Thromboembolism: Natural History, Diagnosis, and Management. Boca Raton, FL: CRC Press, 1987.

2. Goldhaber SZ, Savage DD, Garrison RJ, et al. Risk factors for pulmonary embolism: The Framingham Study. Am J Med 1983;74:1023.

3. Warlow C, Ogston D, Douglas AS. Venous thrombosis following strokes. Lancet 1972;i:1305.

4. McCarthy ST, Robertson D, Turner JJ, Hawkey CJ. Low-dose heparin as a prophylaxis against deep-vein thrombosis after acute stroke. Lancet 1977;ii:800.

5. Weingarden SI. Deep venous thrombosis in spinal cord injury: Overview of the problem. Chest 1992;102(Suppl):636S.

6. Rossi EC, Green D, Rosen JS, et al. Sequential changes in factor VIII and platelets preceding deep vein thrombosis in patients with spinal cord injury. Br J Haematol 1980;45:143.

7. Green D, Rossi EC, Yao JST, et al. Deep vein thrombosis in spinal cord injury: Effect of prophylaxis with calf compression, aspirin, and dipyridamole. Paraplegia 1982;20:227.

8. Walsh PN, Rogers PH, Marder VJ, et al. The relationship of platelet coagulant activities to venous thrombosis following hip surgery. Br J Haematol 1976;32:421.

9. Sue-Ling HM, McMahon MJ, Johnston D, et al. Preoperative identification of patients at high risk of deep venous thrombosis after elective major abdominal surgery. Lancet 1986;1:1173.

10. Stewart GJ. Neutrophils and deep venous thrombosis. Haemostasis 1993;23(Suppl 1):127.

11. Marin HM, Stefanini M. Experimental production of thrombophlebitis. Surg Gynecol Obstet 1960;110:263.

12. Moser KM, LeMoine JR. Is embolic risk conditioned by location of deep venous thrombosis? Ann Intern Med 1981;94:439.

13. Urokinase Pulmonary Embolism Trial (UPET). A national cooperative study. Circulation 1973;47(Suppl 2):1.

14. Browse NL, Thomas ML. Source of non-lethal pulmonary emboli. Lancet 1974;1:258.

15. Weingarden DS, Weingarden SI, Belen J. Thromboembolic disease presenting as fever in spinal cord injury. Arch Phys Med Rehabil 1987;68:176.

16. DiSerio FJ, Parno J, Singer JM. Limitation of impedance plethysmography in assessing efficacy of dihydroergotamine-heparin prophylaxis of deep vein thrombosis. Thromb Res 1985;37:449.

17. Frieden RA, Ahn JH, Pineda HD, et al. Venous plethysmography values in patients with spinal cord injury. Arch Phys Med Rehabil 1987;168:427.

18. Heijboer H, Buller HR, Lensing AWA, et al. A comparison of real-time compression ultrasonography with impedance plethysmography for the diagnosis of deep-vein thrombosis in symptomatic outpatients. N Engl J Med 1993;329:1365.

19. White RH, McGahan JP, Daschbach MM, Hartling RP. Diagnosis of deep-vein thrombosis using duplex ultrasound. Ann Intern Med 1989;111:297.

20. Davidson BL, Elliott CG, Lensing AWA. Low accuracy of color Doppler ultrasound in the detection of proximal leg vein thrombosis in asymptomatic high-risk patients. Ann Intern Med 1992;117:735.

21. Thomas ML. Phlebography. Arch Surg 1972;104:145.

22. Bell WR, Simon TL, Demets DL. The clinical features of submassive and massive pulmonary embolism. Am J Med 1977;62:355.

23. The PIOPED Investigators. Value of the ventilation/perfusion scan in acute pulmonary embolism. Results of the prospective investigation of pulmonary embolism diagnosis (PIOPED). JAMA 1990;263:2753.

24. Bounameaux H, de Moerloose P, Perrier A, Reber G. Plasma measurement of d-dimer as diagnostic aid in suspected venous thromboembolism: an overview. Thromb Haemost 1994;71:1.

25. Raschke RA, Reilly BM, Guidry JR, et al. The weight-based heparin dosing nomogram compared with a "standard care" nomogram. Ann Intern Med 1993;119:874.

26. Hull RD, Raskob GE, Hirsh J, et al. Continuous intravenous heparin compared with intermittent subcutaneous heparin in the initial treatment of proximal-vein thrombosis. N Engl J Med 1986;315:1109.

27. Doyle DJ, Turpie AGG, Hirsh J, et al. Adjusted subcutaneous or intravenous heparin in patients with acute deep vein thrombosis. Ann Intern Med 1987;107:441.

28. Hirsh J, Levine MN. Low molecular weight heparin. Blood 1992;79:1.

29. Hull RD, Raskob GE, Pineo GF, et al. Subcutaneous low-molecular-weight heparin compared with continuous intravenous heparin in the initial treatment of proximal-vein thrombosis. N Engl J Med 1992;326:975.

30. Levine M, Gent M, Hirsh J, et al. A comparison of low-molecular-weight heparin administered primarily at home with unfractionated heparin administered in the hospital for proximal deep-vein thrombosis. N Engl J Med 1996;334:677.

31. Hull RD, Raskob GE, Rosenbloom D, et al. Heparin for 5 days as compared with 10 days in the initial treatment of proximal venous thrombosis. N Engl J Med 1990;322:1260.

32. Hirsh J, Dalen JE, Deykin D, et al. Oral anticoagulants: Mechanism of action, clinical effectiveness, and optimal therapeutic range. Chest 1995;108(Suppl):231S.

33. Lagerstedt CI, Fagher BO, Olsson CG, et al. Need for long-term anticoagulant treatment in symptomatic calf-vein thrombosis. Lancet 1985;2:515.

34. Hull RD, Delmore T, Genton E, et al. Warfarin sodium versus low-dose heparin in the long-term treatment of venous thrombosis. N Engl J Med 1979;301:855.

35. Hull RD, Delmore T, Carter C, et al. Adjusted subcutaneous heparin versus warfarin sodium in the long-term treatment of venous thrombosis. N Engl J Med 1982;306:189.

36. Greenfield LJ, Peyton R, Crute S, Barnes R. Greenfield vena caval filter experience. Arch Surg 1981;116:1451.

37. Greenfield LJ, Stewart JR, Crute S. Improved technique for Greenfield vena cava filter insertion. Surg Gynecol Obstet 1983;156:217.

38. Miller RR, Lies JE, Carretta RF, et al. Prevention of lower extremity venous thrombosis by early mobilization. Ann Intern Med 1976;84:700.

39. Clagett GP, Anderson FA Jr, Heit J, et al. Prevention of venous thromboembolism. Chest 1995;108(Suppl):312S.

40. McKenna R, Galante J, Bachmann F, et al. Prevention of venous thromboembolism after total knee replacement by high dose aspirin or intermittent calf and thigh compression. BMJ 1980;1:514.

41. Hirsh J, Raschke R, Warkentin TE, et al. Heparin: Mechanism of action, pharmacokinetics, dosing considerations, monitoring, efficacy, and safety. Chest 1995;108(Suppl):238S.

42. Green D, Lee MY, Ito VY, et al. Fixed versus adjusted dose heparin in the prophylaxis of thromboembolism in spinal cord injury. JAMA 1988;260:1255.

43. Multicenter Trial. Dihydroergotamine-heparin prophylaxis of postoperative deep vein thrombosis. JAMA 1984;251:2960.

44. Green D, Hirsh J, Heit J, et al. Low molecular weight heparin: a critical analysis of clinical trials. Pharmacol Rev 1994;46:89.

45. Francis CW, Marder VJ, Evarts CM, Yaukoolbodi S. Two-step warfarin therapy. JAMA 1983;249:374.

46. Hull RD, Hirsh J, Jay RM, et al. Different intensities of oral anticoagulant therapy in the treatment of proximal-vein thrombosis. N Engl J Med 1982;307:1676.

47. Bonnar J, Walsh J. Prevention of thrombosis after pelvic surgery by British dextran 70. Lancet 1972;1:614.

48. Turpie AGG, Gent M, Cote R, et al. A low-molecular-weight heparinoid compared with unfractionated heparin in the prevention of deep vein thrombosis in patients with acute ischemic stroke. Ann Intern Med 1992;117:353.

49. Halkin H, Goldberg J, Modan M, Modan B. Reduction of mortality in general medical in-patients by low-dose heparin prophylaxis. Ann Intern Med 1982;96:561.

50. Turpie AGG, Gallus A, Beattie WS, Hirsh J. Prevention of venous thrombosis in patients with intracranial disease by intermittent pneumatic compression of the calf. Neurology 1977;27:435.

51. Nurmohamed MT, van Riel AM, Henkens CMA, et al. Low molecular weight heparin and compression stockings in the prevention of venous thromboembolism in neurosurgery. Thromb Haemost 1996;75:233.

52. Green D, Lee MY, Lim AC, et al. Prevention of thromboembolism after spinal cord injury using low-molecular-weight heparin. Ann Intern Med 1990;113:571.

53. Green D, Chen D, Chmiel JS, et al. Prevention of thromboembolism in spinal cord injury: Role of low molecular weight heparin. Arch Phys Med Rehabil 1994;75:290.

54. Greenfield LJ as quoted in Salzman EW. Low-molecular-weight heparin: Is small beautiful? N Engl J Med 1986;315:957.

55. Green D, Twardowski P, Wei R, Rademaker AW. Fatal pulmonary embolism in spinal cord injury. Chest 1994;105:853.

56. Editorial. Post-thrombotic venous disorders. Lancet 1985;1:1488.

57. Hull RD, Raskob GE, Rosenbloom D, et al. Optimal therapeutic level of heparin therapy in patients with venous thrombosis. Arch Intern Med 1992;152:1589.

58. Lim AC, Roth EJ, Green D. Lower limb paralysis: Its effect on the recanalization of deep-vein thrombosis. Arch Phys Med Rehabil 1992;73:331.

59. Levine MN, Raskob GE, Landefeld S, Hirsh J. Hemorrhagic complications of anticoagulant treatment. Chest 1995;108(Suppl):276S.

60. Levine MN. Complications of anticoagulant and thrombolytic therapy. In J Hirsh, RD Hull (eds), Venous Thromboembolis: Natural History, Diagnosis, and Management. Boca Raton, FL: CRC Press, 1987.

61. Warkentin TE, Levin MN, Hirsh J, et al. Heparin-induced thrombocytopenia in patients treated with low-molecular-weight heparin or unfractionated heparin. N Engl J Med 1995;332:1330.

Chapter 11

Anemia in the Chronically Disabled Patient

David Green and Benjamin T. Esparaz

Anemia is defined as a decrease in circulating hemoglobin. In men and women younger than age 65 years, values less than 12 and 11 g/dl, respectively, are abnormal [1]. With aging, there is a steady decline in the hemoglobin level in normal subjects, so that a hemoglobin value of 12 g/dl is normal in a man over 90 years of age [2].

Prevalance

Anemia is so common in the chronically disabled that it is more the rule than the exception. For example, in an unselected group of 32 elderly amputees admitted to the Rehabilitation Institute of Chicago, 80% had hemoglobin values of less than 12 g/dl and the average hemoglobin value ($\pm$ SD) was 10.5 $\pm$ 2.3 g/dl. These patients had a variety of chronic diseases, including coronary and peripheral vessel atherosclerosis, diabetes, and stump infections. In general, infection, inflammation, and malignancy are the most common disease categories associated with the anemia of chronic disease [3]. Chronic renal and hepatic diseases are also associated with anemia, but the anemia in these disorders has a somewhat different pathogenetic mechanism. Other causes of anemia, such as blood loss, endocrine disorders, and hemolysis, also occur in chronically ill patients and must be distinguished from the anemia of inflammation. In this discussion, we focus mainly on the anemia of inflammation and differentiate it from these other causes of anemia.

Characteristics

The important hematologic terms used in this discussion are defined in Table 11-1. The hemoglobin level in patients with the anemia of inflammation is almost always in the range of 10 $\pm$ 2 g/dl. A more severe anemia usually implies that an additional etiologic factor, such as blood loss, is present. The anemia generally develops within a month after the onset of the chronic illness and is nonprogressive [4, 5]. The red blood cells are normochromic and normocytic, although occasionally there may be mild hypochromia and red blood cell indices are on the low to normal side. The reticulocyte count is inappropriately low for the degree of anemia, indicating that production of red blood cells is impaired. In addition, red blood cell survival studies indicate that there is some increase in cell destruction.

The hallmark of the anemia of inflammation is a reduction in levels of serum iron, which occurs within 48 hours of the onset of an inflammatory process [6, 7]. The serum transferrin value is likewise decreased, but iron stores, as determined by measurements of serum ferritin or visual examination of stained bone marrow smears, are increased. The iron is located predominantly within macrophages rather than in sideroblasts. Iron utilization, measured by determining the incorporation of intravenously injected elemental iron into hemoglobin, is normal, but iron re-utilization, assessed by recording the incorporation of hemoglobin iron into newly synthesized hemoglobin, is abnormal. Iron absorption is also

Table 11-1. Glossary of Hematologic Terms

Red blood cell indices: The *mean corpuscular volume* is determined by dividing the hematocrit by the red blood cell count. High values occur in macrocytic anemias and in conditions in which there are increased numbers of circulating reticulocytes. Low values are seen in iron deficiency anemia and thalassemia. The *mean corpuscular hemoglobin concentration* is determined by dividing the hemoglobin by the hematocrit. High values occur in conditions characterized by spherocytosis, such as congenital and autoimmune hemolytic anemias. Low values occur in iron deficiency and thalassemia.

Reticulocyte count: Normal or elevated values must be interpreted in relationship to the red blood cell count. This is done most simply by multiplying the percentage of reticulocytes by the red blood cell count. Values in excess of 100,000/μL indicate that the bone marrow is compensating for the anemia, whereas lower numbers are characteristic of the anemia of chronic disease and deficiencies of iron, vitamin B_{12}, or folic acid.

Serum iron: This value represents iron bound to transferrin.

Total iron-binding capacity: This value indicates the total amount of circulating transferrin.

Percent saturation: The percentage of transferrin to which iron is bound.

Serum transferrin receptor: The membrane-associated receptor for transferrin that is also found in the circulation; levels are elevated in iron deficiency anemia but not in the anemia of inflammation.

Zinc protoporphyrin: Protoporphyrin is the precursor of heme; when iron metabolism is abnormal, as in iron deficiency, lead poisoning, and the anemia of inflammation, zinc rather than iron is incorporated into protoporphyrin.

Serum ferritin: A circulating and stored iron-protein complex.

Hemosiderin: An aggregate of ferritin molecules visible by light microscopy after Prussian-blue staining.

---

impaired. Other findings are an increase in red cell zinc protoporphyrin, a marker of disturbed iron metabolism [8], and normal levels of serum transferrin receptor, which is reliably increased in iron deficiency anemia [9].

Some characteristic laboratory values in the anemia of inflammation are shown in Table 11-2. According to Schilling [10], the combination of low serum iron and low iron binding capacity with an elevated serum ferritin value is probably the best indicator of the anemia of inflammation. To explain these abnormalities in iron metabolism, normal iron physiology is reviewed and the ways in which chronic disease may alter these pathways is described.

Iron Metabolism

The total body iron content is estimated to be about 3,500 mg in women and 4,000 mg in men. The major fraction of body iron (almost two-thirds) is found in the iron-porphyrin complex of hemoglobin at a concentration of approximately 1 g/kg of red blood cells. The next largest fraction (approximately one-fourth) is stored in the monocyte-macrophage system as ferritin and hemosiderin, and a smaller fraction is present in muscle as myoglobin (approximately 300 mg). The remainder of the essential iron is used in heme and nonheme enzymes for normal cellular function.

Iron is absorbed mainly in the duodenum and proximal jejunum. Iron access is regulated by intestinal mucosal absorption, and iron elimination is regulated by sloughing of epidermal and mucosal cells [11, 12]. Mucosal transferrin binds iron in the gut lumen and transports it across the brush border of the intestinal mucosa. The efficiency of this transport mechanism is increased several-fold when iron stores are depleted by menstruation, abnormal bleeding, increased demands during pregnancy and lactation, and growth spurts. Conversely, absorption is reduced in the presence of excessive iron stores [12–16].

Iron delivery to the cell-surface receptors is initiated by binding of iron to transferrin, forming monoferric and diferric transferrin-iron complexes [6, 12, 17, 18]. These transferrin complexes (mainly diferric) attach to the transferrin receptor cell-surface glycoprotein found on erythroblasts, lymphocytes, connective tissue cells, trophoblastic cells, and other growing cells, including neoplastic cells [19, 20]. An orderly aggregation of several complexes occurs through a lateral movement on the cell membrane, forming larger complexes, which in turn are internalized by endocytosis, a process not unlike the internalization of lipoproteins [6, 21–23]. Iron dissociates from the complex while in the en-

Table 11-2. Characteristic Laboratory Values in the Anemia of Chronic Disease (10 Subjects)

Laboratory Test	Patients Values ± Standard Deviation	Normal Range
Hemoglobulin	9.4 ± 1.4 g/dl	12–15 g/dl
Mean corpuscular hemoglobulin concentration	28 ± 2.5%	32–36%
Serum iron	36 ± 19 µg/dl	50–150 µg/dl
Total iron-binding capacity	250 ± 74 µg/dl	270–400 µg/dl
Iron absorption	5 ± 8%	11–37%
Iron utilization	85 ± 12%	> 75%
Iron re-utilization	36 ± 17%	57–73%

Source: Reprinted with permission from F Haurani, D Green, K Young. Iron absorption in hypoferremia. Am J Med Sci 1965;249:541. Copyright 1965 J.B. Lippincott Company.

docytotic vesicle by acid hydrolysis and becomes incorporated into the cytoplasmic milieu, while the "naked" transferrin, now known as apotransferrin, is returned to the surface and released for another transport cycle [24]. In the erythroblast, this capacity ends when the red blood cell matures and is filled with iron. The process of transport of iron to erythroblast and mature red blood cell is commonly referred to as the anabolic limb of iron utilization.

Mature red blood cells circulate in the vascular system for approximately 120 days. The aged cells are phagocytized by macrophages. The hemoglobin and nonheme iron-containing molecules are degraded and the iron is released and returned to the plasma transferrin to be reused or stored in the monocyte-macrophage system. These iron stores can be mobilized during conditions of increased iron demand. The metabolic pathways of iron are shown in Figure 11-1.

Pathophysiology

Any theory attempting to explain the anemia of inflammation must account for the several characteristic abnormalities of this disorder: the low serum iron, reduced serum transferrin, and increased iron stores; the shortened red blood cell life span; and the absence of a compensatory reticulocytosis.

With regard to the alterations in iron metabolism, inflammation activates macrophages. Quiescent macrophages have a relatively limited ability to bind transferrin, but activated macrophages increase their transferrin receptors dramatically [6]. Transferrin bound to such macrophages must be able to extract their iron. Failure to remove such iron could be the result of increased intracellular concentrations of apoferritin, the synthesis of which is stimulated by interleukin-1, which is a mediator of inflammation [25]. Interleukin-1 also can trigger the release of lactoferrin [26–28]. There is considerable evidence that lactoferrin impairs the transport of iron from macrophages to erythroblasts. Lactoferrin is a transferrin-like protein with a molecular weight of approximately 76,000 daltons [29–31]. It is present in the granules of polymorphonuclear leukocytes [32–34] and released when these cells are mobilized in inflammatory conditions [35, 36]. Lactoferrin binds iron with a greater affinity than transferrin, especially in the acidic environment of inflamed tissues. Lactoferrin successfully competes with transferrin for macrophage iron and also removes iron from iron-transferrin complexes [37]. Because lactoferrin does not transfer iron to erythroblasts [38], hemoglobin production is impaired. The lactoferrin-iron complex binds to receptors on macrophages and thus returns the iron to the macrophages [39]. In support of this lactoferrin theory are the following observations [5, 39]:

1. Neutrophils are required for the development of hypoferremia.
2. During phagocytosis, iron-free lactoferrin is released by neutrophils.

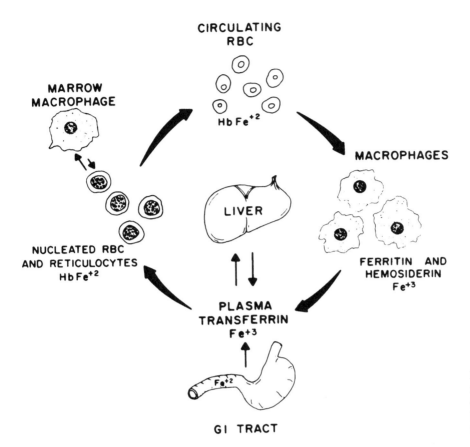

Figure 11-1. The metabolic pathways of iron. (RBC = red blood cell, GI = gastrointestinal.)

3. Under certain conditions, especially in an acidic milieu, lactoferrin can remove iron from transferrin.
4. Only monocytes and macrophages with specific receptors take up the lactoferrin-iron complex.
5. Uptake of this complex by macrophages is much more rapid than the uptake of transferrin.
6. Radiolabeled iron when administered is found mostly in hepatic cells and very little appears in the red blood cells.
7. "Blockade" of the monocyte-macrophage system prevents the hypoferremia of inflammation and reduces uptake of iron-lactoferrin.

Patients with chronic disease have a decreased ability to absorb iron from the gastrointestinal tract [40]. If intestinal cells fail to release iron to plasma transferrin, the iron will be lost when the cells are sloughed. The lactoferrin hypothesis explains the impaired iron absorption, because the lactoferrin-iron receptors are found on the intestinal cell surface [41] and presumably are activated by inflammation.

A moderately shortened red blood cell life span has been recorded in the chronic inflammatory state [4]. Investigators have shown that red blood cell survival in patients with rheumatoid arthritis averages 90 days as compared with 114 days in normal subjects [42]. In other inflammatory disorders, a mean red blood cell survival of 81 days has been demonstrated [43]. It is suggested that increased macrophage and monocyte activity as part of the general inflammatory response results in the premature destruction of minimally abnormal, older red blood cells [4, 44]. This could account for an increase in iron sequestration by the monocyte-macrophage cells. However, the degree of hemolysis is mild and should be well within the compensatory capacity of a normal bone marrow. This leads to the next hypothesis—that erythropoietin production is impaired or the marrow response to erythropoietin is depressed [45, 46]. Previous studies [47] suggested that serum and urinary erythropoietin levels were generally less than expected for the degree of anemia, but more recent investigations [48, 49] have refuted this assertion and shown that the level of the hormone in patients with chronic disease is not significantly different from that of anemic patients without chronic disorders. Furthermore, the marrow response to erythropoietin is impaired only when malignant cells replace the normal bone marrow [50]. Erythropoiesis in the anemia of inflammation can increase when stimulated by hypoxia or cobalt, which indicates that the capacity to respond to a pulse of erythropoietin is retained [51]. The failure of the bone marrow to compensate for the anemia in these patients with chronic disease, despite apparently adequate erythropoietin stimulation, suggests that suppressive factors are at work. Erslev [3] enumerates a number of such marrow suppressants, including prostaglandins, acidic isoferritins, interferons, and tumor necrosis factors, and Faqun et al. [52] reported that inflammatory cytokines in particular could suppress hypoxia-driven erythropoietin production. Since these are products of activated macrophages, they may play an important role in the anemia of patients with chronic inflammatory processes. For example, Means and Krantz [53] showed that recombinant human gamma-interferon inhibited erythroid colony formation; this inhibition could be reversed by increased concentrations of erythropoietin. Finally, depressed protein synthesis due to mild hypothyroidism may exist in some of these patients [54], contributing to the reduced hemoglobin production.

In summary, there appear to be at least four different pathophysiologic mechanisms for the anemia of inflammation: (1) lactoferrin-mediated interference with iron re-utilization from monocyte-macrophage to erythroblast; (2) depression of iron absorption from the gastrointestinal tract that could also be lactoferrin mediated; (3) a shortened red blood cell life span; and (4) suppression of the bone marrow response to erythropoietin by inflammatory cytokines. The underlying theme in all of these disturbances is macrophage activation associated with the chronic inflammatory process. Indeed, if the chronic inflammation undergoes remission, the anemia invariably remits (see Case Management Studies).

Differential Diagnosis

It is incumbent on those caring for patients with chronic disease to accurately diagnose and appropriately treat anemia. It is especially important to differentiate the anemia of inflammation from other anemias, because this anemia is of relatively little clinical significance in that it rarely is severe enough to cause symptoms or demand active transfusion therapy, and it fails to respond to the usual hematinics [1]. The differential diagnosis includes iron deficiency; hypoplastic, macrocytic, and hemolytic anemias; as well as the anemias associated with hepatic and renal disease. Each of these has features that distinguish it from the anemia of inflammation (Figure 11-2).

Iron-Deficiency Anemia

Iron-deficiency anemia may be confused with the anemia of chronic disease because both have a low serum iron, and occasionally the anemia of chronic disease is hypochromic and microcytic. In contrast, iron deficiency anemia has levels of transferrin (total iron-binding capacity) that are increased rather than decreased, serum transferrin receptor is increased, and the percent saturation of the transferrin is usually less than 10%. A second major distinction is that iron stores, as estimated either by serum ferritin or bone marrow iron stain, are decreased in iron deficiency rather than increased as in inflammation. For example, in inflammation ferritin is usually in excess of 60 ng/ml, whereas in iron deficiency it is less than 12 ng/ml. However, in the very elderly or in those with active liver disease, ferritin levels may be raised [55], and serum transferrin receptor may be a more reliable indicator of iron deficiency [9].

The differentiation between the two forms of anemia is critical because, in the case of iron deficiency, the anemia is invariably due to bleeding and the bleeding lesion must be identified and treated.

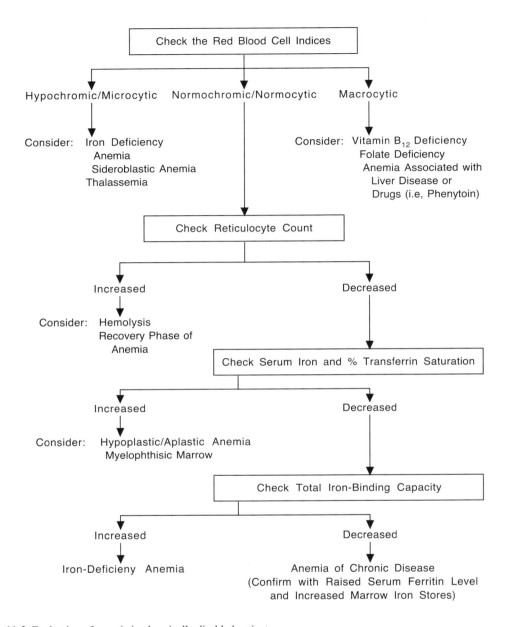

Figure 11-2. Evaluation of anemia in chronically disabled patients.

Furthermore, iron replacement therapy is without benefit if the anemia is due to inflammation. Because patients with inflammatory diseases may also have bleeding lesions, measurements of iron stores and stool examinations for occult blood are an important part of the evaluation of these patients.

Hypoplastic Anemias

Hypoplastic anemias are associated with low reticulocyte counts and increased iron stores. In contradistinction to the anemia of inflammation, however, the serum iron level is increased and the transferrin is almost fully saturated. In addition, there is usually a reduction in the leukocyte and platelet count as well as anemia.

Hypoplastic anemias in patients with inflammation are usually the result of medications, particularly anti-inflammatory, anticonvulsant, and antibiotic drugs. Where doubt exists as to the correct diagnosis, a bone marrow biopsy will demonstrate hypocellularity and increased marrow fat characteristic of hypoplastic anemia. In contrast, the bone marrow of patients with inflammatory diseases is usually normocellular or only mildly hypocellular.

Macrocytic Anemias

Macrocytic anemias occur in patients with liver disease, folic acid or vitamin B_{12} deficiency, and in response to anticonvulsants (i.e., phenytoin) and antimetabolites (i.e., methotrexate). They are distinguished from the anemia of inflammation on a morphologic basis (the latter is normochromic or hypochromic rather than macrocytic) and by the fact that the serum iron is increased and transferrin is iron-saturated. However, the macrocytic anemia accompanying chronic liver disease has many features in common with the anemia of other chronic diseases, including an elevated plasma ferritin value and a chronic unremitting character. Because folate deficiency, due to poor nutrition, may coexist with liver disease in these patients, a trial of folic acid therapy is usually warranted. Many of the other causes of macrocytosis, such as those due to vitamin B_{12} deficiency (pernicious anemia and malabsorption syndrome) or drugs, are readily reversible with appropriate management.

Hemolytic Anemias

Increased red blood cell destruction is associated with a normochromic anemia and an elevated serum ferritin value, but unlike the anemia of inflammation the serum iron and percent iron saturation are increased and there is an absolute increase in reticulocytes. Hemolytic anemias may complicate the course of patients with connective tissue disorders such as systemic lupus erythematosus. They also occur in patients with lymphoma or chronic lymphocytic leukemia, and in patients with *Mycoplasma pneumo-*

niae or cytomegalovirus infections. Occasionally, drugs such as penicillin, quinidine, procainamide, and alpha-methyldopa are the culprits. Successful therapy for the underlying disorder or the use of corticosteroids generally ameliorates the hemolysis and returns the hemoglobin level toward normal.

Anemia of Hepatic and Renal Disease

The anemias of hepatic and renal disease combine many of the features that characterize other anemias. For example, patients with hepatic disorders may have a hypochromic, microcytic anemia and signs of iron deficiency as a result of acute or chronic bleeding from the gastrointestinal tract. Food intake may be impaired with resultant folic acid deficiency and a macrocytic anemia. Others may have hypersplenism secondary to portal hypertension, or abnormalities of the red blood cell membrane due to alterations in cholesterol and phospholipid biosynthesis; in either case the result is increased red blood cell destruction. Finally, there may be only the anemia of inflammation. Likewise, the causes of anemia in patients with impaired renal function may be diverse, including inadequate production of red blood cells due to an absolute or relative lack of erythropoietin, bleeding secondary to uremic gastritis or colitis, or increased red blood cell destruction accompanying severe hypertension. These various mechanisms of anemia must be sorted out and treatment rendered accordingly.

Treatment

An anemia occurring in a patient with a chronic inflammatory disorder or malignant disease should be thoroughly investigated before it is labeled an anemia of chronic disease. It is not uncommon, especially in elderly, chronically debilitated persons, to have nutritional deficiencies, chronic blood loss resulting in concomitant iron deficiency, toxin-induced bone marrow suppression, or malignancy replacing the bone marrow.

Treatment should be directed primarily toward the underlying condition. In the anemia of inflammation, oral iron and parenteral iron dextran are ineffective and simply further increase iron stores. Red blood cell transfusions are indicated in only a few circumstances: for those who manifest clinical evidence of cardiac or cerebral ischemia, become hypotensive and tachycardic with exertion, or require urgent surgery. Blood transfusions may be complicated by transfusion reactions, sensitization to various antigens, and transmission of infectious agents. These hazards must be weighed against the modest benefits of a transient increase in hemoglobin level.

Other therapies designed to stimulate erythropoiesis may also be considered. Androgens, given either orally or parenterally, may increase hemoglobin levels in some patients [56]. However, they also cause fluid retention, cholestatic hepatitis, hirsutism, and hair loss and may be thrombogenic. Cobalt therapy has not been useful [57, 58].

Erythropoietin (EPO) has emerged as an important treatment option for patients with anemia of chronic inflammation. Originally used in the management of the anemia of chronic renal failure [59], EPO was subsequently shown to be effective in increasing hemoglobin levels in patients with a variety of chronic diseases [60, 61]. For example, favorable responses were observed in anemic patients with human immunodeficiency virus (HIV) infection who had levels of endogenous EPO of less than 500 U [62]. The anemia associated with pressure sores was also found to respond satisfactorily [63]. In addition, EPO has been of value in managing the anemia complicating malignant disease and chemotherapy [64].

Resistance to EPO therapy occurs under a number of circumstances [65]. These include inability of the bone marrow to respond to stimulation because of a lack of erythroid precursors due to hypoplasia or fibrosis or because of insufficient nutrients, such as folic acid, vitamin B_{12}, or iron. The latter is most important [66]. Because EPO mobilizes iron from storage sites, supplemental iron therapy may be needed in patients who do not have increased storage iron or who have iron that cannot readily be mobilized—i.e., iron in phagocytes. Other factors contributing to EPO resistance are active infections and uremia; successful control of the infection or increasing the intensity of hemodialysis [67] overcomes the resistance to EPO. Adverse effects from EPO treatment are infrequent, occur almost exclusively in patients with renal failure, and include hypertension and thrombosis when rapid increases in hematocrit raise peripheral vascular resistance and blood viscosity [68]. Last, it is tempting to try to achieve more rapid improvement in the hemoglobin by treating iron-deficiency anemia with EPO as well as iron. While the anemia does resolve sooner with this combination, functional improvement occurs just as quickly with iron alone [69], making it difficult to justify the considerable additional expense of the EPO.

Case Management Studies

Case 1

A 38-year-old man sustained a T12 spinal cord injury with complete motor paraplegia 2 years previously. In the last month, his caregiver had reported an area of induration over the left greater trochanter that has been draining serosanguinous fluid for 2 weeks. On examination, this was found to be a large pressure sore, extending deep to the periosteum. The wound was debrided. Admission laboratory studies revealed a hemoglobin of 9 g/dl, hematocrit of 27, and red blood cell count of 3.3 million per microliter.

1. Calculate the red blood cell indices and state whether the anemia is normochromic, hypochromic, or macrocytic.
2. Based on the history and laboratory findings, would you expect the reticulocyte count to be increased, decreased, or normal?

Other laboratory studies reveal the serum iron to be 19 μg/dl and the total iron binding capacity to be 170 μg/dl. Ferrous sulfate is begun in a dose of 300 mg three times per day. After 3 weeks of treatment, the hemoglobin remains 9 g/dl. Because reconstructive plastic surgery for the pressure sore was contemplated, the patient was transfused with 2 U of packed red cells. During the transfusion, his temperature increased to 105°F and he had rigors. Three days after the transfusion, he was jaundiced, his hemoglobin decreased rapidly back to 9 g/dl, and the surgery was postponed.

3. Before initiating the ferrous sulfate therapy, should any other diagnostic studies have been performed?
4. In iron deficiency, how much of an increase in hemoglobin should be anticipated after 3 weeks of oral iron supplementation?

5. What are the indications for parenteral iron therapy?
6. Was blood transfusion the most appropriate way to increase this patient's hemoglobin level?
7. What are the complications of blood transfusion?
8. How should the anemia be managed at this juncture?

Discussion

In evaluating the causes of anemia in patients with multiple medical problems, a good place to start is with the red cell indices. There are three indices that relate to the size of the red cells and their hemoglobin concentration. The first one is the mean corpuscular volume, or the volume per corpuscle. The volume term is the hematocrit, and the corpuscles are the red cell count. So the mean corpuscular volume would be 27 divided by 0.33, or approximately 82. The normal value is 82–92, so this patient has a normal mean corpuscular volume. The next index is the mean corpuscular hemoglobin, or hemoglobin per corpuscle. The hemoglobin of 9 divided by 0.33 is 27, with a normal range of 27–32. The third index is the mean corpuscular hemoglobin concentration or the concentration of hemoglobin per corpuscle. Now, concentration is mass per unit volume. The mass is the hemoglobin in grams (9) and the volume is the hematocrit (27), or 33. The normal range is 32–36. So in this patient, the mean corpuscular volume, the mean corpuscular hemoglobin, and the mean corpuscular hemoglobin concentration all fall within normal limits. That makes this a normochromic, normocytic anemia.

In iron deficiency, the indices are low, and in deficiencies of folic acid or B_{12}, the values are high. In the anemia of chronic disease, and in most hemolytic anemias, they are usually normal. Although these indices are helpful in categorizing anemia in a general sense, they do not tell you whether the red cells have abnormal shapes or about the distribution of the hemoglobin within the cells, as in target cells, sickle cells, etc. The way to get that information is to examine the blood smear, and this should be a part of every evaluation of an anemic patient. There is also a measure called the red cell distribution width that gives a rough estimate of the heterogeneity of the red cell population.

In the patient under discussion, the smear confirmed a normochromic, normocytic anemia with a red cell distribution width in the normal range. This leads to a consideration of the anemia of chronic disease, and the chronic disease in this case would be the leg infection, which might be a manifestation of osteomyelitis. Other chronic diseases associated with anemia are malignancies, tuberculosis, rheumatoid arthritis, and chronic hepatic or renal disease. The characteristics of anemia of chronic disease include a hemoglobin between 8 and 10 g and reticulocytopenia. Reticulocytes represent regenerating red cell mass. In patients with chronic disease, the regenerative process is impaired. A low reticulocyte count also occurs in iron deficiency anemia, and the anemia of folate and B_{12} deficiency because in all three, a nutrient that the bone marrow needs to make red blood cells is lacking. High reticulocyte counts are observed in individuals who have increased blood destruction or blood loss. In this patient, we would expect the reticulocyte count to be low in association with the anemia of chronic disease.

We are told that his serum iron is 19 and the total iron binding capacity is 170. In the anemia of chronic disease, both the serum iron and the total iron binding capacity are decreased and the percent iron saturation is usually between 10% and 20%. Despite the low serum iron, the iron storage protein, ferritin, is increased, and large amounts of iron may be seen in the bone marrow macrophages; this iron comes from senescent red cells. Normally this iron should be transported to developing erythroblasts by the protein, transferrin, but in the anemia of chronic disease, transferrin levels are greatly decreased. This is why the serum iron is low and the total iron binding capacity reduced.

Differentiating the anemia of chronic disease from iron-deficiency anemia can sometimes be difficult. In iron deficiency, the serum iron is low, but in contrast to the anemia of chronic disease, serum ferritin should also be low and the iron binding capacity should be high. The specificity and sensitivity of these measurements have recently been examined in elderly patients [55]. The investigators found that a low serum iron did not predict iron deficiency, but that a normal or high serum iron almost always meant the individual had abundant iron stores. Also, subjects with a low percent iron saturation were often found to have adequate marrow iron stores. Ferritin, the iron storage protein, was found to increase with age. In iron deficient elderly individuals, ferritin levels were lower than in age-matched cohorts, but were occasionally within the normal range if all ages were grouped together. To be predictive of iron deficiency, ferritin levels need to be below 10 ng/ml, and to be certain iron stores are adequate, ferritin levels should probably exceed 75 ng/ml.

The patient in our example was treated with ferrous sulfate. The response to be expected is a 2-g increase in the hemoglobin in a 3-week period. Failure to achieve this target suggests that iron deficiency is not responsible for the anemia.

Because there was no response to iron, packed red cells were transfused. However, he experienced a transfusion reaction characterized by fever and rigors, and 3 days later he was jaundiced and his hemoglobin was still 9. This suggests that the transfused red cells were hemolyzed; in this process, the cells release their hemoglobin and the hemoglobin binds to the protein, haptoglobin, and the haptoglobin-hemoglobin complex is removed from the circulation by macrophages. Thus, the laboratory signs of a hemolytic transfusion reaction include a decrease in haptoglobin, an increase in plasma hemoglobin and urinary hemosiderin, and an increase in indirect-reacting bilirubin. Patients will also have a positive Coomb's test result, due to recipient antibody attached to the donor cells. In patients having transfusion reactions, the most sensitive indicators are the haptoglobin level and the Coomb's test result. Our patient had a delayed transfusion reaction; this occurs when an individual has been previously sensitized to a red cell antigen but the antibody to that antigen is present in low titer [70]. When the patient is transfused, there is not much antibody, so not many of the transfused red cells are destroyed. However, as antibody titers increase, more cells are hemolyzed, jaundice appears, and anemia recurs.

Other complications of transfusion include the transmission of infectious agents such as hepatitis B, hepatitis C, other hepatitis viruses, human T-cell lymphotropic viruses 1 and 2, HIV-1, HIV-2, cytomegalovirus, Epstein-Barr viruses, and other, as yet undefined viruses. Other infectious agents in blood include *Babesia*, malarial parasites, and *Yersinia*. The latter contaminates stored blood and produces an endotoxin that may be fatal to the recipient.

In view of these dangers of transfusions, we must ask whether the procedure was really indicated in this patient. The most commonly accepted indication for blood transfusion is hemodynamic instability, usually due to surgical or traumatic blood loss. In fact, patients do not need transfusions unless their anemia is severe enough to compromise organ function, i.e., result in cerebral or cardiac ischemia. However, in the rehabilitation setting, one would like to increase the hemoglobin to improve the physical and cognitive function of the patient. This is where erythropoietin may have a role.

In most patients with chronic disease, erythropoietin concentrations are less than those observed in patients with anemia due to other causes, such as iron deficiency [71]. The reasons for this relative deficit in erythropoietin are unknown, but suggest that increasing the levels may improve the anemia. This has proved to be the case in patients with renal disease and those with anemia due to rheumatoid arthritis and the acquired immunodeficiency syndrome [72]. Whether erythropoietin therapy will prove as valuable in the anemias associated with pressure sores, osteomyelitis, and other chronic inflammatory conditions is currently under intense investigation.

Case 2

A 64-year-old woman was referred because of a normochromic, normocytic anemia. She first was seen by her family physician for complaints of weakness, easy fatigability, and occasional tender joints. The tenderness was migratory in pattern and involved the knees, ankles, and elbows. Her past medical, social, and family history were unremarkable. On physical examination, there was slight pallor but no jaundice. There was no hepatosplenomegaly or lymphadenopathy. Her joints were slightly swollen, and pain was elicited with full range of motion. A stool sample was negative for occult blood.

Laboratory studies revealed a hemoglobin of 8.9 g/dl, hematocrit 26.4%, a mean corpuscular volume of 93, a white cell count of 7,100, and a platelet count of 223,000. The blood urea nitrogen was 24 and creatinine was 0.9 (both normal). A review of the peripheral blood film showed a decrease in the number of erythrocytes but normal morphology. The reticulocyte count was 2% (absolute number,

58,000). Additional laboratory determinations included a serum iron of 64 μg/dl, total iron binding capacity of 309 μg/dl, ferritin of 254 ng/ml, B_{12} of 490 pg/ml, and folate of 13 ng/ml (all of these values are within normal limits).

To recapitulate, this patient has joint complaints and a normochromic normocytic anemia. The reticulocyte count is abnormally low for the degree of anemia. Nutritional causes of the anemia are excluded by the normal levels of iron, B_{12}, and folate. The other possible causes for the anemia would be acute blood loss (excluded by the history and physical examination), anemia of uremia (excluded by the normal urea nitrogen and creatinine), endocrine disorders such as hypothyroidism (more commonly the anemia is macrocytic), Addison's disease, or hypopituitarism (not supported by the history or physical examination), marrow aplasia (which would have to be confined to the erythroid elements because the white cells and platelets are normal), and the anemia of inflammation. Pure red cell aplasia is unlikely, because the serum iron is usually elevated in that disorder. Therefore, the anemia of inflammation is the major consideration, and evaluation should proceed to identify the cause of the inflammatory process.

Additional laboratory studies were performed and these revealed an antinuclear antibody titer of 1:160 with a nucleolar pattern; a repeat examination showed a titer of 1:280. A rheumatologic consultant suggested a short trial of corticosteroids (prednisone, 5 mg daily). The joint symptoms promptly subsided; 2 months after starting treatment her hemoglobin had risen to 9.7 g/dl and hematocrit to 28.3%, and at 4 months was 10.5 g/dl and 30.6%. She stated her overall energy level and endurance were much improved. In summary, treatment of this patient's underlying disorder (the rheumatoid arthritis), effected an improvement in both the joint disorder and the anemia.

References

1. Erslev AJ, Gabuzda TG. Pathophysiology of Blood (3rd ed). Philadelphia: Saunders, 1985.
2. Williams WJ. Hematology in the aged. In E Beutler, MA Lichtman, BS Coller, TJ Kipps (eds), Hematology (5th ed). New York: McGraw-Hill, 1995;72.
3. Erslev AJ. Anemia of chronic disorders. In Anemia: Current Issues. Glenside, PA: Toltzis Communications, 1987.
4. Cartwright GE. The anemia of chronic disorders. Semin Haematol 1966;3:351.
5. Lee GR. The anemia of chronic disease. Semin Hematol 1983;20:61.
6. Jandl JH. Blood. Boston: Little, Brown, 1987.
7. Pekarek RS, Bostian KA, Bartelloni PJ, et al. The effects of *Francisella tularensis* infection on iron metabolism in man. Am J Med Sci 1969;258:14.
8. Hastka J, Lasserre JJ, Schwarzbeck A, et al. Zinc protoporphyrin in anemia of chronic disorders. Blood 1993;81:1200.
9. Ferguson BJ, Skikne BS, Simpson KM, et al. Serum transferrin receptor distinguishes the anemia of chronic disease from iron deficiency anemia. J Lab Clin Med 1992;19:385.
10. Schilling RF. Anemia of chronic disease: A misnomer. Ann Intern Med 1991;115:572.
11. Crosby WH. The control of iron balance by the intestinal mucosa. Blood 1963;22:441.
12. Deiss A. Iron metabolism in reticuloendothelial cells. Semin Haematol 1983;20:81.
13. Cavill I, Worwood M, Jacobs A. Internal regulation of iron absorption. Nature 1975;256:328.
14. Crosby WH. Current concepts in nutrition: Who needs iron? N Engl J Med 1977;297:543.
15. Finch CA, Huebers HA. Perspectives in iron metabolism. N Engl J Med 1982;306:1520.
16. Huebers HA, Finch CA. Transferrin: Physiologic behavior and clinical implications. Blood 1984;64:763.
17. Fletcher J, Huehns ER. Function of transferrin. Nature 1968;218:1211.
18. Huebers HA, Finch CA. The physiology of transferrin and transferrin receptors. Physiol Rev 1987;67:520.
19. Jandl JH, Inman JK, Simmons RL, Allen DW. Transfer of iron from serum iron-binding protein to human reticulocytes. J Clin Invest 1959;38:161.
20. Jandl JH, Katz JH. The plasma-to-cell cycle of transferrin. J Clin Invest 1963;42:314.
21. Dautry-Varsat A, Lodish HF. How receptors bring proteins and particles into cells. Sci Am 1984;250:52.
22. Enns CA, Larrick JW, Suomalainen H, et al. Co-migration and internalization of transferrin and its receptor on K562 cells. J Cell Biol 1983;97:579.
23. Hopkins CR, Trowbridge IS. Internalization and processing of transferrin and the transferrin receptor in human carcinoma A431 cells. J Cell Biol 1983;97:508.
24. Veldman A, Van der Heul C, Kroos MJ, Van Eijk HG. Fluorescence probe measurement of the pH of the transferrin microenvironment during iron uptake by rat bone marrow erythroid cells. Br J Haematol 1986;62:155.
25. Koniju AM, Hershko C. Ferritin synthesis in inflammation: I. Pathogenesis of impaired iron release. Br J Haematol 1977;37:7.
26. Kampschmidt RF. Leukocytic endogenous mediator. J Reticuloendothel Soc 1978;23:287.
27. Kluger MJ, Rothenburg BA. Fever and reduced iron: Their interaction as a host defense response to bacterial infection. Science 1979;203:374.

28. Pekarek RS, Wannemacher W Jr., Beisel WR. The effect of leukocyte endogenous mediator (LEM) on the tissue distribution of zinc and iron. Proc Soc Exp Biol Med 1972;140:685.

29. Ainscough EW, Brodie AM, Plowman JE, et al. Studies on human lactoferrin by electron paramagnetic resonance, fluorescence and resonance Raman spectroscopy. Biochemistry 1980;19:4072.

30. Crichton RR. The biochemistry of ferritin. Br J Haematol 1973;24:677.

31. Teuwissen B, Masson PL, Osinski P, Heremans JF. Metal combining properties of human lactoferrin: The possible involvement of tyrosyl residues in the binding sites: Spectrophotometric titration. Eur J Biochem 1972;31:239.

32. Ambruso DR, Johnston RB Jr. Lactoferrin enhances hydroxyl radical production by human neutrophils, neutrophil particulate fractions and an enzymatic generating system. J Clin Invest 1981;67:352.

33. Baggiolini M, deDuve C, Masson PL, Heremans JF. Association of lactoferrin with specific granules in rabbit heterophil leukocytes. J Exp Med 1970;131:559.

34. Bennet RM, Kokocinski T. Lactoferrin content of peripheral blood cells. Br J Haematol 1978;39:509.

35. Kampschmidt RF, Upchurch HF, Johnson HL. Iron transport after injection of endotoxin in rats. Am J Physiol 1965;208:68.

36. Spitznagel JK, Lefell MS. Intracellular and extracellular degranulation of human polymorphonuclear azurophil and specific granules induced by immune complexes. Infect Immunol 1974;10:1241.

37. Van Snick JL, Masson PL, Heremans JF. The involvement of lactoferrin in the hyposideremia of acute inflammation. J Exp Med 1974;140:1068.

38. Brock JH, Esparza I. Failure of reticulocytes to take up iron from lactoferrin saturated by various methods. Br J Haematol 1979;42:481.

39. Van Snick JL, Markowetz B, Masson PL. The binding of human lactoferrin to mouse peritoneal cells. J Exp Med 1976;144:1568.

40. Haurani FI, Green D, Young K. Iron absorption in hypoferremia. Am J Med Sci 1965;249:537.

41. Hershko C, Cook JD, Finch CA. Storage iron kinetics: VI. The effect of inflammation on iron exchange in the rat. Br J Haematol 1974;28:67.

42. Dinant HJ, deMaat CEM. Erythropoiesis and mean red-cell lifespan in normal subjects and in patients with the anemia of active rheumatoid arthritis. Br J Haematol 1978;39:437.

43. Cavill I, Bentley DP. Erythropoiesis in the anemia of rheumatoid arthritis. Br J Haematol 1982;50:583.

44. Cartwright GE, Lee GR. The anemia of chronic disorders. Br J Haematol 1971;21:147.

45. Douglas SW, Adamson JW. The anemia of chronic disorders: Studies of marrow regulation and iron metabolism. Blood 1975;45:55.

46. Mahmood T, Robinson WA, Vautrin R. Granulopoietic and erythropoietic activity in patients with anemias of iron deficiency and chronic disease. Blood 1977;50:449.

47. Ward HP, Kurwick IE, Pisaczyk MJ. Serum level of erythropoietin in anemias associated with chronic infection, malignancy and primary hepatopoietic disease. J Clin Invest 1971;50:332.

48. Schreuder WO, Ting WC, Smith S, Jacobs A. Testosterone, erythropoietin and anemia in patients with disseminated bronchial cancer. Br J Haematol 1984;57:521.

49. Erslev AJ, Wilson J, Caro J. Erythropoietin titers in anemic, nonuremic patients. J Lab Clin Med 1987;109:429.

50. Zucker S, Lysik RM, Friedman S. Diminished bone marrow responsiveness to erythropoietin in myelophthisic anemia. Cancer 1976;37:1308.

51. Lukens JN. Control of erythropoiesis in rats with adjuvant-induced chronic inflammation. Blood 1973;41:37.

52. Faquin WC, Schneider TJ, Goldberg MA. Effect of inflammatory cytokines on hypoxia-induced erthropoietin production. Blood 1992;79:1987.

53. Means RT, Krantz SB. Inhibition of human erythroid colony-forming units by gamma interferon can be corrected by recombinant human erythropoietin. Blood 1991;78:2564.

54. Kaptein EM, Grieb DA, Spencer CA, et al. Thyroxine metabolism in the low thyroxine state of critical nonthyroidal illnesses. J Clin Endocrinol Metab 1981;53:764.

55. Patterson C, Turpie ID, Berger AM. Assessment of iron stores in anemic geriatric patients. J Am Geriatr Soc 1985;33:764.

56. Gardner FH, Pringle JC Jr. Androgens and erythropoiesis. Arch Intern Med 1961;107:846.

57. Weinsaft PD, Bernstein LHT. Cobaltous chloride in the treatment of certain refractory anemias. Am J Med Sci 1955;230:246.

58. Wintrobe MM, Grinstein M, Dubash JJ. The anemia of infection: VI. The influence of cobalt on the anemia associated with inflammation. Blood 1947;2:323.

59. Eschbach JW, Egrie JL, Downing MR, et al. Correction of the anemia of end-stage renal disease with recombinant human erythropoietin. N Engl J Med 1987;316:73.

60. Means RT, Olsen NJ, Krantz SB, et al. Treatment of the anemia of rheumatoid arthritis with recombinant human erythropoietin: Clinical and in vitro results. Blood 1987;70:139a.

61. Means RT, Krantz SB. Progress in understanding the pathogenesis of the anemia of chronic disease. Blood 1992;80:1639.

62. Henry DH, Beall GN, Benson CA, et al. Recombinant human erythropoietin in the treatment of anemia associated with human immunodeficiency virus (HIV) infection and zidovudine therapy. Ann Intern Med 1992;117:739.

63. Turba R, Lewis VL, Green D. Pressure sore anemia: Response to erythropoietin. Arch Phys Med Rehabil 1992;73:498.

64. Henry DH III, Thatcher N. Patient selection and predicting response to recombinant human erythropoietin in anemic cancer patients. Semin Hematol 1996;33(Suppl 1):2.

65. Koury MJ. Investigating erythropoietin resistance. N Engl J Med 1993;328:205.

66. Brugnara C, Colella GM, Cremins J, et al. Effects of subcutaneous recombinant human erythropoietin in normal subjects: Development of decreased reticulocyte hemoglobin content and iron-deficient erythropoiesis. J Lab Clin Med 1994;123:660.

67. Ifudu O, Feldman J, Friedman EA. The intensity of hemodialysis and the response to erythropoietin in patients with end-stage renal disease. N Engl J Med 1996;334:420.

68. Raine AEG. Hypertension, blood viscosity, and cardiovascular morbidity in renal failure: implications of erythropoietin therapy. Lancet 1988;2:97.

69. Green D, Lawler M, Rosen M, et al. Recombinant human erythropoietin: effect on the functional performance of anemic orthopedic patients. Arch Phys Med Rehabil 1996;77:242.

70. Holland PV. Other adverse effects of transfusion. In Petz L, Swisher S (eds), Clinical Practice of Blood Transfusion. New York: Churchill Livingstone, 1981;783.

71. Lukens JN. Control of erythropoiesis in rats with adjuvant-induced chronic inflammation. Blood 1973;41:37.

72. Pincus T, Olssen NJ, Russell IJ, et al. Multicenter study of recombinant human erthropoietin in correction of anemia in rheumatoid arthritis. Am J Med 1990;89:161.

Part VII

Infectious Diseases

Chapter 12
Infections

Michele Till and Peter Pertel

A wide range of infectious diseases are seen in chronically disabled persons. These include urinary tract infections, pneumonia, osteomyelitis, and infected prostheses and cerebrospinal fluid shunts. In addition, the disabled person may have underlying medical conditions that can increase susceptibility for infection. Examples include malignancy, diabetes mellitus, collagen vascular disorders, organ transplant, or the acquired immunodeficiency syndrome (AIDS). New therapies are constantly in development, and management of many diseases is rapidly changing. With new broad-spectrum oral antimicrobials and increased use of indwelling central venous catheters, many diseases that once required lengthy hospital stays can now be managed at home or at extended-care facilities. Although many infections can be managed by the primary care physician, more complicated problems such as aspiration pneumonia, osteomyelitis, AIDS, or infected cerebrospinal fluid shunts usually require a multispecialty team that includes an infectious disease specialist and frequently an orthopedic or neurosurgical consultant.

Because the chronically disabled are at high risk for infections that cause significant morbidity and mortality [1–3], prevention is extremely important. Recently, an alarming increase in the frequency of infections due to antimicrobial-resistant organisms has occurred. Nosocomial as well as community-acquired pathogens, such as *Streptococcus pneumoniae*, *Mycobacterium tuberculosis*, *Staphylococcus aureus*, along with Enterobacteriaceae and species of *Enterococcus*, *Pseudomonas*, and *Candida,* are rapidly developing resistance to previously effective antimicrobial drugs [4–6]. For some pathogens, such as vancomycin-resistant enterococcus, there may be no effective alternative therapy, resulting in high mortality in patients with systemic infections [4, 5]. An active infection control program that can maintain surveillance for and intervene to prevent the spread of resistant organisms is essential [7, 8]. Limiting the inappropriate use of antimicrobials such as cephalosporins and fluoroquinolones that may select for or induce antibiotic resistance is also essential [9–12]. Adherence to proper yet simple hygienic techniques in patient care is more effective and less expensive in controlling infections than any antibiotic [9].

Approach to the Infected Patient

An evaluation of the chronically disabled patient should be well organized and logical. A high index of suspicion for infection should be maintained, even if no fever is present. Fever may not be noted in malnourished or immunocompromised persons or those with neurologic disorders, even in the setting of serious underlying infection. Hypothermia may be the first sign of an overwhelming infection such as sepsis. In addition, an infection may present with only nonspecific signs such as an altered mental status, tachypnea, tachycardia, hypotension, or hypertension. For example, persons with spinal cord injuries may be asymptomatic even with a severe condition such as an acute abdomen or have only

Table 12-1. Initial Evaluation of Febrile Patients

Suspected Site of Infection	Initial Tests
Urinary tract	Complete blood count
	Urinalysis
	Gram's stain and culture of urine
	Blood cultures
Abdomen	Complete blood count
	Serum liver function tests
	Blood cultures
	Urinalysis
	Obstructive abdominal radiographic series
Respiratory tract	Complete blood count
	Chest roentgenogram
	Gram's stain and culture of sputum
	Blood cultures
Soft tissue and bone	Complete blood count
	Wound or bone culture
	Bone roentgenograms
	Blood cultures
Central nervous system	Complete blood count
	Blood cultures
	Computed tomograms of head
	Cerebrospinal fluid cell count
	Cerebrospinal fluid glucose and protein content
	Gram's stain and culture of cerebrospinal fluid

subtle findings including increased muscle spasticity or changes in the appearance of their urine [13]. Failure to consider the possibility of an infectious process may result in significant delays in diagnosis and instituting appropriate therapy.

Similarly, infection is not the only cause of fever. For example, drug fever, especially associated with use of phenytoin and beta-lactam antibiotics, is relatively common [14]. Thromboembolic disease, which is relatively frequent in the chronically disabled, may be an occult source of fever [15]. Central fever has been reported in patients with head trauma or high cervical spinal lesions but is rare and is diagnosed by exclusion [16].

The presence of fever alone should not automatically prompt the clinician to start antimicrobial therapy. It is essential that the patient be thoroughly evaluated with a careful history, physical examination, and appropriate laboratory tests. This initial evaluation, besides possibly revealing the likely etiology of the fever, may be the only opportunity for culture specimens to be collected before antibiotics are started and will help determine the aggressiveness of subsequent management. For example, this evaluation will help decide which patients may be managed in an outpatient or extended-care setting and which others may need to be transferred to an acute care facility [17]. If after a thorough evaluation no cause for the fever is determined and the patient is stable, it may be prudent to withhold antibiotic therapy pending further laboratory and culture data.

The physical examination, including mental status and neurologic evaluation, will aid in the subsequent selection of appropriate laboratory tests. Table 12-1 lists suggested initial tests based on the suspected site of infection. Additional tests, such as serum electrolytes or special radiographic examinations, may be needed. Two easily obtained and extremely helpful tests in evaluating the chronically disabled are the complete blood count and urinalysis. With most significant bacterial infections a leukocytosis with a predominance of neutrophils will be noted, although there are some exceptions. Patients with overwhelming infections such as sepsis may have low white cell counts but other signs of infection are almost always present. Neutropenia caused by chemotherapy or marrow-suppressing medications increases the risk for bacterial infection, especially when the absolute neutrophil count (segmented and band forms) is below 500 cells per microliter [18]. The risk for severe bacterial infections in the febrile neutropenic patient is so great that broad-spectrum antibiotics should be started immediately after obtaining initial cultures [19]. An erythrocyte sedimentation rate is neither specific nor sensitive. An elevated value can be noted with a variety of noninfectious as well as infectious causes. Similarly, a normal value does not exclude most infections [20]. The sedimentation rate may be most useful for measuring response to treatment in diseases such as osteomyelitis.

Patients suspected of having serious infections with potential bacteremia should have blood cultures obtained. Examples include pneumonia, pyelonephritis, endocarditis, meningitis, venous catheter infections, and fever without localizing signs. Subsequent antimicrobial therapy, including route of administration and duration of treatment, will be affected by positive blood culture results. In medically urgent situations such as sepsis, two to three blood cultures should be obtained immediately, before starting empiric antibiotic therapy. Cultures should be obtained as early as possible after the onset of fever. If continuous bacteremia (as with an endovascular infection) is suspected, the timing of the cultures is not critical. If intermittent bacteremia (as with pneumonia or urinary tract infections) is suspected, cultures should be taken randomly over a wide time interval, such as 24 hours, if the patient is hemodynamically stable [21]. Obtaining a single blood culture can be inadequate for detecting bacteremia and can lead to difficulties interpreting positive results with organisms that are often contaminants but may also cause infection [22]. To avoid contamination, the skin must be adequately prepared before drawing blood cultures. Generally, cleansing the skin with 70% alcohol followed by application of an iodine solution is adequate. The iodine should be allowed to dry completely and should not be removed until after the blood has been withdrawn [22]. With standard cultures, 20 ml of blood should be taken from each venipuncture site and distributed between two culture bottles or vials, for isolation of aerobic and anaerobic organisms [21]. The sensitivity of blood cultures is most dependent on the volume of blood sent, so that a minimum of 10 ml per bottle or vial should be obtained [23]. It is not necessary to change the venipuncture needle before inoculating the culture bottles and doing so may increase the risk of needle-stick injury [24]. The blood culture vials should be kept at room temperature during transport to the microbiology laboratory. Immunecompromised patients may require cultures for mycobacteria, fungi, or viruses, in which case special media may be required. Other cultures collected depend on the suspected site of infection and often include sputum and urine cultures in addition to cultures of cerebrospinal fluid, joint fluid, or soft tissue ulcers. Attempts to obtain cultures before starting antibiotics should be made because this may be the only time to identify the organism causing the infection. All cultures should be transported promptly to the microbiology laboratory for processing. Careful follow-up of all culture results must be undertaken so that antimicrobial therapy can be adjusted according to in vitro sensitivities. Studies have demonstrated that patients are often treated with inappropriate antibiotics even though culture results are readily available [25, 26].

Therapy for specific infections are discussed in detail later. Outlined here are some general principles of antimicrobial therapy. Empiric antimicrobial therapy requires selecting drugs active against the most likely organisms causing the infection. Occasionally, this may require the use of more than one medication. Drug choice will be influenced by patient factors such as any history of adverse reactions to medications, prior antibiotic therapy that may have altered the types and sensitivity profiles of suspected organisms, and presence of hepatic and renal insufficiency or other medications that may change the metabolism and clearance of the drug and increase the risk of side effects or decrease efficacy [27]. At each institution, the resistance patterns of common organisms will also influence drug selection. For example, organisms frequently encountered and resistant to commonly used agents include methicillin-resistant *Staphylococcus aureus* and gentamicin-resistant *Pseudomonas aeruginosa* [4, 6]. To help contain costs and slow the development of resistant organisms, institutions may limit the antimicrobials available by the use of drug formularies. Finally, antimicrobial choice will depend on the route of administration and dosing frequency.

Usually medications are less expensive to administer orally than parenterally. Newer medications dosed once or twice a day may also be less expensive than older drugs that must be dosed more frequently. One effective method of reducing antibiotic costs is to have the pharmacy provide information on the costs of administration of the most commonly prescribed agents in the institution.

Urinary Tract Infections

Urinary tract infections are the most common infections in the chronically disabled and represent a significant source of morbidity [2, 3, 28] (see also Chapter 9). They are the most prevalent nosocomial infection, frequently associated with catheterization of the urinary tract [29, 30]. Generally, two groups of persons require long-term catheterization: (1) those with spinal cord injuries or other neurologic diseases affecting bladder function, and (2) those with urinary incontinence.

Persons with neurogenic bladders requiring drainage may be managed with intermittent catheterization regimens. Clean intermittent catheterization has gained widespread acceptance since its introduction [31]. Persons without severe vesicoureteral reflux placed on intermittent catheterization regimens have a low incidence of urinary tract infections despite the frequent presence of asymptomatic bacteriuria [32–35]. Persons requiring indwelling catheters are often elderly nursing home residents with urinary incontinence. Catheterization in these patients prevents soiling and subsequent skin maceration and breakdown. An external condom catheter is an option that may avoid some of the problems associated with an indwelling catheter, but there is still an increased risk of developing bacteriuria and there is no similar option for women [36]. More than 100,000 nursing home residents in the United States have long-term urethral catheters in place [37].

A number of defense mechanisms protect the normally functioning urinary tract from infection [38]. These include the mechanical washout of the upper urinary tracts, the vesicoureteral valve that prevents reflux of urine into the ureters, the antibacterial activity of the bladder mucosa, and the normally acidic urine, and to a lesser degree, high urine osmolality that may inhibit bacterial growth

[39]. Patients with neurogenic bladders have impairments of these normal anatomic and physiologic defenses [38]. Bladder denervation permits overdistension and accumulation of large residual urine volumes that, if allowed to persist for extended periods, promote the growth of bacteria. The high pressures associated with distention can result in mucosal ischemia that can facilitate bacterial tissue invasion. Increased pressures can also result in vesicoureteral reflux, permitting bacteria to reach the upper urinary tracts [40]. Although catheterization effectively drains urine from the bladder, the catheter allows organisms to enter the urinary tract by three pathways: (1) inoculation from the urethra into the bladder at the time of catheterization [41]; (2) migration along the thin film of urethral fluid coating the outside of the catheter [42]; and (3) migration along the internal lumen of a contaminated catheter [43]. Periodically opening the initially sterile system to empty the drainage bag, irrigate the catheter, or collect urine can all result in contamination. Organisms can subsequently multiply to high titers in the collection system before drainage. Even after drainage, organisms may persist in the film of urine coating the inside of the collecting bag and tubing [44].

For infection to occur bacteria must not only gain access to the urinary tract but also colonize the epithelium, multiply, and induce an inflammatory response in the host. The presence of a catheter allows most bacteria to achieve high concentrations in the urine (greater than 10^5 colony-forming units [CFU] per milliliter) within 2 days [45]. In addition, certain strains of bacteria have virulence factors that increase their propensity to cause infection. For example, some gram-negative bacteria express fimbriae that facilitate binding to uroepithelial cells [46]. Also, a glycocalyx that coats the bladder mucosa and surfaces of the catheter and drainage bag can protect bacteria from host defenses [44, 47, 48]. Urease-producing organisms, such as *Proteus* species, elevate the urine pH as a result of splitting urea. With alkalinization of the urine, stones can form that may subsequently function as a nidus of infection [38].

Organisms that colonize the periurethral area and cause urinary tract infections are generally part of the normal fecal flora [49]. Hospitalized patients become colonized with institutional flora, and outbreaks involving highly uropathogenic or antibiotic-

Table 12-2. Organisms Associated with Urinary Tract Infections in Catheterized Patients

Gram-Negative Bacteria	Gram-Positive Bacteria	Yeast
Escherichia coli	Enterococcus faecalis	Candida albicans
Klebsiella pneumoniae	Enterococcus faecium	Candida tropicalis
Proteus mirabilis	Staphylococcus aureus	Torulopsis glabrata
Serratia marcescens	Staphylococcus epidermidis	
Providencia stuartii		
Acinetobacter species		
Enterobacter species		
Citrobacter freundii		
Xanthomonas maltophilia		

resistant organisms may result. Because these organisms can be spread on the hands of health care providers, maintaining good infection control procedures is mandatory [50, 51]. Patients catheterized for more than 30 days will inevitably develop bacteriuria [52]. A wide variety of organisms can be isolated from catheterized patients. The most common organisms include Enterobacteriaceae such as *Escherichia coli* and *Klebsiella pneumoniae*, *Pseudomonas aeruginosa*, and *Enterococcus* species. Isolation of yeast, particularly *Candida albicans*, from the urine of patients who have received antibiotic therapy is not uncommon [53]. Table 12-2 lists organisms associated with urinary tract infections in catheterized patients. Almost all persons requiring long-term catheterization will have at least one organism present at high concentration (greater than 10^5 CFU/ml). Most persons will have at least two organisms and occasionally as many as eight or nine present [52]. As a result, identifying the organism responsible for an infection may be difficult.

Classic symptoms of urinary tract infections such as urinary frequency, urgency, dysuria, and back pain are uncommon in persons with neurogenic bladders. Patients with spinal cord injuries are likely to be asymptomatic or manifest subtle symptoms and signs of infection. Findings that may be seen in these patients include an increased frequency of spontaneous voiding, larger residual volumes, increased muscular spasticity, changes in urine pH, and cloudy or malodorous urine [38]. Some patients exhibit increased sweating associated with autonomic hyperreflexia or report malaise or lethargy [13].

Localizing the anatomic site of a urinary tract infection clinically is difficult. Unfortunately, a practical and reliable method of distinguishing pyelonephritis, cystitis, and colonization has not yet been developed. The gold standard for localizing infection, bilateral ureteral catheterization, is impractical to use in routine clinical settings [54]. Optimal treatment of patients with urinary tract infections requires knowledge of the anatomic sites involved. Cystitis does not require as prolonged or intensive therapy as does pyelonephritis, which is more likely to be associated with bacteremia or renal calculi. An inexpensive method to localize the site of infection is clearly needed in this patient population. White cell casts found on examination of the urine sediment indicates upper tract inflammation and in the setting of a probable infection, may indicate pyelonephritis [55].

Once infection is suspected, the diagnosis is confirmed by analysis and culture of the urine. Although the presence of bacteria in urine at concentrations greater than 10^5 CFU/ml has traditionally confirmed the diagnosis of infection, lower amounts of bacteria are frequently associated with the symptoms and signs of urinary tract infections in both catheterized and noncatheterized persons. Clean-voided urine collected from women with dysuria that contained greater than or equal to 10^2 CFU/ml of bacteria was a sensitive and specific test for infection [56]. In catheterized patients, low-level ($<10^5$ CFU/ml) bacteriuria or candiduria has been shown to progress to concentrations greater than 10^5 CFU/ml approximately 95% of the time, usually within 3 days of the initial culture [45]. These studies suggest that low levels of bacteriuria in a symptomatic patient are consistent with the diagnosis of a urinary tract infection. In fact, a consensus conference sponsored by the National Institute of Disability and Rehabilitation Research defined significant bacteriuria as (1) greater than or equal to 10^2 CFU/ml from persons using intermittent catheterization, (2) greater than or equal to 10^4 CFU/ml in clean-voided specimens from males using comdom catheterization, and (3) any detectable concentration in specimens from persons using indwelling catheterization or from suprapubic aspirates [57].

For accurate results, urine culture specimens should be processed within 1 hour or refrigerated and processed within 24 hours [38]. In patients who can void spontaneously, a clean midstream urine specimen is collected. In patients with chronic indwelling catheters, urine should be aspirated from a catheter port or the tube itself with a sterile syringe. Urine should never be collected from the drainage bag nor should the catheter be disconnected from the bag to collect urine. Although obtaining a urine culture by placing a new sterile catheter may more accurately reflect the organisms in the bladder, it is not certain that this is necessary. Most organisms causing urinary tract infections will be found both in the catheter and the bladder [37]. For patients using intermittent catheterization regimens, a clean midstream catheterized specimen should be collected. For men wearing condom catheters, an accurate culture can be obtained by placing a new external catheter after cleansing the glans penis and collecting the first-voided urine specimen [58]. For incontinent women, careful collection of a clean catch urine specimen may be as accurate as sterile in-and-out catheterization [59].

The urinalysis and Gram's stain are two useful laboratory tools. Finding bacteria on a Gram's stain of unspun urine correlates with concentrations greater than 10^5 CFU/ml on subsequent cultures and may guide empiric antibiotic therapy [60]. Significant pyuria on urinalysis is common in patients with urinary tract infections. In patients who void spontaneously, leukocyte counts greater than 100 cells/mm^3 are associated with infection [61]. In patients with spinal cord injuries, however, the association is less certain. One study reported a relationship between upper tract bacteriuria and leukocyte counts of greater than 200 cells/mm^3.

Many patients without infection, however, had significant pyuria and approximately 25% of patients with documented infection lacked pyuria [62]. Another study examining patients who use intermittent catheterization regimens demonstrated that leukocyte counts varied markedly in aliquots of midstream catheter or terminal catheter urine. The absence of pyuria predicted the absence of gram-negative bacteriuria but pyuria was frequent in sterile specimens. It was also noted that gram-positive organisms produced less of a leukocyte response than gram-negative bacteria or fungi [63]. Most clinical laboratories only report the number of leukocytes per high power microscopic field in spun urine, which is a poorly reproducible test [61]. Thus, the significance of pyuria in a spinal cord injured patient is questionable.

There is often the temptation to treat bacteriuria in asymptomatic persons. Treating asymptomatic bacteriuria, however, has not been shown to effectively reduce the rate of infection and may increase the incidence of resistant organisms [64–69]. An exception may be the treatment of persistent bacteriuria with *Proteus* species that may lead to stone formation and significant morbidity [57]. Patients who have a urinary tract infection should be on appropriate antibiotic therapy before initiating an intermittent catheterization regimen [34]. Bacteriuria in patients on long-term intermittent catheterization is common but prophylactic antibiotic therapy is unwarranted [65]. In the absence of vesicoureteral reflux, bacteriuria may be well tolerated and may resolve spontaneously without specific therapy [34].

Febrile patients with a suspected urinary tract infection should have other possible sources of fever excluded. Initial antimicrobial therapy should target likely pathogens, including Enterobacteriaceae, *Pseudomonas* species, and *Enterococcus* species. The route of administration will depend on the clinical setting. Patients with urosepsis, pyelonephritis, or temperatures greater than or equal to 102°F (38.9°C) should be treated with parenteral antibiotics. Possible regimens include ampicillin, an extended-spectrum penicillin such as piperacillin, a fluoroquinolone, or a third-generation cephalosporin, all frequently used in conjunction with an aminoglycoside. The penicillin-allergic patient may be treated with a fluoroquinolone, aztreonam, or a cephalosporin, although cross-reactivity has been documented [70]. In patients with severe allergic reactions to penicillins, other beta-lactam antibiotics should not be used. Vancomycin should be used to treat gram-positive organisms in penicillin-allergic patients. Parenteral antibiotics can be changed to an appropriate oral agent when the patient is stable and afebrile. In patients who are not severely ill, initial therapy with oral antibiotics including ampicillin, amoxicillin, trimethoprim-sulfamethoxazole, a fluoroquinolone, or a cephalosporin may be used. Not infrequently, patients who are chronically disabled may be infected with organisms that are resistant to most oral antibiotics except some newer agents such as ciprofloxacin. Because of increasing resistance, the use of these antibiotics should be restricted to patients who cannot be treated with other available antimicrobials. After culture results are available, antibiotic therapy should be modified appropriately to minimize cost and spectrum of activity [12]. Obstruction of the urinary tract should be excluded, especially in patients with indwelling catheters.

The usual duration of therapy for symptomatic urinary tract infections is 10–14 days, although patients with recurrences due to the same organism may require longer courses of treatment [71]. If a patient fails to respond to antibiotic therapy or has a rapid recurrence, the presence of urinary tract obstruction, calculi, prostatitis, reflux, or an abscess should be excluded.

Treating infections caused by enterococcus species can be a difficult problem. Localized infections including cystitis can be treated with a single drug such as ampicillin. Serious infections including pyelonephritis and bacteremia require the combination of ampicillin or vancomycin and an aminoglycoside for synergy. Emergence of resistance to ampicillin, vancomycin, and high levels of aminoglycosides has made this pathogen one of the most difficult to treat [72].

Serum levels of aminoglycosides require monitoring to ensure adequate therapeutic levels and to avoid ototoxicity and nephrotoxicity. Often aminoglycoside therapy is initiated with a loading dose followed by maintenance doses adjusted for the level of renal function and the size of the patient [73]. The loading dose of gentamicin and tobramycin is 1.5–2.0 mg/kg. For amikacin the loading dose is 7.5 mg/kg. The loading dose is the same for all patients regardless of renal function. The maintenance dose of gentamicin and tobramycin in a patient with normal renal function (i.e., a creatinine clearance greater than 90 ml/minute) is 1.2–1.7 mg/kg every 8 hours. For amikacin the dose is 5.0 mg/kg every 8–12 hours. Doses must be adjusted in patients with impaired renal function to avoid toxicity. A patient's creatinine clearance can be estimated using the equation of Cockcroft and Gault [74]:

$$\text{Creatinine clearance (ml/min)} = \frac{(140 - \text{age})(\text{weight in kilograms})}{72 \times \text{serum creatinine (mg/dl)}}$$

The result obtained by this formula should be multiplied by 0.85 for women or obese patients. This formula may overestimate the creatinine clearance in patients with decreased muscle mass or use [75]. Patients with creatinine clearances of 50–90, 25–50, and 15–25 ml/min should have the interval between doses extended to every 12, 24, and 36 hours, respectively. In hemodialysis patients, a loading dose of aminoglycoside is given. After each dialysis treatment, maintenance doses of 1.0–2.0 mg/kg for gentamicin and tobramycin and 4.0–7.0 mg/kg for amikacin are infused. These calculations must be considered approximations, and all dosing must be verified by serum levels. Peak levels should be obtained 30 minutes after completion of the infusion. Adequate levels are 4–10 µg/ml for gentamicin and tobramycin and 10–25 µg/ml for amikacin. The lower peak levels should be sufficient to treat urinary tract infections. The trough levels are obtained just before the next infusion. To minimize toxicity, levels of gentamicin and tobramycin should be less than 2 µg/ml and less than 10 µg/ml for amikacin. Generally, drug levels should be checked around the third dose and once weekly thereafter. More frequent determinations may be needed if there are significant changes in the patient's condition or an alteration in the serum creatinine level. Serial serum creatinine levels should be followed and the dose of aminoglycoside reduced or discontinued if the value is increasing. Many other antimicrobial agents, including vancomycin, need to be adjusted for renal insufficiency.

Most cases of candiduria will resolve spontaneously with removal of the catheter or discontinuation of antibiotics [76]. If true cystitis is present, irrigation of the bladder with 200–300 ml amphotericin B at a concentration of 5–10 mg/liter through a triple-lumen catheter and with subsequent cross-clamping for 60–90 minutes over 2 days should be effective. Fluconazole can be used as an alternative.

A dose of 200 mg initially followed by 100 mg a day for 2–4 days should be adequate [77].

Infrequent use of urethral catheters can help prevent urinary tract infections. Behavioral training, medication, surgery, or special clothes and linens may be useful in treating urinary incontinence. If these measures fail, alternatives to indwelling catheters include condom, intermittent, and suprapubic catheterization. None of these alternatives, however, eliminates the risk of bacteriuria and all have other complications associated with their use. When compared with long-term indwelling catheters, intermittent catheterization regimens may reduce the incidence of urinary tract infections and local complications including urethritis, penile and scrotal abscesses, epididymitis, and fistulas, although this is not universally accepted [38, 78]. Although not well studied, one may theorize that suprapubic catheterization may result in easier local care and that the skin surrounding the catheter site would be less likely to be colonized by potential urinary pathogens. It may also decrease the incidence of local urethral complications such as urethritis and strictures [79, 80]. Most urinary diversions involve placement of an ileal conduit. Because of the high rate of upper urinary tract infections associated with urinary diversions, this procedure is of limited use [81].

The development of bacteriuria, although likely in almost all catheterized patients, can be delayed by maintaining a closed and sterile system [82]. Correct instruction for handling the catheter and collection bag is essential. Instillation of antibacterial substances and antibiotics into the drainage bag does not prevent the development of bacteriuria and may select for resistant organisms [83, 84]. Once bacteriuria has developed, draining the bladder or collection bag at short intervals may limit growth to relatively low concentrations [35, 40]. A high level of suspicion for infection will permit early diagnosis and treatment, minimizing complications such as the risk of calculi formation, chronic pyelonephritis, and loss of renal function.

Pneumonia

Pneumonia can result when organisms reach the lungs from one of three mechanisms: (1) inhalation, (2) aspiration, and (3) hematogenous spread. For example, *Mycobacterium tuberculosis* and *Legionella pneumophilia* are usually inhaled, *Streptococcus pneumoniae* and *Haemophilus influenzae* are usually aspirated from a colonized oropharynx, and *Staphylococcus aureus* may be aspirated but may also spread to the lungs hematogenously as in right-sided endocarditis [85]. In hospitalized patients, pneumonia accounts for 10–20% of nosocomial infections and is the leading cause of death due to nosocomial infections [86]. (See also Chapter 17.)

Aspiration is relatively common [87]. Host defenses, however, such as the gag reflex, cough reflex, mucociliary barrier, and local immunity are more than adequate to protect the lungs from infection. If, however, the aspirated organism is highly virulent, normal host defenses are compromised, or a large inoculum reaches the lungs, pneumonia may result [88]. The clinical settings in which significant aspiration occurs are any diseases or processes that reduce the level of consciousness or disrupt the gag and swallowing reflexes. These include neuromuscular disease, head injury, cerebrovascular accidents, seizure disorders, alcoholism, sedation, intubation, and the presence of a nasogastric tube [89]. Persons with spinal cord injury may have a compromised cough along with decreased lung volumes, predisposing them to aspiration, atelectasis, and pneumonia [75].

Three major syndromes result from aspiration: (1) chemical pneumonitis secondary to aspiration of toxic fluids, generally gastric acid; (2) bronchial obstruction secondary to aspiration of particulate matter; and (3) infectious pneumonia [90]. Chemical pneumonitis and mechanical obstruction usually cause acute symptoms [88]. Treatment relies on supportive measures including correction of hypoxemia and fluid support. Bronchoscopy to remove a foreign object may be required with obstruction [91]. Corticosteroid therapy is of no proven benefit in treating chemical pneumonitis [92]. Although chemically damaged lung parenchyma may be more susceptible to bacterial infection, antibiotics should be reserved for cases in which there is evidence of infection such as fever, purulent sputum, leukocytosis, and progressive infiltrates [90]. Early use of antibiotics may not prevent subsequent infections and may select a more resistant bacterial flora [93, 94].

Bacterial aspiration pneumonia is less fulminant than chemical pneumonitis and bronchial obstruc-

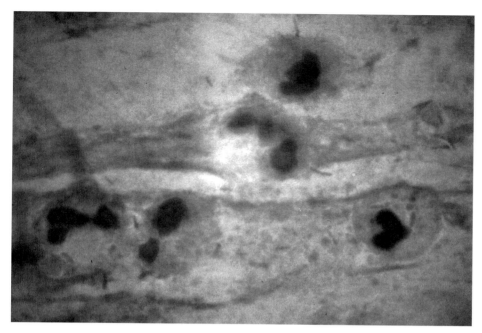

Figure 12-1. Gram's stain of sputum revealing polymorphonuclear cells and gram-negative bacilli in a patient with pneumonia caused by *Pseudomonas aeruginosa*. (Courtesy of Lance Peterson, M.D., Northwestern University Medical School, Chicago.)

tion. Fever and cough productive of purulent sputum in a susceptible host should suggest the diagnosis. Initial symptoms may be minimal or similar to an acute bacterial pneumonia with productive cough, dyspnea, and fever noted [95]. Early, patients will have changes on chest roentgenograms consistent with other forms of bacterial pneumonia. Infiltrates are typically located in dependent areas such as the posterior segments of the upper and lower lobes when persons are supine and the basal segments of the lower lobes when persons are upright [96]. After several days to weeks, tissue necrosis may develop, resulting in abscess or empyema formation. Putrid sputum is seen in about half of patients in this later stage [97, 98]. Aspiration pneumonia may be an insidious process, with persons presenting after weeks or months of weight loss, malaise, low grade fever, and cough. Chest roentgenograms at this time may reveal cavitation, abscess, or empyema. Anemia is typically present [88]. Neoplasm is a diagnostic consideration in these patients.

Although aspiration pneumonia is diagnosed on the basis of clinical presentation, microbiology studies are necessary for determining the etiologic agent. Obtaining adequate sputum samples for both

a Gram's stain and culture is important. Sputum samples should have more than 25 polymorphonuclear cells and less than 10 squamous epithelial cells per high-power microscopic field (Figure 12-1) [99]. In addition, a Gram's stain of the sputum may guide initial antibiotic therapy and help interpret culture results by indicating the predominate organisms in a mixed flora. A sputum smear revealing gram-positive cocci in clusters implies a staphylococcal pneumonia, whereas gram-negative bacilli imply an infection with Enterobacteriaceae or *Pseudomonas* species. A smear with multiple organisms in the setting of a negative sputum culture result implies a pneumonia caused by anaerobes. Similarly, if easily cultured organisms such as *Staphylococcus aureus* and aerobic gram-negative bacilli are not isolated on sputum culture, these bacteria are most likely not involved [100]. If a patient is unable to produce expectorated sputum, bronchoscopy or bronchoalveolar lavage may be of benefit in identifying the causative organisms [101–104]. All patients with suspected pneumonia should have blood cultures obtained.

Aspiration pneumonia is caused by organisms colonizing the oropharynx and occasionally the upper gastrointestinal tract, with the flora for a given person depending on the clinical setting. Aspiration pneumonia tends to be polymicrobial, with anaerobic bacteria predominating [105]. Organisms typically isolated from adults with a community-acquired aspiration pneumonia include *Streptococcus* species, *Bacteroides* species, and other oral anaerobes such as *Peptostreptococcus* and *Peptococcus* species, and to a lesser degree, Enterobacteriaceae [85]. Most hospitalized patients become colonized with institutional flora within several days [106]. These patients, therefore, are at risk for developing pneumonia with organisms such as Enterobacteriaceae, *Pseudomonas* species, *Acinetobacter* species, *Staphylococcus aureus*, and *Legionella* species. Pneumonia in neutropenic patients, in addition to the previously mentioned organisms, may also be caused by *Candida* and *Aspergillus* species [85]. With the continuing epidemic of *Mycobacterium tuberculosis*, this pathogen should be considered in all patients with respiratory infections, especially immunocompromised patients who may have atypical chest roentgenograms. Patients on H2-blocking agents or antacids have increased gastric colonization with aerobic enteric bacteria and may be at increased risk for aspiration pneumonia [107]. Preliminary studies suggest that maintenance of a low gastric pH may reduce the risk of nosocomial pneumonia [108, 109]. Sucralfate, which does not increase the gastric pH, may be an alternative for prophylaxis against stress ulcers [109].

Treatment of aspiration pneumonia is often empiric. For community-acquired aspiration pneumonia, therapy with clindamycin is more efficacious than penicillin G [110, 111]. If gram-negative organisms are suspected in addition to anaerobes, alternatives include ampicillin-sulbactam, cefoxitin, or ticarcillin-clavulanate. Nosocomially acquired aspiration pneumonia requires combination therapy to provide activity against gram-negative bacilli, *Staphylococcus aureus*, and anaerobes. Antibiotics should be selected on the basis of previous therapy and resistance patterns within the facility. Initial therapy should include coverage for *Pseudomonas aeruginosa* with an aminoglycoside and an antipseudomonal third-generation cephalosporin, extended-spectrum penicillin, or imipenem. A high peak serum level of the aminoglycoside is recommended. If *Staphylococcus aureus* is suspected, vancomycin should be added unless methicillin resistance is unlikely, in which case an alternative

such as oxacillin, nafcillin, or clindamycin may be suitable [100]. A newer alternative, piperacillin-tazobactam, offers antipseudomonal and anaerobic coverage [112]. Hypoxemia should be corrected with supplemental oxygen therapy. Bronchial hygiene should be instituted to promote mobilization of secretions. Any loculated fluid collections, such as an empyema, require drainage.

The prognosis depends on the clinical setting. Prompt response to therapy and a good prognosis are seen with community-acquired aspiration pneumonia [113]. Nosocomial-acquired aspiration pneumonia has a higher mortality related to both associated severe underlying disease and infection with aerobic gram-negative bacilli, especially *Pseudomonas aeruginosa* [100, 113].

Prevention of aspiration pneumonia requires recognition of host risk factors. Barium cookie swallow or fluoroscopic examination can document chronic aspiration. Patients chronically aspirating may be helped by speech therapy or positioning. An alternative method of feeding, such as use of a gastrostomy tube, sometimes in conjunction with a tracheostomy or surgical diversion, may need to be considered [89]. Patients with chronic disability should be vaccinated against certain organisms such as *Streptococcus pneumoniae* [114]. Strong emphasis on infection control, particularly in the intensive care setting, may help prevent the dissemination of highly resistant organisms that contribute to the high mortality from nosocomial pneumonia.

Osteomyelitis

Osteomyelitis, one of the most serious complications of severe bone trauma, occurs for a variety of reasons in the chronically disabled [115, 116]. It can result from spread of infection from infected orthopedic appliances or prostheses or from infected pressure sores (see Chapter 13) or ulcers secondary to diabetes mellitus or severe peripheral vascular disease. Hematogenous spread of infection to bone, although more common in children, can occur with bacteremia of any cause and can complicate urinary tract infections, infections associated with venous catheters, or intravenous drug use. Although the outcome of osteomyelitis has improved, chronic disease remains a difficult problem. The prognosis in this disease may continue to improve with advances in surgical techniques and development of new oral antibiotics.

Osteomyelitis is generally classified on the basis of pathogenesis (hematogenous or spread from a contiguous focus), duration of infection (acute versus chronic), extent of bone involvement, and host characteristics (presence of chronic disease or immune suppression) [117, 118]. These classification schemes can help guide management. For example, treatment of acute osteomyelitis requires a shorter course of antimicrobial therapy than that of chronic osteomyelitis. Features of osteomyelitis related to hematogenous infection, spread from a contiguous focus, and vascular insufficiency are discussed in the following section.

An increasing number of cases of hematogenous osteomyelitis are being reported in adults, especially those older than 50 years of age. Although the metaphyses of long bones are frequently involved in children, in adults the vertebral bodies are most commonly affected [119]. Multiple bone involvement may occur in some patients, especially children [120].

The etiologic organism can often be identified by bone biopsy, needle aspiration, or blood culture [121]. Usually only one organism is involved, with over 50% of cases being caused by *Staphylococcus aureus*. Gram-negative bacilli (*Escherichia coli*, *Klebsiella pneumoniae*, *Salmonella* species, *Proteus mirabilis*, and *Pseudomonas aeruginosa*) are found with increasing frequency, particularly in intravenous drug users and patients with urinary tract infections [122, 123]. Intravenous drug users are also at risk for infection with *Candida albicans* [124]. Although organisms isolated from blood cultures typically reflect the cause of the osteomyelitis, this may not be the case in intravenous drug users. A bone biopsy may be required for making a definitive diagnosis [125]. Immunocompromised patients or those receiving long-term antibiotic therapy are at increased risk for osteomyelitis caused by fungi, such as *Candida* or *Aspergillus* [119].

Children with hematogenous osteomyelitis classically present with high fever and systemic toxicity along with local swelling, pain, and limitation of motion of the involved bone [126]. Adults, and especially intravenous drug users, commonly present with few constitutional symptoms and only nonspecific pain of the involved area, often for several months' duration [122]. Vertebral osteomyelitis, the most common site of hematogenous infection in adults, usually presents with local spinal pain of greater than 1 week's duration, with fever only occurring in about half the cases [127]. The diagnosis of osteomyelitis may be overlooked, especially with an occult or transient source of bacteremia, causing delays in appropriate therapy. The erythrocyte sedimentation rate, however, is usually high and is sometimes used to follow response to treatment [128, 129]. Complications of vertebral osteomyelitis include subluxation (especially of the atlantoaxial joint), spinal instability, abscesses, and local extension of infection, all which may lead to significant neurologic deficits [119]. Bony destruction may progress rapidly and epidural abscesses may occur with resulting spinal pain, radicular symptoms, paraparesis, and even paraplegia [129, 130]. Diagnosis is aided by myelography, computed tomography (CT), or magnetic resonance imaging (MRI). MRI provides the best resolution of bone and soft tissue within the axial skeleton [131]. Surgical decompression, debridement, and drainage are essential in patients with neuronal compression, epidural or perivertebral abscesses, or extensive bony involvement [129].

Osteomyelitis secondary to a contiguous source results from the direct inoculation of bone from open fractures or surgery or to the spread of organisms from a nearby source such as an infected decubitus ulcer or odontogenic infection (Figure 12-2) [119, 132, 133]. In the chronically disabled person this type of osteomyelitis often results from major trauma or a chronically infected pressure sore [115, 132]. Although any bone may be involved, long bones of the lower extremity are frequently affected because these are often the site of fracture and open reduction [134]. The skull and mandible can be infected after neurosurgery, oral surgery, or dental infections [133]. The greater trochanter and sacrum are the most frequent sites of osteomyelitis related to pressure sores [135].

More than one organism often causes this type of osteomyelitis. Although *Staphylococcus aureus* is the most common organism isolated, it is frequently part of a mixed infection that may include gram-negative bacilli and even anaerobes [134, 135]. Definitive diagnosis is made by culturing bone. Cultures obtained by swabbing an overlying pressure sore or ulcer have little value due to surface colonization with multiple organisms [136].

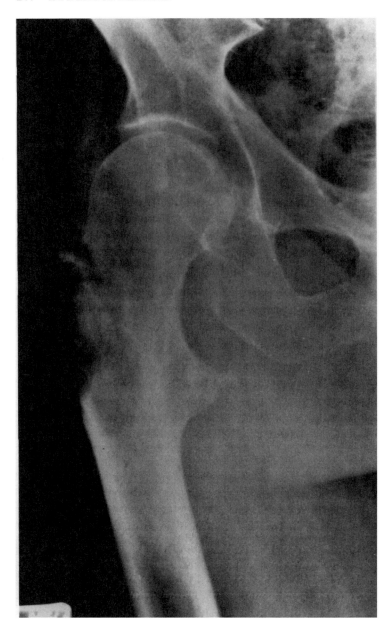

Figure 12-2. Osteomyelitis secondary to a contiguous source of infection. (Reprinted with permission from GL Mandel, RG Douglas Jr, JE Bennett [eds], Principles and Practice of Infectious Diseases [2nd ed]. New York: Wiley, 1985;707.)

One study, however, reported that superficial wound cultures in patients with posttraumatic or postsurgical osteomyelitis isolated the same organisms found at the time of operative debridement in approximately 70% of cases [134]. These superficial cultures, however, also yielded extra organisms not isolated from the bone cultures, making interpretation difficult. Similarly, the value of culturing sinus tract drainage is questionable. One study demonstrated that isolation of *Staphylococcus aureus*, although usually not as a single isolate, from sinus tracts correlated with finding this organism in subsequent bone cultures in approximately 75% of patients. In contrast, isolation of bacteria other than *Staphylococcus aureus* had a low likelihood of predicting the pathogen ultimately cultured from bone.

In addition, not isolating *Staphylococcus aureus* did not exclude it as the cause of osteomyelitis [137]. Because *Staphylococcus aureus* is the most likely cause of osteomyelitis in this setting, isolation of this organism from a sinus tract culture adds little to choosing empiric therapy.

Patients with contiguous osteomyelitis present with local swelling and erythema but may have few systemic symptoms, particularly in chronic or recurrent infections. In chronic or recurrent infections, drainage from a sinus tract is classically seen [138]. Patients with an infected prosthetic joint will generally present with pain and dysfunction or loosening of the prosthesis. Pain with motion implies mechanical loosening, whereas constant pain implies infection. Fever and leukocytosis may be absent but a high (>50 mm/hour) or increasing erythrocyte sedimentation rate is suggestive of infection [139]. Prosthetic joint infections occurring within 3 months of implant are generally considered to be due to contamination at the time of surgery or to postoperative wound infection. Late infections, which occur greater than 1 year after implant, are usually caused by hematogenous seeding from a distant site such as the urinary tract, skin or soft tissue, respiratory tract, or oral cavity [140].

Persons with osteomyelitis associated with vascular insufficiency almost always have underlying diabetes mellitus or peripheral vascular disease. More days are spent in the hospital treating diabetic foot infections that any other complication of diabetes and 13% of patients admitted for diabetic foot problems have osteomyelitis [141–143]. Most patients with osteomyelitis associated with vascular insufficiency are between 50 and 70 years of age and have had diabetes mellitus for at least 2 or more years [144, 145]. The peripheral neuropathy often seen in diabetics increases susceptibility to foot trauma. With both severe vascular disease and diabetes mellitus, poor blood supply results in little or slowed healing of skin lesions. Ulcers may ultimately develop, become infected, and lead to an underlying osteomyelitis [146].

The best method for obtaining cultures is uncertain. One study reported that 62% of cultures obtained by swabbing the ulcer base, 69% obtained by needle aspiration, and 75% by curettage of the ulcer base match those taken from deep tissue culture at the time of amputation [147]. A bone biopsy has the advantage of confirming the diagnosis by histology

as well as providing material for culture [148], although the bone culture may still be contaminated if obtained through infected soft tissue. Also, it may be difficult to distinguish diabetic osteopathy from osteomyelitis based on histology [144]. Most diabetic foot infections including osteomyelitis are polymicrobial and contain more than three organisms [144, 145]. Generally a mixture of gram-positive cocci including enterococci, anaerobic bacteria, and aerobic gram-negative bacilli will be present [144]. The importance of adequate cultures to guide therapy cannot be overstressed.

Patients typically present with local symptoms and signs such as an ulceration, purulent drainage, swelling, erythema, or pain. Infections are often indolent. Fever, leukocytosis, and an elevated sedimentation rate are often absent [144]. However, these studies, as well as blood cultures, should be performed because positive results will aid in diagnosis. Many patients have diminished or absent peripheral pulses and most will have evidence of a sensory neuropathy [146]. The bones most frequently involved are the small bones of the feet such as the metatarsal bones and proximal phalanges (Figure 12-3).

Early studies showed that patients treated with antibiotics alone often had poor outcomes and ultimately required amputation [117, 149]. Better outcomes, however, have been demonstrated with high-dose parenteral antibiotic therapy administered for at least 4 weeks, as long as tissue necrosis or gangrene was absent [144]. One study reported that a 10-week course of culture-guided oral antibiotic therapy after surgical debridement in diabetic patients with suspected pedal osteomyelitis without systemic symptoms may be effective and cost efficient [150].

In acute hematogenous osteomyelitis fewer than one-third of cases will have detectable diagnostic changes on bone roentgenograms within 2 weeks. However, by 4 weeks about 90% will have changes. These include periosteal reaction, cortical irregularity, and permeative destruction [151]. Visualization of a lytic bone lesion requires approximately 50% destruction of the bony matrix [117]. Bone roentgenograms may never reveal an abnormality. CT is more sensitive at detecting discrete areas of bone damage or inflammation in the surrounding tissue. Abnormalities can be visualized earlier on CT than on plain films of bone. In addi-

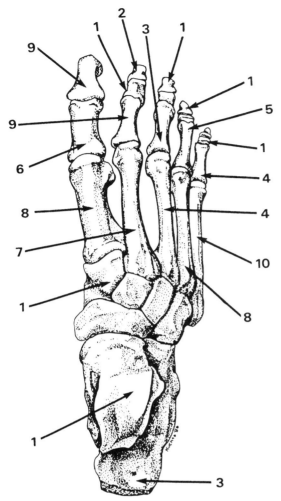

Figure 12-3. Bones involved in 51 patients with diabetic foot osteomyelitis. (Reprinted with permission from DM Bamberger, GP Daus, DN Gerding. Osteomyelitis in the feet of diabetics. Am J Med 1987;83:653. Copyright 1987 Technical Publishing Company.)

tion, CT is useful for evaluating areas difficult to visualize, such as the pelvis [151]. In chromic osteomyelitis, CT is superior for visualizing bony sequestra and cortical destruction. MRI is being used with increasing frequency for diagnosing osteomyelitis and can be an extremely sensitive technique in certain situations. MRI is ideal for detecting bone marrow abnormalities that occur early in the course of osteomyelitis and can help differentiate cellulitis from osteomyelitis. It is su-

perior to CT in this regard [131]. A study using fat-suppressed contrast-enhanced MRI reported that this technique was more sensitive and specific for diagnosing osteomyelitis in cases complicated by conditions such as diabetic neuropathy and pelvic pressure sores [152]. Application of the MRI technique to reveal the difference between the density of bone and its surrounding sequestrum and purulent material is illustrated in Figure 12-4.

The technetium-99m bone scan uses 99mTc-labeled diphosphonates that accumulate preferentially into metabolically active bone [151]. The standard bone scan consists of images obtained 3 hours after injection with the 99mTc. Any disease that increases bone turnover or increases blood flow to the affected area will result in a positive scan result. Examples include osteomyelitis, cellulitis, trauma, and tumor. To enhance the specificity, a three-phase scan is often used. The first phase consists of images obtained during injection of 99mTc and represents the blood flow. The second phase consists of images obtained within 5 minutes and represents blood pooling. The third phase consists of the standard images obtained at 3 hours and represents uptake by bone. With osteomyelitis, all three phases should show uptake in the affected area. With cellulitis, however, uptake in the third phase will be nonfocal and less intense than uptake in the first two phases [153]. Technetium bone scans are sensitive and specific when bone roentgenograms are normal. The specificity drops below 50% with underlying bone abnormalities such as recent surgery, trauma, osteoarthritis, diabetic osteopathy, or tumor [154–156]. False-negative scan results can occur with decreased blood flow to the affected area [151].

In patients with underlying bone disease, a three-phase bone scan followed by either a gallium-67 citrate or indium-111-labeled leukocyte scan may be of benefit. Gallium-67 citrate detects inflammatory processes and has been used in the workup of fevers of unknown origin. Gallium is taken up by leukocytes that localize to areas of infection or inflammation. Some nonspecific bone uptake of gallium may also occur. An indium scan, although more expensive and difficult to perform, may also confirm technetium scan results. Leukocytes obtained from the patient are labeled with ^{111}In and reinjected. As with a gallium scan, the leukocytes subsequently localize to areas with infection or inflammation [151]. Figure 12-5 shows an indium

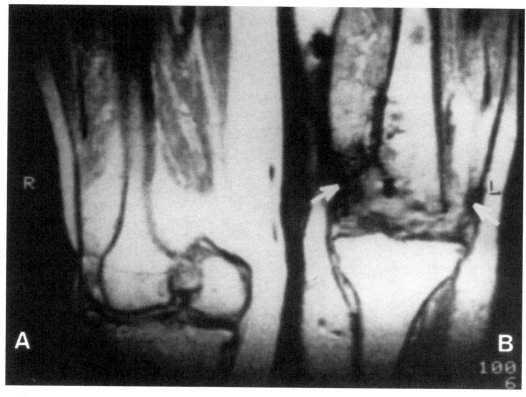

Figure 12-4. A. Magnetic resonance imaging scan of a normal femur. B. Magnetic resonance imaging scan of osteomyelitis of a femur. (Reprinted with permission from LO Gentry. Osteomyelitis: Options for diagnosis and management. J Antimicrob Chemother 1988;21:115. Copyright 1988 Academic Press London, Ltd.)

scan confirming a positive bone scan result in a person who had a prosthetic hip removed because of osteomyelitis and a medullary abscess. With both gallium and indium scans, false-negative results can occur in diseases where less accumulation of leukocytes may be expected, such as chronic osteomyelitis [151]. False-positive scan results can occur with some tumors and noninfectious inflammatory processes [153]. For diagnosing osteomyelitis, a gallium or indium scan is generally compared with a technetium scan. Areas of suspected osteomyelitis should show uptake with both scans. Figure 12-6 shows a negative gallium scan result in a person suspected of having osteomyelitis after the removal of a hip prosthesis. Other scintigraphic tests such as indium-labeled immunoglobulin are being investigated as alternatives to gallium or indium scans because they may be more rapid, less expensive, and expose the patient to less radiation [151]. Despite

the numerous tests available to assist in the diagnosis of osteomyelitis, the diagnosis may remain elusive in some patients, such as those with pressure sores. A bone biopsy may still be required before a definitive diagnosis can be made [153].

Effective therapy for osteomyelitis is poorly defined [120]. Optimal antibiotic regimens and duration of therapy as well as the significance of adequate penetration of the drug into affected bone have not been adequately studied.

Acute osteomyelitis is usually defined as disease of less than 1 month's duration. Studies have shown lower rates of treatment failure with therapy longer than 3–4 weeks [126]. Antimicrobial therapy should be based on a Gram's stain and culture of aspirated material, bone biopsy, or blood. Usually antibiotics are administered parenterally for 4 weeks. The most common isolate, *Staphylococcus aureus*, can be treated with a penicillinase-resistant penicillin such

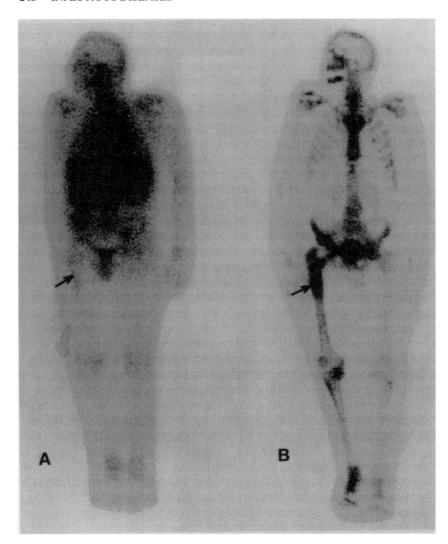

Figure 12-5. A. Technetium-99m scan with activity in the right hip. B. Indium-111 scan confirming infection in the same hip. (Reprinted with permission from LO Gentry. Osteomyelitis: Options for diagnosis and management. J Antimicrob Chemother 1988;21:115. Copyright 1988 Academic Press London, Ltd.)

as oxacillin or nafcillin or with vancomycin, depending on the sensitivity profile of the organism. Serum bactericidal levels can be used to confirm effective killing of the organism by the selected antibiotic regimen [157]. The serum bactericidal level is the highest dilution of the patient's serum that will kill the organism in vitro. Trough levels obtained 30 minutes before the next dose of antibiotic that are greater than or equal to 1:2 correlate with successful outcomes [158]. Acute vertebral osteomyelitis can often be effectively treated with a minimum of 4 weeks of parenteral antibiotics, although longer courses are sometimes necessary [159]. Abscesses,

adjacent joint infection, or extensive bony involvement require surgical drainage or debridement.

Osteomyelitis caused by *Mycobacterium tuberculosis* should be treated with the same regimens used for pulmonary disease, although longer courses are advisable [160].

Chronic osteomyelitis is usually defined as disease for longer than 1 month's duration. In contrast to acute disease, optimal therapy for chronic osteomyelitis is poorly defined. Chronic osteomyelitis is associated with necrotic bone that may sequester organisms. As a result, recurrences have been documented up to 50 years after initial diagnosis [119].

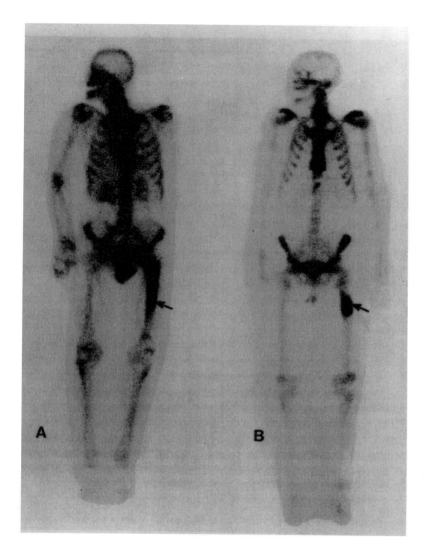

Figure 12-6. A. Gallium-67 scan with negative results for infection in the right hip. B. Technetium-99m scan with activity in the right hip. (Reprinted with permission from LO Gentry. Osteomyelitis: Options for diagnosis and management. J Antimicrob Chemother 1988;21:115. Copyright 1988 Academic Press London, Ltd.)

Successful treatment requires both aggressive surgical debridement and high-dose parenteral antibiotics. The duration of therapy is not clear but 4–6 weeks of parenteral antibiotics followed by 2–3 months of oral antibiotics is reasonable. A review of nearly 500 episodes of osteomyelitis treated between 1980 and 1986 demonstrated that outcome was affected by the type and duration of osteomyelitis and by the organism. Hematogenous osteomyelitis had the best prognosis followed by disease secondary to a contiguous source, whereas osteomyelitis associated with vascular insufficiency had the worst prognosis. Acute osteomyelitis had a much better prognosis than chronic disease. Osteomyelitis caused by *Staphylococcus aureus* had the best outcome followed by infections caused by gram-negative bacilli. Polymicrobial osteomyelitis had the worst outcome. Oral therapy following parenteral antibiotics in 70 cases of chronic osteomyelitis, although not eradicating the causative organism, may have helped to preserve limb function and postpone amputation by suppressing the organism [161].

The effective use of oral antibiotics to treat osteomyelitis has been documented, especially with highly susceptible strains of *Staphylococcus aureus*

[162]. Oral antibiotics with good bone penetration are available and include dicloxacillin and clindamycin for *Staphylococcus aureus* and fluoroquinolones such as ciprofloxacin for gram-negative bacilli [150, 163–165]. Ciprofloxacin is not the drug of choice for gram-positive organisms. For polymicrobial infections, regimens such as ciprofloxacin and clindamycin, trimethoprim-sulfamethoxazole and metronidazole, or amoxicillin-clavulanate may be used.

As with acute osteomyelitis, serum bactericidal levels may be used to confirm adequate killing of the organism by the antibiotic regimen. Peak serum bactericidal levels, drawn 30 minutes after intravenous infusion or 60 minutes after intramuscular injection, that are greater than or equal to 1:16 and trough levels that are greater than or equal to 1:4 are correlated with successful outcomes [158].

The most successful technique for managing prosthetic joint infections is removal of the prosthesis followed by 6 weeks of culture-guided parenteral antimicrobial therapy before placement of a new device. Success rates in excess of 90% can be expected [166–168]. Alternatively, a new device is placed using antibiotic-impregnated cement during the surgery to remove the infected prosthesis. Following surgery, the patient is treated with parenteral antibiotics. Although outcomes are less favorable, success rates of approximately 70–80% can be expected [169–171].

In general, because antimicrobial therapy will be administered for prolonged periods, one must be especially aware of possible side effects and drug interactions that may occur. A serious side effect of antimicrobial therapy, especially ampicillin and clindamycin, is *Clostridium difficile* colitis that requires prompt recognition and management [172].

All patients with chronic osteomyelitis require adequate debridement with removal of all dead and devitalized tissue. Surgical resection of large sequestra, however, creates large defects with resulting instability and risk of pathologic fracture. Complete wound closure should be attempted whenever possible [173]. Grafting of bone into the defect will fail unless the infection is completely eradicated. Acrylic beads containing antibiotics can be used to temporarily fill the dead space. The beads are removed after 3–4 weeks and replaced with cancellous bone [174, 175].

A variety of surgical procedures involving transfer of local or free muscle flaps to fill bony defects and enhance vascular supply have been used [173, 176]. Patients with movement at the site of infection may require mechanical stabilization. Plates, screws, and rods are often used but complicate the treatment of infection. An external fixator, such as the device designed by Ilizarov, can stabilize nonunion and large bony defects with some success [177].

Cerebrospinal Fluid Shunt Infections

Management of hydrocephalus often requires placement of a cerebrospinal fluid shunt. In the United States, approximately 10,000 shunts are placed each year and 6,000 shunts undergo revision [178]. The ventriculoperitoneal shunt is the most common shunt placed. Shunts bypass the protective blood–brain barrier and increase the risk of infection of the central nervous system [179]. Approximately 15% of shunts will become infected, although the rate is higher in low birth weight infants and the elderly [180–182].

Most infections are caused by *Staphylococcus epidermidis* followed by *Staphylococcus aureus.* Gram-negative bacilli account for 5–10% of infections. The most common pathogens causing meningitis, *Haemophilus influenzae, Streptococcus pneumoniae,* and *Neisseria meningitidis,* account for only 5% of cases [183]. The pathogenicity of *Staphylococcus epidermidis* is related to its ability to secrete exopolysaccharide slime or glycocalyxes that facilitate attachment to the shunt and help the organism avoid host defenses and antibiotics [184]. The majority of shunt infections occur within 2 months of surgery and are usually caused by organisms found on the skin that colonize the shunt during placement, such as *Staphylococcus epidermidis* and *aureus* along with diphtheroids [179, 180, 182]. Shunt infections caused by gram-negative bacilli, pneumococci, meningococci, and hemophilus result after hematogenous spread and may occur at any time [180, 185, 186].

Symptoms and signs of cerebrospinal fluid shunt infections are variable although fever is usually present [179]. Patients with early shunt infections may have inflammation along the subcutaneous tract of the shunt [187]. With later infections, nonspecific symptoms and signs predominate, including fever, nausea, emesis, malaise, or other signs of increased intracranial pressure. Shunt malfunction alone is frequently the first sign of infection. Meningeal signs are rare [179]. Involvement of the distal part of a ventriculoperitoneal shunt may result in abdominal symptoms and complications, such as peritonitis, bowel obstruction, and bowel perforation [188, 189]. A subtle manifestation of infection in ventriculovascular shunts is shunt nephritis resulting from immune-complex deposition [190].

Diagnosis of cerebrospinal fluid shunt infections often relies on obtaining fluid by percutaneous aspiration from the shunt reservoir or tubing. Fluid should be sent for a Gram's stain, culture, and cell count. Most patients not receiving antibiotics will have a positive culture result. A negative culture result, however, does not exclude the diagnosis, and culture of the shunt apparatus itself may be needed [181, 191]. Cultures should be obtained whenever a revision is performed on a malfunctioning shunt. Changes in the protein and glucose content and elevations in the cell count of cerebrospinal fluid are usually not pronounced in shunt infections. The median white cell count in one large series was 76 cells/ml [189]. The extent of pleocytosis, however, did correlate with obtaining a positive culture result; approximately 90% of patients with greater than 100 cells/ml had positive culture results. The peripheral white cell count may or may not be elevated [180].

Effective treatment requires antibiotics and usually removal of the infected shunt. High-dose antibiotics are given parenterally and are chosen based on the susceptibility of the causative organism and the ability of the drug to attain adequate levels in the cerebrospinal fluid [192]. Nafcillin or oxacillin is used for susceptible *Staphylococcus* species. For infections with methicillin-resistant strains, vancomycin is used. Although vancomycin penetrates the blood–brain barrier poorly, treatment is often successful. At times, however, intraventricular vancomycin must be added to the regimen [193]. Rifampin penetrates into the cerebrospinal fluid well and may act synergistically with both vancomycin and penicillinase-resistant penicillins. Because antagonistic drug interactions can occur with the addition of rifampin, susceptibility testing may be necessary to confirm synergy [183]. In infections caused by gram-negative bacilli a third-generation cephalosporin, such as ceftriaxone or ceftazidime, should be used [194, 195]. Treatment of some gram-negative organisms, such as *Pseudomonas*

aeruginosa, may require the use of aminoglycosides. Because aminoglycosides do not penetrate into the cerebrospinal fluid, intraventricular administration of these agents must be used. Generally, the aminoglycoside cerebrospinal fluid trough level should be five to ten times the minimum inhibitory concentration of the organism [193]. Antibiotics are continued for 3–4 weeks, until culture results are repeatedly negative.

Antibiotic therapy alone is only effective in certain situations such as when meningitis is the cause of infection [194]. As a result, effective treatment usually requires early removal of the shunt [181]. Use of a temporary external ventricular drain allows for continued ventricular decompression while antibiotics are administered. When the fluid has been sterilized, a new shunt may be placed, usually on the opposite side or into a different anatomic site [195–197]. Treatment with antibiotics and removal of the infected shunt with simultaneous replacement by a new shunt in a different location is less successful and has a high rate of relapse [181].

Human Immunodeficiency Virus Infections

In the United States in 1992, AIDS had become the leading cause of death for men between 25 and 44 years of age. For women in this age group, it was the fourth leading cause of death and increasing rapidly [198]. As the number of persons with AIDS continues to grow, rehabilitation health care providers will play an increasing role in providing care for HIV-infected persons with disabilities.

Although a justifiable cause for concern, few health care workers have been infected with HIV as a result of occupational exposure [199]. The estimated risk for seroconversion after percutaneous exposure to infected fluids, such as blood during a needle stick, is approximately 0.3%. The rate after mucous membrane exposure is unknown but thought to be lower [200]. Occupational risk for infection can be substantially lowered with the proper implementation of precautions to minimize contact with potentially infected body fluids, especially blood. Universal precautions, where the blood and certain body fluids of every person are assumed to be potentially infected, have significantly reduced the potential risk to health care workers [201, 202]. Although no definitive trial has demonstrated conclusively that medications such as zidovudine, which slows HIV replication, will prevent infection after exposure to HIV, experiments in animals and retrospective studies on health-care providers exposed to HIV have shown a benefit to administering zidovudine. Thus, the Centers for Disease Control and Prevention have recommended that zidovudine therapy be initiated after a significant occupational exposure to HIV [203]. Whether recommendations for postexposure prophylaxis will change as resistance to zidovudine becomes more prevalent is unclear.

Despite the intensive research effort devoted to HIV during the past decade, the mechanism of HIV pathogenesis remains poorly understood. When a person is acutely infected with HIV, plasma viremia develops with subsequent infection of lymphocytes and macrophages expressing the CD4 molecule [204]. Within 2–3 months, the recently infected person will develop an antibody response to the virus and become seropositive on serologic test results (such as enzyme immunoassays and Western blots) [205]. Although the combined humoral and cell-mediated host immune response is highly effective at clearing the viremia, it is unable to completely eradicate the infection [206]. Virus persists and replicates within lymphoid organs and tissues [207]. It is at this stage that persons generally experience an extended asymptomatic phase characterized by continued viral replication and a progressive decline in CD4+ cells [208]. The actual mechanism of cell destruction is unclear, but may be related to prolific HIV replication within CD4+ T cells, leading to rapid cell turnover [209, 210]. Once CD4+ cells are depleted, patients are at risk for developing opportunistic infections and malignancies. On the basis of CD4+ cell counts, it is possible to predict diseases a person is at risk for developing [211–215]. For example, most individuals with counts over 500 cells/mm^3 are asymptomatic. Persons with counts between 250 and 500 cells/mm^3 are at risk for developing oral candidiasis, recurrent bacterial infections, and tuberculosis, whereas counts between 100 and 250 cells/mm^3 are associated with Kaposi's sarcoma, lymphoma, recurrent herpes simplex virus infections, and cryptosporidiosis. Persons with severe immunodeficiency—i.e., counts less than 100 cells/mm^3 —are at risk for cytomegalovirus retinitis, esophageal candidiasis, cryptococcosis, toxoplasmosis, *Pneumocystis carinii* pneumonia, and disseminated mycobacterial infections. The major-

ity of HIV-related deaths occur in persons with counts of 50 cells/mm^3 or less [216]. At least 10% of HIV-infected persons have remained asymptomatic with stable CD4+ T-cell counts for more than 8 years [217]. It has been shown that these long-term survivors have low levels of virus and strong virus-specific immune responses [218]. Plasma HIV-1 RNA levels also have prognostic value and can be used to measure the clinical efficacy of therapy directed against HIV [219–221].

Care for HIV-infected persons centers on slowing viral replication and CD4+ cell depletion, preventing opportunistic infections, and treating complications as they arise. Currently approved antiretroviral medications either block the ability of the virus to convert its RNA genome into DNA by inhibiting viral reverse transcriptase (zidovudine, didanosine, zalcitabine, stavudine, and lamivudine) or inhibit the enzyme that is needed for processing the precursor for several structural and functional proteins required for production of infectious virus (saquinavir, indinavir, and ritonavir) [222–226]. Zidovudine, the most studied of the four agents, slows depletion of CD4+ cells, delays progression of disease, and slows progression to death in persons with symptoms [227, 228]. Although the use of this medication for persons with no symptoms and CD4+ cell counts between 200 and 500 cells/mm^3 was controversial [229–231], results of recent trials have demonstrated clinical benefit to starting combination therapy or monotherapy with didanosine in persons with counts less than 500/mm^3 [232, 233]. The combination of zidovudine and lamivudine appears especially promising, with one trial showing pronounced viral supression and an increased CD4+ cell count [220]. The addition of a protease inhibitor may further enhance any therapeutic benefit [224, 225].

Vaccines and antimicrobial prophylaxis are routinely used to decrease the frequency of opportunistic infections. One of the most significant effects on survival in HIV-infected persons was made by the widespread use of antimicrobials such as trimethoprim-sulfamethoxazole to prevent *Pneumocystis carinii* pneumonia. Although other prophylactic measures have had less of an impact [234, 235], many patients will take one or more antimicrobials to prevent opportunistic infections in addition to antiretroviral agents and medications to treat the myriad complications that can arise [236, 237]. Because patients with AIDS take numerous medications, they are at increased risk for drug toxicities, interactions, and allergic reactions and require careful monitoring [238].

Disabling conditions in HIV-infected persons are numerous, including non–HIV-related conditions such as head trauma, spinal cord injury, or strokes [239], and HIV-related conditions such as cardiomyopathy, myositis, chronic lung disease secondary to recurrent infection, or wasting syndrome. Most disabling conditions, however, involve the central and peripheral nervous system and include both neoplasms such as lymphoma and infections such as toxoplasmosis, progressive multifocal leukoencephalopathy, cytomegalovirus radiculopathy or encephalopathy, or herpes simplex virus encephalopathy [240, 241]. In addition, some causes are directly related to the underlying HIV infection such as acute and chronic demyelinating neuropathies, AIDS dementia complex, painful sensory neuropathy, and vacuolar myelopathy [242, 243]. Other complications that occur more frequently and are associated with HIV infection include headaches and seizure disorders, even without underlying opportunistic infections or malignancies [241]. In a given patient, several diseases or processes may be acting in conjunction. For example, peripheral neuropathy secondary to HIV infection may be exacerbated by a vitamin B_{12} deficiency or by one of several neurotoxic medications commonly prescribed such as didanosine or zalcitabine [242]. Although some disabling conditions such as polymyositis tend to occur early in the course of HIV infection, most become manifest during advanced stages of the disease [241].

While an HIV-infected patient is hospitalized, he or she remains at risk for both nosocomial infections such as urinary tract infections, pneumonias, and infections associated with vascular catheters, as well as opportunistic infections and malignancies. In addition, HIV-infected patients with nosocomial bacterial infections may not respond as rapidly to treatment as immunocompetent hosts. The evaluation of an HIV-infected patient with a fever should include a thorough physical examination, blood and urine cultures, serum cell counts and chemistry analysis, and a chest roentgenogram. Additional evaluation should be guided by the results. If an HIV-infected patient does not have a readily identifiable source or does not respond to treatment, a specialist with experience in managing HIV-related illnesses should be consulted. All HIV-infected patients with respiratory symptoms should be placed in isolation until pulmonary infection with *Mycobacterium tuberculosis* is excluded by three negative acid-fast smear results. A high clinical suspicion for tuberculosis should be maintained even with normal chest roentgenograms or changes not typical for tuberculosis [244]. The incidence of tuberculosis is high in HIV-infected persons and transmission from patients with undiagnosed disease to both other patients and health care providers has been well documented [245, 246].

The complicated nature of HIV infection makes a team approach essential for caring for these patients. The rehabilitation specialist will frequently require the assistance of an infectious disease specialist, neurologist, oncologist, psychiatrist, social worker, or dietitian [247]. Consultation with an infectious disease specialist may be especially prudent with the ever increasing use of antiretroviral medications, all of which can produce severe adverse effects.

Drug Fever

The incidence of drug fever is not known but appears to be common in the chronically disabled. Often these patients are receiving multiple medications including anticonvulsants and repeated courses of antibiotics. One study reported that drugs were responsible for fever in approximately 4% of febrile spinal cord–injured patients studied [28]. Although often difficult to distinguish from other possible sources of fever, prompt recognition of drug fever is essential to avoid extensive and costly diagnostic evaluations, needless courses of antibiotics, and prolonged hospitalizations. Drug-induced fever is diagnosed when no other source is present and the fever resolves within 72 hours of stopping the suspected medication [248]. Resolution may be delayed in patients with delayed drug clearance such as from renal or hepatic insufficiency. Drug fever is most often an immunologically mediated hypersensitivity reaction with antigen-antibody complexes and complement stimulating the release of endogenous pyrogens from granulocytes. Drug fever, however, may be idiosyncratic (often due to a genetic defect), pharmacologic (due to endotoxin release from killed cells or bacteria), administration related, or due to altered thermoregulation [249, 250].

Although antimicrobial agents are the most common cause of drug fever, almost any medication can induce fever. Frequently implicated medications include beta-lactam antibiotics and phenytoin. Other drugs such as other anticonvulsants, antineoplastic agents, antihypertensive agents, barbiturates, antiarrhythmic agents, and diuretics have all been noted to cause fever [14]. Medications unlikely to induce fever include corticosteroids, antacids, insulin, digoxin, and diphenhydramine [251]. One review found that the mean time from initiation of the offending drug and onset of fever was 21 days, although the median of 8 days was considerably shorter. This lag time varied considerably from one medication to another [14].

It may be difficult to distinguish drug-induced fever from other possible causes such as infections based on the clinical findings and fever pattern. In one series of 148 cases of drug fever, temperatures ranged from low-grade to over 105°F. Rigors were common and often led to extensive evaluations and empiric antibiotic therapy. Patients, however, generally did not appear toxic. Hypotension as well as relative bradycardia—i.e., a pulse that does not increase by 10 beats per minute for every degree (C) of elevation—were uncommon. Approximately 20% of patients had headaches, myalgias, rash, or eosinophilia. The white blood cell count was often normal and may be a clue to the diagnosis of drug fever [14].

If drug fever is likely, the suspect medication should be stopped immediately. All drugs that are not critical to the management of the patient should also be discontinued because these other medications may sustain the fever by unknown means. Once the fever has resolved, medications can be restarted in a stepwise manner. Corticosteroids are not required unless there is a severe rash, hepatic involvement, or vasculitis. In the rare case that a medication cannot be discontinued due to a life-threatening condition, such as infection with a multidrug resistant organism, treatment with antipyretics, antihistamines and corticosteroids may allow continuation of therapy. In these rare instances, however, an expert in allergy or immunology should be consulted.

Central Fever

Central fever describes fever secondary to disease of the thermoregulatory center of the hypothalamus. Usually lesions in or near the hypothalamus produce hypothermia rather than hyperthermia although persistently or intermittently elevated body temperatures may be seen [16, 252]. Tumors, hemorrhages, degenerative diseases, vascular abnormalities, metabolic disorders, and infectious processes can all affect this area and cause central fever.

Disease of the central nervous system is more likely to cause hyperthermia in children than in adults. Seizure disorders, degenerative brain diseases, chronic heavy metal intoxication, and central nervous system tumors including leukemia have all been associated with fever [253–255].

Unexplained fever in quadriplegic persons has been attributed to an inability to regulate body temperature in response to heating or cooling [256–258]. Although this phenomenon may cause self-limited febrile episodes, a study of spinal cord–injured patients with fever found that fewer than 3% had no etiology identified after careful evaluation. Infections were the most likely source of fever noted [28]. Autonomic hyperreflexia, which can cause flushing and sweating, is common in patients with spinal cord injury above the sixth thoracic vertebra although fever is rare unless an underlying infection is present [259]. In a prospective study of adults with cerebrovascular accidents, approximately 20% developed fever but most had an identifiable pulmonary source, usually a chemical pneumonitis or an infectious pneumonia [260].

In conclusion, central fever is rare in adults. If suspected, the diagnosis is supported by the presence of poikilothermia and endocrine abnormalities including diabetes insipidus. Fever in patients with cerebrovascular accidents or quadriplegia is most often due to an infection. Central fever is a diagnosis of exclusion.

References

1. DeVivo MJ, Black KJ, Stover SL. Causes of death during the first 12 years after spinal cord injury. Arch Phys Med Rehabil 1993;74:248.
2. Whiteneck GG, Charlifue SW, Frankel HL, et al. Mortality, morbidity, and psychosocial outcomes of persons spinal cord injured more than 20 years ago. Paraplegia 1992;30:617.
3. Smith MA, Duke WM. Infections in an acute rehabilitative and chronic population at a large skilled nursing facility. J Am Geriatr Soc 1994;42:45.

4. Cohen ML. Epidemiology of drug resistance: Implications for a post-antimicrobial era. Science 1992;257:1050.

5. Bloom BR, Murray CJL. Tuberculosis: Commentary on a reemergent killer. Science 1992;257:1055.

6. Neu HC. The crisis in antibiotic resistance. Science 1992;257:1064.

7. Maki DG. Control of colonization and transmission of pathogenic bacteria in the hospital. Ann Intern Med 1978;89:777.

8. Broome CV. Preventing the spread of vancomycin resistance—A report from the hospital infection control practices advisory committee prepared by the subcommittee on prevention and control of antimicrobial-resistant microorganisms in hospital: Comment period and public meeting. Federal Register 1994;59:25758.

9. Wenzel RP (ed). Prevention and Control of Nosocomial Infections (2nd ed). Baltimore: Williams & Wilkins, 1993.

10. McGowan JE. Antimicrobial resistance in hospital organisms and its relation to antimicrobial use. Rev Infect Dis 1983;5:1033.

11. Sanders CC. Chromosomal cephalosporinases responsible for multiple resistance to newer beta-lactam antibiotics. Annu Rev Microbiol 1987;41:573.

12. Joshi N, Milfred D. The use and misuse of new antibiotics. Arch Intern Med 1995;155:569.

13. Ditunno JF, Formal CS. Chronic spinal cord injury. N Engl J Med 1994;330:550.

14. Mackowiak PA, LeMaistre CF. Drug fever: A critical appraisal of conventional concepts. Ann Intern Med 1987;106:728.

15. Weingarden SI, Weingarden DS, Belen MD. Fever and thromboembolic disease in acute spinal cord injury. Paraplegia 1988;26:35.

16. Wolff SM, Fauci AS, Dale DC. Unusual etiologies of fever and their evaluation. Ann Rev Med 1975;26:277.

17. Fried TR, Gillick MR, Lipsitz LA. Whether to transfer? Factors associated with hospitalization and outcome of elderly long-term care patients with pneumonia. J Gen Intern Med 1995;10:246.

18. Pizzo PA. Management of fever in patients with cancer and treatment-induced neutropenia. N Engl J Med 1993;328:1323.

19. Hughes WT, Armstrong D, Bodey GP, et al. Guidelines for the use of antimicrobial agents in neutropenic patients with unexplained fever. J Infect Dis 1990;161:381.

20. Bedell SE, Bush BT. Erythrocyte sedimentation rate. Am J Med 1985;78:1001.

21. Chandrasekar PH, Brown WJ. Clinical issues of blood cultures. Arch Intern Med 1994;154:841.

22. Aronson MD, Bor DH. Blood cultures. Ann Intern Med 1987;106:246.

23. Mermel LA, Maki DG. Detection of bacteremia in adults: Consequences of culturing an inadequate volume of blood. Ann Intern Med 1993;119:270.

24. Leisure MK, Moore DM, Schwartzman JD. Changing the needle when inoculating blood cultures: A no-benefit and high-risk procedure. JAMA 1990;264:2111.

25. Arbo MDJ, Snydman DR. Influence of blood culture results on antibiotic choice in the treatment of bacteremia. Arch Intern Med 1994;154:2641.

26. Gross PA, Barrett TL, Dellinger EP. Quality standard for the treatment of bacteremia. Clin Infect Dis 1994;18:428.

27. Moellering RC. Principles of anti-infective therapy. In GL Mandell, JE Bennett, R Dolin (eds), Principles and Practice of Infectious Diseases (4th ed). New York: Churchill Livingstone, 1995;199.

28. Sugarman B, Brown D, Musher D. Fever and infection in spinal cord injury patients. JAMA 1982;248:66.

29. Hale RW, Hooton TM, Culver DH, et al. Nosocomial infections in U.S. hospitals, 1975–1976: Estimated frequency by selected characteristics of patients. Am J Med 1981;70:947.

30. Garibaldi RA, Brodine S, Matsumiya S. Infections among patients in nursing homes. Policies, prevalence and problems. N Engl J Med 1981;305:731.

31. Lapides J, Diokno AC, Silber SJ, et al. Clean, intermittent self-catheterization in the treatment of urinary tract disease. J Urol 1972;107:458.

32. King RB, Carlson CE, Mervine J, et al. Clean and sterile intermittent catheterization methods in hospitalized patients with spinal cord injury. Arch Phys Med Rehabil 1992;73:798.

33. Dionka AC. Clean intermittent catheterization in UTI management. Infect Urol 1988;1:3, 13.

34. McGuire EJ, Savastano JA. Long-term follow-up of spinal cord injury patients managed by intermittent catheterization. J Urol 1983;129:775.

35. Dionka AC, Sonda LP, Hollander JB, et al. Fate of patients started on clean intermittent self-catheterization therapy 10 years ago. J Urol 1983;129:1120.

36. Sotolongo JR, Koleilat N. Significance of asymptomatic bacteriuria in spinal cord injury patients on condom catheter. J Urol 1990;143:979.

37. Warren JW. Catheter-associated urinary tract infections. Infect Dis Clin North Am 1987;1:823.

38. Stover SL, Lloyd LK, Waites KB, et al. Neurogenic urinary tract infection. Neurol Clin 1991;9:741.

39. Kaye D. Antibacterial activity of human urine. J Clin Invest 1968;47:2374.

40. Wu YC. Total bladder care for the spinal cord injured patient. Ann Acad Med 1983;12:387.

41. Helmholz HF. Determination of the bacterial content of the urethra: A new method with results of a study of 82 men. J Urol 1950;64:158.

42. Kass EH, Schneiderman LJ. Entry of bacteria into the urinary tracts of patients with inlying catheters. N Engl J Med 1957;256:556.

43. Kunin CM, McCormack RC. Prevention of catheter-induced urinary-tract infections by sterile closed drainage. N Engl J Med 1966;274:1155.

44. Nickel JC, Gristina P, Costerton JW. Electron microscopic study of an infected Foley catheter. Can J Surg 1985;28:50.

45. Stark RP, Maki DG. Bacteriuria in the catheterized patient. What quantitative level of bacteriuria is relevant? N Engl J Med 1984;311:560.

46. Iwahi T, Abe Y, Nakao M, et al. Role of type 1 fimbriae in the pathogenesis of ascending urinary tract infection induced by *Escherichia coli* in mice. Infect Immunol 1983;39:1307.

47. Ladd TI, Schmiel D, Nickel JC, et al. The use of a radiorespirometric assay for testing the antibiotic sensitivity of catheter-associated bacteria. J Urol 1987;138:1451.

48. Cox AJ, Hukins DWL, Sutton TM. Infection of catheterised patients: Bacterial colonisation of encrusted Foley catheters shown by scanning electron microscopy. Urol Res 1989;17:349.

49. Garibaldi RA, Burke JP, Britt MR, et al. Meatal colonization and catheter-associated bacteriuria. N Engl J Med 1980;303:316.

50. Sanderson PJ, Rawal P. Contamination of the environment of spinal cord injured patients by organisms causing urinary tract infection. J Hosp Infect 1987;10:173.

51. Ehrenkranz NJ, Alfonso BC. Failure of bland soap handwash to prevent hand transfer of patient bacteria to urethral catheters. Infect Control Hosp Epidemiol 1991;12:654.

52. Warren JW, Muncie HL, Berquist EJ, et al. Sequelae and management of urinary tract infection in the patient requiring chronic catheterization. J Urol 1981;125:1.

53. Hamory BH, Wenzel RP. Hospital-associated candiduria: Predisposing factors and review of the literature. J Urol 1978;120:444.

54. Stamey TA, Govan DE, Palmer JM. The localization and treatment of urinary tract infections: The role of bactericidal urine levels as opposed to serum levels. Medicine 1965;44:1.

55. Sobel JD, Kaye D. Urinary tract infections. In GL Mandell, JE Bennett, R Dolin (eds), Principles and Practice of Infectious Diseases (4th ed). New York: Churchill Livingstone, 1995;662.

56. Stamm WE, Counts GW, Running KR, et al. Diagnosis of coliform infection in acutely dysuric women. N Engl J Med 1983;307:463.

57. Consensus Statement from the National Institute on Disability and Rehabilitation Research. The prevention and management of urinary tract infections among people with spinal cord injuries. J Am Paraplegia Soc 1992;15:194.

58. Ouslander JG, Greengold BA, Silverblatt FJ. An accurate method to obtain urine for culture in men with external catheters. Arch Intern Med 1987;147:286.

59. Ouslander JG, Schapira M, Schnelle JF. Urine specimen collection from incontinent female nursing home residents. J Am Geriatr Soc 1995;43:279.

60. Kunin CM. Diagnostic methods. In CM Kunin (ed), Detection, Prevention and Management of Urinary Tract Infections. Philadelphia: Lea & Febiger, 1987;195.

61. Stamm WE. Measurement of pyuria and its relation to bacteriuria. Am J Med 1983;75:53.

62. Hooton TM, O'Shaughnessy EJ, Clowers D, et al. Localization of urinary tract infection in patients with spinal cord injury. J Infect Dis 1984;150:85.

63. Gribble MJ, Puterman ML, McCallum NM. Pyuria: Its relationship to bacteriuria in spinal cord injured patients on intermittent catheterization. Arch Phys Med Rehabil 1989;70:376.

64. Maynard FM, Diokno AC. Urinary infection and complications during clean intermittent catheterization following spinal cord injury. J Urol 1984;132:943.

65. Mohler JL, Cowen DL, Flanigan RC. Suppression and treatment of urinary tract infection in patients with an intermittently catheterized neurogenic bladder. J Urol 1987;138:336.

66. Nicolle LE, Bjornson J, Harding GKM, et al. Bacteriuria in elderly institutionalized men. N Engl J Med 1983;309:1409.

67. Abrutyn E, Mossey J, Berlin JA, et al. Does asymptomatic bacteriuria predict mortality and does antimicrobial treatment reduce mortality in elderly ambulatory women? Ann Intern Med 1994;120:827.

68. Nicolle LE, Hayhew WJ, Bryan L. Prospective randomized comparison of therapy and no therapy for asymptomatic bacteriuria in institutionalized elderly women. Am J Med 1987;83:27.

69. Gribble MJ, Puterman ML. Prophylaxis of urinary tract infection in persons with recent spinal cord injury: A prospective, randomized, double-blind, placebo-controlled study of trimethoprim-sulfamethoxazole. Am J Med 1993;95:141.

70. Saxon A, Beall GN, Rohr AS, et al. Immediate hypersensitivity reactions to beta-lactam antibiotics. Ann Intern Med 1987;107:204.

71. Turck M, Ronald AR, Petersdorf RG. Relapse and reinfection in chronic bacteriuria. II. The correlation between site of infection and pattern of recurrence in chronic bacteriuria. N Engl J Med 1968;278:422.

72. Moellering RC. The enterococcus: A classic example of the impact of antimicrobial resistance on therapeutic options. J Antimicrob Chemother 1991;28:1.

73. Bennett WM, Aronoff GR, Golper TA, et al. Drug Prescribing in Renal Failure (2nd ed). Philadelphia: American College of Physicians, 1991.

74. Cockcroft DW, Gault MH. Prediction of creatinine clearance from serum creatinine. Nephron 1976;16:31.

75. Schmitt J, Midha M, McKenzie N. Medical complications of spinal cord disease. Neurol Clin 1991;9:779.

76. Sanford JP. The enigma of candiduria: Evolution of bladder irrigation with amphotericin B for management. From anecdote to dogma and a lesson from Machiavelli. Clin Infect Dis 1993;16:145.

77. Johnson JR. Should all catheterized patients with candiduria be treated? Clin Infect Dis 1993;17:814.

78. DeWire DM, Owens RS, Anderson GA, et al. A comparison of the urological complications associated with long-term management of quadriplegics with and without chronic indwelling urinary catheters. J Urol 1992;147:1069.

79. Schiotz HA, Malme PA, Tanbo TG. Urinary tract infections and asymptomatic bacteriuria after vaginal plastic surgery. A comparison of suprapubic and transurethral catheters. Acta Obstet Gynecol Scand 1989;68:453.

80. Hammarsten J, Lindqvist K. Suprapubic catheter following transurethral resection of the prostate: A way to decrease the number of urethral strictures and improve the outcome of operations. J Urol 1992;147:648.

81. Schmidt JD, Hawtrey CE, Flocks RH, et al. Complications, results, and problems of ileal conduit diversions. J Urol 1973;109:210.

82. Wong ES. Guideline for prevention of catheter-associated urinary tract infections. Am J Infect Control 1983;11:28.

83. Gillespie W, Jones J, Teasdale C, et al. Does the addition of disinfectant to urine drainage bags prevent infection in catheterized patients? Lancet 1983;1:1037.

84. Thompson RL, Haley CE, Searcy MA, et al. Catheter-associated bacteriuria: Failure to reduce attack rates using periodic installations of a disinfectant into urinary drainage systems. JAMA 1984;251:747.

85. Donowitz GR, Mandell GL. Acute pneumonia. In GL Mandell, JE Bennett, R Dolin (eds), Principles and Practice of Infectious Diseases (4th ed). New York: Churchill Livingstone, 1995;619.

86. Gross PA, Neu HC, Aswapokee P, et al. Deaths from nosocomial infections: Experience in a university hospital and a community hospital. Am J Med 1980;68:219.

87. Huxley EJ, Viroslav J, Gray WR, et al. Pharyngeal aspiration in normal adults and patients with depressed consciousness. Am J Med 1978;64:564.

88. Finegold SM. Aspiration pneumonia. Rev Infect Dis 1991;13(S9):S737.

89. Miller FR, Eliachar I. Managing the aspirating patient. Am J Otolaryngol 1994;15:1.

90. Bartlett JG, Gorbach SL. The triple threat of aspiration pneumonia. Chest 1975;68:560.

91. Zavala DC, Rhodes ML. Foreign body removal: A new role for the fiberoptic bronchoscope. Ann Otol Rhinol Laryngol 1975;84:650.

92. Wolfe JE, Bone RC, Ruth WE. Effects of corticosteroids in the treatment of patients with gastric aspiration. Am J Med 1977;63:719.

93. Arms RA, Dines DE, Tinstman TC. Aspiration pneumonia. Chest 1974;65:136.

94. Petersdorf RG, Curtin JA, Hoeprich PD, et al. A study of antibiotic prophylaxis in unconscious patients. N Engl J Med 1957;257:1001.

95. Bartlett JG. Anaerobic bacterial infections of the lung. Chest 1987;6:901.

96. Lode H. Initial therapy in pneumonia. Am J Med 1986;80(S5c):70.

97. Bartlett JG, Finegold SM. Anaerobic pleuropulmonary infections. Medicine 1972;51:413.

98. Kline BS, Berger SS. Pulmonary abscess and pulmonary gangrene. Arch Intern Med 1935;56:753.

99. Murray PR, Washington JA. III. Microscopic and bacteriologic analysis of expectorated sputum. Mayo Clin Proc 1975;50:339.

100. Scheld WM, Mandell GL. Nosocomial pneumonia: Pathogenesis and recent advances in diagnosis and therapy. Rev Infect Dis 1991;13(S9):S743.

101. Chastre J, Fagon JY, Soler P, et al. Diagnosis of nosocomial bacterial pneumonia in intubated patients undergoing ventilation: Comparison of the usefulness of bronchoalveolar lavage and the protected specimen brush. Am J Med 1988;85:499.

102. Faling LJ. New advances in diagnosing nosocomial pneumonia in intubated patients: Part I. Am Rev Respir Dis 1988;137:253.

103. Chastre J, Fagon J-Y, Bornet-Lesco M, et al. Evaluation of bronchoscopic techniques for the diagnosis of nosocomial pneumonia. Am J Respir Crit Care Med 1995;152:231.

104. Kollef MH, Bock KR, Richards RD, et al. The safety and diagnostic accuracy of minibronchoalveolar lavage in patients with suspected ventilator-associated pneumonia. Ann Intern Med 1995;122:743.

105. Bartlett JG, Finegold SM. Anaerobic infections of the lung and pleural space. Am Rev Respir Dis 1974;110:56.

106. Johanson WG, Pierce AK, Sanford JP. Changing pharyngeal bacterial flora of hospitalized patients: Emergence of gram-negative bacilli. N Engl J Med 1969;281:1137.

107. duMoulin GC, Hedley-Whyte J, Paterson DG, et al. Aspiration of gastric bacteria in antacid-treated patients: A frequent cause of postoperative colonisation of the airway. Lancet 1982;1:242.

108. Daschner F, Kappstein I, Engels I, et al. Stress ulcer prophylaxis and ventilation pneumonia: Prevention by antimicrobial cytoprotective agents? Infect Control Hosp Epidemiol 1988;9:59.

109. Tryba M. Risk of acute stress bleeding and nosocomial pneumonia in ventilated intensive care unit patients: Sucralfate vs. antacids. Am J Med 1987;83(S3B):117.

110. Levison ME, Mangura CT, Lorbes B, et al. Clindamycin compared with penicillin for the treatment of anaerobic lung abscess. Ann Intern Med 1983;98:466.

111. Gudiol F, Manresa F, Palleras R, et al. Clindamycin vs. penicillin for anaerobic infections: High rate of penicillin failures associated with penicillin-resistant *Bacteroides melaninogenicus*. Arch Intern Med 1990;150:2525.

112. Piperacillin/tazobactam. Med Lett Drugs Ther 1994;36:7.

113. Bartlett JG. Treatment of anaerobic pleuropulmonary infections. Ann Intern Med 1975;83:376.

114. Darouiche RO, Groover J, Rowland J, et al. Pneumococcal vaccination for patients with spinal cord injury. Arch Phys Med Rehabil 1993;74:1354.

115. Sugarman B. Osteomyelitis in spinal cord injury. Arch Phys Med Rehabil 1984;65:132.

116. Brennan PJ, DeGirolamo MP. Musculoskeletal infections in immunocompromised hosts. Orthop Clin North Am 1991;22:389.

117. Waldvogel FA, Medoff G, Swartz MN. Osteomyelitis: A review of clinical features, therapeutic considerations, and unusual aspect. N Engl J Med 1970;282:198, 260, 316.

118. Cierny G, Mader JT, Pennick H. A clinical staging system of adult osteomyelitis. Contemp Orthop 1985;10:17.

119. Waldvogel FA, Vasey H. Osteomyelitis: The past decade. N Engl J Med 1980;303:360.

120. Sexton DJ, McDonald M. Osteomyelitis: Approaching the 1990s. Med J Aust 1990;153:91.

121. Wisneski RJ. Infectious disease of the spine. Diagnostic and treatment consideration. Orthop Clin North Am 1991;22:491.

122. McHenry MC, Alfidi RJ, Wilde AH, et al. Hematogenous osteomyelitis: A changing disease. Cleve Clin Q 1975;42:125.

123. Sapico FL, Montgomerie JZ. Vertebral osteomyelitis in intravenous drug abusers: Report of three cases and review of the literature. Rev Infect Dis 1980;2:196.

124. Holzman RS, Bishko F. Osteomyelitis in heroin addicts. Ann Intern Med 1971;75:693.

125. Levine DP, Sobel JD. Infections in intravenous drug abusers. In GL Mandell, JE Bennett, R Dolin (eds), Principles and Practice of Infectious Diseases (4th ed). New York: Churchill Livingstone, 1995;2696.

126. Dich VQ, Nelson JD, Haltalin KC. Osteomyelitis in infants and children: A review of 163 cases. Am J Dis Child 1975;129:1273.

127. Musher DM, Thorsteinsson SB, Minuth JN, et al. Vertebral osteomyelitis: Still a diagnostic pitfall. Arch Intern Med 1976;136:105.

128. Sapico FL, Montgomerie JZ. Vertebral osteomyelitis. Infect Dis Clin North Am 1990;4:539.

129. Hitchon PW, Osenbach RK, Yuh WTC, et al. Spinal infections. Clin Neurosurg 1992;38:373.

130. Heary RF, Hunt CD, Wolansky LJ. Rapid bony destruction with pyogenic vertebral osteomyelitis. Surg Neurol 1994;41:34.

131. Tehranzadeh J, Wang F, Mesgarzadeh M. Magnetic resonance imaging of osteomyelitis. Crit Rev Diag Imag 1992;33:495.

132. Darouiche RO, Landon GC, Kilma M, et al. Osteomyelitis associated with pressure sores. Arch Intern Med 1994;154:753.

133. Topazian RG. Osteomyelitis of the jaws. In RG Topazian, MH Goldberg (eds), Oral and Maxillofacial Infections (3rd ed). Philadelphia: Saunders, 1994;251.

134. Perry CR, Pearson RL, Miller GA. Accuracy of cultures of material from swabbing of the superficial aspect of the wound and needle biopsy in the preoperative assessment of osteomyelitis. J Bone Joint Surg 1991;73A:745.

135. Sugarman B, Hawes S, Musher DM, et al. Osteomyelitis beneath pressure sores. Arch Intern Med 1983;143:683.

136. Rudensky B, Lipschits M, Isaacsohn M, et al. Infected pressure sores: Comparison of models for bacterial identification. South Med J 1992;85:901.

137. Mackowiak PA, Jones SR, Smith JW. Diagnostic value of sinus-tract cultures in chronic osteomyelitis. JAMA 1978;239:2772.

138. Gruber HE. Bone and the immune system. Proc Soc Exp Biol Med 1991;197:219.

139. Hamblen DL. Diagnosis of infection and the role of permanent excision arthroplasty. Orthop Clin North Am 1993;24:743.

140. Maderazo EG, Judson S, Pasternak H. Late infections of total joint prostheses. A review and recommendations for prevention. Clin Orthop 1988;229:132.

141. Gibbons GW, Eliopoulos GM. Infection of the diabetic foot. In GP Kozak, CS Hoar, JL Rowbotham, et al (eds), Management of Diabetic Foot Problems. Philadelphia: Saunders, 1984;97.

142. Lipsky BA, Pecoraro RE, Wheat LJ. The diabetic foot: Soft-tissue and bone infection. Infect Dis North Am 1990;4:409.

143. Kozak GP, Rowbotham JL. Diabetic foot disease: A major problem. In GP Kozak, CS Hoar, JL Rowbotham, et al (eds), Management of Diabetic Foot Problems. Philadelphia: Saunders, 1984;1.

144. Bamberger DM, Daus GP, Gerding DN. Osteomyelitis in the feet of diabetic patients. Long-term results, prognostic factors, and the role of antimicrobial and surgical therapy. Am J Med 1987;83:653.

145. Fierer J, Daniel D, Davis C. The fetid foot: Lower-extremity infections in patients with diabetes mellitus. Rev Infect Dis 1979;1:210.

146. Brodsky JW, Schneidler C. Diabetic foot infections. Orthop Clin North Am 1991;22:473.

147. Sapico FL, Witte JL, Canawati HN, et al. The infected foot of the diabetic patient: Quantitative microbiology and analysis of clinical features. Rev Infect Dis 1984;6(S1):S171.

148. White LM, Schweitzer ME, Deely DM, et al. Study of osteomyelitis: Utility of combined histologic and microbiologic evaluation of percutaneous biopsy samples. Radiology 1995;197:840.

149. Benton GS, Kerstein MD. Cost effectiveness of early digit amputation in the patient with diabetes. Surg Gynecol Obstet 1985;161:523.

150. Eckman MH, Greenfield S, Mackey WC. Foot infections in diabetic patients. Decision and cost-effectiveness analyses. JAMA 1995;273:712.

151. Wegener WA, Alavi A. Diagnostic imaging of musculoskeletal infection. Roentgenography; gallium, indium-labeled white blood cell, gammaglobulin, bone

scintigraphy; and MRI. Orthop Clin North Am 1991;22:401.

152. Morrison WB, Schweitzer ME, Bock GW, et al. Diagnosis of osteomyelitis: Utility of fat-suppressed contrast-enhanced MR imaging. Radiology 1993;189:251.

153. Rosenthall L. Radionuclide investigation of osteomyelitis. Curr Opin Radiol 1992;4:62.

154. Brown ML, Collier D, Fogelman I. Bone scintigraphy: Part 1. Oncology and infection. J Nucl Med 1993;34:2236.

155. Littenberg B, Mushlin AI, and the Diagnostic Technology Assessment Consortium. Technetium bone scanning in the diagnosis of osteomyelitis: A meta-analysis of test performance. J Gen Intern Med 1992;7:158.

156. Al-Sheikh W, Sfakianakis GN, Mnaymneh W, et al. Subacute and chronic bone infections: Diagnosis using In-111, Ga-67 and Tc-99m MDP bone scintigraphy, and radiography. Radiology 1985;155:501.

157. Reller LB, Stratton CW. Serum dilution test for bactericidal activity. II. Standardization and correlation with antimicrobial assays. J Infect Dis 1977;136:196.

158. Weinstein MP, Stratton CW, Hawley HB, et al. Multicenter collaborative evaluation of a standardized serum bactericidal test as a predictor of therapeutic efficacy in acute and chronic osteomyelitis. Am J Med 1987;83:218.

159. Sapico FL, Montgomerie JZ. Pyogenic vertebral osteomyelitis: Report of nine cases and review of the literature. Rev Infect Dis 1979;1:754.

160. Perez-Stable EJ, Hopewell PC. Current tuberculosis treatment regimens: Choosing the right one for your patient. Clin Chest Med 1989;10:323.

161. Ingram C, Eron LJ, Goldenberg RI, Morrison AJ, et al. Antibiotic therapy of osteomyelitis in outpatients. Med Clin North Am 1988;72:723.

162. Bell SM. Further observations on the value of oral penicillins in chronic staphylcoccal osteomyelitis. Med J Aust 1976;2:591.

163. Peterson LR, Lissack LM, Canter K, et al. Therapy of lower extremity infections with ciprofloxacin in patients with diabetes mellitus, peripheral vascular disease, or both. Am J Med 1989;86:801.

164. Gentry LO, Rodriguez GG. Oral ciprofloxacin compared with parenteral antibiotics in the treatment of osteomyelitis. Antimicrob Agents Chemother 1990;34:40.

165. Gentry LO. Oral antimicrobial therapy for osteomyelitis. Ann Intern Med 1991;114:986.

166. Callaghan JJ, Salvati EA, Brause DM, et al. Reimplantation for salvage of the infected hip. In The Hip: Proceedings of the 14th Open Scientific Meeting of the Hip Society. St. Louis: Mosby, 1986;65.

167. Windsor RE, Insall JN, Urs WK, et al. Two-stage reimplantation for the salvage of total knee arthroplasty complicated by infection. J Bone Joint Surg 1990;72A:272.

168. Salvati EA, Chekofsky KM, Brause BD, et al. Reimplantation in infection. Clin Orthop 1982;170:62.

169. Buchholz HW, Elson R, Engelbrecht E. Management of deep infection of total hip replacement. J Bone Joint Surg 1981;63B:342.

170. Carlsson AS, Josefsson G, Lindberg L. Revision with gentamicin-impregnated cement for deep infection in total hip arthroplasties. J Bone Joint Surg 1978;60A:1059.

171. Buchholz HW, Elson R, Lodenkamper H. The infected joint implant. In B McKibbin (ed), Recent Advances in Orthopedics. Edinburgh: Churchill Livingstone, 1979;139.

172. Stiefeld SM, Graziani AL, MacGregor RR, et al. Toxicities of antimicrobial agents used to treat osteomyelitis. Orthop Clin North Am 1991;22:439.

173. Cierny G, Mader JT. Adult chronic osteomyelitis. Orthopedics 1984;7:1557.

174. Henry SL, Seligson D, Mangino P, et al. Antibiotic-impregnated beads. Part I: Bead implantation versus systemic therapy. Orthop Rev 1991;20:242.

175. Popham GJ, Mangino P, Seligson D, et al. Antibiotic-impregnated beads. Part II: Factors in antibiotic selection. Orthop Rev 1991;20:331.

176. May JW, Jupiter JB, Gallico GG, et al. Treatment of chronic osteomyelitis bone wounds. Microvascular free tissue transfer: A 13-year experience in 96 patients. Ann Surg 1991;214:241.

177. Green SA. Osteomyelitis. The Ilizarov perspective. Orthop Clin North Am 1991;22:515.

178. Croll TP, Greiner DG, Schut L. Antibiotic prophylaxis for the hydrocephalic dental patient with a shunt. Pediatr Dent 1979;1:81.

179. Walters BC. Cerebrospinal fluid shunt infection. Neurosurg Clin North Am 1992;3:387.

180. Schoenbaum SC, Gardner P, Shillito J. Infections of cerebrospinal fluid shunts: Epidemiology, clinical manifestations, and therapy. J Infect Dis 1975;131:543.

181. Walters BC, Hoffman HJ, Hendrick EB, et al. Cerebrospinal fluid shunt infections: Influences on initial management and subsequent outcome. J Neurosurg 1984;60:1014.

182. George R, Leibrock L, Epstein M. Long-term analysis of cerebrospinal fluid shunt infections: A 25-year experience. J Neurosurg 1979;51:804.

183. Gardner P, Leipzig T, Phillips P. Infections of central nervous system shunts. Med Clin North Am 1985;69:297.

184. Johnson GM, Lee DA, Regelman WE, et al. Interference with granulocyte function by *Staphylococcus epidermidis* slime. Infect Immunol 1986;54:13.

185. Keucher TR, Mealey J. Long-term results after ventriculoatrial and ventriculoperitoneal shunting for infantile hydrocephalus. J Neurosurg 1979;50:179.

186. Raimondi AJ, Robinson JS, Kuwamura K. Complications of ventriculo-peritoneal shunting and a critical comparison of the three-piece and one-piece systems. Child Brain 1977;3:321.

187. Haines SJ, Taylor F. Prophylactic methicillin for shunt operations: Effect on incidence of shunt malfunction and infection. Child Brain 1982;9:10.

188. Brook I, Johnson N, Overturf GD, et al. Mixed bacterial meningitis: A complication of ventriculo- and lumboperitoneal shunts. J Neurosurg 1977;47:961.

189. Forward KC, Fewer MD, Stiver HG. Cerebrospinal fluid shunt infections: A review of 35 infections in 32 patients. J Neurosurg 1983;59:725.

190. Wald SL, McLaurin RL. Shunt-associated glomerulonephritis. Neurosurgery 1978;3:146.

191. Bayston R, Spitz L. Infective and cystic causes of malfunction of ventriculoperitoneal shunts for hydrocephalus. Z Kinderchir 1977;22:419.

192. Mates S, Glazer J, Shapiro K. Treatment of cerebrospinal fluid shunt infections with medical therapy alone. Neurosurgery 1982;11:781.

193. Wen DY, Bottini AG, Hall WA, et al. The intraventricular use of antibiotics. Neurosurg Clin North Am 1992;3:343.

194. Rennels MB, Wald ER. Treatment of *Hemophilus influenzae* type B meningitis in children with cerebrospinal fluid shunts. J Pediatr 1980;97:424.

195. James HE, Walsh JW, Wilson HD, et al. The management of cerebrospinal fluid shunt infections: A clinical experience. Acta Neurochir 1981;59:157.

196. Mori K, Raimondi AJ. An analysis of external ventricular drainage as a treatment for infected shunts. Child Brain 1975;1:243.

197. Scarff TB, Nelson PB, Reigel DH. External drainage for ventricular infection following cerebrospinal fluid shunts. Child Brain 1978;4:129.

198. Centers for Disease Control and Prevention. Update: Mortality attributable to HIV infection among persons age 25-44 years—United States, 1991 and 1992. MMWR 1993;42:869.

199. Centers for Disease Control and Prevention. Healthcare workers with documented and possible occupationally acquired AIDS/HIV infection, by occupation, reported through March 1993, United States. HIV/AIDS Surveillance Report 1993; May:13.

200. Tokars JI, Marcus R, Culver DH, et al. Surveillance of HIV infection and zidovudine use among health care workers after occupational exposure to HIV-infected blood. The CDC Cooperative Needlestick Surveillance Group. Ann Intern Med 1993;118:913.

201. Wong ES, Stotka JL, Chinchilli VM, et al. Are universal precautions effective in reducing the number of occupational exposures among health care workers? A prospective study of physicians on a medical service. JAMA 1991;265:1123.

202. Fahey BJ, Koziol DE, Banks SM, et al. Frequency of nonparenteral occupational exposures to blood and body fluids before and after universal precautions training. Am J Med 1991;90:145.

203. Centers for Disease Control and Prevention. Case-control study of HIV seroconversion in health-care workers after percutaneous exposure to HIV-infected blood—France, United Kingdom, and United States, January 1988–August 1994. MMWR 1995;44:929.

204. McDougal JS, Mawle A, Cort SP, et al. Cellular tropism of the human retrovirus HTLV-III/LAV. I. Role of T cell activation and expression of the T4 antigen. J Immunol 1985;135:3151.

205. Centers for Disease Control and Prevention. Update: Serologic testing for antibody to human immunodeficiency virus. MMWR 1988;36:833.

206. Daar ES, Moudgil T, Meyer RD, et al. Transient high levels of viremia in patients with primary human immunodeficiency virus type 1 infection. N Engl J Med 1991;324:961.

207. Pantaleo G, Graziosi C, Demarest JF, et al. HIV infection is active and progressive in lymphoid tissue during the clinically latent stage of disease. Nature 1993;362:355.

208. Fauci AS, Schnittman SM, Poli G, et al. NIH conference: Immunopathogenic mechanisms in human immunodeficiency virus (HIV) infection. Ann Intern Med 1991;114:678.

209. Wei X, Ghosh SK, Taylor ME, et al. Viral dynamics in human immunodeficiency virus type 1 infection. Nature 1995;373:117.

210. Ho DD, Neumann AU, Perelson AS, et al. Rapid turnover of plasma virions and CD4 lymphocytes in HIV-1 infection. Nature 1995;373:123.

211. Crowe SM, Carlin JB, Stewart KI, et al. Predictive value of CD4 lymphocyte numbers for the development of opportunistic infections and malignancies in HIV-infected persons. J Acquir Immune Defic Syndr 1991;4:770.

212. Nightingale SD, Byrd LT, Southern PM, et al. Incidence of *Mycobacterium avium-intracellulare* complex bacteremia in human immunodeficiency virus-positive patients. J Infect Dis 1992;165:1082.

213. Phair J, Munoz A, Detels R, et al. The risk of *Pneumocystis carinii* pneumonia among men infected with human immunodeficiency virus type 1. N Engl J Med 1990;322:161.

214. Pertel P, Hirschtick R, Phair J, et al. Risk of cytomegalovirus retinitis in persons infected with the human immunodeficiency virus. J Acquir Immune Defic Syndr 1992;5:1069.

215. Hirschtick RE, Glassroth J, Jordan MC, et al. Bacterial pneumonia in persons infected with the human immunodeficiency virus. N Engl J Med 1995;333:845.

216. Yarchoan R, Venzon DJ, Pluda JM, et al. CD4 count and the risk for death in patients infected with HIV receiving antiretroviral therapy. Ann Intern Med 1991;115:184.

217. Learmont J, Tindall B, Evans L, et al. Long-term symptomless HIV-1 infection in recipients of blood products from a single donor. Lancet 1992;340:863.

218. Cao Y, Qin L, Zhang L, et al. Virologic and immunologic characterization of long-term survivors of human immunodeficiency virus type 1 infection. N Engl J Med 1995;332:201.

219. Mellors JW, Kingsley LA, Rinaldo CR, et al. Quantitation of HIV-1 RNA in plasma predicts outcome after seroconversion. Ann Intern Med 1995;122:573.

220. Eron JJ, Benoit SL, Jemsek J, et al. Treatment with lamivudine, zidovudine, or both in HIV-positive patients with 200 to 500 CD4+ cells per cubic millimeter. N Engl J Med 1995;333:1662.

221. O'Brien WA, Hartigan PM, Martin D, et al. Changes in plasma HIV-1 RNA and CD4+ lymphocyte counts and the risk of progression to AIDS. N Engl J Med 1996;334:426.

222. Greene WC. The molecular biology of human immunodeficiency virus type 1 infection. N Engl J Med 1991;324:308.

223. Bartlett JG. Mini review: antiretroviral therapy in HIV-infected patients: update. Infect Dis Clin Pract 1994;3:340.

224. Collier AC, Coombs RW, Schoenfeld DA, et al. Treatment of human immunodeficiency virus infection with saquinavir, zidovudine, and zalcitabine. N Engl J Med 1996;334:1011.

225. Gulick R, Mellors J, Havlir D, et al. Potent and sustained antiretroviral activity of indinavir (IDV) in combination with zidovudine (ZDV) and lamivudine (3TC). Presented at the Third National Conference on Human Retroviruses and Opportunistic Infections, Washington, DC, 1996. Abstract LB7.

226. Markowitz M, Saag M, Powderly WG, et al. A preliminary study of ritonavir, an inhibitor of HIV-1 protease, to treat HIV-1 infection. N Engl J Med 1995;333:1534.

227. Fischl MA, Richman DD, Grieco MH, et al. The efficacy of azidothymidine (AZT) in the treatment of patients with AIDS and AIDS-related complex: A double-blind, placebo-controlled trial. N Engl J Med 1987;317:185.

228. Richman DD, Fischl MA, Grieco MH, et al. The toxicity of azidothymidine (AZT) in the treatment of patients with AIDS and AIDS-related complex: A double-blind, placebo-controlled trial. N Engl J Med 1987;317:192.

229. Sande MA, Carpenter CC, Cobbs CG, et al. Antiretroviral therapy for adults HIV-infected patients. Recommendations from a state-of-the-art conference. National Institute of Allergy and Infectious Diseases State-of-the-Art Panel on Anti-Retroviral Therapy for Adult HIV-Infected Patients. JAMA 1993;270:2583.

230. Volberding PA, Lagakos SW, Koch MA, et al. Zidovudine in asymptomatic human immunodeficiency virus infection. N Engl J Med 1990;322:941.

231. Seligmann M, Warrell DA, Aboulker JP, et al. Concorde: MRC/ANRS randomised double-blind controlled trial of immediate and deferred zidovudine in symptom-free HIV infection. Lancet 1994;343:871.

232. Gazzard B. Further results from the European/Australian delta trial. Presented at the Third National Conference on Human Retroviruses and Opportunistic Infections, Washington, DC, 1996. Abstract LD5a.

233. National Institutes of Health. ACTG 175: Executive summary. September 14, 1995.

234. Gallant JE, Moore RD, Chaisson RE. Prophylaxis for opportunistic infections in patients with HIV infection. Ann Intern Med 1994;120:932.

235. Bartlett JG. Prevention of opportunistic infections in human immunodeficiency virus-infected patients. Infect Dis Clin Prac 1994;3:260.

236. Lane HC, Laughon BE, Falloon J, et al. Recent advances in the management of AIDS-related opportunistic infections. Ann Intern Med 1994;120:945.

237. Smith GH. Treatment of infections in the patient with acquired immunodeficiency syndrome. Arch Intern Med 1994;154:949.

238. Lee BL. Drug interactions and toxicities in patients with AIDS. In MA Sande, PA Volberding (eds), The Medical Management of AIDS (4th ed). Philadelphia: Saunders, 1994;161.

239. Meythaler JM, Cross LL. Traumatic spinal cord injury complicated by AIDS related complex. Arch Phys Med Rehabil 1988;69:219.

240. So YT, Olney RK. Acute lumbosacral polyradiculopathy in acquired immunodeficiency syndrome: Experience in 23 patients. Ann Neurol 1994;35:53.

241. Brew BJ. Central and peripheral nervous system abnormalities. Med Clin North Am 1992;76:63.

242. Brew BJ. HIV-1-related neurological disease. J Acquir Immune Defic Syndr 1993;6(S1):S10.

243. Robertson KR, Hall CD. Human immunodeficiency virus-related cognitive impairment and the acquired immunodeficiency syndrome dementia complex. Semin Neurol 1992;12:18.

244. Long R, Maycher B, Scalini M, et al. The chest roentgenogram in pulmonary tuberculosis patients seropositive for human immunodeficiency virus type 1. Chest 1991;99:123.

245. Dooley SW, Villarino ME, Lawrence M, et al. Nosocomial transmission of tuberculosis in a hospital unit for HIV-infected patients. JAMA 1992;267:2632.

246. Beck-Sague C, Dooley SW, Hutton MD, et al. Hospital outbreak of multidrug-resistant *Mycobacterium* tuberculosis infections: Factors in transmission to staff and HIV-infected patients. JAMA 1992;268:1280.

247. Levinson SF, O'Connell PG. Rehabilitation dimensions of AIDS: A review. Arch Phys Med Rehabil 1991;72:690.

248. Young EJ, Fainstein V, Musher DM. Drug-induced fever: Cases seen in the evaluation of unexplained fever in a general hospital population. Rev Infect Dis 1982;4:69.

249. Rousch MK, Nelson KM. Understanding drug-induced febrile reactions. Am Pharm 1993;NS33:39.

250. Mackowiak PA. Southwestern internal medicine conference: Drug fever: Mechanisms, maxims and misconception. Am J Med Sci 1987;294:275.

251. Lipsky BA, Hirschmann JV. Drug fever. JAMA 1981;245:851.

252. Wolff SM, Adler RC, Buskirk ER, et al. A syndrome of periodic hypothalamic discharge. Am J Med 1964;36:956.

253. McClung HJ. Prolonged fever of unknown origin in children. Am J Dis Child 1972;124:544.

254. Lohr JA, Hendley JO. Prolonged fever of unknown origin. Clin Pediatr 1977;16:768.

255. Pizzo PA, Lovejoy FH, Smith DH. Prolonged fever in children: Review of 100 cases. Pediatrics 1975;55:468.

256. Weber M. Two cases of lesions of the cervical portion of the spinal marrow, exhibiting the phenomena of heatstroke. Trans Clin Soc Lond 1868;1:163.

257. Guttmann L, Silver J, Wyndham CH. Thermoregulation in spinal man. J Physiol 1958;142:406.

258. Holmes G. Spinal injuries in warfare. BMJ 1915;1:815.

259. Colachis SC. Autonomic hyperreflexia with spinal cord injury. J Am Paraplegia Soc 1992;15:171.

260. Przelomski MM, Roth RM, Glickman RA, et al. Fever in the wake of a stroke. Neurology 1986;36:427.

Chapter 13
Pressure Sores

Victor L. Lewis, Jr.

When soft tissue is compressed between bone and a subjacent hard surface, blood flow is cut off and tissue death occurs. The minimum time necessary for tissue death may be 1–2 hours [1]. The volume of dead tissue is greatest next to the bone and least at the skin surface, creating, as the wound demarcates, a volcano-shaped defect with bone at the base [2], usually requiring professional management.

Because of the importance of pressure in causing the tissue death, the tissue defect is commonly called a pressure sore or ulcer. Many such sores have occurred with the patient lying on the back in the decubitus position. The term *decubitus ulcer* is then used synonymously with pressure sore, although the position characteristically produces sores of the postsacral and heel, scapula, and occiput areas only.

The sites of the bony prominence most at risk for pressure ulceration are, in order of frequency of ulcer occurrence, the ischial tuberosity, the sacrum and coccyx, and the greater trochanter of the femur [3]. The ischial tuberosity is uncovered by the inferior edge of the gluteus maximus muscle in the seated position, when it is most at risk for ulceration. The sacrum, coccyx, and trochanter are not covered by muscle and are at risk whenever direct pressure is applied. Areas similarly at risk, but less frequently injured, are the occiput, scapula, elbow, knee, and medial and lateral malleoli.

Pathophysiology

Areas of soft tissue breakdown have been graded by depth grade I–IV [4]. Superficial skin losses are graded I and II, subcutaneous wounds are grade III, and deep wounds exposing bone are grade IV. Superficial ulcers may be caused by abrasion of the skin in sliding or transferring, folding of insensate skin, bruising or hematoma in transferring or falling, abrasion by unpadded buttons or garments, and other minor trauma. These injuries usually occur in denervated tissue because the patient is unaware of the trauma or absence of protective sensation, or cannot control movement due to paralyses, spasticity, or weakness.

Pressure ulcers are distinguished from neurotrophic, venous, arterial, vasculitic, and neoplastic ulcers. Neurotrophic ulcers occur on the heels and under the metatarsal heads of the feet of diabetic patients with peripheral neuropathy. The cause is unrecognized trauma from footwear and compression of soft tissue caused by loss of the metatarsal arch. Venous ulcers occur on the leg at sites of communicating vessels between the superficial and deep venous systems. The affected legs show superficial varicose veins, hyperpigmentation, and subcutaneous fibrosis.

Arterial and vasculitic ulcers also occur on the lower extremity rather than about the pelvis. Arterial ulcers in innervated patients are painful and associated with signs of arteriosclerotic peripheral vascular disease, such as weak pulses, hair loss, and thin skin.

Diagnosis of soft tissue complications of arteriosclerotic peripheral vascular disease in paraplegic patients is usually delayed because of the absence of claudication and leg pain. Patients with risk factors for arterial disease should be examined for physical findings of arterial disease including absence of pulses, hair loss, and skin temperature changes [5]. The ulcers associated with collagen disease may or may not occur over the courses of arteries and veins, are associated with exacerbations of the disease, and occur with loss of end circulation of small vessels.

Prophylaxis

The least expensive and easiest way to treat pressure sores is to prevent them [6–8]. The lack of good animal models for human pressure sores makes possible only estimates of the minimum requirements to produce breakdown. Animal studies indicate this is 2 hours of pressure [1]. Healthy insensate persons must use a mirror to check all pressure areas daily. They must follow a program of pressure releases. Areas showing redness, firmness, or erosion indicating an episode of ischemia must be protected from pressure until all signs of injury recede.

Patients who cannot turn or check themselves must be repositioned at least every 2 hours and checked daily for areas of redness, induration, and breakdown. Urinary incontinence and diarrhea, which damage the skin, must be controlled by catheterization, diet, and medication [9]. When acute malnutrition has been unavoidable, flotation beds limit pressure on compromised tissue [10].

Wound Evaluation

To decide on appropriate treatment of an open wound, a decision must first be made about its cause. When, by location and appearance, a diagnosis of pressure sore is made, its depth and the nature of the material at the wound base must be ascertained. Depth is determined by debridement, the removal of devitalized tissue. Debridement is accomplished by sharp instrument removal of tissue when the care givers have access to instruments, and pain control is adequate. Debridement may be accomplished more slowly by use of enzymes in the home or less skilled care facility [11].

After the decision has been made that there is dead tissue, surgical consultation is appropriate. Wounds with devitalized tissue are not ready for interval dressing changes. These wounds require debridement.

The best place for initial debridement is usually the operating room, where light and instruments are available for complete wound care. Toilette debridement of the unreconstructable patient is performed at the bedside.

Wound bacteriology is determined at debridement. Biopsy cultures at the interface of the living and dead tissue are obtained to try to determine true pathogens. Wounds about the pelvis are usually contaminated by a mixed aerobic and anaerobic coliform flora, which can be qualitatively identified by swab culture but most of which play no role in wound infection.

The majority of pressure sores, in spite of their content of dead tissue contaminated by coliform bacteria, are not invasively infected. Occasionally, especially in badly debilitated patients with serious intercurrent illnesses such as diabetes mellitus, a rapidly spreading gangrene caused by *Bacteroides melaninogenicus* and *Proteus* species may occur [12–14]. These infections require aggressive primary and secondary debridement of all involved tissue and may present major reconstructive challenges. A description of the appropriate antibiotics for treating pressure sores, gangrene, and osteomyelitis, if present, is found in Chapter 12.

If debridement establishes the presence of a grade IV pressure sore, after initial treatment the wound base will be bone. Because the periosteum has been destroyed by the pressure necrosis, and the bone surface exposed to coliform bacteria, tests are frequently performed to determine whether the bone is infected [15]. Classic papers on the treatment of pressure sores have not [16], however, stressed the treatment of bone, and the pathologic correlation between radiologic and laboratory diagnoses and the final ostectomy is not always stated. In one prospective series [15], the erythrocyte sedimentation rate and white blood cell count, bone biopsy, plain radiograph, bone scan, and computed tomography were compared with the pathologist's diagnosis on the final ostectomy specimen submitted at operative reconstruction. An elevated erythrocyte sedimentation rate of 120 mm/hour and a plain film of the pelvis [17] interpreted as positive for osteomyelitis were good predictors of final pathology. Bone biopsy was useful but more predictive of the absence than the presence of osteomyelitis. Double- or triple-phase technetium bone scan and computed tomography did not correlate well with the final pathologic state in this series. Indium bone scans have not been extensively evaluated in the diagnosis of the status of bone underlying pressure sores.

After debridement, interval dressings are used for wound care. If debris remains, sodium hypochlorite solution (full-strength Dakin's solution) [18, 19] is used until the wound is completely clean. When the wound is clean, it is dressed with saline [20]. The liquid is applied to roll gauze in all large wounds, so that loose sponges are not lost in the wound. Daily physical therapy in a setting where a joint movement program can be combined with whirlpool wound irrigation is useful. Systemic antibiotics are not used prophylactically. Cellulitis, indicated by surrounding tissue redness, warmth, induration, and fever after debridement, is treated with antibiotics, determined by biopsy culture. Occasionally a topical antimicrobial, either mafenide acetate or silver sulfadiazine [21], is indicated to treat an infected, ischemic wound. Recent work [22] suggests a future role in growth factors and other topical agents in the healing of wounds, including pressure sores.

Evaluation for Reconstruction

When a clean, granulating grade IV wound has been established, a decision must be made about the necessity and appropriateness of operative reconstruction (Table 13-1). Sores in innervated patients, which occur acutely, such as backboard-induced sacral sores during patient transfer, can usually be managed by debridement, interval dressings, and nutritional repletion with the expectation that the sores will heal without flap reconstruction. Sores that occur during acute debilitating illnesses can be similarly managed, with the expectation that they will heal by granulation, contraction, and epithelialization [23]. Only occasionally is an operation necessary to provide a durable soft tissue coverage, in the previously described circumstances.

Some individuals with deep pressure sores are not candidates for surgical reconstruction because of short life expectancy or medical conditions that make it unlikely that they can withstand an operation. Recent data, however, suggest that some nursing home patients, previously not considered reconstructive candidates, may benefit from flap repairs [24].

Table 13-1. Conditions Optimized Before Surgery

Problem	Status
Wound bed	Clean and granulating
Underlying bone	Appropriate laboratory and radiographic tests obtained
Nutrition	Positive nitrogen balance
Spasticity	Controlled or minimized
Contractures	Released or minimized
Urosepsis	Treated
Anemia and volume contracture	Corrected
Soft tissue calcification	Planned resection
Diarrhea	Controlled
Smoking	Discontinued
Intercurrent illnesses	Stabilized
Coagulation profile	Evaluated

Patients with grade IV pressure sores related to acute or chronic spinal cord injury, myelomeningocele, syringomyelia, spinal cord tumor, and other lesions, and who have a long life expectancy, physically are candidates for surgical reconstruction. Associated psychiatric status must be assessed separately [25].

Preparation for surgery includes evaluation and treatment of anemia and coagulation abnormalities, nutritional depletion, spasticity [26], joint contraction, soft tissue calcification, urinary calculi or sepsis, and stabilization of underlying medical problems. The treatment of soft tissue calcification, anemia, and urinary tract problems is discussed elsewhere in this book. Joint contracture that is not relieved by physiotherapy may require an orthopedic procedure for joint and ligament release [27]. Open pressure sores may aggravate existing spasticity, especially at dressing changes [28]. Thus, spasticity refractory to medication and neurostimulator control may be improved by wound closure. Preoperative control of spasticity by cord section or phenol injection is unacceptable to most patients at present, because patients have been encouraged by new research to hope that functional cord restoration may become possible.

The most important contributor to wound healing is the state of nutrition. Useful preoperative evaluations include the total lymphocyte count, serum albumin and transferrin levels, urinary nitrogen study, and the anergy antigen battery [29]. The transferrin level should be greater than 180 mg/dl and the lymphocyte count greater than 1,500 cells/μl. Skin tests should show reactivity to the common antigens, such as purified protein derivative, mumps, *Candida*, and streptokinase-streptodornase. When patients are nonreactive, there is an increased incidence of wound infection or sepsis and possibly death [8, 30].

With regard to nutritional status, the 24-hour urinary nitrogen determination is useful in determining protein requirement and balance [29]. A nutrition support service can prescribe a diet and supplementation to place the patient in positive nitrogen balance. Diarrhea, caused by hyperosmolar nutritional supplements, antibiotics, or gastroenteritis, must be controlled before operation.

Patients are counseled that cigarette smoking exposes them to carbon monoxide and nicotinic acid, both of which are vasoconstrictors that may complicate flap reconstruction [31]. However, patients are not refused reconstruction if they will not stop smoking.

Intercurrent illnesses require careful consideration in patient selection. Patients with hypoprothrombinemia caused by warfarin therapy must have their prothrombin times brought to less than 1.2 times the control value. Anticoagulation can be continued until just before surgery by the administration of heparin, which is stopped 6–8 hours preoperatively. Warfarin treatment may also be resumed at this time. Corticosteroid-dependent conditions such as collagen disease have a significant risk of failure of primary healing. The multiple problems associated with insulin-dependent diabetes increase operative and wound healing risk. Iliofemoral arteriosclerosis may involve vessels supplying the key pedicles necessary for reconstruction [5]. When the risk-benefit ratio has been optimized, and the patient accepts the operation, there is a reconstructive procedure of choice for each major pressure sore area and alternate procedures for secondary reconstruction or flap failure [32]. When seeking to return a patient to full-seated tolerance, split-thickness skin grafts are seldom durable. Split-thickness skin graft applied to granulating bone has no padding, and quickly erodes. Direct advancement suture of the wound margins usually can only be accomplished with tension, especially of the deep layers, leading to dehiscence, requiring secondary closure.

Closure thus routinely requires tissue movement for bulky, tension-free tissue replacement [33]. The tissue movements, or flaps, combine muscle with the overlying fat and skin in musculocutaneous units [34]. This type of flap optimizes blood supply, because the muscles are fed by named, identifiable, vessels; supplies a higher oxygen concentration to the underlying bone, which may help heal chronic osteomyelitis; may adhere better to bone, because muscle seems to heal to bone better than fat, limiting shear and recurrence; and provides more bulk, which may limit the ischemic effect of pressure and, hence, recurrence. However, when abused, muscle tolerates warm ischemia less well than skin. The traditional flaps of skin and fat, randomly dependent on the blood supply at their base, are still treatment alternatives and make excellent secondary choices.

Surgical Management

Sacral Area

Primary Choice

The primary choice is the gluteus maximus advancement [35] or rotation [36] myocutaneous flap (Figure 13-1 and Table 13-2). Blood supply is excellent from the superior and inferior gluteal vessels, either or both of which will support the flap. It can be used unilaterally or bilaterally and can be rerotated. The advancement flap may leave a midline scar, which can break down. The gluteus maximus cannot be sacrificed in the ambulatory patient, but must be split, or the origin resutured to the opposite gluteus to prevent hip instability [37].

Secondary Choices

Rerotation of the gluteus maximus flap is a secondary choice. For the upper sacral area, the transverse lumbar [38], thoracolumbar-sacral [39], and combined gluteus latissimus flap are secondary choices. For the coccygeal area, the tensor fascia lata [40], gluteal thigh [41], and Limberg flaps can be used. The traditional inferiorly based buttock flap is available as a primary or secondary procedure or as a split flap from either side.

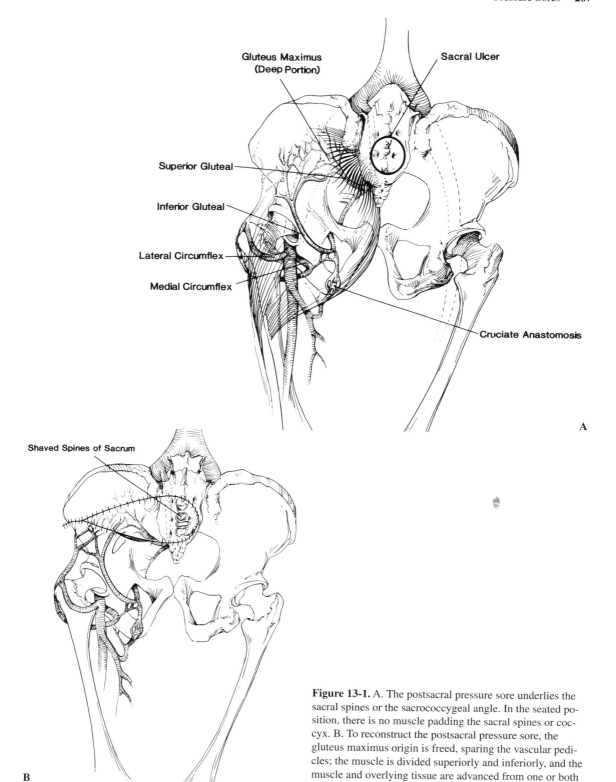

Gluteus Maximus
(Deep Portion)

Sacral Ulcer

Superior Gluteal

Inferior Gluteal

Lateral Circumflex

Medial Circumflex

Cruciate Anastomosis

A

Shaved Spines of Sacrum

B

Figure 13-1. A. The postsacral pressure sore underlies the sacral spines or the sacrococcygeal angle. In the seated position, there is no muscle padding the sacral spines or coccyx. B. To reconstruct the postsacral pressure sore, the gluteus maximus origin is freed, sparing the vascular pedicles; the muscle is divided superiorly and inferiorly, and the muscle and overlying tissue are advanced from one or both sides to the midline.

Table 13-2. Primary and Secondary Reconstruction of Sacral, Ischial, and Trochanteric Pressure Sores

Site	Procedure of Choice Primary Reconstruction	Alternate Procedures Secondary Reconstruction
Sacrum	Gluteus maximus advancement of rotation flap	Rerotation gluteus flap Transverse lumbar or upper back flap Traditional rotation flap Gluteal thigh flap Limberg flap Tensor fascia lata musculocutaneous flap
Ischium	Hamstring V-Y myocutaneous flap	Inferior gluteus maximus myocutaneous flap Medially based posterior thigh flap Tensor fascia lata musculocutaneous flap Gracilis musculocutaneous flap
Trochanter	Tensor fascia lata musculocutaneous flap	Vastus lateralis muscle flap and skin graft Rectus femoris muscle flap and skin graft Gluteus medius-tensor fascia lata musculocutaneous flap Bipedicled skin flap

Ischial Area

Primary Choice

The hamstring V-Y myocutaneous flap [42, 43] is the first choice for ischial reconstruction (Figure 13-2). The skin island is large, and readvancement is possible. A partial version of the flap has been described for medial or smaller lesions [44].

The inferior gluteus maximus myocutaneous flap [45] includes the lower edge of the gluteus maximus muscle and a triangle of overlying skin and fat. The donor defect can be closed in a V-Y fashion. Flap advancement requires lateral division of the gluteus maximus muscle, and this cannot be done in the ambulatory patient.

Secondary Choices

The gluteal thigh flap has an excellent blood supply from the descending branch of the inferior gluteal artery [41] and covers the ischium and perineum without use of a muscle. The medially based posterior tight flap is reliable and bulky [46]. Residual space beneath the flap can be filled by turning over the lateral hamstrings. The tensor fascia lata flap tip will reach the area. The gracilis musculocutaneous flap also reaches the area [47].

Trochanteric Area

Primary Choice

The tensor fascia lata musculocutaneous flap, either as a V-Y [48, 49] or a rotation flap [40] (Figure 13-3), is the primary choice for this area. The single dominant pedicle from the lateral circumflex branch of the profunda femoris vessels is high in the thigh. The flap is long and can be reused, and the proximal muscle-containing area is bulky.

Secondary Choices

The secondary choices are the vastus lateralis muscle flap [50] and skin graft, rectus femoris [51] muscle flap, gluteus medius-tensor fascia lata musculocutaneous flap [52], and bipedicled skin flap [46]. Of these, by far the best choice is the vastus lateralis, which should be reserved for this purpose or to fill a large Girdlestone arthroplasty defect.

Management of Underlying Bone

How to treat the underlying bone is based on the results of the preoperative laboratory studies and radiographs. If preoperative studies indicate osteo-

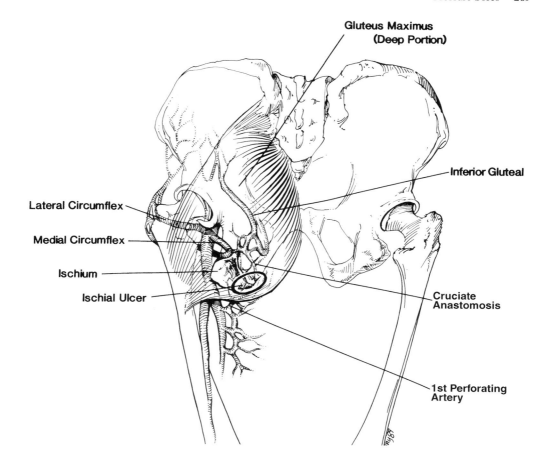

Gluteus Maximus
(Deep Portion)

Inferior Gluteal

Lateral Circumflex

Medial Circumflex

Ischium

Ischial Ulcer

Cruciate
Anastomosis

1st Perforating
Artery

A

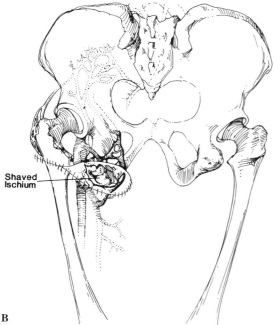

Shaved
Ischium

B

Figure 13-2. A. The location of the ischial pressure ulcer
underlying the ischial tuberosity. The gluteus maximus
muscle does not underlie the tuberosity in the seated position. However, the gluteus maximus is adjacent and available for reconstruction. B. The gluteus maximus
musculocutaneous flap slides medially to cover the shaved
ischial tuberosity. Clinically, the closed donor site defect
does not overlie the femur.

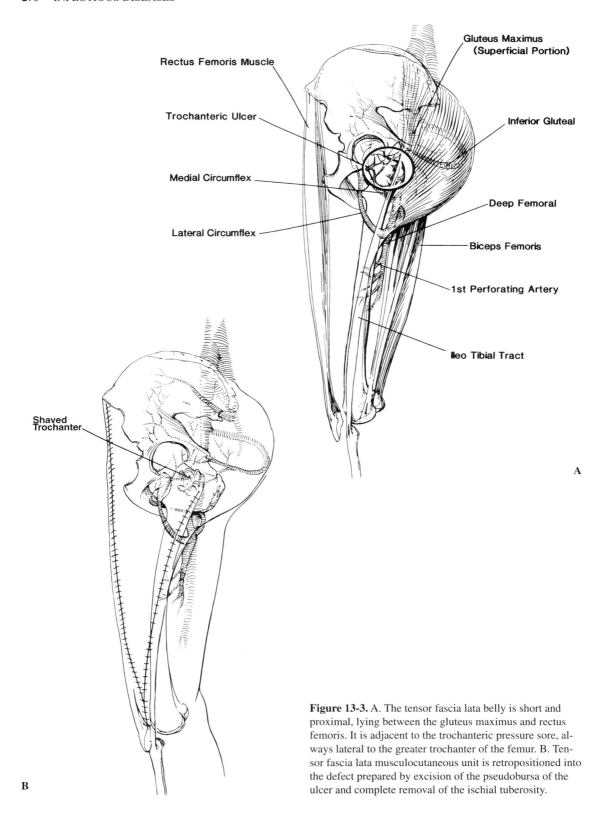

Rectus Femoris Muscle

Gluteus Maximus
(Superficial Portion)

Trochanteric Ulcer

Inferior Gluteal

Medial Circumflex

Deep Femoral

Lateral Circumflex

Biceps Femoris

1st Perforating Artery

Ileo Tibial Tract

A

Shaved
Trochanter

B

Figure 13-3. A. The tensor fascia lata belly is short and proximal, lying between the gluteus maximus and rectus femoris. It is adjacent to the trochanteric pressure sore, always lateral to the greater trochanter of the femur. B. Tensor fascia lata musculocutaneous unit is retropositioned into the defect prepared by excision of the pseudobursa of the ulcer and complete removal of the ischial tuberosity.

myelitis is probable, an aggressive ostectomy is performed and the cut edges as well as the central specimen examined for infection [53]. An aggressive ostectomy in the sacral area includes removal of the sacral spines and surface, with coccygectomy. Aggressive ostectomy in the ischial area is a total ischiectomy. Aggressive ostectomy of the trochanteric area is complete trochanterectomy. The area of the hip joint is inspected to be sure the joint is not eroded and contaminated. If the joint is open, Girdlestone arthroplasty [54] is necessary and a flail hip will result.

When osteomyelitis is not suspected for sacral sores, the coccyx is left in place if the sacrococcygeal joint is not violated and contaminated. Only the spines underlying the wound are removed. When preoperative studies do not indicate osteomyelitis of the ischium, only the ischial tuberosity is removed. The ischial body is preserved to prevent pelvic tilt and the creation of a perineal pressure point under the pubis. Even in cases when osteomyelitis is not suspected in trochanteric ulcers, complete trochanterectomy is performed to eliminate the bony prominence and prevent recurrence of trochanteric pressure sores.

The operative blood loss for an ostectomy and major flap reconstruction is anticipated to be 250–1,500 ml. Preoperatively, anemia is corrected either by transfusion or the administration of recombinant erythropoietin [55]. Intraoperatively, blood is closely monitored. Denervated patients, particularly quadriplegics, cannot compensate for blood loss by vasoconstriction. When blood loss reaches 500 ml, the anticipated additional blood loss is estimated and the patient considered for transfusion.

The minimum postoperative bed confinement is 2 weeks, followed by gradual remobilization in the rehabilitation setting. In many spinal cord centers bed rest is 3–6 weeks. Patients at bed rest receive passive physiotherapy of uninvolved joints, intermittent compression of the legs to prevent thromboembolism, and Foley catheter bladder drainage. The bowel program, performed by the staff, is begun 3 days after operation. Preoperative bowel preparation is omitted to prevent diarrhea after the operation.

The patient remains in Clinitron therapy [56] until transferred to a hospital bed for remobilization. The Clinitron keeps the patient from turning. Other systems (e.g., low air loss therapy and water mattresses) also are satisfactory. When ready for sit-ting, the patient is transferred to bed and checked for range of motion in the joints proximate to the repair and for orthostatic hypotension. The patient with adequate joint range and without orthostatic hypotension is allowed to sit for 15 minutes and then placed in bed, and the flap is checked for erythema and marginal dehiscence. If the tissues tolerate the pressure, gradual remobilization begins, with the sutures in place for the first week of sitting to prevent minor skin edge separation. Full seated tolerance is achieved 6–7 weeks after surgery.

Reconstruction of pressure sores is not uncomplicated. Failure of primary healing can be expected in a minimum of 10–15% of cases [57]. Early postoperative problems are dehiscence, hematoma, and wound infection. Each requires treatment of its cause, wound repreparation, and secondary closure. All prolong immobilization and hospitalization. In terms of time and expense, it is usually not worthwhile to expect secondary healing of a dehisced flap with dressings alone. The observation has been made that the frequency of failure of primary healing increases with the duration of denervation, particularly after approximately 7 years.

Late complications of pressure sores include recurrence, development of new sores, and squamous cell carcinoma. The reasons for recurrence or new sores include depression and self-destructive personalities, alcohol and drug abuse, cushion and wheelchair defects, falls and injuries, inadequate attendant care, and urinary and bowel incontinence. Each factor deserves investigation and correction before a secondary operation is performed. Patients with multiple pressure sore recurrences after adequate operative reconstruction and rehabilitation are refractory and do not benefit from repeated operations [29, 58].

Marjolin's ulcer may occur in sores left open for long periods, usually 20 or more years. The diagnosis [59–61] is suspected by the growth of exophytic tumor at the wound edges, although this does not always occur. Biopsy of suspicious areas in chronic wounds is appropriate. The usual diagnosis is squamous cell carcinoma. Treatment is wide resection and flap reconstruction of the defect, frequently with contemporaneous regional node dissection. The prognosis is not good. Most patients die of metastatic cancer within 2 years in spite of adequate local control. Chemotherapy and radiation therapy have not been palliative.

References

1. Daniel RK, Wheatley D, Priest D. Pressure sores and paraplegia: An experimental model. Ann Plast Surg 1985;15:41.

2. Nola GT, Vistnes LM. Differential response of skin and muscle in the experimental production of pressure sores. Plast Reconstr Surg 1980;66:728.

3. Vasconez LO, Schneider WJ, Jurkiewicz MJ. Pressure sores. Curr Probl Surg 1987;14:1.

4. Shea JD. Pressure sores: Classification and management. Clin Orthop 1975;112:89.

5. Yokoo KM, Kronon M, Lewis VL Jr, et al. Delayed diagnoses of peripheral vascular disease in spinal cord injury patients. Presented at the Annual Meeting of the American Spinal Injury Association, San Diego, CA, May 1992.

6. Griffin ER. Decubitus ulcers, prevention and management: A review. Military Med 1982;147:369.

7. Linder RM, Upton J. The prevention of pressure sores. Surg Rounds 1983;6:42.

8. Pressure sores in adults: Prediction and prevention. U.S. Department of Health and Human Services, Agency for Health Care Policy and Research, Rockville, MD, May 1992.

9. Allman RM, Laprade CA, Noel LB, Walker IM, et al. Pressure sores among hospitalized patients. Ann Intern Med 1986;105:337.

10. Lewis VL Jr. Operative Repair. In N Bergstrom, MA Bennett, CE Carlson, et al (eds), Treatment of Pressure Ulcers, Clinical Practice Guideline, Number 15. AHCPR Publication No. 95-0652. Rockville, MD: Agency for Health Care Policy and Research, Public Health Service, U.S. Department of Health and Human Services, December 1994.

11. Rao DB, Sane PG, Georgier BL. Collagenase in the treatment of dermal and decubitus ulcers. J Am Geriatr Soc 1975;23:22.

12. Galpin JE, Chow AW, Bayer AS, Guze LB. Sepsis associated with decubitus ulcers. Am J Med 1976;61:346.

13. Lewis VL Jr, Myers MB, Griffith BH. Early diagnosis of crepitant nonclostridial gangrene caused by *Bacteroides melaninogenicus*. Plast Reconstr Surg 1978;62:276.

14. Myers MB, Cherry G, Bornside BB, Bornside GH. Ultraviolet red fluorescence of *Bacteroides melaninogenicus*. Appl Microbiol 1969;17:760.

15. Lewis VL Jr, Bailey MH, Pulawski G, et al. The diagnosis of osteomyelitis in patients with pressure sores. Plast Reconstr Surg 1988;81:229.

16. Conway H, Griffith BH. Plastic surgery for closure or decubitus ulcers in patients with paraplegia based on experience with 1,000 cases. Am J Surg 1956;91:946.

17. Hendrix RW, Calenoff L, Lederman RB, Neiman HL. Radiology of pressure sores. Radiology 1981;138:351.

18. Kozol RA, Gillies C, Elgebaly SA. Effects of sodium hypochlorite (Dakin's solution) on cells of the wound module. Arch Surg 1988;123:420.

19. Smith RF, Blasi D, Dayton SL, Chipps DD. Effects of sodium hypochlorite on the microbial flora of burns and normal skin. J Trauma 1974;14:983.

20. Rogers DM, Blouin GS, O'Leary JP. Providone iodine wound irrigation and wound sepsis. Surg Gynecol Obstet 1983;157:426.

21. Kucan JO, Robson MC, Heggers JP, Ko F. Comparison of silver sulfadiazine, povidone-iodine, and physiologic saline in the treatment of chronic pressure ulcers. J Am Geriatr Soc 1981;29:232.

22. Phillips LG, Abdullah KM, Geldner PO, et al. Applications of basic fibroblast growth factor may reverse diabetic wound healing impairment. Ann Plast Surg 1993;31:331.

23. Morgan JE. Topical therapy of pressure ulcers. Surg Gynecol Obstet 1975;141:945.

24. Sugler EL, Lavizzo-Mourey R. Management of stage III pressure ulcers in moderately demented nursing home residents. J Gen Intern Med 1991;6:507.

25. Disa JJ, Carlton JM, Goldberg NH. Efficacy of operative cure in pressure sore patients. Plast Reconstr Surg 1992;89:272.

26. Richardson RR, Cerullo LJ, McLone DG, et al. Percutaneous epidural neurostimulation in modulation of paraplegic spasticity. Acta Neurochir 1979;49:235.

27. Haher JN, Haher TR, Devlin VJ, Schwartz J. The release of flexion contractures as a prerequisite for the treatment of pressure sores in multiple sclerosis: A report of ten cases. Ann Plast Surg 1983;11:246.

28. Hall PA, Young JV. Autonomic hyperreflexia in spinal cord injured patients: Trigger mechanism—Dressing changes of pressure sores. J Trauma 1983;23:1074.

29. Kenney JB, Edgerton MT, Edlich RF. Recurrent pressure sores: Evaluation and treatment. Contemp Orthop 1984;8:51.

30. Mullen JL. Consequences of malnutrition in the surgical patient. Surg Clin North Am 1981;61:465.

31. Rees TD, Liverett DM, Guy CL. The effect of cigarette smoking on skin-flap survival in the face lift patient. Plast Reconstr Surg 1984;73:911.

32. Stal S, Serure A, Donovan W, Spira M. The perioperative management of the patient with pressure sores. Ann Plast Surg 1983;11:347.

33. Ger R, Levine SA. The management of decubitus ulcers by muscle transposition. Plast Reconstr Surg 1976;58:419.

34. Fisher J, Woods JB. Experimental comparison of bone revascularization by musculocutaneous and cutaneous flaps. Plast Reconstr Surg 1987;79:87.

35. Ramirez OM, Ramasastry SS, Granuck MS, et al. A new surgical approach to closure of large lumbosacral meningomyelocele defects. Plast Reconstr Surg 1987;80:799.

36. Baek SM, Williams GD, McElhinney AJ, Simon BE. The gluteus maximus myocutaneous flap in the management of pressure sores. Ann Plast Surg 1980;6:471.

37. Ramirez OM, Orlando JC, Hurwitz DJ. The sliding gluteus maximus myocutaneous flap: Its relevance in ambulatory patients. Plast Reconstr Surg 1984;74:68.

38. Hill HL, Brown RG, Jurkiewicz MJ. The transverse lumbosacral back flap. Plast Reconstr Surg 1984;62:177.

39. Vyas C, Binns JH, Wilson AM. Thoracolumbar-sacral flaps in the treatment of sacral pressure sores. Plast Reconstr Surg 1980;65:159.

40. Nahai F, Silveston JS, Hill ML. The tensor fascia lata in myocutaneous flap. Ann Plast Surg 1978;1:372.

41. Hurwitz DJ, Swartz WM, Mathes SJ. The gluteal thigh flap: A reliable, sensate flap for the closure of buttock and perineal wounds. Plast Reconst Surg 1981;68:521.

42. Hurteau JE, Bostwick J, Nahai F, et al. V-Y advancement of hamstring musculocutaneous flap for coverage of ischial pressure sores. Plast Reconstr Surg 1981;68:539.

43. Kroll SS, Hamilton S. Multiple and repetitive uses of the extended hamstring V-Y myocutaneous flap. Plast Reconstr Surg 1989;84:296.

44. Bailey MH, Lewis VL, Smith J, Sullivan M. Improved surgical management of the ischial pressure sore. Plast Surg Forum 1987;10:86.

45. Scheflan M, Nahai F, Bostwick, J. Gluteus maximus island musculocutaneous flap for closure of sacral and ischial ulcers. Plast Reconstr Surg 1981;68:533.

46. Griffith BH. Flaps for closure of pressure sores. In WC Grabb, MB Myer (eds), Skin Flaps. Boston: Little, Brown, 1975.

47. Wingate GB, Friedland JA. Repair or ischial pressure ulcers with gracilis myocutaneous island flaps. Plast Reconstr Surg 1978;62:245.

48. Lewis VL Jr, Cunningham BL, Hugo NE. The tensor fascia lata V-Y retroposition flap. Ann Plast Surg 1981;6:34.

49. Paletta CE, Freedman B, Shehadi S. The V-Y tensor fascia lata musculocutaneous flap. Plast Reconstr Surg 1989;88:852.

50. Dowden RV, McCraw JB. The vastus lateralis muscle flap: Technique and applications. Ann Plast Surg 1980;4:396.

51. Bhagwat BM, Pearl RM, Laub DR. Uses of the rectus femoris myocutaneous flap. Plast Reconstr Surg 1978;62:698.

52. Little JW, Lyons JR. The gluteus medius tensor fasciae latae flap. Plast Reconstr Surg 1983;71:366.

53. Daroviche RO, Landon GC, Klima M, et al. Osteomyelitis associated with pressure sores. Arch Intern Med 1994;154:753.

54. Evans GRD, Lewis VL, Manson PN. Hip joint communication with pressure sores—The refractory wound and the role of Girdlestone arthroplasty. Plast Reconstr Surg 1993;91:288.

55. Turba R, Lewis VL, Green D. Pressure sore anemia: Response to erythropoietin. Arch Phys Med Rehabil 1992;73:498.

56. Dolezal R, Cohen M, Schultz RC. The use of Clinitron therapy unit in the immediate postoperative care of pressure ulcers. Ann Plast Surg 1985;14:33.

57. Basson MD, Burney RE. Defective wound healing in patients with paraplegia and quadriplegia. Surg Gynecol Obstet 1982;155:9.

58. Rogers J, Wilson LF. Preventing recurrent tissue breakdowns after "pressure sore" closures. Plast Reconstr Surg 1975;56:419.

59. Grotting JC, Bunkis J, Vascontez LO. Pressure sore carcinoma. Ann Plast Surg 1987;18:527.

60. Yarkony GM, Berkwits L, Lewis VL Jr. Marjolin's ulcer complicating a pressure ulcer. Case report and literature review. Arch Phys Med Rehabil 1986;67:831.

61. Stankard CE, Cruse CW, Wells KE, Karl R. Chronic pressure sore carcinoma. Ann Plast Surg 1993;30:274.

Part VIII

Neurology

Chapter 14

Spasticity: Mechanisms and Management

John R. McGuire and William Z. Rymer

Spasticity, which refers to abnormal stretch reflex behavior, is a disabling component of upper motor neuron lesions. Brain injury, stroke, spinal cord injury, cerebral palsy, and multiple sclerosis are common causes of spasticity. Clinically, spasticity is easy to recognize but can be difficult to quantify and treat. The pathophysiology of spasticity is complex and controversial, which makes research in this area challenging. This chapter reviews definitions, mechanisms, measurement, and treatment of spasticity.

Definitions and Characteristics

It is important to differentiate spasticity from rigidity because both are associated with increased resistance to passive movement. Lance [1] described spasticity as a "motor disorder characterized by a velocity dependent increase in tonic stretch reflexes (muscle tone) with exaggerated tendon jerks, resulting from hyperexcitability of the stretch reflex, as one component of the upper motor neuron syndrome." Thus, to understand spasticity, one must understand upper and lower motoneuron pathways, the components of muscle tone, and the mechanisms of the stretch reflex. In contrast, rigidity is a velocity independent, bidirectional (flexion/extension) phenomenon, associated with tremor, bradykinesia, or other extrapyramidal signs.

Upper Versus Lower Motoneuron Pathways

The lower motoneuron (LMN) includes the anterior horn cell, its nerve root, and peripheral nerve up to the neuromuscular junction. LMN lesions are associated with weakness, hyporeflexia, and muscle atrophy. Guillain-Barré syndrome, polio, radiculopathies, and peripheral nerve injuries are common disorders that affect LMNs.

The upper motoneuron (UMN) system consists of all the pathways above the anterior horn cell, including the brain, brain stem, and spinal cord. Clinically, hyperreflexia, along with weakness, differentiates UMNs from LMNs. Also, UMN lesions can result in a syndrome that can be manifested as positive and negative symptoms (Table 14-1) [2–5]. Positive symptoms or abnormal behaviors, such as clonus, especially at the ankle, can interfere with ambulation and the proper fit of orthotics. Physiologically, clonus is the result of the effects of Ia afferent synaptic input (from muscle spindle primary endings) on hyperexcitable motoneurons. The clasp-knife reflex involves the central actions of unmyelinated and small myelinated high threshold mechanoreceptors that inhibit reflex activity in extensor muscles. These reflexes are released with spinal cord lesions influencing descending reticulospinal pathways, traversing the dorsolateral funiculus of the spinal cord [6].

The goal of managing UMN lesions involves decreasing the number of abnormal behaviors (reflex re-

Table 14-1. Characteristics of Upper Motor Neuron Lesions

Abnormal behaviors (positive symptoms)
Reflex release phenomena
Hyperactive proprioceptive reflexes (clasp-knife, Babinski sign, clonus)
Increased resistance to stretch
Relaxed cutaneous reflexes (flexor spasms)
Loss of precise autonomic control (dysreflexia in SCI)
Performance deficits (negative symptoms)
Decreased dexterity and mobility
Paresis/weakness
Fatigability

Table 14-2. Possible Mechanisms of Spasticity

A. Increased motor neuronal excitability
1. Excitatory synaptic input is enhanced
2. Inhibitory synaptic input is reduced
3. Changes in the intrinsic electrical properties of the neuron
B. Enhanced stretch-evoked synaptic excitation of motor neurons
1. Gamma efferent hyperactivity
2. Excitatory interneurons more sensitive to muscle afferent

lease phenomena, hyperactive proprioceptive reflexes, etc.) to improve function if the performance deficits (weakness, fatigability, etc.) are not overwhelming.

Pattern of Spasticity Depends on Lesion Location

The location of the lesion within the UMN system will influence the pattern of spasticity and other associated phenomena. Cerebral spasticity affects primarily antigravity muscles, lower limb extensors, and upper limb flexors. Flexor spasms are rare and there are less clasp-knife phenomena and clonus. Cerebral "shock," a period of hyporeflexia, thought to be caused by loss of tonic facilitation from descending pathways, can last 2–3 weeks. Autonomic phenomena are typically absent with cerebral lesions [7].

In contrast to cerebral lesions, spasticity from spinal cord lesions tends to produce a flexor pattern in lower limbs. Flexor spasms, clasp-knife phenomena, and clonus are more common with spinal cord lesions. Spinal shock can last up to 16 weeks and autonomic dysreflexia is common [7]. The differences between cerebral and spinal spasticity may be related to loss of key descending pathways with spinal cord lesions and to the potential structural reorganization of the cord in spinal injury.

Muscle Tone

Muscle tone refers to the resistance one feels with passive movement of the limb. The intrinsic me-

chanical, elastic properties of muscle and connective tissue form one key component of muscle tone. The tonic stretch reflexes are a second, and probably the most important, component of muscle tone and are discussed in the following section. The tonic stretch reflex is mediated by the excitatory central actions of spindle receptors (primary and secondary endings). These central excitatory effects are countered by inhibitory central actions of the Golgi tendon organ afferents via inhibitory (Ib) interneurons [8].

Mechanisms

The mechanism of spasticity is complex and controversial. Hyperactive stretch reflex mechanisms are largely responsible for spasticity and not changes in the passive muscle properties [5]. Whether alterations in stretch reflex behavior are due to a lower threshold or increased gain of the stretch reflex or a combination of the two is currently under investigation [9–11].

The stretch reflex may become hyperactive by increased excitability of the motoneuronal pool or by enhanced stretch-evoked synaptic excitation of motoneurons (Table 14-2) [5]. Increased motoneuronal excitability may be the result of enhanced excitatory synaptic input by segmental afferents, regional excitatory interneurons, or descending pathways. Alternatively, reduced inhibitory synaptic input by Renshaw cell recurrent inhibition, Ia inhibitory interneurons, or Ib afferent fibers could

Table 14-3. Measurement of Spasticity

A. Clinical scales
1. Modified Ashworth:
   0 = no increase in tone
   1 = slight increase in tone (catch and release)
   +1 = slight increase in tone
       (catch + minimal resist <½ ROM)
   2 = marked increase in tone through most ROM
   3 = considerable increase in tone,
       passive ROM difficult
   4 = rigid in flexion and extension
2. Brunnstrom scale
3. Fugl-Meyer scale
B. Electrophysiologic testing
1. H-reflex, H/M ratio, F-wave
2. Tonic vibration reflex (TVR)
C. Biomechanical
1. Pendulum test
2. Servo-controlled motor-driven device

also cause increased excitability of the motoneuronal pool [5, 12]. Changes in the intrinsic electrical properties of the neuron by changes in passive membrane electrical properties or changes in voltage-sensitive membrane conductance could also make the motoneuron more excitable but has limited support in the literature [13, 14]. Enhanced stretch-evoked synaptic excitation of motoneurons could be caused by gamma efferent hyperactivity [15–17] or excitatory interneurons becoming more sensitive to muscle afferent input by collateral sprouting [18], denervation hypersensitivity [19, 20], or a decrease in presynaptic inhibition [21, 22].

There is limited experimental evidence that supports altered net descending excitation as the cause of spasticity in cerebral injury; however, the origins of spinal spasticity are much less obvious. Most likely, the mechanism of spinal spasticity is due to a combination of these factors, but further study is needed.

Measurement of Spasticity

Quantifying spasticity is as difficult as understanding its mechanism. Clinical, electrophysiologic, and biomechanical techniques have been used (Table 14-3).

The modified Ashworth scale [23] is a widely used clinical scale that provides a qualitative measure of spasticity. The Brunnstrom scale [24] is useful in describing motor recovery after stroke because it incorporates spasticity with muscle synergy patterns but lacks specificity for spasticity. The Fugl-Meyer scale [25], although not specific for spasticity, can be a useful method of measuring both physical and functional motor recovery. Although useful at the bedside, these clinical scales are only qualitative measures of spasticity and tend to lack inter-rater reliability.

Electrophysiologic tests (Table 14-3) such as the H-reflex and tonic vibration reflex offer more quantifiable measures of spasticity but are technically limited and tend to correlate poorly with the intensity of spasticity [26–29].

The biomechanical techniques (Table 14-3) offer a more reliable measure of spasticity but are also limited. The pendulum test can be used to access spasticity in the quadriceps and hamstring muscles by measuring knee movement with an electrogoniometer and tachometer as the limb sways from a fully extended position over the edge of a table [30–32]. This technique is limited by the dominant inertial components of the lower limb and may not accurately reflect the reflex components of spasticity [33, 34]. Despite these limitations, there is generally good correlation between trials, and the pendulum test can be done using isokinetic exercise equipment [35].

In our laboratory, we quantify spasticity using a servo-controlled motor-driven device with position and torque sensors. This device passively stretches the limb while recording the electromyographic (EMG) activity of the spastic muscle [36, 37]. By correlating the increase in torque with the onset of the EMG activity one can derive an estimate of the threshold of the stretch reflex. This onset is a reflection of the degree of spasticity. Thus, a shift to the left of the torque-angle relation would indicate a reduced threshold of the stretch reflex or increased tone. Likewise a shift to the right would indicate increased threshold of the stretch reflex or decreased tone. This technique is an effective means of quantifying spasticity for research purposes but has limited usefulness at the bedside because it is time consuming and technically difficult [38].

Treatment

Before initiating any treatment for spasticity, it is important to remember the potential benefits of

Table 14-4. Treatment of Spasticity

Conservative/preventive
   Eliminate source of nociception, treat UTI, fecal
      impaction, pressure sores, HO
Positioning
   Foam pads, modular wedge system, WC seating
      systems, prone standers, custom molded system
Physical modalities/interventions
   ROM/therapeutic exercise
   Orthosis, splinting/casting
   Heat: hydrocollator pack, paraffin, whirlpool,
      ultrasound
   Cold: local, generalized, cooling spray
   EMG biofeedback
   Electrical stimulation: agonist, antagonist?
Medications
   Baclofen, diazepam
   Dantrolene sodium, clonidine
   Investigational: progabide, tizanidine, THC
Chemical blocks
   Local anesthetics
   Phenol, botulinum toxin
Surgery
   Intrathecal baclofen
   Tendon transfers/lengthening
   Rhizotomy: anterior/posterior
   Cordotomy: T-myelotomy

spasticity. Increased extensor tone in the legs may help a patient stand or assist with transfers. Reflex activity may help preserve muscle bulk and retard osteoporosis [39]. When spasticity interferes with function, hygiene, or becomes painful, then a therapeutic intervention is warranted (Table 14-4).

Successful management depends on establishing treatment goals—e.g., improving hand function by reducing the spasticity in wrist and finger flexors, improving ambulation by reducing spasticity in ankle planter flexors, or facilitating hygiene by reducing hip or shoulder adductor spasticity. A pyramid approach [40] is an effective model for managing spasticity but each treatment must be individualized. Each day it is important to establish the base of treatment by eliminating sources of nociception. For example, treating urinary tract infections, fecal impactions, pressure sores, heterotopic ossification, fractures, ingrown toenails, and reducing anxiety will reduce spasticity [41]. Also observe how the patient

is positioned in bed and in the wheelchair. Proper positioning with foam pads, modular wedge systems, or custom molded seating systems can improve a patient's alignment and symmetry, which can relax spastic muscles and potentially improve function [42].

Physical Modalities and Interventions

Physical modalities and therapeutic interventions should be considered next. These techniques may be effective by relaxing or fatiguing the spastic muscle directly, general relaxation, or by facilitation of antagonist muscles.

Range of motion exercises to spastic limbs are essential to preventing limb contractures and may help to reduce tone. "Carry-over" from range of motion exercises may be caused by changes in the musculotendinous unit or plastic changes in the central nervous system [43]. There is some evidence to suggest these prolonged effects may be the result of reduced Ca^{++} influx into motoneurons, leading to reduced transmitter release [44, 45].

Therapeutic exercise, such as neurodevelopmental treatment, places patients in reflex-inhibiting postures. These positions can elongate the spastic muscle and temporarily reduce tone and help promote voluntary movement [46]. A properly fitted orthosis, splinting, or casting can also produce a tonic stretch of the spastic muscle that may decrease the reflex activity and help maintain alignment [47–50]. Even though the exact mechanism is not known, prolonged stretch of a spastic muscle may reduce tone by decreasing the sensitivity of the spindle to stretch by resetting the threshold of the stretch reflex [51].

Heat and cold are common modalities used for temporary relief of a spastic limb. Hydrocollator pack, paraffin, whirlpool, and ultrasound can be used as a local source of heat or for general relaxation. Deep heat such as ultrasound has been shown to reduce tone by decreasing spindle sensitivity and increasing collagen extensibility [52]. Cold, localized with a cooling spray or generalized, may temporarily reduce spasticity by decreasing muscle spindle firing and slowing nerve conduction velocity [53–61]. These techniques seem to be most effective for local treatment of muscle spasms and not for generalized spasticity.

Table 14-5. Neurotransmitters

Excitatory
Aspartate, glutamine, substance P
Inhibitory
Glycine
Presynaptic inhibition
GABA

EMG biofeedback has been used to reduce tone by either direct relaxation of the spastic muscle or facilitating antagonist muscle recovery. This technique has had mixed success in published reports owing to a wide range of experimental protocols and different patient populations [62–65]. More controlled studies are needed to establish the effectiveness of this modality.

Electrical stimulation of either agonist or antagonist muscle has been reported to temporarily reduce tone [66–72]. Previous studies using electrical stimulation have been poorly controlled and typically have used either the Ashworth scale or the pendulum test to quantify spasticity. Using a servo-controlled motor-driven device to quantify spasticity in our laboratory, there was a significant delay in the onset of the stretch reflex or reduction in tone after cutaneous stimulation of the antagonist dermatome. These reductions of the stretch reflex response lasted up to 50 minutes following 5–10 minutes of stimulation, whereas stimulation of the spastic muscle itself or antagonist muscle stimulation produced an earlier onset of the stretch reflex or an increase in tone [73–75]. Although the mechanism is not entirely clear, these beneficial effects may be due to reciprocal inhibition of the stretch reflex. Additional studies are being done to further delineate which stimulation parameters and stimulus locations will be the most effective at reducing spasticity.

Medications

Medications can be used as the next line of potential treatment but are limited by potential side effects. Baclofen, diazepam, and dantrolene sodium are the most widely used medications. Baclofen and diazepam act centrally and dantrolene sodium works peripherally at the level of the muscle.

Baclofen is a gamma-aminobutyric acid (GABA) analogue that unlike GABA, can easily cross the blood–brain barrier and bind to the GABA B receptor, which presynaptically interferes with the release of excitatory neurotransmitters [76–78] (Table 14-5). Baclofen has been more effective in spasticity due to spinal cord lesions rather than cortical or subcortical lesions [43]. It is effective in reducing flexor spasms and increasing range of motion [79, 80]. Although usually well tolerated, side effects include muscle weakness, sedation, hypotonia, ataxia, confusion, and hallucinations [81, 82]. Seizures and hallucinations have been reported with sudden withdrawal [83]. The dosage of baclofen starts at 10 mg/day, with a maximum recommended dose of 80 mg/day, in divided doses. Some patients have tolerated higher doses (up to 120 mg/day).

Diazepam, or other benzodiazepines, enhances presynaptic inhibition in the spinal cord and at supraspinal levels by potentiating the postsynaptic effects of GABA [76, 84]. Benzodiazepines act at the brain stem reticular formation, which may be more sensitive to the drug's effects, and spinal polysynaptic pathways [85, 86]. Typically diazepam is added to baclofen after an adequate trial of baclofen fails to relieve spasticity. Common side effects include sedation and reduced memory, attention, and motor coordination [87]. These potential side effects make diazepam more appropriate for patients with spinal cord injuries rather than those with cortical lesions. The dosage of diazepam starts at 2 mg/day, with a maximum of 60 mg/day [43, 88]. Ketazolam, a benzodiazepine, and clorazepate, a benzodiazepine analogue, have also been used to treat spasticity [89–91].

Dantrolene sodium is recommended for cerebral spasticity because it is the only medication that works at the level of the muscle, but it is limited by potential side effects [43, 85, 88]. Dantrolene reduces the release of calcium from the sarcoplasmic reticulum, which is important for the activation myosin-ATPase, thus weakening muscle contraction [85]. Dantrolene affects fast twitch muscles more than slow twitch, and fortunately has little effect on cardiac or smooth muscle [92]. The major side effect of dantrolene is weakness, which limits its usefulness in stroke patients [88]. Other side effects include hepatotoxicity (<1%), mild sedation, dizziness, diarrhea, nausea, and vomiting. The dosage starts at 25–50 mg/day, with a maximum recommended dose of 400 mg/day, in divided doses [92]. Liver enzyme levels should be checked regularly and the drug stopped if abnormalities develop.

Clonidine, an alpha$_2$-agonist, has had mixed success in the treatment of spinal spasticity [93, 94]. Clonidine reduces the sympathetic outflow from the brain and brain stem and may inhibit afferent input to the spastic reflex arc at the substantia gelatinosa of the dorsal horns [88]. A dosage of 0.1–0.4 mg/day has been used orally or, more conveniently, with a transdermal patch. Side effects include postural hypotension, depressed mood, syncope, nausea, and vomiting.

Investigational drugs such as progabide, tizanidine, tetrahydrocannabinol (THC), and glycine have had limited success in the literature. Progabide, a GABA agonist that binds to both A and B receptors, reduced tone in patients with multiple sclerosis without improving function but was limited by a high incidence of side effects including elevated liver enzymes (30%), weakness, and fever [95–97]. Tizanidine, a central alpha$_2$-agonist may inhibit spinal polysynaptic pathways by facilitating the release of glycine. Several studies have compared tizanidine to baclofen with similar effectiveness [98–106], although tizanidine was more sedating but caused less weakness than baclofen. Both tizanidine and baclofen are more effective at reducing tone in extensor muscles than flexors. One study compared tizanidine to diazepam in cerebral spasticity and found improved walking distance and less sedation than diazepam [107]. Sedation may be the limiting factor in using this medication for cerebral spasticity. THC, the active component of marijuana, has been reported to reduce spasticity [108]. A study of nine patients with multiple sclerosis showed reduction in spasticity with 10 mg THC compared with control subjects, without the patients feeling "high" [109]. Preliminary reports using glycine, an important inhibitory neurotransmitter, have demonstrated subjective improvements in spasticity [110, 111]. Another study using threonine, a precursor of glycine, has offered encouraging results [112]. Additional controlled studies using these agents are needed to fully evaluate their potential effectiveness.

Chemical Neurolysis

Chemical blocks of peripheral nerves or muscles may be used to temporarily reduce spasticity in a specific muscle or group of muscles. Commonly used agents include phenol, local anesthetics, and more recently botulinum toxin [113].

Temporary blocks such as lidocaine or bupivacaine can also be used to help distinguish contracture from spasticity, improve brace fitting, facilitate serial casting, or evaluate whether a longer acting agent would be beneficial. Although the pharmacologic effect of these agents is only several hours [114], the functional effect may last for weeks if the block is combined with a consistent stretching program and bivalved casting or splinting. It is important to monitor the patient's skin for pressure effects from casting as the effects of the block wear off.

Phenol (2–6% solution) injections of peripheral nerves or muscles has been an effective method of reducing spasticity and typically last 3–6 months. This technique has been shown to improve gait, sitting positioning, and reduce painful spasms and clonus [115–126]. Phenol has a higher incidence of painful dysesthesias (2–32%), which can be minimized by avoiding mixed nerves. Other potential side effects of phenol include loss of useful motor function or muscle imbalance, edema, infection, and deep venous thrombosis [114].

Recent reports using botulinum toxin to weaken spastic muscle have had encouraging results [127–129]. Botulinum toxin inhibits the release of acetylcholine at the neuromuscular junction and has primarily been used for strabismus, torticollis, and facial dystonias [130–134]. The initial effect is not seen for several days but may last for 3–4 months [135]. Possible side effects include weakness of adjacent muscles, transient fatigue, and nausea [136]. Further study is needed to evaluate the long-term effectiveness of botulinum toxin in the treatment of spasticity.

Surgical Management

Surgical procedures are typically reserved for those patients who have not responded to the usual medications or as a "last resort." The most successful is intrathecal baclofen, which was recently approved by the U.S. Food and Drug Administration for the treatment of spasticity caused by multiple sclerosis or spinal cord injury [137, 138]. It involves the infusion of the drug into the subarachnoid space from a subcutaneously implanted pump. The programmable pump is about the size of a hockey puck (7.5 cm diameter and 2.8 cm thick) and is implanted in the lateral abdomen. Direct infusion of baclofen into the cerebrospinal fluid increases its concentration 50 times [139, 140]. Several placebo-controlled studies have demonstrated dramatic reductions in muscle tone and spasms with a low incidence of side effects [141–147]. The most common side effects were drowsiness, nausea, weakness, hypotension, and headache, which usually resolved with reducing the dosage. Overdose can cause seizures, coma, or respiratory depression. Other possible complications include pump failure and infection [148–150]. Because of the potential side effects this intervention should be reserved for those patients who have not responded to oral baclofen.

Orthopedic procedures such as tendon transfers or lengthening have been more successful in the lower extremities. In particular the split anterior tibial transfer in combination with an Achilles tendon lengthening has demonstrated success at improving equinovarus deformity in hemiplegia and improving gait [151–154]. Given the complex nature of upper limb function, tendon transfers have been less successful. Obturater neurectomy combined with iliopsoas myotomy can be used to improve positioning and hygiene in patients with severe hip adductor and hip flexor spasticity [40].

Selective posterior rhizotomy, primarily in the lumbosacral areas, has been used in cerebral palsy patients with a low incidence of recurrence [155, 156]. Again this technique is limited to only the severe cases of spasticity. Percutaneous rhizotomies using a radiofrequency needle have also been used successfully with few complications [157–159]. Cordotomy or myelotomy are the last resort for the most severe cases of spasticity and are rarely done [160–163].

Case Management Study

One year previously, a 29-year-old man sustained a brain injury in a motor vehicle collision. He initially received extensive inpatient therapy and was eventually transferred to a skilled nursing facility. He was seen in our outpatient clinic because of increased pain in his right arm and leg and difficulty with hygiene, wheelchair positioning, and transfers.

Physical examination revealed isolated movement of his left arm and leg with no volitional movement and markedly increased tone of his right arm and leg. He had flexion contractures of the right elbow, wrist, and fingers. His right hip was adducted and flexed. There were also flexion contractures of both knees and the left hip. Initial evaluation included x-ray films, which revealed heterotopic ossification in both hips.

He was started on a low dose of dantrolene with only a slight reduction in tone. Higher doses were limited by increased daytime drowsiness. He had difficulty sleeping at night because of spasms, which were reduced with an evening dose of diazepam. A low dose of baclofen was also tried with only a slight improvement in tone reduction. He continued to be limited by marked increased tone of his right arm and both hips and knees. To further evaluate range of motion in the right arm and both legs and to facilitate casting, temporary nerve blocks with local anesthetics were done. An epidural block with local anesthetic was done to evaluate range of motion at both hips and knees. We have used this technique in previous patients to help distinguish the degree of range of motion limited by heterotopic ossification, joint contracture, and spasticity.

After the patient's epidural block, there continued to be limited range of motion at both hips and only 10 degrees of improved knee extension. Because of this, it was decided that the surgical approach would be more effective than motor point or additional nerve blocks. The patient eventually underwent surgery for removal of the heterotopic ossification and release of the hamstrings and hip adductors. After the surgery he had improved range of motion at both hips and knees with improved sitting balance and reduced spasms.

A brachial plexus block with a local anesthetic was done to evaluate his right arm. This revealed improved range of motion at the right elbow, wrist, and fingers. Because of this, it was felt that a motor point block with a longer-acting agent would be appropriate. His right wrist and finger flexors, pronator teres, brachialis, pectoralis major, and brachial radialis were all injected with a total dose of 400 units botulinum toxin. After 2–3 days, he had improved range of motion of his right arm and reduced pain. The injection also helped facilitate hygiene and splinting.

This case study illlustrates how the management of spasticity in a complicated patient involves an interdisciplinary approach based on patient-specific goals. Achieving these goals required proper evaluation, splinting, oral medication, and the use of temporary nerve blocks, longer-acting motor point blocks, and surgical procedures. In this patient, as in other patients, the temporary nerve blocks were useful in evaluating the potential effectiveness of longer-acting agents such as botulinum toxin, and to help guide the surgical approach.

Conclusion

Despite the complex nature of spasticity, successful management is crucial to improving function and quality of life in patients with UMN lesions. More research is needed to help understand the pathophysiology of spasticity so that more effective treatments can be identified. A standardized method of quantifying spasticity is needed so that therapeutic interventions can be evaluated with multicenter trials. Stepped care or a pyramidal approach, with a clear understanding of the patient's goals followed by the use of a wide range of rehabilitation resources, is crucial to the successful management of spasticity. As with other medical or surgical interventions, potential side effects must be weighed against potential benefits.

References

1. Lance JW. Symposium synopsis. In RG Feldman, RR Young, WP Koella (eds), Spasticity: Disordered Motor Control. Chicago: Year Book, 1980;487.
2. Landau WM. Spasticity: What is it? What is it not? In RG Feldman, RR Young, WP Koella (eds), Spasticity: Disordered Motor Control. Chicago: Year Book, 1980;17.
3. Shahani BT, Young RR. The flexor reflex in spasticity. In RG Feldman, RR Young, WP Koella (eds), Spasticity: Disordered Motor Control. Chicago: Year Book, 1980;287.
4. Young RR, Wierzbicka MD. Behavior of single motor units in normal subjects and in patients with spastic paresis. In PJ Delwaide, RR Young (eds), Clinical Neurophysiology in Spasticity: Contribution to Assessment and Pathophysiology. Amsterdam: Elsevier, 1985;27.
5. Katz RT, Rymer WZ. Spastic hypertonia mechanisms and measurement. Arch Phys Med Rehabil 1989;70:144.
6. Rymer WZ, Houk JC, Crago PE. Mechanisms of the clasp-knife reflex studied in an animal model. Exp Brain Res 1979;37:93.
7. Whitlock JA. Neurophysiology of spasticity. In MB Glenn, J Whyte (eds), Practical Management of Spasticity in Children and Adults. Philadelphia: Lea & Febiger, 1990;8.
8. Gordon J, Ghez C. Muscle receptors and spinal reflexes: The stretch reflex. In ER Kandel, JH Schwartz, TM Jessell (eds), Principles of Neural Science (3rd ed). New York: Elsevier, 1991;564.
9. Lee WA, Boughton A, Rymer WZ. Absence of stretch reflex gain enhancement in voluntarily activated spastic muscle. Exp Neurol 1987;98:317.
10. Powers RK, Campbell DL, Rymer WZ. Stretch reflex dynamics in spastic elbow flexor muscles. Ann Neurol 1989;25:3242.
11. Powers RK, Marder-Meyer J, Rymer WZ. Quantitative relations between hypertonia and stretch reflex threshold in spastic hemiparesis. Ann Neurol 1988;23:115.
12. Pierrot-DesiDigny E, Mazieres L. Spinal mechanisms underlying spasticity. In PJ Delwaide, RR Young (eds), Clinical Neurophysiology in Spasticity: Contribution to Assessment and Pathophysiology. Amsterdam: Elsevier, 1985;63.
13. Hochman S, McCrea DA. The effect of chronic spinal transection on homonymous Ia EPSP rise times in triceps surae motoneurons in the cat. Abstr Soc Neurosci 1987;186:12.
14. Hounsgard J, Hultborn H, Jesperson B, Kiehr O. Intrinsic membrane properties causing a bistable behavior of alpha-motoneurons. Exp Brain Res 1984;55:391.
15. Dietrichson P. Phasic ankle reflexes in spasticity and parkinsonian rigidity. The possible role of the fusimotor system. Acta Neurol Scand 1971;47:22.
16. Dietrichson P. Tonic ankle reflexes in parkinsonian rigidity and spasticity. The possible role of the fusimotor system. Acta Neurol Scand 1971;47:163.
17. Rushworth G. Spasticity and rigidity: An experimental study and review. J Neurol Neurosurg Psychiatry 1960;23:99.
18. Rodin BE, Sampogna SL, Kruger L. An examination of intraspinal sprouting in dorsal root axons with the tracer horseradish peroxidase. J Comp Neurol 1983;215:187.
19. Nygren LG, Fuxe K, Gosta J, Olson L. Functional regeneration of 5-hydroxytryptamine nerve terminals in the rat spinal cord following 5,6-dihydroxytryptamine induced degeneration. Brain Res 1974;78:377.
20. Nygren LG, Olson L. On spinal noradrenaline receptor supersensitivity: Correlation between nerve terminal densities and flexor reflexes various times after intracisternal 6-hydroxydopamine. Brain Res 1976;116:455.
21. Burke D, Ashby P. Are spinal "presynaptic" inhibitory mechanisms suppressed in spasticity? J Neurol Sci 1972;15:321.
22. Iles JF, Roberts RC. Presynaptic inhibition of monosynaptic reflexes in the lower limbs of subjects with upper

motoneuron disease. J Neurol Neurosurg Psychiatry 1986;49:937.

23. Bohannon RW, Smith MB. Interrater reliability on a modified Ashworth scale of muscle spasticity. Phys Ther 1987;67:206.

24. Brunnstrom S. Movement Therapy in Hemiplegia. New York: Harper & Row, 1970.

25. Fugl-Meyer AR, Jaasko L, Leyman I, et al. The post-stroke hemiplegic patient: A method for evaluation of physical performance. Scand J Rehabil Med 1975;7:13.

26. Delwaide PJ. Contribution of human reflex studies to the understanding and management of the pyramidal syndrome. In BT Shahani (ed), Electromyography in Central Nervous System Disorders: Central EMG. Boston: Butterworth, 1984.

27. Delwaide PJ. Electrophysiological testing of spastic patients: Its potential usefulness and limitations. In PJ Delwaide, RR Young (eds), Clinical Neurophysiology in Spasticity: Contributions to Assessment and Pathophysiology. Amsterdam: Elsevier, 1985.

28. Ashby P, Verrier M, Carleton S, Somerville J. Vibratory inhibition of the monosynaptic reflex and presynaptic inhibition in man. In RG Feldman, RR Young, WP Koella (eds), Spasticity: Disordered Motor Control. Chicago: Year Book, 1980.

29. Chan CWY. Some techniques for the relief of spasticity and their physiological basis. Physiother Can 1986;38:85.

30. Wartenberg R. Pendulousness of the legs as a diagnostic test. Neurology 1951;1:18.

31. Boczko M, Mumenthaler M. Modified pendulousness test to assess tonus of thigh muscles in spasticity. Neurology 1958;8:846.

32. Bajd T, Vodovnik L. Pendulum testing of spasticity. J Biomed Eng 1984;6:9.

33. Bajd T, Bowman RG. Testing and modeling of spasticity. J Biomed Eng 1982;4:90.

34. Burke D, Gillies JD. Hamstrings stretch reflex in human spasticity. J Neurol Neurosurg Psychiatry 1971;34:231.

35. Bohannon RW. Variability and reliability of the pendulum test for spasticity using a Cybex II isokinetic dynamometer. Phys Ther 1987;67:659.

36. Powers RK, Campbell DL, Rymer WZ. Stretch reflex dynamics in spastic elbow flexor muscles. Ann Neurol 1989;25:32.

37. Powers RK, Marder-Meyer J, Ryrner WZ. Quantitative relations between hypertonia and stretch reflex threshold in spastic hemiparesis. Ann Neurol 1988;23:115.

38. Katz RT, Rovai G, Brait C, Rymer WZ. Objective quantification of spastic hypertonia: Correlation with clinical findings. Arch Phys Med Rehabil 1992;73:339.

39. Gans BM, Glenn MB. Introduction. In MB Glenn, J Whyte (eds), Practical Management of Spasticity in Children and Adults. Philadelphia, Lea & Febiger, 1990;1.

40. Merritt J. Management of spasticity in spinal cord injury. Mayo Clinic Proc 1981;56:614.

41. Pierce DS, Nickel VH. The Total Care of Spinal Cord Injuries. Boston: Little, Brown, 1977;86.

42. Guttman L. Spinal Cord Injury—Comprehensive Management and Research. Oxford: Blackwell Scientific, 1976;517.

43. Katz RT. Management of spasticity. Am J Phys Med Rehabil 1988;67:108.

44. Castellucci VF, Kandel ER. A quantal analysis of the synaptic depression underlying habituation of the gill-withdrawal reflex in *Aplysia*. Proc Natl Acad Sci USA 1974;71:5004.

45. Castellucci VF, Carew TJ, Kandel ER. Cellular analysis of long-term habituation of the gill withdrawal reflex of *Aplysia californica*. Science 1978;202:1306.

46. Bobath B. Adult Hemiplegia: Evaluation and Treatment. London: Heinemann, 1970.

47. Kaplan N. Effect of splinting on reflex inhibition and sensorimotor stimulation in treatment of spasticity. Arch Phys Med Rehabil 1962;43:565.

48. Booth BJ, Doyle M, Montgomery J. Serial casting for the management of spasticity in the head-injured adult. Phys Ther 1983;63:1960.

49. McPherson JJ, Becker AH, Franszczak N. Dynamic splint to reduce the passive component of hypertonicity. Arch Phys Med Rehabil 1985;66:249.

50. Collins K, Oswald P, Burger G, Nolden G. Customized adjustable orthoses: Their use in spasticity. Arch Phys Med Rehabil 1985;66:397.

51. Otis JC, Root L, Kroll MA. Measurement of plantar flexor spasticity during treatment with tone-reducing casts. J Pediatr Orthop 1985;5:682.

52. Giebler KB. Physical modalities. In MB Glenn, J Whyte (eds), Practical Management of Spasticity in Children and Adults. Philadelphia: Lea & Febiger, 1990;118.

53. Levine MG, Kabat H, Knott M, Voss DE. Relaxation of spasticity by physiological techniques. Arch Phys Med Rehabil 1954;35:214.

54. Hartviksen K. Ice therapy in spasticity. Acta Neurol Scand 1962;38(Suppl 3):79.

55. Miglietta O. Evaluation of cold in spasticity. Am J Phys Med 1962;41:148.

56. Miglietta O. Electromyographic characteristics of clonus and influence of cold. Arch Phys Med Rehabil 1964;45:508.

57. Knutsson E. On effects of local cooling upon motor functions in spastic paresis. Prog Phys Ther 1970;1:124.

58. Mecomber SA, Herman RM. Effects of local hypothermia on reflex and voluntary activity. Phys Ther 1971;51:271.

59. Miglietta O. Action of cold on spasticity. Am J Phys Med 1973;52:198.

60. Lightfoot E, Verrier M, Ashby P. Neurophysiological effects of prolonged cooling of the calf in patients with complete spinal transection. Phys Ther 1975;55:251.

61. Chan CWY. Some techniques for the relief of spasticity and their physiological basis. Physiother Can 1986;38:85.

62. Basmajian JV. Biofeedback in rehabilitation: A review of principles and practices. Arch Phys Med Rehabil 1981;62:469.

63. Wolf SL, Binder-MacLeon SA. Electromyographic biofeedback applications to the hemiplegic patient: Changes in upper extremity neuromuscular and functional status. Phys Ther 1983;63:1393.

64. Wolf SL, Binder-MacLeod SA. Electromyographic biofeedback applications to the hemiplegic patient: Changes in lower extremity neuromuscular and functional status. Phys Ther 1983;63:1404.

65. DeBacher G. Biofeedback in spasticity control. In JV Basmajian (ed), Biofeedback: Principles and Practice for Clinicians (3rd ed). Baltimore: Williams & Wilkins, 1989;141.

66. Alfieri V. Electrical treatment of spasticity. Scand J Rehabil Med 1982;14:177.

67. Bajd T, Gregoric M, Vodovnik L, Benko H. Electrical stimulation in treating spasticity resulting from spinal cord injury. Arch Phys Med Rehabil 1985;66:515.

68. Hines AE, Crago PE, Billian C. Functional electrical stimulation for the reduction of spasticity in the hemiplegic hand. Biomed Sci Instrum 1993;29:259.

69. Vodovnik L, Bowman BR, Winchester P. Effects of electrical stimulation on spinal spasticity. Scand J Rehabil Med 1984;19:29.

70. Vodovnik L, Stefanovska A, Bajd T. Effects of stimulation parameters on modification of spinal spasticity. Med Biol Eng Comput 1987;25:439.

71. Robinson CJ, Kett NA, Bolam JM. Spasticity in spinal cord injured patients: Short term effects of electrical stimulation. Arch Phys Med Rehabil 1988;69:598.

72. Robinson CJ, Kett NA, Bolam JM. Spasticity in spinal cord injured patients: Initial measures and long term effects of surface electrical stimulation. Arch Phys Med Rehabil 1988;69:862.

73. Given JD, Dewald JPA, McGuire JR, Heckman CJ, et al. Changes in stretch reflex threshold in spastic muscle as a result of electrical stimulation. Soc Neurosci Abstr 1991;17:1033.

74. Given JD, Dewald JPA, McGuire JR, Buchanan TS, et al. Evidence for changes in muscle mechanical properties and stretch reflex characteristics in spastic hemiparetic stroke. Soc Neurosci Abstr 1992;18:1411.

75. Dewald JPA, Given JD, Rymer WZ. Significant reductions in upper limb spasticity in hemiparetic stroke using cutaneous levels of electrical stimulation. Soc Neurosci Abstr 1993;19:990.

76. Davidoff RA. Antispasticity drugs: Mechanisms of action. Ann Neurol 1985;17:107.

77. Faigle JW, Keberle H, Degen PH. Chemistry and pharmacokinetics of baclofen. In RG Feldman, RR Young, WP Koella (eds), Spasticity: Disordered Motor Control. Chicago: Year Book, 1980.

78. Koella WP. Baclofen: Its general pharmacology and neuropharmacology. In RG Feldman, RR Young, WP Koella (eds), Spasticity: Disordered Motor Control. Chicago: Year Book, 1980.

79. Duncan GW, Shahani BT, Young RR. An evaluation of baclofen treatment for certain symptoms in patients with spinal cord lesions. Neurology 1976;26:441.

80. Sachais BA, Logue JN, Carey MS. Baclofen, a new antispastic drug. Arch Neurol 1977;34:422.

81. Hattab JR. Review of European clinical trials with baclofen. In RG Feldman, RR Young, WP Koella (eds), Spasticity: Disordered Motor Control. Chicago: Year Book, 1980.

82. Knutsson E, Lindblom U, Martensson A. Lioresal and spasticity. Acta Neurol Scand 1972;48(Suppl 51):449.

83. Terrence DV, Fromm GH. Complications of baclofen withdrawal. Arch Neurol 1981;38:588.

84. Costa E, Guidotti A. Molecular mechanisms in the receptor action of benzodiazepines. Annu Rev Pharmacol Toxicol 1979;19:531.

85. Young RR, Delwaide PJ. Drug therapy: Spasticity. N Engl J Med 1981;304:28, 96.

86. Tseng T, Wang S. Locus of action of centrally acting muscle relaxants diazepam and tybamate. J Pharmcol Exp Ther 1971;178:350.

87. Glenn MB. Antispasticity medications in the patient with traumatic brain injury. J Head Trauma Rehabil 1986;1:71.

88. Whyte J, Robinson KM. Pharmacologic management. In MB Glenn, J Whyte (eds), Practical Management of Spasticity in Children and Adults. Philadelphia: Lea & Febiger, 1990;201.

89. Basmajian JV, Shankardass K, Russell D, et al. Ketazolam treatment for spasticity: Double-blind study of a new drug. Arch Phys Med Rehabil 1984;65:698.

90. Basmajian JV, Shankardass K, Russell D. Ketazolam once daily for spasticity: Double-blind cross-over study. Arch Phys Med Rehabil 1986;67:556.

91. Lossius R, Dietrichson P, Lunde PKM. Effect of clorazepate in spasticity and rigidity: A quantitative study of reflexes and plasma concentrations. Acta Neurol Scand 1985;71:190.

92. Pinder RM, Brogden RN, Speight TM, Avery GS. Dantrolene sodium: A review of its pharmacological properties and therapeutic efficacy in spasticity. Drugs 1977;13:3.

93. Nance PW, Shears AH, Nance DM. Clonidine in spinal cord injury. Can Med Assoc J 1985;133:41.

94. Donovan WH, Carter RE, Rossi CD, et al. Clonidine effect on spasticity: A clinical trial. Arch Phys Med Rehabil 1988;69:193.

95. Mondrup K, Pedersen E. The effect of the GABA-agonist, progabide, on stretch and flexor reflexes and on voluntary power in spastic patients. Acta Neurol Scand 1984;69:191.

96. Mondrup K, Pedersen E. The clinical effect of the GABA-agonist, progabide, on spasticity. Acta Neurol Scand 1984;69:200.

97. Rudick RA, Breton D, Krall RL. The GABA-agonist progabide for spasticity in multiple sclerosis. Arch Neurol 1987;44:1033.

98. Newman PM, Nogues M, Newman PK, et al. Tizanidine in the treatment of spasticity. Eur J Clin Pharmacol 1982;23:31.

99. Lapierre Y, Bouchard S, Tansey C, et al. Treatment of spasticity with tizanidine in multiple sclerosis. Can J Neurol Sci 1987;14:513.

100. Corston RN, Johnson F, Godwin-Austen RB. The assessment of drug treatment of spastic gait. J Neurol Neurosurg Psychiatry 1981;44:1035.

101. Hassan N, McLellan DL. Double-blind comparison of single doses of DS103-282, baclofen, and placebo for suppression of spasticity. J Neurol Neurosurg Psychiatr 1980;43:1132.

102. Heazlewood V, Symoniw P, Maruff P, et al. Tizanidine-initial pharmacokinetic studies in patients with spasticity. Eur J Clin Pharmacol 1983;25:65.

103. Smolenski C, Muff S, Smolenski-Kautz S. A double-blind comparative trial of a new muscle-relaxant, tizanidine (DS102282), and baclofen in the treatment of chronic spasticity in multiple sclerosis. Curr Med Res Opin 1981;7:374.

104. Bass B, Weinshenker B, Rice GPA, et al. Tizanidine versus baclofen in the treatment of spasticity in patients with multiple sclerosis. Can J Neurol Sci 1988;15:15.

105. Hoogstraten MC, van der Ploeg RJO, Van der Burg W, et al. Tizanidine versus baclofen in the treatment of multiple sclerosis patients. Acta Neurol Scand 1988;7:224.

106. Stein R, Nordal HJ, Oftedal SI, et al. The treatment of spasticity in multiple sclerosis: A double-blind clinical trial of a new anti-spastic drug tizanidine compared with baclofen. Acta Neurol Scand 1987;75:190.

107. Bes A, Eysette M, Pierrot-Deseilligny E, et al. A multi-centre, double-blind trial of tizanidine, a new antispastic agent, in spasticity associated with hemiplegia. Curr Med Res Opin 1988;10:709.

108. Malec J, Harvey RF, Cayner JJ. Cannabis effect on spasticity in spinal cord injury. Arch Phys Med Rehabil 1982;63:116.

109. Petro DJ, Ellenberger C. Treatment of human spasticity with delta-9-tetrahydrocannabinol. J Clin Pharmacol 1981;21:413S.

110. Stern P, Bokonjic R. Glycine therapy in 7 cases of spasticity. Pharmacology 1974;12:117.

111. Barbeau A. Preliminary study of glycine administration in patients with spasticity. [Abstract.] Neurology 1974;24:392.

112. Barbeau A, Roy M, Chouza C. Pilot study of threonine supplementation in human spasticity. Can J Neurol Sci 1982;9:141.

113. Glenn MB. Nerve blocks. In MB Glenn, J Whyte (eds). Practical Management of Spasticity in Children and Adults. Philadelphia: Lea & Febiger, 1990;227.

114. Ritchie JM, Greene NM. Local anesthetics. In AG Gilman, LS Goodman, LS Rall, F Murad (eds), Goodman and Gilman's The Pharmacological Basis of Therapeutics (7th ed). New York: Macmillan, 1985;302.

115. Awad EA. Intramuscular neurolysis for stroke. Minn Med 1972;8:711.

116. Brattsrom M, Morik U, Svantesson G. Electromyographic studies of peripheral nerve block with phenol. Scand J Rehabil Med 1970;2:17.

117. Copp EP, Harris R, Keenan J. Peripheral nerve block and motor point block with phenol in the management of spasticity. Proc R Soc Med 1970;63:937.

118. Copp EP, Keenan J. Phenol nerve and motor point block in spasticity. Rheum Phys Med 1972;11:287.

119. DeLateur BJ. A new technique of intramuscular phenol neurolysis. Arch Phys Med Rehabil 1972;53:179.

120. Halpern D, Meelhuysen FE. Phenol motor point block in the management of muscular hypertonia. Arch Phys Med Rehabil 1966;47:659.

121. Katz J, Knott LW, Feldman DJ. Peripheral nerve injections with phenol in the management of spastic patients. Arch Phys Med Rehabil 1967;48:97.

122. Khalili AA, Betts HB. Peripheral nerve block with phenol in the management of spasticity: Indications and complications. JAMA 1967;200:1155.

123. Moritz U. Phenol block of peripheral nerves. Scand J Rehabil Med 1973;5:160.

124. O'Hanlan JT, Galford HR, Bosley J. The use of 45% alcohol to control spasticity. Va Med Monthly 1969;96:429.

125. Petrillo CR, Chu DS, Davis SW. Phenol block on the tibial nerve in the hemiplegic patient. Orthopedics 1980;3:871.

126. Spira R. Management of spasticity in cerebral palsied children by peripheral nerve block with phenol. Dev Med Child Neurol 1971;13:164.

127. Borg-Stein J, Pine ZM, Miller J, Brin M. Botulinum toxin for treatment of spasticity in multiple sclerosis. [Abstract.] Am J Phys Med Rehabil 1992;71:251.

128. Das TK, Park DM. Botulinum toxin in treatment spasticity. Br J Cerebral Palsy 1989;43:401.

129. Snow U, Tsui JKC, Bhatt MH, et al. Treatment of spasticity with botulinum toxin: A double blind study. Ann Neurol 1990;28:512.

130. Borodic GE, Cozzolino D. Blepharospasm and its treatment, with emphasis on the use of botulinum toxin. Plast Reconstr Surg 1989;83:546.

131. Botulinum toxin for ocular muscle disorders. Med Lett Drugs Ther 1990;32:100.

132. Greene P, Kang U, Fahn S, et al. Double-blind, placebo controlled trial of botulinum toxin for the treatment of spasmodic torticollis. Neurology 1990;40:1213.

133. Jankovic J, Brin MF. Therapeutic use of botulinum toxin. N Engl J Med 1991;324:1186.

134. Schwartz KS, Jankovic J. Predicting the response to botulinum toxin injections for the treatment of cervical dystonia. [Abstract.] Neurology 1990;40(Suppl 1):382.

135. Borg-Stein J, Stein J. Update on pharmacology: Pharmacology of botulinum toxin and implications for use in disorders of muscle tone. J Head Trauma Rehabil 1993;8:103.

136. Greene P, Kang U, Fahn S, et al. Double-blind, placebo controlled trial of botulinum toxin for the treatment of spasmodic torticollis. Neurology 1990;40:1213.

137. Muller H, Zierski J, Dralle D, Borner U, et al. The effect of intrathecal baclofen on electrical muscle activity in spasticity. J Neurol 1987;234:348.

138. Hankey GJ, Steward-Wynne EG, Perlman D. Intrathecal baclofen for severe spasticity. Med J Aust 1986;145:465.

139. Faigle JW, Keberle H. The chemistry and kinetics of Lioresal. Postgrad Med J 1972;48(Suppl):9.

140. Muller H, Zierski J, Dralle D, et al. Pharmacokinetics of intrathecal baclofen. In H Muller, J Zierski, RD Penn (eds), Local Spinal Therapy of Spasticity. Berlin: Springer, 1988;253.

141. Coffey R, Cahill D, Steers W, et al. Intrathecal baclofen for intractable spasticity of spinal origin: Results of a long-term multicenter study. J Neurosurg 1993;78:226.

142. Loubser PG, Narayan R, Sandin KJ, et al. Continuous infusion of intrathecal baclofen: Long term effects on spasticity in spinal cord injury. Paraplegia 1991;29:48.

143. Ochs G, Struppler A, Meyerson BA, et al. Intrathecal baclofen for long term treatment of spasticity: A multicenter study. J Neurol Neurosurg Psychiatry 1989;52:933.

144. Parke B, Penn RD, Savoy SM, Corcos D. Functional outcome after delivery of intrathecal baclofen. Arch Phys Med Rehabil 1989;70:30.

145. Penn RD. Intrathecal baclofen for severe spasticity. Ann NY Acad Sci 1988;531:157.

146. Penn RD, Kroin JS. Long-term intrathecal baclofen infusion for treatment of spasticity. J Neurosurg 1987;66:181.

147. Penn RD, Savoy SM, Corcos D, et al. Intrathecal baclofen for severe spinal spasticity. N Engl J Med 1989;320:1517.

148. Delhaas EM, Brouwers JRB. Intrathecal baclofen overdose: Report of 7 events in 5 patients and review of the literature. Int J Clin Pharmacol Ther Toxicol 1991;29:274.

149. Muller H, Zierski J. Long-term intrathecal baclofen infusion. In CD Marsden (ed), Treating Spasticity: Pharmacological Advances. Toronto: Hans Huber, 1989;55.

150. Teddy P, Jamous A, Gardner B, et al. Complications of intrathecal baclofen delivery. Br J Neurosurg 1992;6:115.

151. Waters RL, Perry J, Garland DE. Surgical correction of gait abnormalities following stroke. Clin Orthop 1978;131:54.

152. Keenan MAE. The orthopedic management of spasticity. J Head Trauma Rehabil 1987;2:62.

153. Craig CL, Zimbler S. Orthopedic procedures. In MB Glenn, J Whyte (eds), Practical Management of Spasticity in Children and Adults. Philadelphia: Lea & Febiger, 1990;268.

154. Waters RL, Frazier J, Garland DE, et al. Electromyographic gait analysis before and after operative treatment for hemiplegic equinus and equinovarus deformity. J Bone Joint Surg [Am] 1982;64:284.

155. Fasano VA, Broggi G, Barolat-Romana G, Sguazzi A. Surgical treatment of spasticity in cerebral palsy. Child Brain 1978;4:289.

156. Sindou M, Mifsud JJ, Boisson D, Goutelle A. Selective posterior rhizotomy in the dorsal root entry zone for treatment of hyperspasticity and pain in the hemiplegic upper limb. Neurosurgery 1986;18:587.

157. Herz DA, Parsons KC, Pearl L. Percutaneous radiofrequency foramenal rhizotomies. Spine 1983;8:729.

158. Kennemore D. Radiofrequency neurotomy for peripheral pain and spasticity syndromes. Contemp Neurosurg 1983;5:1.

159. Kasdon DL, Lathi E. A prospective study of radiofrequency rhizotomy in the treatment of post-traumatic spasticity. Neurosurgery 1984;15:526.

160. Ivan LP. Longitudinal (Bischof's) myelotomy. In HH Schmidek, WH Sweet (eds), Operative Neurosurgical Techniques: Indications, Methods, and Results. New York: Grune & Stratton, 1982;1163.

161. Benedetti A, Colombo F. Spinal surgery for spasticity (46 cases). Neurochirurgia 1981;24:195.

162. Laitinen L, Singounas E. Longitudinal myelotomy in the treatment of spasticity of the legs. J Neurosurg 1971;35:536.

163. Kasdon DL. Controversies in the surgical management of spasticity. Clin Neurosurg 1986;33:523.

Chapter 15
Autonomic Dysreflexia

Christina Marciniak and David Chen

Autonomic dysreflexia (AD) is an aberrant auto-nomic response that occurs in persons with lesions above the sympathetic outflow from the spinal cord, generally above the sixth thoracic vertebra (T-6). Sympathetic hyperactivity predominates over the parasympathetic activity following noxious stimula-tion below the level of the spinal cord injury (SCI). Although cases of AD have been described in the setting of pure progressive autonomic failure [1] and brain stem or cerebellar tumor resection [2, 3], it is overwhelmingly a disturbance seen in the tetraplegic or high paraplegic population. A variety of terms have been used to describe this phenomenon, in-cluding sympathetic hyperreflexia [4], paroxysmal neurogenic hypertension [5], hypertensive auto-nomic crisis, and autonomic hyperreflexia [6–15].

During episodes of AD a constellation of clinical changes results from hyperactivity of the autonomic nervous system. Patients with clinical features consis-tent with AD were described as early as 1860 by Hilton [16] and 1890 by Bowlby [17]. Head and Riddock de-scribed these same findings in 1917 in the numerous persons with SCIs in World War I [18]. Guttman and Whitterage subsequently provided detailed observa-tions of the clinical manifestations of AD [19]. Because of the severe consequences of untreated episodes, prompt diagnosis and management are paramount.

Pathophysiology

The central autonomic network is a regulatory sys-tem involving control of visceromotor, neuroen-docrine, complex motor, and pain-modulating con-trol mechanisms. Areas of the telencephalon, dien-cephalon, and brain stem control preganglionic sympathetic and parasympathetic visceromotor out-puts. The nucleus tractus solitarius in the medulla re-lays viscerosensory afferents of the glossopharyngeal as well as the vagus nerves. This area initiates the medullary reflexes controlling cardiovascular, respi-ratory, and autonomic afferents as well as providing viscerosensory inputs to other central autonomic ner-vous system regions [20].

Spinal afferents follow the sympathetic trunk, re-laying both nociceptive and nonnociceptive informa-tion to the central autonomic network as well as interacting in segmental spinal autonomic reflexes. The principal output of the central nervous system is via the preganglionic sympathetic neurons in the in-teromediolateral cell column (T2 to L1 segments of the spinal cord) and parasympathetic output carried by the vagus nerve and the sacral spinal cord [20].

Following spinal cord injuries at or above the T6 level, transmission of impulses from the vasomotor center to the interomediolateral cell column (inner-vating splanchnic vascular beds and lower limbs) is interrupted. Immediately after the injury, patients experience "spinal shock": sympathetic nervous system activity is reduced, muscles are flaccid, and muscle stretch reflexes are absent. Bladder and bowel activity is reduced because of diminished sacral parasympathetic activity [21]. Blood pressure is decreased, most likely because of a reduction in sympathetic vasomotor activity as evidenced by re-duced plasma norepinephrine and epinephrine lev-

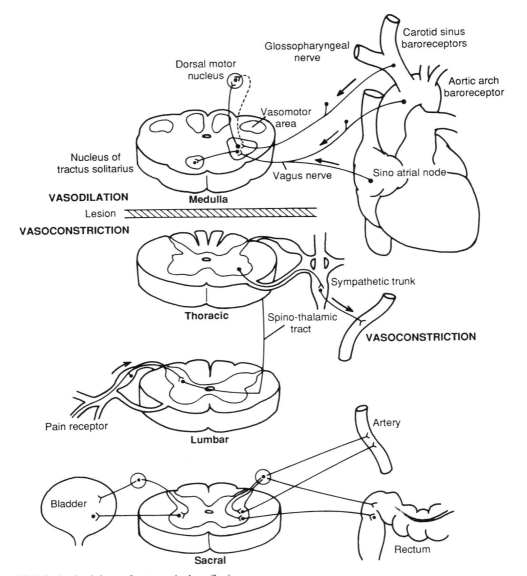

Figure 15-1. Pathophysiology of autonomic dysreflexia.

els. Orthostatic hypotension may be severe because of the lack of reflex sympathetic vasoconstrictor activity [22]. Norepinephrine and 5-hydroxytryptamine are reduced in areas below the level of the spinal cord transection in the sympathetic lateral column and the ventral horn. These amines act as inhibitory neurotransmitters; their decrease may allow facilitation of the cord below the SCI [23].

Within weeks to months after the SCI, reflex cord activity returns. The cardiovascular and other sympathetically mediated changes seen with AD may then occur. Following the onset of noxious, proprioceptive, or other sensory stimuli below the level of the SCI, impulses travel to the spinal cord, synapsing within the dorsal columns and spinothalamic tract, as well as with multilevel infrasegmental sympathetic neurons in the interomediolateral cell column, reflexively activating them [23] (Figure 15-1). The resultant sympathetic discharge leads to peripheral and splanchnic vasoconstriction with profound elevations in blood pressure. The sudden increase in blood pressure is sensed by the intact carotid and aortic baroreceptors. Impulses traveling via cranial nerves X and XI transmit information to brain stem centers. Central activation of the vagus nerve excites cholinergic receptors of the heart with resultant bradycardia [24]. Blocked at the level of the SCI, inhibitory fibers from the vasomotor center, although activated, can only affect sympathetic activity above the SCI. Thus, vasodilation occurs above the SCI but vasoconstriction continues unchecked below that level. Studies of catecholamine metabolism have found lower resting levels of plasma norepinephrine and epinephrine in tetraplegics [25]. Following the onset of bladder stimulation, an increase in blood pressure results in increased norepinephine but not epinephrine levels. Norepinephrine is a transmitter at sympathetic adrenergic nervous terminals and its increase reflects increased sympathetic nervous activity [5]. Plasma prostaglandins (PGE2) are elevated during and following episodes of AD [26] and may be in part responsible for release of catecholamines [27]. PGE2 also may be responsible for the headache seen with AD [26]. Dopamine beta-hydroxylase activity increases [28, 29] as well, indicating increased release of catecholamines from the adrenal medulla and nerve endings [27]. Alpha-adrenergic blockers such as phenoxybenzamine can suppress the symptoms, confirming the impression of a sympathetic origin for the hypertension [27].

When nonhypertensive doses of tritiated norepinephrine are infused in patients with SCIs, more tritium is retained than in healthy controls. Following infusion of larger hypertensive doses, plasma norepinephrine concentrations are inappropriately high, which is indicative of an increased response to exogenous catecholamines or denervation hypersensitivity [5]. Thus, exaggerated spinal reflexes predominate in the development of AD; however, the absence of inhibitory supraspinal influences also probably plays a role [30, 31].

Studies of continuous ambulatory blood pressure monitoring have found that in patients with SCI who have recently experienced AD, greater coefficients of variation in diastolic blood pressure and heart rate may be seen as compared with persons with SCI without AD and normal control subjects. Systolic blood pressure in persons with SCI with AD is also more variable than in normal subjects [32]. These findings confirm the impression that owing to reduced basal sympathetic nervous system activity below the SCI, exaggerated cardiovascular responses to adrenergic stimulation may be responsible for AD [32].

Demographics

In a retrospective review of 444 patients with SCI at level T6 or above, Lindan found 48% of patients exhibited AD, although a greater prevalence was found in cervical (60%) than thoracic (20%) spinal injuries [33]. Kurnick reported an incidence of 85% in his patient population with similar injury levels [34].

Patients may exhibit signs of AD as early as 1 month postinjury [35]. The majority of patients, however, experience onset of these episodes 3–6 months after injury following the period of spinal shock. Ninety-two percent of patients susceptible to the disorder had their first episode by 1 year, although first attacks have been reported as late as 3–12 years postinjury [33, 35].

Attacks tend to decrease in frequency with time although individual episodes may still be as severe. Signs and symptoms in children are similar, though blood pressure elevations tend to be less severe and hyperhidrosis is not commonly seen [35]. Ninety-two percent of patients in Lindan's series continued to experience AD as long as 20 years after the injury [33].

Clinical Features

Episodes of AD may be triggered by a wide variety of stimuli below the level of the SCI. Stimuli arising from the bladder or other pelvic structures are the most common precipitants. In a series of 105 cases of AD, 84 were brought about by bladder distention or insertion of a urinary catheter [33]. Bladder distention results in significant elevations in systolic blood pressure and pulse pressure [23, 36, 37]. Peaks in blood pressure correlate with elevations in detrusor pressure [38]. Bladder spasms, urinary tract infections, epididymitis, or distention of the bladder during evaluations such as cystometrograms may have the same effect [15, 34, 38–40]. AD at the time of cystoscopy was found in 70% of patients with SCIs at the level of T7 or above [40]. AD during cystometrograms may occur either as a consequence of catheter insertion or bladder filling. Deliberate bladder distension to induce AD to enhance performance by elite tetraplegic athletes has recently been reported [41]. Hyperreflexic bladders may begin contracting at low volumes [42]. Catheter insertion under ultrasonographic control may prevent catheter-induced AD [42]. Ileal conduit loopography is also associated with AD [43]. Misoprostol was reported to produce AD in a tetraplegic patient, presumably as a result of prostaglandin effects on increasing detrusor tone [44]. Rectal examination or distention of the rectum with an impaction, flatulence, at the time of a bowel program, or with an enema may trigger AD [18, 33]. Conditions of the rectal areas such as hemorrhoids and anal fissures also provide sufficient stimulation to begin an episode of AD.

Recurrent AD in association with menstruation was found to resolve with removal of a large ovarian cyst [45]. Occult intra-abdominal processes such as appendicitis, chronic cholecystitis, erosive gastritis, and intestinal volvulus may have symptoms of AD at presentation that aid in detection of the pathologic condition [46]. Testicular torsion [47], pressure on the testicles and glans penis [48], and sexual intercourse in women [49] and men [47] have all been reported to cause AD.

Many cutaneous and proprioceptive stimuli have been described as triggers as well. Ingrown toenails, pressure sores [33], cold exposure [34], high temperature, sunburns [39], and tight clothing including abdominal supports or shoes have all been reported to cause the syndrome. Even dressing changes for pressure sores may produce AD [50] and require premedication before the treatments. Passive stretching at the hip joint with range of motion has been reported to produce AD episodes [35, 51], as have changes in bed positioning [35]. Three cases of AD brought on by transfers into the wheelchair were found to be due to recurrent dislocation of the hip [52]. AD with lower extremity manipulation was also seen in the setting of a femur fracture [53].

Patients at risk for AD should be carefully monitored during functional electrical stimulation. Ashley et al. monitored cardiopulmonary responses to functional electrical stimulation–assisted hydraulic resistance training in 10 high SCI subjects and found that immediately on stimulation, piloerection was seen and systolic blood pressure increased, accompanied by a decrease in heart rate as compared with able-bodied control subjects [6]. Surgery or other therapeutic procedures may result in AD. Extracorporeal shock wave lithotripsy is frequently accompanied by hypertension in patients undergoing this treatment for renal and ureteral calculi [9, 54, 55]. Removal of renal stones via open or percutaneous procedures may have the same effect [8, 56]. Upper extremity surgery [12], and orthopedic procedures [53, 57] may produce AD. The syndrome may occur during recovery from anesthesia [58]. AD has been caused by electroejaculation for the collection of semen for fertility studies or artificial insemination [59], as well as with the use of intrathecal neostigmine for ejaculation [60].

Although pulmonary embolism occurs in 5–14% of acute SCI patients, pulmonary embolism has only rarely been reported to precipitate an episode of AD [10]. The low frequency of occurrence may be related to the timing of acute pulmonary emboli in this setting, which generally occur during the first 4 months following SCI, during the phase of spinal shock [10].

In susceptible women, AD may occur during labor in up to two-thirds of women [13, 61–66]. Symptoms of AD appear simultaneously with labor, though this may be difficult to perceive or distinguish from abdominal spasms. Hypertension from AD needs to be distinguished from pre-eclampsia, which is not increased in this population [67]. Catecholamine release may produce uterine artery vasoconstriction, reducing uterine blood flow and resulting in fetal distress. Continuous monitoring of blood pressure during labor is mandatory in this population [68]. Other consequences of pregnancy that may lead to AD in the woman with SCI include impaired voiding with increased residual urine volume [66] and urinary tract infections [64].

Curiously, AD has also been reported in response to orthostatic challenge. Three SCI subjects who had an initial decrease in blood pressure on becoming upright with use of a tilt table, were then noted to develop hyperhidrosis and hypertension. Symptoms resolved with lying down and patients responded to treatment with mineralocorticoids [69]. Presumably these changes were generated by hypotension-induced sympathetic impulses from blood vessels [69].

Following the introduction of noxious, proprioceptive, or other sensory stimuli below the SCI level, sympathetic adrenergic activity increases. Vasoconstriction of venous and arterial beds results in marked elevations in blood pressure. Increases in blood pressure to 300 mm Hg (50–150 over baseline) and 220 diastolic (40–80 over baseline) have been reported [34, 35, 70]. Carotid and aortic baroreceptor activation occurs in response to the hypertension and, via the vagus nerve, may result in a reduced heart rate. This decrease, however, is inadequate to lower blood pressure significantly [21]. Bradycardia (<60 beats per minute) is considered a characteristic of AD, but is not frequently seen. In patients with lesions above the level of T1, cardiac sympathetic tone may predominate, leading to tachycardia [35]. As the blood pressure increases, patients experience a throbbing headache, bitemporal, bifrontal, or occipital in location [35]. This headache is seen in up to 56% of patients and is thought to be due to either dilatation of cerebral blood vessels or elevations in prostaglandin E_2 [71]. Excessive sweating above and around the spinal cord level occurs from sympathetic cholinergic activity. Neck flushing and congestion of nasal passages are also frequent features [35]. Neurologic deficits include lethargy, visual blurring, aphasia, seizures, blindness, and coma [33, 35]. Ocular findings include mydriasis and lid lag due to compensatory sympathetic discharge above the cord lesion [72]. Prominence of the papillae of the skin and piloerection are seen as a result of stimulating sympathetic postganglionic fibers to the skin [35]. A metallic taste, dyspnea, nausea, and penile erection have also been reported [19, 33, 35].

Laboratory Features

Because of the classic clinical features and characteristic setting in which AD occurs, laboratory evaluations are not generally required. Prompt identification of the precipitating factor and treatment of the condition is usually the primary focus. Chest radiography during episodes of autonomic hyperreflexia show cardiomegaly [19, 70]. This is caused by redistribution of blood from peripheral blood vessels. Electroencephalography during AD does not show any specific changes.

A variety of findings have been reported on electrocardiography. Atrial fibrillation has been reported in association with AD [73, 74]. The vagal stimulation seen in response to the hypertension produces a decreased atrial refractory period, increasing the

rate of atrial repolarization and predisposing to the initiation of atrial fibrillation [75]. Recognition of this finding is important because drugs used in the treatment of AD (guanethidine, nifedipine, and ganglionic blockers) alter atrioventricular node conduction. Use of these drugs may lead to an increase in ventricular response rate in the presence of atrial fibrillation. Other findings on electrocardiography include premature ventricular contractions, premature atrial contractions, bigeminy, first- and second-degree atrioventricular block, and T and U wave changes [19, 76].

Differential Diagnosis

Conditions sharing similar clinical features with AD include toxemia of pregnancy, pheochromocytoma, posterior fossa neoplasms, migraine headaches, cluster headaches, and primary hypertension [35]. Pheochromocytoma can be distinguished from AD, however, because the pallor and vasoconstriction below the level of the SCI in association with facial flushing would be uncharacteristic. Marked elevations in catecholamines would be seen in the setting of pheochromocytoma and are not found in AD [14]. Cluster headaches, although they may produce nasal congestion, sweating, and flushing, generally produce unilateral flushing and headaches. A history of prior episodes may be helpful in cluster or migraine headaches [35]. Posterior fossa neoplasms may produce urinary catecholamines mimicking pheochromocytoma; however, features associated with this neoplasm include a different pattern of neurologic deficits, papilledema, and frequent bradycardia. Toxemia of pregnancy results in more persistent hypertension that does not return to normal after removal of a trigger stimulus [35].

Complications

Untreated AD may produce significant morbidity and even death. Seizures have been reported in association with episodes of AD [35, 77, 78]. The seizure may occur in the absence of an intracranial pathologic condition as determined by computed tomography of the brain [78].

Intracranial and subarachnoid hemorrhage may also be precipitated by the hypertension [77, 79, 80] although this is uncommon. In a survey of the Veterans' Affairs Spinal Cord Injury Center and the Department of Health and Human Services Regional Centers, 14 cases of cerebral hemorrhage in this SCI population were identified [79]. Of 3,000 cases of intracranial hemorrhage, 3 cases were encountered secondary to AD. Intracerebral hemorrhage has been described in a patient in labor with AD [61]. In an experimental model of SCI [81] increased intracranial pressure with partial disruption of the blood–brain barrier occurs, altering the cerebral vessel integrity. These changes may increase the risk of hemorrhage in the period shortly after spinal cord trauma [81]. AD occurring after reconstruction procedures may lead to hemorrhage at the surgical site [82].

Pulmonary edema and heart failure may result from the sympathetic discharge. The acute increase in peripheral vascular resistance and hypertension produces a shift in circulating blood volume from the periphery to the low-resistance pulmonary venous and ultimately pulmonary arterial bed. Pulmonary edema results [83]. Arrowood recorded an increase in pulmonary capillary wedge pressure followed by florid pulmonary edema in a tetraplegic with a history of cardiac disease [84]. Death has only rarely been reported [33, 79]. In Lindan's series, an incidence of 0.2% was found [33].

Management

The management and treatment of AD involves both nonpharmacologic and pharmacologic interventions, depending on the circumstances and likely stimulating factors in each case.

General Measures

The management of an acute episode of AD generally focuses on reducing the elevated blood pressure, and identifying and removing the episode-provoking stimulus. The initial action taken is to raise the patient's head of the bed or sit the patient upright and monitor the blood pressure at intervals of approximately 5 minutes. Any tight clothing and footwear, restraints or straps, as from a drainage legbag, should be removed or loosened.

Once these general measures are taken, attention should focus on identifying the noxious stimulus. In most cases, finding and removing or alleviating the stimulus will resolve the episode, often quickly, and without the use of any pharmacologic agents. As bladder distention is the most common episode-provoking stimulus, bladder catheterization should be performed, or if an indwelling catheter is present, checking the tubing for obstruction, irrigating, or changing the catheter should be done. If fecal impaction is suspected, care should be taken before performing a rectal examination or in attempting manual removal, because the procedure itself can exacerbate the episode. The use of lidocaine jelly as lubricant should be considered when attempting manual disimpaction to decrease any nociceptive stimuli from the procedure. Lidocaine jelly may also be useful when applied to irritated skin in cases where an ingrown toenail is identified and suspected of being the etiologic factor. A thorough skin examination may be necessary to determine the presence of decubitus ulcers, pressure areas, or other skin lesions that may initiate an episode of AD. In the event that the cause of the episode is not readily identified and removed, and the blood pressure remains elevated, the use of pharmacologic agents is indicated. In addition, if the hypertension is severe, generally considered a diastolic blood pressure exceeding 100 mm Hg, immediate treatment with a pharmacologic agent should be instituted.

Pharmacologic Agents

The use of pharmacologic intervention in the treatment of an acute episode of AD is aimed primarily at decreasing the severe hypertension that is responsible for the acute symptoms and that may lead to more severe sequelae. For this reason, antihypertensive agents account for most of the drugs that are used in the treatment of AD. Table 15-1 lists some of the most commonly recommended pharmacologic agents and dosages used in the management of AD. In general, it is recommended that short-acting antihypertensive agents be used. The reasoning for this is that once the cause of the episode is identified and removed, a dramatic decrease in blood pressure usually occurs, and if a long-acting agent is used, this may result in prolonged hypotension. With the use of any pharmacologic agent, blood pressure should be closely monitored.

Table 15-1. Pharmacologic Agents for the Treatment of Autonomic Dysreflexia

Drug	Acute Episodes	Prophylaxis/Recurrent Episodes
Ganglionic blockers		
Mecamylamine	2.5–5.0 mg PO	5.0 mg tid
Trimethaphan	0.1–1.0 mg/min IV	
Pentolinium		20–40 mg PO qid
Alpha-adrenergic blockers		
Phentolamine	5–10 mg IV push	
Phenoxybenzamine		30–60 mg PO bid
Guanethidine		2.5–25 mg PO daily
Prazosin		1.0 mg twice a day PO
Vasodilators		
Nifedipine	10 mg PO/SL	10–30 mg PO tid
Nitroprusside	0.5–1.5 µg/kg/min IV	
Amyl nitrate	30-sec inhalation	
Hydralazine	10 mg slow IV push	
Diazoxide	100–150 mg IV push	
Other		
Clonidine		0.1–0.2 mg bid

Ganglionic blocking agents, including mecamylamine and trimethaphan, have been reported to be among the most effective agents in treating hypertension during AD [4, 11, 85]. These agents act by inhibiting both sympathetic adrenergic and cholinergic discharges [86]. Mecamylamine may be given in oral doses of 2.5–5.0 mg, and may be repeated during an episode, if needed [85]. Trimethaphan is effective when given intravenously [9, 87]. Side effects of the ganglionic blocking agents include visual disturbance, dry mouth, constipation, urinary retention, decreased sweating, and hypotension [86].

Alpha-adrenergic blocking agents, including phentolamine and phenoxybenzamine, have been noted to be variably effective [88]. Phenoxybenzamine is a long-acting oral agent that is effective in treating hypertension primarily due to excess of circulating catecholamines [11]. It has also been noted to have a relaxation effect on the bladder wall musculature [89]. This may explain its benefit in preventing AD when given before the performance of procedures that may result in bladder distention. Side effects of the alpha-adrenergic blocking agents include postural hypotension, tachycardia, nasal congestion, and anejaculation [89].

Pharmacologic agents whose mechanism of action is primarily by vasodilation are probably the most commonly used and effective drugs in treating an acute episode of AD. Nifedipine, a calcium channel blocker, is one of the most commonly used agents in treating AD [89]. It is a potent peripheral arterial vasodilator that is rapidly absorbed after oral or sublingual administration. A dose of 10 mg is generally sufficient to achieve a rapid reduction in blood pressure. In addition, nifedipine may be given repeatedly at the same dose if the hypertension returns. Side effects that may limit its use include headache, tachycardia, dizziness, fatigue, nausea, and orthostatic hypotension.

Nitrates are direct-acting vasodilators whose primary action is dilation of the venous system [89]. Intravenous nitroglycerin and nitroprusside are effective in treating hypertension due to AD, but are usually reserved for the most severe cases that do not respond to other interventions. Sublingual nitroglycerin and inhaled amyl nitrate are other shorter acting forms of nitrates that may be used. Another form of nitrate, nitroglycerin ointment, is increasing in popularity as a treatment agent. Although there is little written information regarding its use in AD, we and other authors have found nitroglycerin ointment effective in rapidly lowering blood pressure, with the added benefit that the ointment can be removed immediately, if needed, without long-lasting effects.

In more severe episodes of AD or those that do not respond to more commonly used agents, two other agents are also available. Hydralazine, a direct-acting arterial vasodilator, may be given in a dose of 10 mg by slow intravenous injection [88]. Its onset of action is usually delayed, and side effects include tachycardia and increased cardiac output. Diazoxide, also a direct-acting arterial vasodilator, is very effective in reducing severe hypertension. It can be administered rapidly in intravenous boluses of 100–150 mg. Side effects include sodium retention, hyperglycemia, nausea, vomiting, and tachycardia. It is also recommended that an intravenous diuretic, such as furosemide, 40–80 mg, or bumetanide, 0.5–1.0 mg, be given before administering diazoxide, to enhance its antihypertensive effects and counteract sodium and water retention.

Prevention

The key to the management of recurrent episodes and preventing episodes of AD is identifying those factors or stimuli that have triggered or are likely to trigger an attack, and taking steps to avoid them. Despite these measures, recurrent episodes may occur and the use of pharmacologic agents is often required for prophylaxis.

General Measures and Education

Patient and family education are vital components in the management of recurrent episodes and in attempts at preventing future occurrences. Information regarding the condition, common symptoms, common causes, and general treatment measures should be explained to the patient and family. A medical alert card (Figure 15-2) explaining the condition and information regarding symptoms, causes, and treatment can be carried on the person. With proper knowledge of this condition and a handy card containing this information, the patient can assist other health care providers or persons unfamiliar with the condition in the treatment of an acute or recurrent episode.

General measures to prevent recurrent episodes focus on the more common causes of AD. Maintaining regular bladder and bowel programs, and attention to good skin and nail care serve as the foundation for prevention.

Rehabilitation Institute of Chicago

AUTONOMIC DYSREFLEXIA
ALERT CARD

(Autonomic Hyperreflexia)
This cardholder has a spinal cord injury and is at risk for a condition known as Autonomic Dysreflexia. Unless this condition is treated quickly, it could lead to convulsions, stroke or death from high blood pressure. See the inside of this card for proper treatment of Autonomic Dysreflexia. (Autonomic Hyperreflexia).

SYMPTOMS: severe pounding, headache, goosebumps, sweating, flushing, stuffy nose, anxiousness, "not feeling right," high blood pressure.

COMMON CAUSES: full bladder, full bowel, skin sore, ingrown toenails, tight clothing, could be annoying stimulus the body reacts to.

TREATMENT:

1. SIT UP, remove abdominal binder, elastic stockings, tight clothing.
2. Check urine output:
   For an indwelling catheter, if little or no output:
   a. check all tubing for kinks, or full bag.
   b. flush catheter. if no fluid returns or if unable to flush then.
   c. change catheter.

   For intermittent catheter program:
   a. catheterize this person IMMEDIATELY.
   b. if amount of urine is greater then 500 cc (16 ounces), stop cathing for 5 minutes, then continue to catheterize.
3. Check bowels for fullness:
   a. insert anesthetic ointment or gel if available, into rectum/ bowel.
   b. gently remove stool, if present.
4. Check skin for sores, ingrown toenails - apply anesthetic ointment or gel.
5. If all above treatments fail and symptoms continue:
   a. go to the nearest emergency room.
   b. give them this card.
   c. this hypertension should be treated medically.

THIS IS A MEDICAL EMERGENCY

Figure 15-2. Medical alert card for autonomic dysreflexia. (Courtesy of the Rehabilitation Institute of Chicago.)

Pharmacologic Agents

In patients who continue to experience recurrent episodes of AD despite adhering to these general measures, prophylactic use of a pharmacologic agent may be indicated.

The use of topical anesthetics, such as lidocaine jelly for urethral catheterizations or dibucaine ointment during the performance of bowel programs, are simple measures that may be sufficient to minimize the stimuli that accompanies these procedures and prevent AD.

Several of the drugs that may be used in the treatment of acute episodes have also been reported to be effective in preventing recurrent episodes of AD. Phenoxybenzamine has been reported to be beneficial in preventing recurrent episodes in doses ranging from 30–100 mg/day [88], although several investigators have recently questioned its effectiveness [90]. It should be noted that studies in rats have shown that long-term administration of phenoxybenzamine is associated with an increase in gastrointestinal tumor formation [90].

More selective alpha$_1$-blocking agents, such as prazosin and terazosin, have recently been reported to be effective prophylactic agents without the side effects commonly associated with other alpha-adrenergic blocking agents [89, 91]. Treatment with prazosin is usually begun at a dose of 1 mg daily given at night, and may be increased to 1 mg twice a day. Terazosin has the advantage and convenience of once a day dosing. Side effects of both agents include first dose hypotension, syncope, drowsiness, dizziness, palpitations, headache, and easy fatigability, although they are reportedly less with terazosin [89].

The ganglionic blocking agents, mecamylamine and pentolinium, have been used to prevent recurrent episodes of AD. Mecamylamine appears to be effective in preventing recurrences at dosages less than those ordinarily used for treatment of hypertension, thus minimizing its side effects [85]. Mecamylamine is probably the preferred ganglionic blocker because of its more uniform and predictable absorption and blood pressure response, and fewer side effects [88].

Guanethidine, a sympathetic adrenergic blocking agent, has been suggested as an available alternative in the management of AD. Dosages ranging from 2.5–25 mg/day have been recommended [4, 11]. Side effects, including diarrhea and postural hypotension, tend to be cumulative because of the long half-life of the agent. In addition, it should be noted that paradoxical hypertension may occur when used concomitantly with sympathomimetic agents.

Other drugs have been suggested to prevent AD. Clonidine, a central alpha-adrenergic agonist, has been reported by several authors to be effective in preventing AD in persons with SCI [50, 92]. The drug may be administered orally usually in doses of 0.1–0.2 mg twice daily. A transdermal patch is also available that is applied once weekly and may deliver the medication in a more uniform, steady manner. Propantheline bromide (Pro-Banthine) and oxybutynin are two other agents that may be useful in preventing AD, primarily in those persons where the episode-provoking stimuli is uninhibited bladder contractions. Both drugs have anticholinergic properties, but in addition, oxybutynin also has direct smooth muscle relaxing properties. Side effects of these agents include constipation, urinary retention, dry mouth, and decreased sweating.

Special Situations

As discussed previously, practically any noxious stimuli below the neurologic level of injury may provoke an acute episode of AD. This raises the issue of situations where diagnostic or therapeutic interventions are required that may trigger AD. Certain steps may be taken and pharmacologic agents administered prior to a procedure in an attempt at preventing the occurrence of AD or minimizing the severity of an acute episode. Special circumstances where AD may be anticipated include the performance of diagnostic procedures and surgery and during labor and delivery.

Diagnostic Procedures and Surgery

A number of invasive diagnostic and therapeutic procedures have been reported to provoke episodes of AD in persons with SCIs, including cystoscopy [40, 93], cystometry [94], electroejaculation [59], and extracorporeal shock wave lithotripsy [54]. Surgery, including orthopedic, neurosurgical, and urologic procedures, may produce AD in certain individuals. The incidence of AD during surgery has been reported to be less in patients receiving regional or general anesthesia, compared with local anesthesia [58]. In fact, the use of spinal anesthesia has been reported by a number of authors to be highly effective in preventing AD, with few complications [94–96].

Despite the use of local, regional, or general anesthesia, episodes may occur during surgical procedures. The use of halothane may be more effective in preventing AD when general anesthesia is used, and as an effective means of treating hypertension when it occurs intraoperatively [96, 97].

In addition, several of the pharmacologic agents previously mentioned for management of acute episodes may be used intraoperatively, if necessary, and there have been suggestions about using them preoperatively to prevent episodes. Nifedipine appears to be effective when administered preoperatively and when AD occurs during urologic procedures such as cystoscopy and extracorporeal shock wave lithotripsy [54, 93]. The dose used is usually 10 mg orally preoperatively, and 10–20 mg orally or sublingually when an episode occurs during a procedure.

Other previously discussed agents that may be effective include the ganglionic blockers, such as mecamylamine (2.5 mg orally 20–30 minutes before a procedure), the alpha-blockers, such as phentolamine (40 mg intravenously before a procedure), and in more severe cases, the vasodilators, trimethaphan (0.5–1.0 mg/minute intravenously), diazoxide, and hydralazine (5–10 mg intravenous bolus) [85, 88, 98]. In addition, it has been reported that chlorpromazine, an alpha-adrenergic blocking agent, may be beneficial both prophylactically or for treatment during a surgical procedure when administered intravenously or intramuscularly [99].

The use of topical or local anesthesia has been suggested in procedures where urethral or bladder instrumentation is required, but because the muscle proprioceptive receptors are not blocked, bladder distention may still result in AD.

Labor and Delivery

AD may occur in pregnant women with SCIs as a result of the stimulation from uterine contractions during labor and delivery. Knowledge and awareness of this condition by those delivering the obstetric care is vital in order to provide proper care for the patient and fetus.

To ensure proper treatment, AD must be differentiated from pre-eclampsia. Hypertension caused by AD is episodic and manifested by transient increases in blood pressure during uterine contractions and resolution between contractions. In contrast, the hypertension in pre-eclampsia tends to persist until delivery.

General measures that may be taken to prevent AD include the use of an indwelling catheter to prevent bladder distention, especially during the later stages of pregnancy including labor, and the use of topical anesthetics during manual examinations when assessing the progress of labor. Maternal blood pressure and cardiac rhythm should be monitored and may require the use of intra-arterial monitoring. Fetal heart rate monitoring should be employed to identify fetal distress, which may occur as a result of AD or its treatment [100].

In terms of treatment, it has been suggested that reserpine may be given before the delivery date in order to prevent the occurrence of AD [101]. Regional anesthesia, more specifically via epidural anesthesia, appears to be the treatment of choice for the prevention and management of AD during labor and delivery [61, 63, 66, 102].

If the use of epidural anesthesia is not adequate in controlling the hypertension, several of the pharmacologic agents previously described for acute management may be used. The use of hydralazine, calcium channel blockers, diazoxide, nitroglycerin, phentolamine, or ganglionic blockers such as trimethaphan have been suggested [61, 94].

If AD cannot be controlled, delivery by cesarean section may be the most expedient method of management, and result in the prompt cessation of the syndrome [62, 65, 66, 100].

Case Management Study

A 30-year-old man sustained an SCI in a motor vehicle crash 3 months earlier with residual C7 complete tetraplegia. He had been undergoing inpatient rehabilitation for the past 6 weeks and had been relatively free of medical complications. One evening while in bed, he complained of the sudden onset of a severe, bitemporal pounding headache. He reported no precipitating symptoms or aura. In addition, the patient reported mild nasal congestion and facial and neck sweating. Vital signs were notable for a pulse of 105 and blood pressure of 160/110. On physical examination, he was noted to be in moderate distress and discomfort from the headache, his face and neck were flushed and diaphoretic, and cardiac and chest examination findings were only notable for tachycardia. Below the shoulder, his skin was pale and cool to the touch. His skin was otherwise intact, with no evidence of pressure sores or skin irritation. His neurologic examination findings were unchanged.

What is the differential diagnosis and what immediate treatment measures would you institute?

Discussion

In the clinical setting described, the diagnosis of septicemia might have been considered, blood and urine cultures obtained, and antibiotic treatment started, or the possibility of a cardiovascular event might have led to the administration of antihypertensive medication. However, the first consideration should be autonomic dysreflexia. The initial treatment measures in this patient included raising the head of the bed to put the patient in a more upright, sitting position, removing his abdominal binder, and loosening his clothing. Using dibucaine ointment as an anesthetic lubricant to minimize further stimuli, rectal examination was done to determine whether there was stool in the rectal vault; none was found. Bladder catheterization was performed and 700 ml of urine was obtained. Minutes after the bladder was emptied, the patient reported a significant decrease in the severity of the headache and his blood pressure decreased to 115/70. Fifteen minutes later, the patient reported resolution of the headache, and his blood pressure had returned to baseline values. No further treatment measures were needed.

This patient had experienced an episode of AD. In this case, the noxious stimuli that triggered the episode was bladder distention. In retrospect, the patient reported that he had accidentally forgotten to catheterize several hours before the event, which resulted in the excess urine volume and bladder distention. Although bladder distention is the most common stimulus for AD, other common forms of stimuli, such as rectal impaction, tight fitting clothes, pressure sores, and ingrown toenails, should also be considered. As in most episodes, treatment and resolution of AD in this case primarily focused on identifying and alleviating the provoking stimulus and did not require any pharmacologic intervention.

References

1. Mitsui T, Kawai H, Taguchi E, Miyamoto H, et al. Autonomic hyperreflexia in pure progressive autonomic failure: A case report. Neurology 1993;43:1823.
2. Cameron SJ, Doig A. Cerebellar tumors presenting with clinical features of phaeochromocytoma. Lancet 1970;1:492.
3. Finestone HM, Teasell RW. Autonomic dysreflexia after brainstem tumor resection. Am J Phys Med Rehabil 1993;72:395.
4. Young JS. Use of guanethidine in control of sympathetic hyperreflexia in persons with clinical and thoracic cord lesions. Arch Phys Med Rehabil 1963;44:204.
5. Mathius CJ, Christensen NJ, Corbett JL, et al. Plasma catecholamines during paroxysmal neurogenic hypertension in quadriplegic man. Circ Res 1976;39:204.
6. Ashley EA, Laskin JJ, Olenik LM, et al. Evidence of autonomic dysreflexia during functional electrical stimulation in individuals with spinal cord injuries. Paraplegia 1993;31:593.
7. Brian JE, Clark RB, Quirk JG. Autonomic hyperreflexia, cesarean section and anesthesia: A case report. J Reprod Med 1988;33:645.
8. Chang C, Chen M, Chang L. Autonomic hyperreflexia in spinal cord injury patient during percutaneous nephrolithotomy for renal stone: A case report. J Urol 1991;146:1601.
9. Chen L, Castro AD. Autonomic hyperreflexia during extracorporeal shock-wave lithotripsy (ESWL) in quadriplegic patients. Can J Anesth 1989;36:604.
10. Colachis SS. Autonomic hyperreflexia in spinal cord injury associated with pulmonary embolism. Arch Phys Med Rehabil 1991;72:1014.
11. Colachis SS. Autonomic hyperreflexia with spinal cord injury. J Am Paraplegia Soc 1992;15:171.
12. Greene ES, Seltzer JL. Autonomic hyperreflexia during upper extremity surgery. Can Anaesth Soc J 1981;28:268.
13. Katz VL, Thorp JM, Cefalo RC. Epidural analgesia and autonomic hyperreflexia: A case report. Am J Obstet Gynecol 1990;162:471.
14. Manger WM, Davis SW, Chu D. Autonomic hyperreflexia and its differentiation from pheochromocytoma. Arch Phys Med Rehabil 1979;60:159.
15. Mew LG. Autonomic hyperreflexia. Ann Emerg Med 1981;10:151.
16. Hilton J. Pain and the therapeutic influence of mechanical and physiological rest in accidents and surgical diseases. Lancet 1860;2:401.
17. Bowlby AA. The reflexes in cases of injury to the spinal cord. Lancet 1890;1:1071.
18. Head H, Riddock G. The automatic bladder, excessive sweating and some other reflex conditions in gross injuries of the spinal cord injuries of the spinal cord. Brain 1917;40:188.
19. Guttman L, Whitteridge D. Effects of bladder distention on autonomic mechanisms after spinal cord injuries. Brain 1947;70:361.
20. Benarroch EE. The central autonomic network: Functional organization, dysfunction and perspective. Mayo Clin Proc 1993;68:988.
21. Mathius CJ, Frankel HL. Clinical manifestations of malfunctioning sympathetic mechanisms in tetraplegia. J Auton Nerv Syst 1983;7:303.
22. McLeod JG, Tuck RR. Disorders of the autonomic nervous system: Part 1. Pathophysiology and clinical features. Ann Neurol 1987;21:419.

23. Cole TM, Kottke FJ, Olson M, et al. Alterations in cardiovascular control in high spinal myelomalacia. Arch Phys Med Rehabil 1967;48:359.

24. Naftchi NE. Mechanism of autonomic dysreflexia. Contributions of catecholamine and peptide neurotransmitters. Ann NY Acad Sci 1990;579:133.

25. Mathius CJ, Christensen NJ, Corbett JL, et al. Plasma catecholamines, plasma renin activity and plasma aldosterone in tetraplegic man, horizontal and tilted. Clin Sci Mol Med 1975;49:291.

26. Naftchi NE, Demeny M, Lowman EW, Tuckman J. Hypertensive crisis in quadriplegic patients. Circulation 1978;57:336.

27. Claus-Walker J, Halstead LS. Metabolic and endocrine changes in spinal cord injury: II (section 1). Consequences of patient decentralization of the autonomic nervous system. Arch Phys Med Rehabil 1982;63:569.

28. Frankel HL, Guttman L, Paeslack V. Cardiac irregularities during labour in paraplegic women. Paraplegia 1965;3:144.

29. Mathius CJ, Smith SD Frankel HL, Spaulding JM. Dopamine B-hydroxylase release during hypertension sympathetic nervous overactivity in man. Cardiovasc Res 1976;10:176.

30. Frankel HL, Mathius CJ. Cardiovascular aspects of autonomic dysreflexia since Guttman and Whitteridge. Paraplegia 1979;17:46.

31. Wallin G. Abnormalities of sympathetic regulation after cervical cord lesions. Acta Neurochir (Wien) 1986;36:123.

32. Krum H, Howes LG, Brown DJ, Louis WJ. Blood pressure variability in tetraplegia patients with autonomic hyperreflexia. Paraplegia 1989;27:284.

33. Lindan R, Joiner E, Freehafer AA, Hazel C. Incidence and clinical features of autonomic dysreflexia in patients with spinal cord injury. Paraplegia 1980;18:285.

34. Kurnick NB. Autonomic hyperreflexia and its control in patients with spinal cord lesions. Ann Intern Med 1956;44:678.

35. Kewralramani LS. Autonomic dysreflexia in traumatic myelopathy. Am J Phys Med 1980;59:1.

36. Roussan MS, Abramson AS, Lippmann HI, D'Oronzio G. Somatic and autonomic responses to bladder filling in patients with complete transverse myelopathy. Arch Phys Med Rehabil 1966;47:450.

37. Wurster RD, Randall WC. Cardiovascular responses to bladder distention in patients with spinal transection. Am J Physiol 1975;228:1288.

38. Thyberg M, Ertzgaard P, Gylling M, Granerus G. Blood pressure response to detrusor pressure elevation in patients with reflex urinary bladder after a cervical or high thoracic spinal cord injury. Scand J Rehabil Med 1992;24:187.

39. Johnson B, Thomason R, Pallares V, Sandove MS. Autonomic hyperreflexia review. Mil Med 1975;140:345.

40. Snow JC, Siderpoulos HP, Kripke BJ, et al. Autonomic hyperreflexia during cystoscopy in patients with high spinal cord injuries. Paraplegia 1977-78;15:327.

41. Wheeler G, et al. Testosterone, cortisol, and catecholamine responses to exercise stress and autonomic dysreflexia in elite quadriplegic athletes. Paraplegia 1994;32:292.

42. Perkash I, Friedland GW. Catheter-induced hyperreflexia in spinal cord injury patients: Diagnosis by sonographic voiding cystourethrography. Radiology 1986;159:453.

43. Barbaric ZL. Autonomic dysreflexia in patients with spinal cord lesions. Complication of voiding cystourethrography and ilial loopography. AJR Am J Roentgenol 1976;127:293.

44. Valdyanathan S, Krishnan KR. Misoprostol associated autonomic dysreflexia in a traumatic tetraplegic patient. Paraplegia 1996;34:121.

45. Komar VN, Mullican CN. Ovarian cyst and autonomic dysreflexia. Arch Phys Med Rehabil 1989;70:547.

46. Charney KJ, Juler GH, Comarr AE. General surgery problems in patients with spinal cord injuries. Arch Surg 1975;110:1083.

47. Scott MD, Morrow JW. Phenoxybenzamine in neurogenic bladder dysfunction after spinal cord injury: Autonomic dysreflexia. J Urol 1978;119:483.

48. Sell GH, Naftchi NE, Lorman EW, Rusk MA. Autonomic hyperreflexia and catecholamine metabolites in spinal cord injury. Arch Phys Med Rehabil 1972;53:415, 424.

49. McGuire EJ, Wagner FM, Weiss RM. Treatment of autonomic dysreflexia with phenoxybenzamine. J Urol 1976;115:53.

50. Hall PA, Young JV. Autonomic hyperreflexia in spinal cord injured patients: Trigger mechanism—Dressing changes of pressure sores. J Trauma 1983;23:1074.

51. McGarry J, Woolsey RM, Thompson CW. Autonomic hyperreflexia following passive stretching to the hip joint. Phys Ther 1982;62:30.

52. Graham GP, Dent CM, Evans PD, McKibbin B. Recurrent dislocation of the hip in adult paraplegics. Paraplegia 1992;30:587.

53. Givre S, Freed HA. Autonomic dysreflexia: A potentially fatal complication of somatic stress in quadriplegics. J Emerg Med 1989;7:461.

54. Kabalin JN, Lennon S, Gill HS, et al. Incidence and management of autonomic dysreflexia and other intraoperative problems encountered in spinal cord injury patients undergoing extracorporeal shock wave lithotripsy without anesthesia on a second generation lithotriptor. J Urol 1993;149:1064.

55. Stowe DF, Bernstein JS, Madsen KE, et al. Autonomic hyperreflexia in spinal cord injured patients during extracorporeal shock wave lithotripsy. Anesth Analg 1989;68:788.

56. Raeder JC, Gisvold SE. Perioperative autonomic hyperreflexia in high spinal cord lesions: A case report. Acta Anaesthesiol Scand 1986;30:672.

57. Jane MJ, Freehafer AA, Hazel C, et al. Autonomic dysreflexia: A cause of morbidity and mortality in ortho-

pedic patients with spinal cord injury. Clin Orthop 1982;169:151.

58. Schonwald G, Fish KJ, Perkash I. Cardiovascular complications during anesthesia in chronic spinal cord injured patients. Anesthesia 1981;55:550.

59. Frankel HL, Mathias CJ. Severe hypertension in patients with high spinal cord lesions undergoing electro- ejaculation-management with prostaglandin E_2. Paraplegia 1980;18:293.

60. Rossier AB, Ziegler WL, Duchosal PW, Meylan J. Sexual functions and dysreflexia. Paraplegia 1971;9:51.

61. McGregor JA, Meeuwsen J. Autonomic hyperreflexia: A mortal danger for spinal cord damaged women in labor. Am J Obstet Gynecol 1985;151:330.

62. Nath M, Vivian JM, Cherny WB. Autonomic hyperreflexia in pregnancy and labor: A case report. Am J Obstet Gynecol 1979;134:390.

63. Stirt JA, Marco A, Conklin KA. Obstetric anesthesia for a quadraplegic patient with autonomic hyperreflexia. Anesthesia 1979;51:560.

64. Tabsh KM, Brinkman CR, Reff RA. Autonomic dysreflexia in pregnancy. Obstet Gynecol 1982;60:119.

65. Verduyn WH. Spinal cord injured women, pregnancy and delivery. Paraplegia 1986;24:231.

66. Wanner MB, Rageth CJ, Zäch GA. Pregnancy and autonomic hyperreflexia in patients with spinal cord lesions. Paraplegia 1987;25:482.

67. Robertson DN. Pregnancy and labour in the paraplegic. Paraplegia 1972;10:209.

68. Spielman FJ. Parturient with spinal cord transection. Complications of autonomic hyperreflexia. Obstet Gynecol 1984;64:147.

69. Khurana RK. Orthostatic hypotension induced autonomic dysreflexia. Neurology 1987;37:1221.

70. Arieff AJ, Tigay EL, Pyzek SW. Acute hypertension induced by urinary bladder distention. Arch Neurol 1962;67:248.

71. Naftchi NE, Tuchman J. Hypertensive crisis in spinal man. Am Heart J 1979;97:536.

72. Wayne EM, Vukov JG. Eye findings in autonomic hyperreflexia. Ann Ophthalmol 1977;9:41.

73. Forrest GP. Atrial fibrillation associated with autonomic dysreflexia in patients with tetraplegia. Arch Phys Med Rehabil 1991;72:592.

74. Pine ZM, Miller SD, Alonso JA. Atrial fibrillation associated with autonomic dysreflexia. Am J Phys Med Rehabil 1991;70:271.

75. Nadeau RA, Roberge FA, Bilittle J. Role of the sinus node in the mechanism of cholinergic atrial fibrillation. Circ Res 1970;27:129.

76. Kendrick WW, Scott JW, Jouseat Botterell EH. Reflex sweating and hypertension in traumatic transverse myelitis. Treat Serv Bull 1953;8:437.

77. Kursh ED, Freehafer A, Persky L. Complications of autonomic dysreflexia. J Urol 1977;118:70.

78. Yarkony GM, Katz RT, Wu Y. Seizures secondary to autonomic dysreflexia. Arch Phys Med Rehabil 1986;67:834.

79. Eltorai I, Kim R, Vulpe M, et al. Fatal cerebral hemorrhage due to autonomic dysreflexia in a tetraplegic patient: Case report and review. Paraplegia 1992;30:355.

80. Hanowell LH, Wilmot C. Spinal cord injury leading to intracranial hemorrhage. Crit Care Med 1988;16:911.

81. Albin MS, Leonide B, Wolfe S. Brain and lungs at risk in cervical cord transection. Surg Neurol 1985;24:191.

82. Wackwitz DL, Engber WD, Bruskewitz R. Autonomic dysreflexia: A cause of postoperative hemorrhage. J Bone Joint Surg [Am] 1982;64:297.

83. Kiker JD, Woodside JR, Jelinek GE. Neurogenic pulmonary edema associated with autonomic dysreflexia. J Urol 1982;128:1038.

84. Arrowood JA, Mohant PK, Thamas MD. Cardiovascular problems in the spinal cord injury patient. Physical Medicine and Rehabilitation: State of the Art Reviews 1987;1:443.

85. Braddom RL, Johnson EW. Mecamylamine in control of hyperreflexia. Arch Phys Med Rehabil 1969;50:448.

86. Taylor P. Agents acting at the neuromuscular junction and autonomic ganglia. In AG Gilman, TW Rall, AS Nies, P Taylor (eds), Goodman and Gilman's The Pharmacological Basis of Therapeutics (8th ed). New York: Macmillan, 1990;166.

87. Nieder RM, O'Higgins JW, Aldrete JA. Autonomic hyperreflexia in urologic surgery. JAMA 1970;213:867.

88. Erickson RP. Autonomic hyperreflexia: pathophysiology and medical management. Arch Phys Med Rehabil 1980;61:431.

89. Braddom RL, Rocco JF. Autonomic dysreflexia: A survey of current treatment. Am J Phys Med Rehabil 1991;70:234.

90. Lindan R, Leffler EJ, Kedia KR. A comparison of the efficacy of an alpha-1-adrenergic blocker in the slow calcium channel blocker in the control of autonomic dysreflexia. Paraplegia 1985;23:34.

91. Chancellor MB, Erhard MJ, Hirsch IH, Stass WE. Prospective evaluation of terazosin for the treatment of autonomic dysreflexia. J Urol 1994;151:111.

92. Wright KC, Agre JC, Wilson BC, Theologides A. Autonomic dysreflexia in a paraplegic man with catecholamine-secreting neuroblastoma. Arch Phys Med Rehabil 1986;67:566.

93. Dykstra DD, Sidi AA, Anderson LC. The effect of nifedipine on cystoscopy-induced autonomic hyperreflexia in patients with high spinal cord injuries. J Urol 1987;138:1155.

94. Trop CS, Bennett CJ. Autonomic dysreflexia and its urological implications: A review. J Urol 1991;146:1461.

95. Broecker BH, Hranowsky N, Hackler RH. Low spinal anesthesia for the prevention of autonomic dysreflexia in the spinal cord injury patient. J Urol 1979;122:366.

96. Lambert DH, Deane RS, Mazuzan JE. Anesthesia and the control of blood pressure in patients with spinal cord injury. Anesth Analg 1982;61:344.

97. Alderson JD, Thomas DG. The use of halothane anesthesia to control autonomic hyperreflexia during transurethral surgery in spinal cord injury patients. Paraplegia 1975;13:183.

98. Sizemore GW, Winternitz WW. Autonomic hyperreflexia—Suppression with alpha-adrenergic blocking agents. N Engl J Med 1970;282:795.

99. McGuire EJ, Rossier AB. Treatment of acute autonomic dysreflexia. J Urol 1983;129:1185.

100. Greenspon JS, Paul RH. Paraplegia and quadriplegia: Special consideration during pregnancy and labor and delivery. Am J Obstet Gynecol 1986;155:738.

101. Saunders D, Yeo J. Pregnancy and quadriplegia—The problem of autonomic dysreflexia. Aust NZ J Obstet Gynaecol 1968;8:152.

102. Abouleish E. Hypertension in a paraplegic parturient. Anesthesiology 1980;53:348.

Chapter 16

Pain

James C. Erickson III

Pain is a universal experience of all creatures. The basic function of nociception is protective for the organism, to avoid noxious stimuli, such as fire or penetration by a sharp object, or to rest quietly until broken bones or internal injuries heal. There is always a psychological component of pain in adult humans, who may interpret the painful intrusion on their lives with fear, anger, anxiety, and depression. Disabled persons have unique problems because of altered or severe limitations of locomotion, dexterity, sensation, and visceral functions. Their emotional responses to these physical changes are the same as other persons with pain of benign and malignant causes without the functional disabilities. Effective pain management for disabled persons usually requires a comprehensive strategy rather than simply prescribing analgesic drugs, a series of injections, or surgical invasions. A physically disabled patient needs a well-coordinated variety of treatment modalities intended to achieve maximum physical and psychological rehabilitation.

Physiology of Pain

Treating patients who suffer from chronic pain requires a basic knowledge of the physiology of pain perception, transmission, and modulation. Knowledge of the complex chemical and electrical events in the central nervous system (CNS) has leaped ahead during recent years. Although an extensive review of the physiology of pain is beyond the purpose of this chapter, basic knowledge and recent research and clinical experience are discussed.

A stimulus that is sufficiently intense to elicit pain activates receptors in the periphery that are sensitive to thermal, chemical, or mechanical alterations of the normal milieu. Pain and temperature sensations are conducted from the cutaneous receptors through the small-diameter myelinated axons of A delta nerves and the unmyelinated C fibers. Transmission of afferent impulses in A delta nerves averages 6–20 m/second, whereas C fibers conduct more slowly at a rate of 0.5–2.0 m/second. The speed of transmission of impulses involving proprioception, motor, and reflex functions in the thicker, more heavily myelinated A alpha, beta, and gamma nerves far exceeds that of the nociceptive nerves.

The A delta nerves respond to two types of nociception. The mechanothermal nociceptors respond to heat as well as mechanical stimuli. All of the heat-sensitive receptors respond to temperatures greater than 45–47°C, whereas some react to skin temperatures below pain threshold and some also respond to cooling. The mechanoreceptors are sensitive to tissue damage caused by sharp and pointed objects. Both of these myelinated nociceptors have the property of sensitization, in which repeated stimulations cause progressively greater responses, as demonstrated by increased intensity of axonal discharges as well as the subjective reactions of individuals undergoing psychophysiologic tests.

C fibers are the most numerous component of peripheral afferent nerves, and of these approximately 90% are nociceptors. They are sensitive to thermal, mechanical, and chemical stimuli applied to skin. Transduction is the process by which nociceptors are stimulated by noxious phenomena. Peripheral tissue injury has been found to cause the release of chemicals that mediate the initial phases of inflammation. End products, which include prostaglandins E_2 and I_1 and thromboxane, are released, sensitizing the peripheral C fiber nerve endings to the action of bradykinin, the leukotrienes, and histamine. In addition, the receptors themselves seem to release substance P, which enhances nociception and activates further release of histamine from mast cells. These neuropeptides play a role in tissue repair as well as the defense response.

Most afferent nerves enter the spinal cord through the dorsal nerve root, with their cell bodies lying in the dorsal root ganglion. Approximately 30% of the axons of ventral roots are unmyelinated C fibers whose cell bodies also lie within the dorsal root ganglion. The primary nociceptors synapse directly with a variety of cells in the dorsal horn of the spinal cord. These cells are projection neurons, which relay messages to higher cerebral centers; excitatory interneurons, which conduct the nociceptive message to other projection neurons or nearby interneurons; or inhibitory neurons, whose role is the modification of nociceptive impulses. Some excitatory interneurons mediate spinal reflex responses via synapses with motoneurons in the ventral horn. These cell bodies and the afferent nerve endings from dorsal horn cell bodies are arranged in lamina as described by Rexed [1], with the A delta nociceptive fibers synapsing with interneurons in laminae I and V and C fibers in lamina II.

The organization of synapses of primary afferent neurons and the secondary interneurons (projection, excitatory, and inhibitory neurons) is exceedingly complex. The endings of the primary nociceptive neurons often extend rostrocaudad from one to three levels within the spinal cord, with connecting interneurons creating a vast arborization with the secondary connecting neurons. Within the dorsal horn are found the neurotransmitter substances that have been the subjects of much conjecture and research during the last two decades. Neuropeptides and nonpeptides either enhance the transmission of nociception (substance P, cholecystokinin, angiotensin II, and somatostatin) or diminish the intensity of transmitted painful stimuli. The endorphins and enkephalins act on the special opioid receptor cells, with serotonin and gamma-aminobutyric acid (GABA) enhancing the

modulation. Opioid receptors are found in especially high density in lamina I (the marginal zone), lamina II (substantia gelatinosa), and lamina V and are designated as μ, δ, κ, ε, and σ, each having affinity for different opioid substances, whether endogenous or systemically administered chemicals. The intricacies of the opioid receptor systems and the endorphins are thoroughly explored in an excellent review by Yaksh [2].

The majority of projection neurons from the dorsal horns cross to the contralateral ventral and lateral spinothalamic tracts, forming the ascending nociceptive pathways to thalamic nuclei. Ipsilateral ascending pain pathways to the intralaminar thalamic nuclei are largely conductors from C fiber nociceptors. The axons of the spinoreticular neurons lie in close apposition to spinothalamic pathways and are believed to project to both sides of the brain stem reticular formation, resulting in further modification of pain transmission. Descending control of nociceptive transmission arises in the periaqueductal gray matter, and rostroventral matter of the medulla via projections into laminae I, II, and V of the spinal cord. Serotonin, which inhibits nociceptive cells in the dorsal horn, is produced by selective stimulation of the rostroventral matter. In addition, electrostimulation of the periaqueductal gray matter and rostroventral matter produces analgesia, and the microinjection of minute doses of morphine into those structures also creates effective analgesia.

Naloxone applied to the same structures causes a reversal of morphine-induced analgesia. Thus, experimental work and limited clinical application of midbrain stimulation have led the way for advances in antinociceptive therapy. Fields's [3] lucid descriptions of the peripheral nociceptive anatomy and physiology, pain pathways of the CNS, and CNS mechanisms for control of pain transmission are worthy of further study.

The thalamus provides the last CNS area for nociceptive modulation, as synapses from ascending connecting axons and the myriad midbrain and pontine reticular connections finally synapse with tertiary neurons that project to sensory areas of the cortical postcentral gyrus. It is here that pain perception occurs, influenced by input from the endless ramifications and interneuronal network of the brain.

The neuroanatomy, physiology, and pharmacology of nociception are extremely complex, as suggested in the previous paragraphs. Pain treatment is further complicated by the many neuronal and humoral influences on the system, plus the complexities of the pathologic processes. Disabled patients who have cerebral and spinal cord lesions present especially challenging questions for the investigators and therapists. An appreciation of the nociceptive system enables them to devise treatment strategies with greater prospects of success than the employment of simplistic methods.

Evaluation of Pain Syndromes

A comprehensive historical survey is vital. A history of the pain complaint must include details of the character of pain at the time of onset, the temporal relationship to the related injury, and the changes as the pain syndrome evolved to that presented. The apparent sites of original and referred pains must be identified. The impact on the patient's lifestyle, such as the ability to pursue vocational goals and the effect on his or her family must be considered, as well as the severity of the disability. The physician should become sensitive to patients' use of hyperbole and extravagant descriptors of pain [4]. A complete systemic review must be conducted for past medical ailments and allergies, surgical operations, and familial conditions that may affect the patient's care (pharmacogenetic problems such as malignant hyperpyrexia) and other important information. Reports from referring physicians or those who have treated the patient in the recent and distant past may reveal important clinical information. All laboratory data must be gathered and collated.

A meticulous physical examination is vital. Neurologic assessment must include estimations of altered muscle strength, sensory perception of sharp and cold sensations, proprioception, and the presence or absence of normal and abnormal deep tendon and pathologic reflexes. Additional investigations, such as tests of somatosensory evoked potential, may be invaluable.

Radiologic imaging contributes greatly to the knowledge and understanding of clinical problems and therapeutic planning. Recent developments of sophisticated imaging techniques have enhanced our knowledge and the effectiveness of treatment to a remarkable degree during recent years. Computed tomographic (CT) scanning and magnetic resonance imaging (MRI) have made tremendous contributions to the diagnosis and visualization of internal pathology, thus avoiding surgical explorations in many patients.

Psychological evaluation is usually indicated in victims of chronic pain and is best directed by a psychiatrist or psychologist, although the primary physician is usually responsible for requesting consultation by these specialists. It is often helpful to order a psychometric test, such as the Minnesota Multiphasic Personality Index, although this is usually within the purview of the mental health practitioner. Administration of the McGill Pain Questionnaire may also be instructive in evaluation procedures [4].

Differential nerve blocks are helpful in evaluation of the etiology of pain and the estimation of the relative importance of the psychological effect. Anesthesiologists who are interested in the management of pain will usually perform these injections, which consist of a simulated or placebo nerve block, a sympathetic ganglion or plexus block, and a somatosensory nerve or plexus block.

Significant relief of pain by a simulated block indicates the presence of an important psychological component of the pain complaint but does not automatically indicate factitious injury, malingering, or faking of the pain. The majority of patients in pain have a psychological response, and their personal experiences are genuine. To classify a person's complaint as being "real" or "not real" is denigrating and reveals a lack of insight by the therapist. Positive responses to placebo procedures are experienced by about 33% of normal subjects tested in a variety of situations [5], whereas 55% of patients with chronic pain of a variety of causes were significantly relieved by placebo injections [6]. There is an ever present danger of overemphasizing the positive placebo response, with consequent lessening of the therapist's investment in diagnostic and therapeutic efforts on behalf of the victim of the pain. When pain relief is accomplished by placebo, intensified evaluation of socioeconomic and psychological aspects of the patient's milieu is indicated.

Placebo medication administered orally or parenterally may provide the desired relief in patients whose psychological component far exceeds the nociceptive portion of their complaint. Although this may be instructive to the therapist who is planning the therapeutic strategy, the continued use of placebo medication as a pacifier only delays delivery of effective treatment and convinces the patient of the necessity of this "medication." The practice of prescribing placebo medication for prolonged therapy should be avoided.

Relief of pain by blockade of a sympathetic ganglion, such as the stellate or lumbar sympathetic ganglia for the upper or lower extremities, respectively, signals the presence of reflex sympathetic dystrophy or a sympathetic mediated pain syndrome. This condition develops after direct injuries to peripheral nerves and plexuses, as well as following cerebral and spinal insults. The pain is usually out of proportion to the apparent injury and can be especially aggravating to patients. Other abnormalities are seen with reflex sympathetic dystrophy syndrome, such as trophic changes of the skin and nails, variable temperature and coloration of the skin, extreme sensitivity to touch, and demineralization of osseous structures in the area (Sudeck's atrophy).

An effective sensory nerve blockade should create analgesia and comfort in the painful area. The somatosensory blockade will also relieve sympathetic mediated pains, and thus it is usually carried out during a separate session from the sympathetic block when used diagnostically.

There are two techniques for administering differential nerve blocks: the anatomic and pharmacologic methods. The anatomic approach refers to the blockade of specific nerves or plexuses that serve the painful site using local anesthetic drugs. As an example, pain of an upper extremity may be evaluated by injection of a local anesthetic into the brachial plexus to test somatosensory response, and a stellate ganglion block will affect sympathetic mediated pain. Simulated (placebo) blocks may be administered in the same anatomic areas. The pharmacologic method usually involves injection of ascending concentrations of dilute solutions of local anesthetics into the epidural or intrathecal spaces, especially for low back, hip, or lower extremity pains [7]. Pain relief following injection of a small volume of saline signifies a placebo response. If the patient's complaint persists, a dilute solution of procaine hydrochloride or lidocaine hydrochloride is then injected to effect a sympathetic blockade. This should cause the lower extremities to become warm but preserve sensory and motor function. If pain is relieved, reflex sympathetic dystrophy syndrome or sympathetic mediated pain is indicated. A series of lumbar paravertebral or epidural sympathetic blocks may be prescribed as part of the patient's therapy. Persistence of pain after injection of the dilute local anesthetic should be followed by similar injections of more concentrated solutions of the anesthetics to block sensory and motor function.

If pain persists after effective neural blockade is completed, a central pain syndrome or "encephalization" of the pain pattern is assumed. This frequently occurs in patients with paraplegia, quadriplegia, hemiplegia, and injuries to major plexuses and nerves, in whom normal afferent sensation is permanently lost. Such patients are not candidates for neurosurgical destructive procedures or neurolytic injections. Such invasive procedures will not be beneficial, will expose the victim to increased hazard, and may result in development of more severe pain. Many patients have been referred for consultation whose pain was aggravated by aggressive neurodestructive procedures. Meticulous evaluation should enable one to avoid such errors.

The presence of abnormal coagulation or of infection at proposed injection sites presents strong contraindications to the execution of such procedures. Nerve blocks administered to patients who are receiving anticoagulant drugs may result in dangerous hemorrhage into deep tissue planes or the epidural space from uncontrolled bleeding. The insertion of needles through infected tissue may spread infection wherever the needle is inserted, whether at deep fascial levels or in epidural or intrathecal spaces. Such potential disasters must be considered whenever nerve blocking procedures are undertaken.

Specific Pain Problems of the Disabled

Cerebral and spinal cord damage often causes deafferentation, which implies the extensive loss of sensory functions. Patients who have suffered from cerebral damage (from strokes, brain tumors, or trauma), or who have spinal myelopathy at almost any level, may have pain in distal areas, where sensation and normal nociception are lost. This neuropathic pain may become severe and cause great distress to the person whose lifestyle has already been severely disrupted. The pain may be characterized as a burning sensation but is often described as constricting, squeezing, and vise-like and may present in the thorax, abdomen, perineum, and lower extremities in paraplegia, with the arms included in quadriplegia. Beric and coworkers [8] investigated patients presenting with "central dysesthesia syndrome" and determined that the ventral spinothalamic pathways were destroyed but that residual dorsal column system input contributed to misinterpretation of stimuli at the thalamic level where the spinothalamic and dorsal column systems converge. They reported no beneficial effects from membrane stabilizers (carbamazepine and phenytoin), tricyclic antidepressants (amitriptyline), neurolytic and surgical rhizotomies, and epidural dorsal column stimulators. Most of those who had rhizotomies and epidural stimulators developed more severe discomfort. The patients usually reported a delay of weeks to a few months before the development of pain. The investigators opined that future hopes lay in avoidance of the syndrome by research efforts aimed at prevention of the sensory reorganization that leads to the dysesthesias and pain.

Patients become especially distressed by deafferentation pain and often question the possibility of relief by amputation of the painful area. Self-mutilation behaviors in rats have been provoked by complete and partial surgical denervation of the forelimbs. Rabin and colleagues [9] reported autotomy or destruction and subsequent amputation of the denervated portions of limbs by gnawing. Latency from denervation to the first self-attack was several days to 6 weeks. This phenomenon mimics the severity of distress of human patients and their intense desire to seek relief by any means, however drastic it may seem. Surgical ablation of sensory nerves, interruption of spinal tracts, and amputations of limbs do not relieve the chronic pain but merely add further mutilation.

My experience with differential blocks with local anesthetics has repeatedly revealed the ineffectiveness of peripheral and intrathecal neural blockade in patients with deafferentation pain syndrome. Placebo injections afforded temporary relief in 60% of these patients, whereas sympathetic and sensory blocks were almost universally ineffective. The perceived relief of pain following the placebo usually lasted 1 or 2 days, although about 10% enjoyed relative comfort for weeks to months. The management of these patients evolved to the prescription of membrane stabilizers, nonsteroidal anti-inflammatory analgesics, and vigorous efforts to engage the person in occu-

pational and physical therapeutic planning and psychological strategies.

Pain at the level of myelopathy following spinal cord destruction seems to occur with relative frequency. Complaints of unrelenting constriction and tight sensations occurring unilaterally or bilaterally at and immediately below the level of spinal cord destruction are also extremely aggravating. Pain and temperature perceptions are absent in the painful zones, which occur immediately below normally innervated dermatomes. Peripheral nerve blocks administered to a few of these patients have only raised the level of their pain complaint to the uppermost edge of the new analgesic area. This portion of the paraplegic patient's pain may be caused by dysesthesias due to overlapping dermatomes in the incompletely denervated areas and is analogous to the findings of Beric and associates [8]. Therapy for such complaints is similar to that mentioned previously.

Spinothalamic tractotomy is occasionally selected as the antinociceptive surgical procedure for patients whose pain is unilateral and usually of malignant etiology. Immediate relief of the original pain may be accomplished, but dysesthesic pain may develop after a latent period of several weeks to months. This operation is now almost entirely restricted to patients whose expected longevity ensures that pain will not return to plague their remaining days. When cordotomies are performed for benign pain syndromes, dysesthetic or deafferentation pain is a frequent sequel. Treatment is similar to that described previously.

Hemiplegia following cerebrovascular accidents results in similar pain syndromes that occur less frequently but are equally resistant to therapy. Peripheral somatosensory and sympathetic nerve blocks are ineffective unless there is a distinct reflex sympathetic dystrophy syndrome, when sympathetic nerve blocks may provide relief.

Patients who are not severely disabled often suffer from dysesthesias and pain in deafferentiated or amputated parts of the body. Postamputation phantom limb pain is similar in many respects, and the variety of nerve blocks and surgical procedures that are tried is ample testimony to their ineffectiveness. The complaints generated by meralgia paresthetica are also similar, in that the zone innervated by the lateral femoral cutaneous nerve is anesthetic and "tight" but is constantly painful. Nerve blocks with local anesthetics with or without corticosteroids may benefit some of these patients. This author has seen patients with loss of normal sensation in other discrete anatomic areas who have suffered severe discomfort and distress, often developing depression neuroses. Trauma to digital nerves may cause numbness of part of a finger or thumb. Prolonged pressure on supraorbital or greater occipital nerves may cause distressing dysesthesias of the forehead and scalp. In these examples, as with other anatomic sites of denervation, pain treatment with local anesthetic injections and expectant waiting may result in the relief of the abnormal sensation. These patients should become actively engaged in rehabilitation therapy conceived to encourage activity with a realistic effort to regain as much function as possible. Coincident depression or other psychological reactions must be addressed simultaneously if an optimal therapeutic result is to be obtained.

Reflex Sympathetic Dystrophy

Reflex sympathetic dystrophy syndrome usually develops after injury to a peripheral nerve, although it may occur in hemiplegic or hemiparetic persons following strokes. The incident of injury may be trivial or may follow an upper or lower extremity fracture. The severity of the subjective pain may be out of proportion to the appearance of the involved limb, and patients characteristically guard it from seemingly innocuous contact and may become obsessed with the need to protect the area. The pains seem to be maintained by efferent hyperactivity of the sympathetic nervous system in the region affected and are usually relieved by regional blockade of the sympathetic ganglion or plexus involved. In most cases, a series of three to six sympathetic blocks may provide prolonged or permanent relief. The syndrome is poorly understood and may be labeled as any of the following:

Causalgia
Minor causalgia
Sudeck's atrophy (involving osteoporosis)
Posttraumatic osteoporosis
Shoulder-hand syndrome
Leriche's posttraumatic pain syndrome
Reflex sympathetic dystrophy
Postinfarction sympathetic dystrophy
Sympathetic mediated pain

In addition to the intense pain and cutaneous hypersensitivity or allodynia, trophic changes of the

skin, nails, and hair develop, with temperature changes and hyperhidrosis. Atrophy and immobility of the limb follow unless appropriate therapy is begun within several weeks to months of the onset. Timely use of sympathetic regional blocks usually is effective in treating the syndrome and permits rehabilitation procedures to begin to restore flexibility, strength, and normal function [10]. Precise explanations of the cause of reflex sympathetic dystrophy syndrome are still lacking, although it is believed that a vicious cycle of self-perpetuating pain is established. Efferent sympathetic hyperactivity causes vasoconstriction, trophic deterioration, and pain, which triggers afferent nociceptive units, with a reflex arc developing in the rostral segments of the thoracic spinal cord. This cycle and the arc have been compared to an electrical short circuit. The analogy seems to be especially appropriate when we observe the prompt benefits of switching off the sympathetic hyperactivity by blocking the involved nerves.

Other therapeutic modalities may be effective in mild reflex sympathetic dystrophy syndrome. Oral or systemic administration of corticosteroids, oral therapy with propranolol, and hypnotherapy may be tried. Regional perfusion of the involved limb with an alpha-adrenergic blocking agent (guanethidine, reserpine) has enjoyed popularity [11]. In this procedure, the drug is injected intravenously after isolation of the limb's circulation behind an arterial tourniquet, but because of the lack of consistent and prolonged improvement, the technique has lost favor with many therapists. A well-conceived program of physical therapy is always essential for the return to satisfactory function. The best strategy is to arrange for physical therapy sessions to follow within a few hours of the administration of the sympathetic blocks, while maximum comfort persists.

Many patients are referred with diagnoses of reflex sympathetic dystrophy syndrome because of complaints of persistent, burning pain. Careful evaluation may reveal a lack of the typical signs of this syndrome, such as an absence of allodynia, trophic changes, edema, and impaired function. Such patients deserve meticulous evaluation rather than subjecting them to nerve blocks in a routine manner. Neuralgias caused by herpes zoster or other infectious organisms or traumatic or chemical neuritis may be the offending agents. Mistaken diagnoses of reflex sympathetic dystrophy syndrome may be made when neural entrapment is caused by scarring or constricting fibrous tissue. The relief of purported reflex sympathetic dystrophy syndrome following resection and repair of an ulnar nerve [12] and correction of an inadequate carpal tunnel release [13] are reported.

The shoulder pain of hand-shoulder syndrome seen in hemiplegic patients is usually caused by paralysis of shoulder girdle musculature and subsequent separation of the glenohumeral joint, resulting in painful stretching of the bicipital tendon. Sympathetic regional blocks are not effective, but the application of a well-designed, supportive sling provides effective relief.

An excellent example of the phenomenon was presented by a 65-year-old man who suffered a right-sided stroke that left him hemiplegic. About 4 months after the cerebrovascular accident he developed pain, swelling, and discoloration of the flaccid, paralyzed right hand and arm. The arm was hypesthetic to all sensory testing, with obvious pain during range of motion exercises. The hand and fingers were tender, edematous (sausage fingers), and the skin mottled and cooler than the opposite side. Conservative treatments with physical therapy, analgesics, and oral cortisone were not effective. A series of stellate ganglion blocks were begun, with physical therapy sessions immediately afterward. After four injections (in 2 weeks) the pain and edema of the hand and forearm were gone, but he still complained of shoulder pain. Re-evaluation of the shoulder revealed a gap of about 2.0 cm between the head of the humerus and the acromion process. Loss of muscle tone of the shoulder girdle allowed the weight of the arm to pull relentlessly whenever he was erect. Orthopedic consultation could not promise significant improvement from surgery. A firm supportive sling provided excellent relief when he stood or sat erect. Rehabilitation progressed well and he was discharged with no need for analgesic medications.

Management with Pharmacologic Agents

The initial intervention for patients who suffer persistent pain usually consists of the administration of analgesic drugs. Patients often take the initiative, as advised by the usual hyperbole of television and magazine advertisements, and select a nonsteroidal anti-inflammatory agent to use or abuse according to their responses, expectations, and the efficacy of the chemical agent. Typical advertisements promise prompt and complete relief of pain, and many patients expect and tolerate nothing less than this ideal. To make the issue more complex, physicians usually prescribe analgesics to be taken "prn." This is the abbreviation for the Latin phrase, *pro re nata*, which means "according to circumstances." Consequently, drugs are usually taken only when pain is relatively severe. It is far more effective to prescribe a realistic dose of an appropriately potent analgesic to be taken on a time-contingent basis in order to maintain an effective blood level. The intent might be phrased "to maintain a reasonable degree of *comfort*," rather than to treat pain.

The evaluation of pathologic situations and the causes of intractable pain often require intensive and prolonged investigation. Analgesic drugs should be provided while studies are progressing, as well as during the various phases of rehabilitation for patients with disabling conditions. The oral route should be used unless swallowing function and airway maintenance are jeopardized, as in obtunded patients, or if abnormal gastrointestinal function precludes this route. The parenteral administration of analgesic drugs to impatient persons who can eat and drink is poor management and may contribute to the development of addiction. The use of powerful narcotics is appropriate for pain of an acute nature but is rarely justified for chronic pain syndromes, such as those seen in disabled patients as described earlier.

Aspirin and all the other nonsteroidal anti-inflammatory drugs except acetaminophen are especially useful in the presence of bone and joint pains because of their interruption of prostaglandin synthesis. Many newer nonsteroidal anti-inflammatory agents, such as ibuprofen, naproxen, diclofenac, diflunisal, and ketorolac have been tried in lieu of aspirin and have proved effective as well as expensive. When these drugs do not provide adequate pain relief, aspirin or acetaminophen may be combined with one of the weaker narcotics, such as codeine, oxycodone, and propoxyphene. The additive effects of the two dissimilar drugs may provide sufficient pain control if the prescription is individualized according to the patient's age, habitus, and the existing pathology. Tylenol No. 3 (acetaminophen, 325 mg, with codeine, 30 mg) is one of the most frequently prescribed preparations. Percocet and Darvocet contain acetaminophen and oxycodone or propoxyphene, respectively. The use of such combinations enables one to avoid overdosing with a single agent, and to also avoid toxic or undesirable secondary effects. Aspirin and all other nonsteroidal anti-inflammatory drugs except acetaminophen may cause abnormal platelet function. When nerve block procedures are planned, the use of these drugs should be discontinued and a normal bleeding time ascertained. The concomitant use of heparin and coumarin anticoagulants precludes most nerve block procedures. In addition, coumarin plus dosing with most of the nonsteroidal agents causes an exaggerated response in prolongation of the prothrombin time. Table 16-1 is a list of various analgesics, with the nonsteroidal agents followed by the narcotics, from weak to more potent. Another liability of the nonsteroidal anti-inflammatory drugs is gastric irritation and occasional bleeding, which may become severe. Combinations of any of the nonsteroidal agents and weak or strong narcotics have proven to be the most effective means to control pain for many patients.

Patients whose pain syndromes cannot be controlled, or at least ameliorated, by even the most potent drugs are often the victims of the psychological component of their pain syndrome. The usual aberration is a depression neurosis, which patients often deny. The addition of a tricyclic antidepressant drug will frequently enhance pain control so that rehabilitation therapy can begin in earnest and high doses of narcotics can be reduced. Doxepin, nortriptyline, and amitriptyline have an effective antinociceptive effect by modification of pain transmission in the spinal cord [3]. In addition, a chronic pain syndrome may become a "psychological equivalent" of a depression neurosis and thus be responsive to antidepressant medication. Small doses (10–25 mg) of the previously mentioned medications are often effective, although I avoid amitriptyline because of its prolonged latency and the frequency of troublesome side effects.

Case Management Study

A 68-year-old man with Guillian-Barré syndrome became able to function weakly and feed himself but was virtually incapacitated by constant pain in the coc-

cygeal area whenever he sat in a wheelchair. He demanded three Tylenol No. 3 tablets every 2 or 3 hours and had nocturnal insomnia. His wife accompanied him throughout each day, even while he was hospitalized, in her efforts to comfort him. The patient was sent to the Pain Management Service for a nerve block of the coccyx. Evaluation revealed an intelligent, debilitated man who complained of severe pain and projected a mien of abject depression. He tolerated sitting for only 5 minutes, while watching the clock. Examination was unremarkable except for his weeping and protestations while palpating near the coccyx. When his attention was diverted, he offered no complaint and conversed easily. A differential block series was planned, with the initial injection being the simulated block—a placebo procedure. He almost immediately experienced great relief and was more comfortable when supine and for a few extra minutes when sitting. Doxepin was begun at 25 mg at bedtime and the Tylenol No. 3 doses were set on a time-contingent program. The doxepin dosage was increased rapidly to 150 mg while the analgesic combination was reduced in quantity with increased intervals between doses. Physical therapy was intensified. He improved rapidly and made even greater progress after his physiatrist diplomatically convinced his wife to take a vacation from her self-imposed nursing duties for several days. He was soon discharged, taking only the tricyclic antidepressant, and with ongoing interventions with a psychiatrist and physical therapist.

Benzodiazepines are often prescribed for anxious and depressed patients. Diazepam (Valium) enhances the depression of chronic pain patients and must be discontinued, although not abruptly. Patients who are habituated to large quantities of diazepam must be weaned gradually in order to avoid a troublesome reaction to the withdrawal. Meanwhile, analgesic and antidepressant medication should be started in adequate doses to ease the patient's anguish and to permit physical therapy and other rehabilitation activities to proceed.

Sudden, lightning-like, or stabbing paroxysmal pains are typical complaints of patients suffering from deafferentation syndromes resulting from damage to any portion of the peripheral or central nervous system. Phenytoin (Dilantin) and carbamazepine (Tegretol) have been tried because of their membrane-stabilizing and anticonvulsant effects. Although all patients do not gain significant benefit, some will volunteer the information that

Table 16-1. Common Analgesics

Drug	Dosage	Dosage Interval (hrs)	Comments
Mild pain			
Acetylsalicylic acid (aspirin)	650 mg PO	4–6	Analgesic, antipyretic, and anti-inflammatory; affects platelet activity
Acetaminophen (Tylenol)	650 mg PO	4–6	Weak analgesia; overdose may be hepatotoxic
Mild to moderate pain			
Ibuprofen (Motrin, Advil)	400 mg PO	4–6	Similar to aspirin; available over the counter
Naproxen (Naprosyn)	375–500 mg PO	8–12	Similar to aspirin; liquid suspension available
Diflunisal (Dolobid)	500 mg PO	8–12	Less gastrointestinal upset than aspirin
Diclofenac (Voltaren)	40–75 mg PO	12	Similar to aspirin; preparations are enteric coated
Indomethacin (Indocin)	25–50 mg PO	6–8	Potent analgesia; higher incidence of side effects
Ketorolac (Toradol)	10 mg PO	8	Limited to 2 wks; risk of gastric bleeding
Moderate to distressing pain			
Propoxyphene (Darvon)	100 mg PO	4	65 mg = 650 mg of aspirin; related to methadone
Codeine	60 mg PO	4	Equipotent to aspirin, 650 mg; same liabilities as morphine
Oxycodone (Percodan)	5–10 mg PO	4	Similar to codeine
Severe pain			
Ketorolac (injection)	30–60 mg IM	12	As potent as morphine, 8–10 mg; risk of gastric bleeding
Meperidine (Demerol)	50–100 mg IM	2–3	Least analgesia of this group; oral dosing is often unsatisfactory
Hydromorphone (Dilaudid)	1.5 mg IM	3–4	Potent analgesic; good gastrointestinal absorption
Levorphanol (Levo-Dromoran)	2 mg IM		
	4 mg PO	4–5	Potent analgesia; little euphoria
Morphine	10 mg IM	3–4	
	60 mg PO	4–5	The standard; new oral forms offer improved absorption and effectiveness
Methadone	10 mg IM	4–5	
	20 mg PO	5–6	Potent analgesia; least euphoria; useful in drug detoxification

their pain is still present but is significantly reduced and no longer plays a dominant role in their lives.

The physician who seeks to treat disabled patients with chronic pain and other persons who perceive themselves to be disabled by pain must try to maintain a comprehensive attitude and to create a therapeutic plan that satisfies the needs of both the nociceptive and the psychological problems. The two components of pain are inseparable.

Conclusion

Pain in a disabled person must be evaluated with the same care as in functionally able patients. Familiarity with the anatomy, physiology, and pharmacology of the nervous system, and particularly the ramifications of nociception, is needed for the creation of effective treatment plans. The psychological component of pain must also be addressed and treated during the rehabilitation program if an optimal restoration of function is to be gained. Diagnostic and prognostic differential regional blocks and therapeutic sympathetic and somatic nerve blocks have significant roles in enhancing the effectiveness of rehabilitation and evaluating the pain pattern. Neuropathic or deafferentation pain presents a challenge, which still requires research into the neuropharmacology of nociception. The judicious use of nonnarcotic analgesics, in combination with the weaker narcotics, tricyclic antidepressants, and membrane stabilizers, should enable patients to undertake their rehabilitation therapy in greater comfort and with positive expectations of success.

References

1. Rexed B. A cytoarchitectonic atlas of the spinal cord in the cat. J Comp Neurol 1952;96:415.
2. Yaksh TL. Opioid receptor systems and the endorphins: A review of their spinal organization. J Neurosurg 1987;67:157.
3. Fields HL. Pain. New York: McGraw-Hill, 1987.
4. Melzack R. The McGill Pain Questionnaire: Major properties and scoring methods. Pain 1975;1:277.
5. Evans FJ. The placebo response in pain reduction. Adv Neurol 1974;4:289.
6. Erickson JC. Differential nerve blocks and the evaluation of intractable pain. In Abstracts of Scientific Papers. 1974 Annual Meeting, American Society of Anesthesiologists, 1974;169.
7. Winnie AP, Collins VJ. Differential neural blockade in pain syndromes of questionable etiology. Med Clin North Am 1968;52:123.
8. Beric A, Dimitrijevic MR, Lindblom U. Central dysesthesia syndrome in spinal cord injury patients. Pain 1988;34:109.
9. Rabin AG, Anderson EG. Autotomy following limb denervation: Effects of previous exposure to neurectomy. Pain 1985;21:105.
10. Lofstrom JB, Lloyd JW, Cousins MJ. Sympathetic neural blockade of upper and lower extremity. In MJ Cousins, PO Bridenbaugh (eds), Neural Blockade in Clinical Anesthesia & Management of Pain. Philadelphia: Lippincott, 1980.
11. Miller RD, Munger WL, Powell PE. Chronic pain and local anesthetic neural blockade. In MJ Cousins, PO Bridenbaugh (eds), Neural Blockade in Clinical Anesthesia & Management of Pain. Philadelphia: Lippincott, 1980.
12. Campbell JN, Raja SN, Meyer RA. Painful sequelae of nerve injury. In R Dubner, GF Gebhardt, MR Bond (eds), Proceedings of the Vth World Congress on Pain. Amsterdam: Elsevier, 1988.
13. Erickson JC. Evaluation and management of autonomic dystrophies of the upper extremity. In JM Hunter, LH Schneider, EJ Mackin, JA Bell (eds), Rehabilitation of the Hand. St. Louis: Mosby, 1978.

Part IX
Pulmonary

Chapter 17
Pulmonary Disorders

James I. Couser, Jr., and James Sliwa

Respiratory problems are becoming increasingly commonplace among patients undergoing rehabilitation and are frequent causes of transfer back to acute care services from rehabilitation [1]. In some individuals, respiratory impairment may be the primary disability, whereas in others it may be a comorbidity following a stroke, spinal cord injury, or other physical impairment. In either case, physicians and allied health personnel providing care to this population should have an understanding of the evaluation and treatment of typical respiratory disorders.

This chapter is divided into three sections. The first focuses on the pathophysiology, diagnosis, and management of patients who are disabled by chronic obstructive pulmonary disease (COPD). The second section presents the general clinical approach to prevention, recognition, and treatment of pulmonary complications, which are common causes of morbidity and mortality in rehabilitation patients with restrictive physiologic impairment due to neurologic, neuromuscular, and chest wall disorders. The third section addresses specific respiratory problems that are unique to patients with stroke and spinal cord injury.

Chronic Obstructive Pulmonary Disease

COPD is a disorder characterized by cough, sputum production, dyspnea, expiratory airflow limitation, and impaired gas exchange. Predominantly a disease of cigarette smokers, COPD is estimated to affect nearly 15 million Americans and is the fifth leading cause of death in the United States [2]. The death rate from COPD has risen by 22% in the past decade, and the mortality 10 years after diagnosis is greater than 50% [3]. Compared with the general population, patients with COPD are twice as likely to rate their health as only fair or poor and nearly twice as likely to report limitations in daily activities [4]. In the United States, individuals with COPD are second only to persons with coronary heart disease in Social Security disability payments made for severe disease. In 1986 COPD was responsible for more than 17 million physician office visits [5], and there is epidemiologic evidence that the prevalence of COPD is increasing worldwide, particularly in elderly individuals [6].

Pathophysiology

There are two types of COPD—chronic bronchitis and emphysema. Although overlap among these two types is common, airflow obstruction is the hallmark of COPD and may be caused by both functional and structural abnormalities. In addition, up to two-thirds of patients with COPD have hyperreactive airways suggesting an asthmatic component [7]. Expiratory airflow obstruction in COPD is usually the result of one or more of the following mechanisms: (1) intraluminal secretions; (2) bronchial wall thickening; (3) smooth muscle hypertrophy and bronchoconstriction; and (4) loss of airway supporting structure. The first three mechanisms contribute to an increase in airway re-

315

sistance in patients with COPD whereas the fourth leads to a loss of elastic recoil of the lungs.

Chronic airflow obstruction leads to air trapping and lung hyperinflation. The increase in total lung volume results in shortening of the vertical muscle fibers of the diaphragm. As a result, the diaphragm is placed at a mechanical disadvantage and inspiratory work of breathing is increased. Chronic hypercapnia may develop in patients who have a combination of high inspiratory load from increased airway resistance and inspiratory muscle weakness [8], whereas hypoxemia develops in patients with COPD because of ventilation-perfusion ($\dot{V}/\dot{Q}$) mismatching. In emphysema, there may be well-ventilated areas with poor perfusion because of destruction of the pulmonary capillaries (high $\dot{V}/\dot{Q}$ areas), whereas in chronic bronchitis, airflow obstruction may lead to reduced ventilation in regions where perfusion is maintained (low $\dot{V}/\dot{Q}$ areas). In patients with mixed disease, both high and low $\dot{V}/\dot{Q}$ areas may be seen [9]. Chronic hypoxemia may result in changes in the pulmonary vasculature leading to pulmonary hypertension and right-sided heart failure.

Most patients with COPD eventually experience a decrease in their ability to perform physical activities. The pathophysiologic mechanisms that contribute to reduced exercise tolerance include (1) decreased ventilatory capacity; (2) hypoxemia; (3) respiratory muscle dysfunction; and (4) right ventricular dysfunction due to pulmonary hypertension [5].

Diagnosis

The usual initial symptom in COPD is the gradual onset of exertional dyspnea. Productive cough with clear sputum is another common symptom. Patients may also complain of wheezing, which results from turbulent flow through airways that may be narrowed by intraluminal secretions or bronchospasm. Almost all patients with COPD have a history of cigarette smoking and often do not seek medical attention until symptoms begin to interfere with daily activities.

Physical examination findings are often normal until airflow limitation is severe [10]. Patients with marked dyspnea usually have an increased respiratory rate and use accessory muscles of respiration. Signs of hyperinflation include a barrel-shaped chest with reduced diaphragmatic excursion on percussion and auscultation. There may be diminished intensity of breath sounds, expiratory wheezing, and a prolonged expiratory time. Jugular venous distension, an increase in the pulmonic component of the second heart sound (P2), a murmur of tricuspid insufficiency, and peripheral edema all suggest severe disease associated with pulmonary hypertension and right ventricular failure.

Although history and physical examination findings are highly suggestive, the diagnosis of COPD is confirmed by spirometry. A reduction in the forced expiratory volume in 1 second (FEV_1) associated with a reduction in the ratio of FEV_1 to forced vital capacity (FVC) to less than 70% are typical findings. The American Thoracic Society suggests that the diagnosis of COPD in elderly individuals requires reduction in FEV_1 and FEV_1/FVC less than two standard deviations from the mean value as well as a consistent history, physical examination findings, and other confirmatory laboratory data [11]. The severity of airway obstruction is based on the percentage of predicted FEV_1; a mild defect is diagnosed when the percentage of predicted FEV_1 is less than 80 and greater than or equal to 65, a moderate defect when the percentage of predicted FEV_1 is less than 65 and greater than or equal to 50, and a severe defect when the percentage of predicted FEV_1 is less than 50. Residual volume and total lung capacity are often increased in COPD, particularly in emphysematous patients. Inspiratory muscle strength (PI_{max}) may be reduced because of the effects of hyperinflation on diaphragm function. Single-breath diffusing capacity is usually normal in chronic bronchitis but reduced in emphysema.

Measurements of oxygen saturation and arterial blood gases are not useful in diagnosing COPD. However, to help assess adequacy of oxygenation in patients with moderate or severe COPD, oximetry should be done at rest and with activity. Arterial blood gas analysis may be useful in more severely obstructed patients (FEV_1 <50% predicted) to determine adequacy of ventilation ($PaCO_2$) and acid-base status.

The chest roentgenogram with mild airflow obstruction may appear normal but frequently shows hyperlucent lung fields and flattened diaphragms in severely limited patients. Prominence of the central pulmonary arteries may suggest the development of pulmonary hypertension. Other laboratory tests that may be helpful in the evaluation of patients with COPD include a hemoglobin level to assess for

Table 17-1. Selected Inhaled Bronchodilators

Agent	Delivery System	Duration of Action (hrs)	Dose
Ipratropium bromide	MDI	6–8	2–6 puffs every 6 hrs
	Nebulized solution	6–8	0.5 mg every 6 hrs
Metaproterenol	MDI	3–4	2–4 puffs every 3–4 hrs
	Nebulized solution	3–4	0.3 ml every 3–4 hrs
Albuterol	MDI	4–6	2–4 puffs every 4–6 hrs
	Nebulized solution	4–6	2.5 mg every 4–6 hrs
	Dry powder inhaler	4–6	200 µg every 4–6 hrs
Pirbuterol	MDI (breath actuated)	4–6	2 puffs every 4–6 hrs
Salmeterol*	MDI	10–12	2 puffs every 12 hrs

MDI = metered dose inhaler.
*Not currently approved for chronic obstructive pulmonary disease.

polycythemia in chronically hypoxemic patients, and a serum bicarbonate level to look for evidence of metabolic compensation for chronic respiratory acidosis in severely obstructed patients. Gram's staining of sputum samples may be useful in patients with productive cough to assess purulence and the need for antibiotics; however, sputum culture rarely adds useful information.

Management

The principal goals in management of patients with COPD are to minimize and prevent progression of airflow limitation, to correct hypoxemia, and to improve functional status [12]. The most important strategy to prevent progression of airflow limitation is smoking cessation. The rate of decline in lung function in smokers can be slowed with smoking cessation so that it approaches that of nonsmokers [13]. Nicotine replacement therapy, support groups, and behavior modification programs may help motivated individuals to stop smoking. Other preventive measures include a pneumococcal vaccination, currently recommended for all patients with COPD [14], and annual prophylactic vaccination against influenza.

Bronchodilators

The first line of medical therapy for COPD is the inhalation of bronchodilator aerosols (Table 17-1). A variety of bronchodilator delivery systems are available, including the metered dose inhaler (MDI), MDI with large volume spacer device, breath-actuated devices, and the jet and ultrasonic nebulizer. There are considerable data that suggest that if appropriate technique is used, MDIs are as effective as nebulizers in delivering aerosolized medication [15, 16]. Unfortunately, many patients are unable to use their MDIs correctly [17], and many physicians are unable to demonstrate appropriate technique to their patients [18]. The addition of a spacer device to the MDI improves aerosol delivery to the distal airways and reduces oropharyngeal and laryngeal deposition of medication. This is particularly important when inhaled corticosteroids are being used to prevent oropharyngeal candidiasis and hoarseness. A number of breath-actuated devices are currently available, including the dry powder inhaler. This device requires a rapid inhalation technique that may be difficult for weak or elderly patients. In some patients who have difficulty with MDIs or breath-actuated devices, it may be appropriate to deliver aerosolized bronchodilators with a jet or ultrasonic nebulizer. During acute episodes of airflow obstruction, some COPD patients experience greater improvement in symptoms using a nebulizer than an MDI [6].

Anticholinergic Agents

Ipratropium bromide has become the drug of first choice in the medical treatment of COPD. It is a quaternary anticholinergic agent that is poorly absorbed and does not usually cause significant atropine-like side effects. Although its onset of action is slower than beta-adrenergic agonists, ipratropium provides a greater peak bronchodilator effect and a more sustained duration of action [19]. The recommended dose of ipratropium bromide is two puffs four times a day; however, this dose may be doubled or tripled for maximal benefit in severely obstructed patients without notable side effects [12, 20]. Recently, ipratropium has become available as an inhalant solution and can be nebulized in a dose of 0.5 mg in saline every 4–6 hours or as needed.

Beta-Adrenergic Agonists

Before the introduction of ipratropium bromide, beta-adrenergic agonists were the mainstay of bronchodilator treatment for COPD. These agents produce bronchial smooth muscle relaxation by stimulating adenyl cyclase. A variety of formulations are available as MDIs, inhalant solutions for nebulization, or oral preparations. Because of their rapid onset of action, beta-agonists are the preferred method of treating acute symptoms of COPD. Recommended doses (2–4 puffs three or four times a day) may result in suboptimal bronchodilation and inadequate control of symptoms, and it may be necessary to double the number of puffs in order to achieve the goals of therapy [21]. Combination therapy with beta-adrenergic agonists and ipratropium bromide does not achieve greater bronchodilation than maximal doses of either agent alone [22]; however, by combining these medications in lower doses it may be possible to produce a comparable benefit and minimize side effects. Oral beta-agonists are no more effective than inhaled therapy and are associated with a high incidence of side effects, particularly tremor. These agents should only be used in patients who are unable to use inhaled therapy.

Theophylline

The role of theophylline in the treatment of COPD is controversial, and its mechanism of action is poorly understood. It is a relatively weak bronchodilator when compared with inhaled anticholinergic or beta-adrenergic drugs. However, when used in combination with either ipratropium bromide [23] or a beta-agonist [24], theophylline appears to have an additive bronchodilator effect. In addition, long-acting theophylline preparations have been shown to reduce overnight declines in FEV_1 and morning respiratory symptoms in patients with COPD [25]. Most clinicians favor the addition of oral theophylline in patients with COPD whose symptoms are not adequately controlled with inhaled bronchodilators [12, 21]. Initially, a low dose of long-acting theophylline (100–200 mg/day) should be used for several days to enhance patient tolerance. This dose can gradually be increased as tolerated, aiming for a therapeutic blood level of 8–12 mg/liter. Potential side effects include gastrointestinal symptoms, tremulousness, and insomnia. Other potentially beneficial effects of theophylline in COPD are improved collateral ventilation, respiratory muscle function, and mucociliary clearance [26].

Corticosteroids

A trial of systemic corticosteroids is often recommended for patients with severe COPD who continue to have disabling symptoms despite maximal therapy with inhaled bronchodilators and theophylline [12, 21, 23]. Oral corticosteroids can produce a significant objective and subjective benefit in some patients with COPD [27]. The potential benefits of long-term corticosteroid therapy must be weighed against its well-known side effects. If a therapeutic trial of corticosteroids is undertaken, a dose of 0.5 mg/kg per day of prednisone or its equivalent should be given for 2–3 weeks. If there is significant objective improvement (>25% increase in FEV_1 as determined by spirometry before and after initiation of treatment), the medication is tapered to the lowest dose that maintains improvement in lung function and symptomatic benefit. Without documented objective improvement, continued treatment with systemic corticosteroids cannot be justified. There is little evidence to suggest that alternate-day steroids or inhaled steroids are beneficial in patients with COPD [21, 28].

Adjunctive Therapy for Chronic Obstructive Pulmonary Disease

Antibiotics and Mucolytics

The routine use of antibiotics for COPD exacerbations is controversial [29]. Exacerbations may be in-

Table 17-2. Criteria for Medicare Reimbursement for Home Oxygen

---

1. Acceptable primary diagnosis
   Emphysema, chronic obstructive bronchitis
   Chronic obstructive pulmonary disease, chronic obstructive asthma
   Interstitial disease
       and
2. PaO_2 ≤55 mm Hg or SaO_2 ≤88%
       or
1. Acceptable primary diagnosis
       and
2. PaO_2 = 56–59 mm Hg or SaO_2 = 89–91%
       and
3. Evidence of cor pulmonale (P pulmonale on ECG, polycythemia, or congestive heart failure)

PaO_2 = partial pressure of arterial oxygen; SaO_2 = arterial oxygen saturation; ECG = electrocardiogram.

fectious and result from either viral or bacterial pathogens. When patients with COPD develop acute symptoms of dyspnea associated with increased sputum quantity and purulence, antibiotic therapy produces earlier resolution of symptoms [30]. Amoxicillin, trimethoprim-sulfamethoxazole, or tetracycline should be prescribed for a 7- to 10-day period.

A number of pharmacologic treatments have been tried to control excess sputum production in COPD. However, the value of these approaches remains unproven. In one recent randomized, double-blind, placebo-controlled study, iodinated glycerol (60 mg four times daily) improved cough frequency and severity, chest discomfort, ease in raising sputum, and the patient's assessment of his or her overall condition [31]. A trial of iodinated glycerol may be warranted in patients with excessive sputum that they are unable to clear.

Oxygen

Long-term oxygen therapy improves survival in hypoxemic patients with COPD [32, 33]. This beneficial effect appears to be mediated by reduction in secondary pulmonary hypertension [34]. Benefits of long-term oxygen are greatest if it is used at least 18 hours per day, but most hypoxemic patients require oxygen continuously (24 hours per day). Some patients have adequate oxygenation at rest but desaturate during exercise or sleep. In these individuals, oxygen supplementation has been shown to improve daytime performance when used with exertion [35], and improve sleep quality while reducing pulmonary artery pressure when administered at night [36, 37]. The Medicare criteria for reimbursable oxygen supplementation are shown in Table 17-2.

Three systems are in common use for home oxygen therapy: oxygen concentrators, compressed gas oxygen, and liquid oxygen. Oxygen concentrators are electrically powered, extract oxygen from air, and supply oxygen in standard liter flow. They are the least expensive form of oxygen delivery but their size and weight limit their portability. In the event of a power failure, an alternate source of oxygen (usually compressed gas) must be available.

Compressed gas cylinders store oxygen and come in variety of sizes. Large H cylinders that weigh more than 200 lb are generally used for home oxygen. This volume of gas lasts about 2.4 days at a flow rate of 2 liters/minute. Smaller E (18 lb), D (9 lb), and C (7 lb) tanks are available for portable use; however, tank weight is still limiting for most patients. Recently, a lightweight aluminum and fiberglass cylinder weighing only 4 lb has become available but its practicality is limited because of low storage capacity. At a flow rate of 2 liters/minute, the oxygen lasts only 1 hour. Other disadvantages of compressed gas are the need for frequent home visits by the home care company to replenish the oxygen supply and the complexity of transfilling oxygen from the large H cylinder to smaller portable units.

Table 17-3. Guidelines for Home Oxygen Delivery Systems*

Condition	System
Sedentary, bed bound, or homebound patients	Oxygen concentrator, backup compressed gas cylinder
Ambulatory patients who rarely get out (physician visits)	Oxygen concentrator, supplemental cylinders on a stroller
Ambulatory patients who leave home several times a week	Liquid oxygen with lightweight ambulatory units

*Based on recommendations from Third Consensus Conference on Home Oxygen Therapy. New problems in supply, reimbursement, and certification of medical necessity for long-term oxygen therapy. Am Rev Respir Dis 1990;142:721.

Liquid oxygen systems are particularly useful for ambulatory patients because of superior portability. The stationary-reservoir liquid oxygen units are more convenient, store more oxygen, and are more manageable than H cylinders. Larger amounts of liquid oxygen can be stored in smaller, more lightweight containers that are easier to fill from larger reservoirs. The major disadvantage of liquid oxygen is its cost for both the home care company and the patient.

When prescribing a home oxygen therapy system for patients with COPD, a number of considerations must be taken into account, including storage capacity, weight, bulk, size, cost, availability, transfillability, range of the portable unit, and condition of the patient. A major goal of therapy is patient mobility, so it is important to provide patients with the least encumbering system that will meet their needs. The standard of care should be for the patient to be ambulatory if possible [38, 39]. Some guidelines for home oxygen therapy are provided in Table 17-3 [40].

Pulmonary Rehabilitation

The goals for pulmonary rehabilitation in patients with COPD are to maximize functional capacity and improve quality of life. Pulmonary rehabilitation programs provide education, respiratory, physical, and occupational therapy, exercise training, and psychosocial support. These programs benefit many patients, regardless of the extent of their disease [41, 42], and reduce respiratory symptoms, anxiety, depression, and the need for hospital and medical care [43]. In addition, pulmonary rehabilitation has been shown to improve exercise performance and quality of life [44]. Patients generally participate in these programs as outpatients, although severely limited patients may benefit from an inpatient program [41].

Restrictive Ventilatory Disorders

Patients with neuromuscular and skeletal disorders, stroke, and brain injury are at increased risk for pulmonary complications owing to restriction in pulmonary function from respiratory muscle weakness and mechanical problems with the lungs or chest wall (Table 17-4). For example, respiratory failure is the most common cause of death in patients with severe myopathies, kyphoscoliosis, and anterior horn cell disorders [45–47], whereas bacterial pneumonia is the leading nonneurologic cause of death after stroke [48, 49] and spinal cord injury [50]. Pneumonia is also a common, often fatal, complication in patients with brain injury [51].

Pathophysiology

Discussion of the specific pathophysiology of respiratory impairment associated with each of the conditions in Table 17-4 is beyond the scope of this chapter; however, some general statements are appropriate.

Respiratory muscle weakness is the major cause of serious respiratory complications in rehabilitation patients with restrictive impairments. Expiratory muscle weakness markedly reduces cough effectiveness. As a result, these patients develop retained secretions, macroatelectasis and microatelectasis, and frequent lower respiratory tract

Table 17-4. Some Neuromuscular and Skeletal Diseases That Cause Respiratory Impairment

Location	Disease
Cerebral cortex/brain stem	Stroke
	Brain injury
Spinal cord/anterior horn cell	Spinal cord injury
	Amyotrophic lateral sclerosis
	Poliomyelitis
	Postpolio syndrome
Peripheral nerves	Guillain-Barré syndrome
	Phrenic nerve injury
	Peripheral neuropathies
	Infectious
	Diabetes mellitus
	Chronic alcoholism
Neuromuscular junction	Myasthenia gravis
	Botulism
	Organophosphate poisoning
Muscle	Muscular dystrophies
	Myopathies
Skeletal	Kyphoscoliosis
	Obesity
	Ankylosing spondylitis
	Fibrothorax/thoracoplasty
	Flail chest

infections. Because the inspiratory muscles perform most of the work of breathing, weakness of these muscles frequently leads to hypercapnic respiratory failure. Reduced inspiratory muscle contractility is associated with reductions in tidal volume, increased dead space ventilation, alveolar collapse, loss of lung and chest wall elasticity, $\dot{V}/\dot{Q}$ mismatching, and worsening hypoxemia [52]. Reduction in pulmonary and chest wall compliance occurs, even in the absence of kyphoscoliosis [53]. As inspiratory muscle weakness progresses, alveolar hypoventilation and hypercapnia develop.

The ventilatory response to hypoxemia and hypercapnia is reduced in the presence of respiratory muscle weakness and altered chest mechanics. It is unclear if this reduction is the result of alteration in the respiratory center drive [54] or other mechanisms such as decreased chemoreceptor responsiveness to acute increases in $PaCO_2$ in the face of chronically increased cerebrospinal fluid bicarbonate concentrations [52]. Alveolar hypoventilation is particularly common during sleep in patients with

respiratory muscle weakness because of the decrease in minute ventilation and the increase in diaphragmatic workload that are known to occur [55].

Sleep apnea is another common problem in patients with kyphoscoliosis [56], stroke [57], postpolio syndrome [58], muscular dystrophy [59], and spinal cord injury [60]. The mechanisms for sleep apnea in patients with neuromuscular and skeletal disorders are not clear but may be related to upper airway muscle dysfunction, loss of airway protective reflexes, and normal loss of muscle tone, particularly during rapid eye movement sleep [55]. Stroke patients with brain stem lesions may be particularly susceptible to sleep apnea if there is respiratory center damage [57].

Clinical Evaluation of Patients with Restrictive Disorders

Respiratory symptoms in disabled patients with restrictive impairment are often minimal, particularly when these patients are nonambulatory. The most common symptom is fatigue [47]. Other symptoms include dyspnea on exertion, productive cough, and generalized muscle weakness. Daytime somnolence, morning headache, and impaired concentration are often associated with alveolar hypoventilation, hypercapnia, and sleep apnea. These symptoms may be harbingers for severe ventilatory failure.

Patients with restrictive disorders typically develop a rapid, shallow breathing pattern. Other pertinent physical examination findings may include dyssynchronous movement of the abdomen or thorax, marked kyphosis, scoliosis, or both, accessory muscle use, reduced or absent diaphragmatic excursion, and findings suggestive of right-sided heart failure (jugular venous distension, increased P2, and peripheral edema). It is useful to observe a spontaneous or voluntary cough during the physical examination to assess cough strength and effectiveness.

Restriction in pulmonary function is defined by a reduction in total lung capacity [11]. Lung volume measurement is often not practical for disabled patients, however, and a number of simple, dependable, and reproducible parameters can be done portably to assess severity of impairment and to follow the progression of disease and response to therapy. The most valuable of these is the vital capacity (VC), which is related to respiratory muscle strength and pulmonary compliance [61]. Ventilatory impairment may develop insidiously as VC decreases in slowly progressive disorders. In normal adults, the VC averages 50 ml/kg. Secretion clearance is impaired when VC decreases below 30 ml/kg, and ventilatory failure occurs at a VC of 10 ml/kg [59].

Maximum static mouth pressures will detect abnormalities at an early stage of acute or chronic respiratory muscle weakness and may be even more sensitive than the VC [62]. PI_{max} and maximum expiratory pressure (PE_{max}) can be measured simply and reproducibly at the bedside. A PI_{max} of –70 cm H_2O and a PE_{max} of 100 cm H_2O are considered normal. A normal $PaCO_2$ generally cannot be maintained with a PI_{max} of less than –20 cm H_2O, and an ineffective cough is typically seen when PE_{max} decreases below 40 cm H_2O [46].

Arterial blood gas analysis should be done in patients with a VC, PI_{max}, or PE_{max} less than or equal to 50% of predicted because these values correlate with onset of hypercapnia [47, 61]. In individuals with less severe abnormalities, noninvasive pulse oximetry may be used to assess oxygenation. If the SaO_2 decreases below 90%, an arterial blood gas determination should be obtained.

Polysomnography may be helpful in detecting sleep disordered breathing in patients with respiratory muscle weakness and should be done in patients with excessive fatigue, daytime somnolence, morning headache, and daytime hypercapnia. Sleep studies are also useful in the assessment and treatment of patients who may be candidates for nocturnal ventilatory support because appropriate levels of continuous positive airway pressure and noninvasive ventilation can be titrated in this monitored setting.

General Approach to the Management of Disabled Patients with Restrictive Ventilatory Disorders

Patients with respiratory dysfunction due to neuromuscular and skeletal disorders have limited reserve to compensate for acute illness. Relatively minor disturbances such as upper respiratory infections may precipitate acute respiratory failure in these individuals. Strategies aimed at preventing aspiration and retained secretions should be initiated in patients with respiratory muscle weakness. Chest physical therapy, frequent suctioning, incentive spirometry, cough assist maneuvers, and other forms of respiratory therapy may help reverse secretion-related complications such as mucus plugging and atelectasis. Bronchoscopy may be indicated when other methods fail.

Oxygen

Low-flow oxygen therapy should be used in hypoxemic patients with restrictive disorders to improve dyspnea and exercise tolerance and to prevent development of pulmonary hypertension and cor pulmonale. Although the multicenter oxygen trials [32, 33] focused on patients with COPD, it is generally assumed that the beneficial effects seen in these studies also apply to patients with restrictive disorders. Oxygen therapy should be titrated carefully in a monitored setting in these individuals because the ventilatory response to oxygen and carbon dioxide may be blunted. Respiratory depression with worsening hypercapnia and respiratory acidosis may occur rarely [63].

Respiratory Muscle Training

Respiratory muscle training has been shown to increase strength and endurance in patients with kyphoscoliosis [64], muscular dystrophy [65], and spinal cord injury [66]. It is not clear, however, that these improvements translate into improved dyspnea and functional capacity [67]. Studies in patients with COPD suggest that benefit is not achieved unless a sufficient load (25–35% of PI_{max}) is placed on the respiratory muscles during training [68, 69]. Some authors have warned that vigorous respiratory muscle training may be inappropriate and hazardous in patients with severe respiratory muscle weakness and hypercapnia [59].

Most studies have focused on training of the inspiratory muscles. Little is known about the effects of expiratory muscle training that might be particularly beneficial in patients with weak cough. Estenne and coworkers showed that pectoralis muscle training led to improved expiratory muscle function in a small group of tetraplegic patients [70]. This type of training should increase effectiveness of cough and might reduce the incidence of pulmonary infections in disabled individuals. Further study must be done before respiratory muscle training can be routinely recommended in patients with restrictive ventilatory impairments.

Assisted Ventilation

As respiratory muscle weakness becomes advanced in high spinal cord injury patients or in some disabled individuals who do not recover sufficiently from acute respiratory failure, lung restriction and alveolar hypoventilation may not allow survival without some form of ventilatory support. A variety of noninvasive methods are available for individuals with chronic respiratory failure. Detailed discussion of these is beyond the scope of this chapter and they have been reviewed elsewhere [47, 71, 72]. Current interest has focused on the use of nasal positive pressure ventilation (NPPV) in both acute and chronic forms of respiratory failure. NPPV has been shown to improve daytime symptoms and gas exchange while relieving nocturnal oxygen desaturation in patients with restrictive thoracic disorders [73]. It may also prolong survival and improve quality of life [52].

NPPV is less bulky and more portable than most types of negative pressure ventilation (i.e., iron lung, poncho wrap, or tortoise shell ventilators), its application may be simpler in severely disabled patients, and it causes less musculoskeletal discomfort in patients with chest wall deformities [72, 74]. NPPV also avoids the severe oxygen desaturation from upper airway obstruction during sleep that is seen in some patients using negative pressure ventilators [74, 75]. There are preliminary data to suggest that NPPV may be more effective than negative pressure ventilation in reducing diaphragmatic activity and providing respiratory muscle rest [76, 77].

Patients who are being considered for chronic noninvasive ventilatory support must be carefully selected. In general, the best candidates are those with slowly progressive conditions such as postpolio syndrome or kyphoscoliosis; they should have intact upper airway function and minimal secretions; they should be capable of spontaneous ventilation without support for sustained periods; and they should be motivated to succeed because adaptation to noninvasive support may take prolonged periods of time [72, 78].

Invasive ventilation with permanent tracheostomy has been advocated for patients who require ventilatory support for more than 16 hours a day [79]. Carefully selected patients with chronic respiratory failure can be managed at home. Factors to be assessed in determining the feasibility of home ventilation are (1) the underlying disease causing respiratory failure; (2) medical stability; (3) patient and family desires about continued care; and (4) availability of home care resources [80]. Comprehensive guidelines have been published for appropriate management of disabled patients requiring continuous ventilatory support [80].

Speech is an important consideration for chronically ventilated patients and should not be overlooked. It is possible for many ventilated patients with tracheostomy tubes to swallow and speak, provided their oropharyngeal muscle strength is adequate. Cuffless tubes may be used if tidal volumes are increased on the ventilator to compensate for leaks [81], and one-way valves may also be used to facilitate speech [82].

Special Problems

Pneumonia After Stroke

Pneumonia is a common and potentially life-threatening complication of stroke, accounting for up to 40% of deaths occurring more than 8 days after stroke [83]. A number of factors contribute to increased risk for pneumonia after stroke. The most important are dysphagia and aspiration of oropharyngeal material due to swallowing dysfunction. Other risk factors include depressed sensorium, impaired gag and cough reflexes, inadequate hydration, immobility, decreased cough strength because of expiratory muscle weakness on the involved side, and iatrogenic causes such as sedating medications and feeding tubes.

Aspiration of material into the tracheobronchial tree is the most common cause of pneumonia in stroke patients. Aspiration is often unsuspected and may be detected with videofluoroscopy in up to 50% of patients after stroke [84]. Clinical variables that may help predict the risk of aspiration after stroke include bilateral or brain stem strokes with cranial nerve involvement, abnormal cough, abnormal gag, and dysphonia [85]. Although aspiration of oropharyngeal contents does not always lead to pneumonia, it is thought to be an important risk factor in the pathogenesis of bacterial pneumonia [86].

A number of physiologic abnormalities in the swallowing mechanism may contribute to aspiration following stroke (see Chapter 8). Veis and Logemann used videofluorography to identify swallowing defects after stroke. All patients who aspirated had disorders involving the pharyngeal phase of the swallow, the most important of which was a delayed swallowing reflex. Reduced pharyngeal peristalsis was the next most frequent disorder, followed by reduced tongue control. Seventy-five percent of patients had more than one abnormality in the swallowing mechanism [87].

Aspiration pneumonia following stroke is frequently preventable and a number of preventive strategies should be employed in stroke patients. A high index of suspicion is necessary, and risk factors for aspiration outlined previously should be sought. A careful bedside assessment of swallowing by a speech or swallowing therapist should be done, although bedside clinical evaluation is frequently inadequate to detect significant silent aspiration [88]. Videofluoroscopy is often necessary in the evaluation of the swallowing mechanism and can help target specific therapy [89]. It is best if the swallowing therapist is present during this study because management strategies can be tested that include positioning of the patient, texture and consistencies of feedings, and motor treatments [90].

It is frequently necessary to avoid oral feeding after stroke until swallowing function has been adequately assessed. If there is significant swallowing dysfunction, enteral feeding support may be indicated to ensure adequate caloric and nutritional intake during the rehabilitation process. The choice of tubes for feeding may be influenced by available medical and surgical expertise, the advantages of bolus versus continuous feeding, and long-term care issues in a given individual [91].

The diagnosis of aspiration pneumonia may be difficult to confirm in stroke patients (see Chapter 12). Initially, most patients present with mild signs and symptoms that may include low-grade fever, cough, and increased sputum production, but clinical features may be atypical [92]. Cough strength may be reduced after stroke so symptoms and signs such as confusion, fever, and increased respiratory rate may be the only indications of early respiratory infection [93] and should prompt Gram's staining and culture of sputum as well as chest radiography. The precise location of the infiltrate is usually dependent on the position of the patient at the time of aspiration. If patients are supine when they aspirate, infiltrates are usually seen in the superior segment of the right lower lobe or the posterior segment of the upper lobes, whereas if the patient aspirates while upright or semirecumbant, the infiltrates are usually seen in the basal segments of the lower lobes [94].

Once the stroke survivor has returned to the community, aspiration pneumonia is usually caused by anaerobic mouth flora [95]. Penicillin G is the drug of choice for community-acquired aspiration pneumonia because of its activity against these organisms and *Streptococcus pneumoniae*. Treatment should be continued for 10–14 days. Alternative antibiotics include clindamycin and first- and second-generation cephalosporins. If the pneumonia occurs in the hospital setting, as is often the case during rehabilitation following stroke, it is usually the result of enteric gram-negative bacilli [96]. The combination of an antipseudomonal penicillin and an aminoglycoside is generally recommended, although a number of alternative regimens may be effective including a third-generation cephalosporin with an aminoglycoside, or a parenteral quinolone in combination with clindamycin or a third-generation cephalosporin. The duration of parenteral therapy for hospital-acquired aspiration pneumonia is usually 10–14 days.

Other measures that may be helpful in the management of stroke patients with aspiration pneumonia include administration of supplemental oxygen for hypoxemia, chest physical therapy to help promote secretion clearance in patients with weak cough, and bronchodilators if airflow obstruction is present. Postural drainage may be effective if individuals produce more than 30 ml of sputum per day [97]. Early mobilization and exercise may reduce cardiopulmonary dysfunction associated with acute pneumonia [98], and appropriate positioning can enhance secretion clearance as well as oxygen transport [99].

Spinal Cord Injury

Despite significant improvements in survival, respiratory complications remain a major problem in the population with traumatic spinal cord injuries, with as many as two-thirds of these patients experiencing such a complication [100]. Pneumonia is the leading cause of death after spinal cord injury [50], whereas atelectasis, ventilatory failure, and pulmonary embolism are common causes of morbidity [100]. Ongoing preventive measures, careful surveillance, prompt diagnosis, and appropriate treatment of respiratory complications are necessary in these patients in order to minimize morbidity and mortality.

In the individual with a spinal cord injury, the extent of respiratory compromise is related to the level of injury and the extent of associated respiratory muscle paralysis. Patients at risk for respiratory complications are those with cervical and high thoracic to midthoracic spinal cord injuries. Patients with injuries at the first cervical level have no inspiratory or expiratory muscle function and are dependent on ventilators. Although individuals with injuries between C2 and C5 may also require ventilatory support, the need decreases as the cord level proceeds caudad. Injuries to the cervical cord result in impairment of all or most of the expiratory muscle function. The diaphragm is usually completely innervated with lesions below C5 so inspiratory function is preserved; however, expiratory forces remain reduced so cough can be ineffective.

In the early postinjury period, patients often suffer from "spinal shock," which is manifested as a flaccid paralysis, and the level of injury may appear higher than it actually is [101]. Patients must be carefully monitored during this period because cord levels may ascend transiently due to edema and lead to acute respiratory failure requiring mechanical ventilation. Pulmonary function during this period is markedly reduced, with FVC ranging from 25–30% in those in whom it can be measured (C4) [102]. Spinal shock resolves slowly over days to months, and as flaccid paralysis is replaced with spasticity, pulmonary function improves. In mid- (C3 to C6) and lower cord injuries (C6 to midthoracic), the FVC doubles from initial values. By 5 months postinjury, it will be 50–60% of predicted [103]; however, this can be influenced by body posture. In the sitting position, gravitational pull on the abdominal contents decreases diaphragmatic excursion and thus increases the work of breathing. The use of abdominal binders can increase vital capacity and improve ventilatory capacity in marginal patients by maintaining the diaphragm in an elevated position.

Optimal management of all patients with spinal cord injury requires a multidisciplinary team-oriented approach in both the acute and chronic setting in order to prevent pulmonary complications. Respiratory problems such as mucus plugging, atelectasis, and pulmonary emboli may not be recognized as quickly in patients with spinal cord injuries as they are in normally innervated individuals. Comprehensive management requires careful attention to aggressive secretion removal and measures to improve vital capacity.

Secretion removal in patients with spinal cord injuries may be facilitated in a variety of ways. Frequent suctioning and chest percussion are time-honored methods. Manually assisted cough, when performed correctly, can quadruple spontaneous expiratory pressure and improve efficacy of cough [104]. This maneuver requires a trained assistant in order to be effective. It is also likely that patients are unable to cough as often as is necessary [105]. Mechanical exsufflation has recently been shown to provide cough peak expiratory flow that was greater than that produced by manually assisted cough [106]. This method also requires a trained care provider. Another recently reported technique is functional electrical stimulation. This technique employs an abdominal binder with attached electrodes that stimulate contraction of the abdominal muscles. Spontaneous expiratory pressure [107] and cough peak expiratory flows [105] can be increased significantly using this method and it has the potential advantage of self-administration. When other methods fail, bronchoscopy may be indicated for some patients with high cervical spine injuries and mucus plugging with atelectasis. Repeated bronchoscopies for secretion clearance are expensive and impractical, however.

Traditional measures designed to increase vital capacity in patients with spinal cord injuries include incentive spirometry, intermittent positive pressure breathing, and deep breathing exercises. There is controversy about the benefits of these maneuvers [108], but most authors recommend incentive spirometry or regular deep breathing exercises for those patients who can participate in these activities. Inspiratory muscle training has been shown to reduce symptoms, increase inspiratory muscle strength and endurance, and protect against fatigue in quadriplegia [109]. Such training is accomplished by breathing through resistance. It must be maintained indefinitely because gains are quickly lost if training is stopped. It has also recently been shown that training the clavicular portion of the pectoralis major muscle with repetitive isometric contraction can lead to improved expiratory muscle function in tetraplegics, thus potentially increasing cough effectiveness and reducing the prevalence of bronchopulmonary infections in these patients [110].

Conclusion

In summary, obstructive lung disease and restrictive ventilatory disorders are common in disabled individuals. Even though these conditions are usually chronic and progressive, strategies aimed at prevention of complications, early recognition and treatment of worsening airflow obstruction and respiratory muscle weakness, pulmonary rehabilitation, and assisted ventilation in carefully selected patients can reduce morbidity and mortality and improve functional capacity in the disabled.

References

1. Stineman MG, Williams SV. Predicting in-patient length of rehabilitation stay. Arch Phys Med Rehabil 1990;71:881.
2. Redline S. The epidemiology of COPD. In NS Cherniack (ed), Chronic Obstructive Pulmonary Disease. Philadelphia: Saunders, 1991;225.
3. Burrows B, Bloom JW, Traver GA, Cline MG. The course and prognosis of chronic airway obstruction in a sample from the general population. N Engl J Med 1987;317:1309.
4. Feinleib M, Rosenberg HM, Collins JG, et al. Trends in COPD morbidity and mortality in the United States. Am Rev Respir Dis 1989;140:S9.
5. Higgins MW, Thom T. Incidence, prevalence, and mortality: Intra- and intercountry differences. In MJ Hensley, NA Saunders (eds), Clinical Epidemiology of Chronic Obstructive Pulmonary Disease. New York: Marcel Dekker, 1989;23.
6. Mahler DA. Chronic obstructive pulmonary disease. In DA Mahler (ed), Pulmonary Disease in the Elderly Patient. New York: Marcel Dekker, 1991;159.
7. Owens GR. Public screening for lung disease: Experience with the NIH Lung Health Study. Am J Med 1991;91(Suppl 4A):37S.
8. Begin P, Grassino A. Inspiratory muscle dysfunction and chronic hypercapnea in chronic obstructive pulmonary disease. Am Rev Respir Dis 1991;143:905.
9. Wagner PD. Effects of COPD on gas exchange. In NS Cherniack (ed), Chronic Obstructive Pulmonary Disease. Philadelphia: Saunders, 1991;73.
10. Stubbing DG, Mathur PN, Roberts RS, Campbell EJM. Some physical signs in patients with chronic airflow obstruction. Am Rev Respir Dis 1982;125:549.
11. Medical Section of the American Lung Association. Lung function testing: Selection of reference values and interpretive strategies. Am Rev Respir Dis 1991;144:1202.
12. Ferguson GT, Cherniack RM. Management of chronic obstructive pulmonary disease. N Engl J Med 1993;328:1017.
13. Dockery DW, Speizer FE, Ferris BG, et al. Cumulative and reversible effects of lifetime smoking on simple tests of lung function in adults. Am Rev Respir Dis 1988;137:286.
14. Centers for Disease Control. Pneumococcal polysaccharide vaccine. MMWR 1989;38:64, 73.
15. Summer W, Elston R, Tharpe L, et al. Aerosol bronchodilator delivery methods. Relative impact on pulmonary function and cost of respiratory care. Arch Intern Med 1989;149:618.
16. Bowton DL, Goldsmith WM, Haponik EF. Substitution of metered dose inhalers for handheld nebulizers: Success and cost savings in a large, acute-care hospital. Chest 1992;101:305.
17. Allen SC, Prior A. What determines whether an elderly patient can use a metered dose inhaler correctly? Br J Dis Chest 1986;80:45.
18. Guidry GG, Brown WD, Stogner SW, George RB. Incorrect use of metered dose inhalers by medical personnel. Chest 1992;101:31.
19. Braun SR, McKenzie WN, Copeland C, et al. A comparison of the effect of ipratropium and albuterol in the treatment of chronic obstructive airway disease. Arch Intern Med 1989;149:544.
20. Karpel JP. Bronchodilator responses to anti-cholinergic and beta-adrenergic agents in acute and stable COPD. Chest 1991;99:871.
21. Medical Section of the American Lung Association. Standards for the diagnosis and care of patients with chronic obstructive pulmonary disease. Am J Respir Crit Care Med 1995;152:577.
22. Easton PA, Jadue C, Dhingra S, Anthonison NR. A comparison of the bronchodilating effects of a beta-2 adrenergic agent (albuterol) and an anti-cholinergic agent (ipratropium bromide), given by aerosol alone or in sequence. N Engl J Med 1986;315:735.
23. Chapman KR. Therapeutic algorithm for chronic obstructive pulmonary disease. Am J Med 1991;91(Suppl 4A):17S.
24. Filuk RB, Easton PA, Anthonison NR. Responses to large doses of salbutamol and theophylline in patients with chronic obstructive pulmonary disease. Am Rev Respir Dis 1985;132:871.
25. Martin RJ, Pak J. Overnight theophylline concentrations and effects on sleep and lung function in chronic obstructive pulmonary disease. Am Rev Respir Dis 1992;145:540.
26. Ziment I. Pharmacologic therapy of obstructive airway disease. Clin Chest Med 1990;11:461.
27. Mandella LA, Manfreda J, Warren CPW, Anthonison NR. Steroid response in stable chronic obstructive pulmonary disease. Ann Intern Med 1982;96:17.
28. Shim CS, Williams MH Jr. Aerosol beclomethasone in patients with steroid-responsive chronic obstructive pulmonary disease. Am J Med 1985;78:655.
29. Nicotra MB, Rivera M, Awe RJ. Antibiotic therapy in acute exacerbations of chronic bronchitis: A controlled study using tetracycline. Ann Intern Med 1982;97:18.

30. Anthonison NR, Manfreda J, Warren CPW. Antibiotic therapy in exacerbations of chronic obstructive pulmonary disease. Ann Intern Med 1987;106:196.

31. Petty TL. The National Mucolytic Study: Results of a randomized, double-blind, placebo-controlled study of iodinated glycerol in chronic obstructive bronchitis. Chest 1990;97:75.

32. Nocturnal Oxygen Therapy Trial Group. Continuous or nocturnal oxygen therapy in hypoxemic chronic obstructive lung disease: A clinical trial. Ann Intern Med 1980;93:391.

33. Medical Research Council Working Party. Long-term domiciliary oxygen therapy in chronic hypoxic cor pulmonale complicating chronic bronchitis and emphysema. Lancet 1981;1:681.

34. Timms RM, Khaja FU, Williams GW, et al. Hemodynamic response to oxygen therapy in chronic obstructive pulmonary disease. Ann Intern Med 1985;102:29.

35. Bye PTP, Esau SA, Levy RD, et al. Ventilatory muscle function during exercise in air and oxygen in patients with chronic airflow limitation. Am Rev Respir Dis 1985;132:236.

36. Fletcher EC, Miller J, Divine GW, et al. Nocturnal oxyhemoglobin desaturation in COPD patients with arterial oxygen tensions above 60 mm Hg. Chest 1987;92:604.

37. Fletcher EC, Luckett RA, Goodnight-White S, et al. A double-blind trial of nocturnal supplemental oxygen for sleep desaturation in patients with chronic obstructive pulmonary disease and a daytime PaO_2 above 60 mm Hg. Am Rev Respir Dis 1992;145:1070.

38. Conference on Home Oxygen Therapy. Problems in prescribing and supplying oxygen for Medicare patients. Am Rev Respir Dis 1986;134:340.

39. Second Conference on Home Oxygen Therapy. Further recommendations for prescribing and supplying long-term oxygen therapy. Am Rev Respir Dis 1988;138:745.

40. Third Consensus Conference on Home Oxygen Therapy. New problems in supply, reimbursement, and certification of medical necessity for long-term oxygen therapy. Am Rev Respir Dis 1990;142:721.

41. Foster S, Lopez D, Thomas HM. Pulmonary rehabilitation in COPD patients with elevated PCO_2. Am Rev Respir Dis 1988;138:1519.

42. Neiderman MS, Clemente PH, Fein AM, et al. Benefits of a multidisciplinary pulmonary rehabilitation program: Improvements are independent of lung function. Chest 1991;99:798.

43. Make BJ. Pulmonary rehabilitation: Myth or reality? Clin Chest Med 1986;7:519.

44. Moser KM, Bokinsky GE, Savage RT, et al. Results of a comprehensive rehabilitation program: Physiologic and functional effects on patients with chronic obstructive pulmonary disease. Arch Intern Med 1980;140:1596.

45. Inkley SR, Oldenburg FC, Vignos PJ Jr. Pulmonary function in Duchenne muscular dystrophy related to stage of disease. Am J Med 1974;56:297.

46. Kelly BJ, Luce JM. The diagnosis and management of neuromuscular diseases causing respiratory failure. Chest 1991;99:1485.

47. Bach JR. Pulmonary rehabilitation in neuromuscular disorders. Semin Respir Med 1993;14:515.

48. Bounds JV, Weibers DO, Whisnant JP, Okazaki H. Mechanisms and timing of deaths from cerebral infarction. Stroke 1981;12:474.

49. Silver FL, Norris JW, Lewis AJ, Hachinski VC. Early mortality following stroke: A prospective review. Stroke 1984;15:492.

50. Devivo MJ, Black KI, Stover SL. Causes of death during the first 12 years after spinal cord injury. Arch Phys Med Rehabil 1993;74:248.

51. Demling R, Riessen R. Pulmonary dysfunction after cerebral injury. Crit Care Med 1990;18:768.

52. Grippi MA, Fishman AP. Respiratory failure in structural and neuromuscular disorders involving the chest bellows. In AP Fishman (ed), Pulmonary Diseases and Disorders (2nd ed). New York: McGraw-Hill, 1988;2299.

53. Estenne M, Heilporn A, Delhez L, et al. Chest wall stiffness in patients with chronic respiratory muscle weakness. Am Rev Respir Dis 1983;128:1002.

54. Baydur A. Respiratory muscle strength and control of ventilation in patients with neuromuscular disease. Chest 1991;99:330.

55. Aldrich MS. Neurologic aspects of sleep apnea and related respiratory disturbances. Otolarnygol Clin North Am 1990;23:761.

56. Mezon BL, West P, Israels J, Kryger M. Sleep breathing abnormalities in kyphoscoliosis. Am Rev Respir Dis 1980;122:617.

57. Askenasy JJM, Goldhammer I. Sleep apnea as a feature of bulbar stroke. Stroke 1988;19:637.

58. Steljes DG, Kryger MH, Kirk BW, Millar TW. Sleep in postpolio syndrome. Chest 1990;98:133.

59. Smith PEM, Calverly PMA, Edwards RHT, et al. Practical problems in the respiratory care of patients with muscular dystrophy. N Engl J Med 1987;316:1197.

60. Bonekat HW, Anderson G, Squires J. Obstructive disordered breathing during sleep in patients with spinal cord injury. Paraplegia 1990;28:392.

61. Braun NMT, Arora NS, Rochester DF. Respiratory muscle and pulmonary function in polymyositis and other proximal myopathies. Thorax 1983;38:616.

62. Black LF, Hyatt RE. Maximal static respiratory pressures in generalized neuromuscular disease. Am Rev Respir Dis 1971;103:641.

63. Johanson WG Jr, Peters JI. Respiratory failure: Pathophysiology and treatment. In JF Murray, JA Nadel (eds), Textbook of Respiratory Medicine. Philadelphia: Saunders, 1988;2017.

64. Hornstein S, Inman S, Ledsome JR. Ventilatory muscle training in kyphoscoliosis. Spine 1987;12:859.

65. Dimarco AF, Kelling J, Sajovic M, et al. The effects of inspiratory resistive training on respiratory muscle

function in patients with muscular dystrophy. Muscle Nerve 1985;8:284.

66. Gross D, Ladd H, Riley E, et al. The effect of training on strength and endurance of the diaphragm in quadriplegia. Am J Med 1980;68:27.

67. Fernandez E, Tanchoc-Tan M, Make BJ. Methods to improve respiratory muscle function. Semin Respir Med 1993;14:446.

68. Larson JL, Kim MJ, Sharp JT, Larson DA. Inspiratory muscle training with a pressure threshold breathing device in patients with chronic obstructive pulmonary disease. Am Rev Respir Dis 1988;138:689.

69. Harver A, Mahler DA, Daubenspeck JA. Targeted inspiratory muscle training improves respiratory muscle function and reduces dyspnea in patients with chronic obstructive pulmonary disease. Ann Intern Med 1989;111:117.

70. Estenne M, Knoop C, Vanvaerenbergh J, et al. The effect of pectoralis muscle training in tetraplegic subjects. Am Rev Respir Dis 1989;139:1218.

71. Hill NS. Clinical application of body ventilators. Chest 1986;90:897.

72. Meyer TJ, Hill NS. Noninvasive positive pressure ventilation to treat respiratory failure. Ann Intern Med 1994;120:760.

73. Hill NS, Eveloff SE, Carlisle CC, Goff SG. Efficacy of nocturnal nasal ventilation in patients with restrictive thoracic disease. Am Rev Respir Dis 1992;145:365.

74. Ellis ER, Bye PT, Bruderer JW, Sullivan CE. Treatment of respiratory failure during sleep in patients with neuromuscular disease. Positive pressure ventilation through a nose mask. Am Rev Respir Dis 1987;135:148.

75. Hill NS, Redline S, Carskadon MA, et al. Sleep disordered breathing in patients with Duchenne muscular dystrophy using negative pressure ventilators. Chest 1992;102:1656.

76. Belman MJ, Soo Woo GW, Kuei JH, Shadmehr R. Efficacy of positive vs negative pressure ventilation in unloading the respiratory muscles. Chest 1990;98:850.

77. Carrey Z, Gottfried SB, Levy RD. Ventilatory muscle support in respiratory failure with nasal positive pressure ventilation. Chest 1990;97:150.

78. Gay PC, Patel AM, Viggiano RW, Hubmayr RD. Nocturnal nasal ventilation for treatment of patients with hypercapnic respiratory failure. Mayo Clin Proc 1991;66:695.

79. Branthwaite MA. Assisted ventilation 6. Noninvasive and domiciliary ventilation: Positive pressure techniques. Thorax 1991;46:208.

80. O'Donohue WJ, Giovannoni RM, Goldberg AI, et al. Long-term mechanical ventilation: Guidelines for management in the home and at alternate community sites. Chest 1986;90(Suppl):1S.

81. Bach JR, Alba AS. Tracheostomy ventilation: A study of efficacy with deflated cuffs and cuffless tubes. Chest 1990;97:679.

82. Passy V. Passy-Muir tracheostomy speaking valve. Otolaryngol Head Neck Surg 1986;95:247.

83. Brown M, Glassenberg M. Mortality factors in patients with acute stroke. JAMA 1973;224:1493.

84. Horner J, Massey EW. Silent aspiration following stroke. Neurology 1988;38:317.

85. Kelly BJ, Luce JM. The diagnosis and management of neuromuscular disease causing respiratory failure. Chest 1991;99:1485.

86. Huxley EJ, Viroslav J, Gray WR, Pierce AK. Pharyngeal aspiration in normal adults and patients with depressed consciousness. Am J Med 1978;64:564.

87. Veis SL, Logemann JA. Swallowing disorders in persons with cerebrovascular accidents. Arch Phys Med Rehabil 1984;66:372.

88. Splaingard ML, Hutchins B, Sultan LD, Chaudhuri G. Aspiration in rehabilitation patients: Videofluoroscopy vs bedside clinical assessment. Arch Phys Med Rehabil 1988;69:637.

89. Chen MYM, Ott DJ, Peele VN, Gelfand DW. Oropharynx in patients with cerebrovascular disease: Evaluation with videofluoroscopy. Radiology 1990;176:641.

90. Robinson KM, Siegler EL, Streim JE. Medical emergencies in rehabilitation medicine. In JA DeLisa (ed), Rehabilitation Medicine: Principles and Practice. Philadelphia: Lippincott, 1993;783.

91. Garrison SJ, Rolak LA. Rehabilitation of the stroke patient. In JA DeLisa (ed), Rehabilitation Medicine: Principles and Practice. Philadelphia: Lippincott, 1993;801.

92. Brott T. Prevention and management of medical complications of the hospitalized elderly stroke patient. Clin Geriatric Med 1991;7:475.

93. Garibaldi RA, Neuhaus EG, Nurse BA. Infections in the elderly. In JW Rowe, RW Besdine (eds), Geriatric Medicine. Boston: Little, Brown, 1988;302.

94. Bartlett JG. Anaerobic bacterial infections of the lung. Chest 1987;91:901.

95. Bartlett JG, Finegold SM. Anaerobic infections of the lung and pleural space. Am Rev Respir Dis 1974;100;56.

96. Neiderman MS. Nosocomial pneumonia in the elderly. In MS Neiderman (ed), Respiratory Infections in the Elderly. New York: Raven, 1991;207.

97. Cochrane G, Webber B, Clarke S. Effects of sputum on pulmonary function. BMJ 1977;2:1181.

98. Orlava OE. Therapeutic physical culture in the complex treatment of pneumonia. Phys Ther Rev 1959;39:153.

99. Dean E, Ross J. Discordance between cardiopulmonary physiology and physical therapy: Toward a rational basis for practice. Chest 1992;101:694.

100. Jackson AB, Groomes TE. Incidence of respiratory complications following spinal cord injury. Arch Phys Med Rehabil 1994;75:270.

101. Mansel JK, Norman JR. Respiratory complications and management of spinal cord injuries. Chest 1990;97:1446.

102. Maurer JR. Respiratory issues in quadriplegics and high paraplegics. Pulmonary Perspectives 1994;11:6.

103. Ledsome JR, Sharp JM. Pulmonary function in acute cervical cord injury. Am Rev Respir Dis 1981;124:41.

104. Kirby NA, Barnerias MJ, Siebens AA. An evaluation of assisted cough in quadriplegics. Arch Phys Med Rehabil 1966;47:705.

105. Jaeger RJ, Turba RM, Yarkony GM, Roth EJ. Cough in spinal cord injured patients: Comparison of three methods to produce cough. Arch Phys Med Rehabil 1993;74:1358.

106. Bach JR. Mechanical insufflation-exsufflation: Comparison of peak expiratory flows with manually assisted and unassisted coughing techniques. Chest 1993;104:1553.

107. Linder SH. Functional electrical stimulation abdominal binder to enhance cough in quadriplegia. Chest 1993;103:166.

108. Polatty RC, McElaney MA, Marcelino V. Pulmonary complications in the spinal cord injury patient. Physical Medicine and Rehabilitation: State of the Art Reviews 1987;1:353.

109. Gross D, Ladd HW, Riley EJ, et al. The effect of training on strength and endurance of the diaphragm in quadriplegia. Am J Med 1980;68:27.

110. Estenne M, Knoop C, VanVaerenbergh J, et al. The effect of pectoralis muscle training in tetraplegic subjects. Am Rev Respir Dis 1989;139:1218.

Part X

Rheumatology

Chapter 18

Rheumatologic Problems

Rowland W. Chang

The rehabilitation of the severely disabled often requires the use of limbs that are weak or spastic or the overuse of limbs that are not affected by the disabling process. In either event, optimal functioning of the joints and periarticular structures is important in the performance of bed mobility, transfers, ambulation, and the activities of daily living. Preexisting rheumatologic conditions can complicate standard rehabilitation therapy for stroke, head trauma, spinal cord injury, and so on. For instance, the functional goals of a stroke patient with preexisting rheumatoid arthritis may need to be set at a lower level than those of a patient who is otherwise healthy. Furthermore, the choice of a walking aid will now have to take into account painful and potentially unstable upper extremity joints.

In addition to preexisting disease, musculoskeletal problems can result from the disabling condition or the rehabilitation process. These conditions as well as the approach to musculoskeletal issues in the chronically disabled are discussed in this chapter. Information and approaches to the rehabilitation of persons with rheumatic diseases can be found elsewhere [1–3].

Evaluation

The diagnosis and treatment of musculoskeletal conditions are greatly facilitated by the specification of relatively few descriptive parameters (Table 18-1). The goal of the clinical assessment (i.e., history and physical examination) and diagnostic tests (e.g., radiographs and blood tests) is to characterize the variables of the presenting problem. Although precise diagnosis still may be elusive, at least a plan of therapy can be derived while the patient is followed over time.

History

The history is an important means of characterizing rheumatic complaints. Acute conditions can be distinguished from subacute or chronic problems. Local ailments or systemic disease can be identified. Some sense can be gained of whether the articular or periarticular structures are involved. Inflammatory processes can be differentiated from noninflammatory (e.g., degenerative) processes.

Important elements of a rheumatologic history include the following:

1. Where are the symptoms located (in the joint, tendon, muscle, bursa)?
2. Has there been any detectable swelling in the joints, tendon sheaths, or bursae? Swelling may be a manifestation of an inflammatory condition.
3. Are the symptoms of pain or stiffness made worse after joint, tendon, or muscle use (suggestive of a noninflammatory process) or after prolonged immobility (suggestive of inflammatory conditions)?
4. Is there early morning stiffness? More than 2 hours of morning stiffness suggests an inflammatory condition. Less than 1 hour characterizes degenerative problems.

Table 18-1. Questions to Be Answered
by a Rheumatologic Workup

1. Is the problem acute, subacute, or chronic?
2. Is the problem generalized or localized?
3. Is the problem articular, periarticular, or nonarticular?
4. Is the problem inflammatory or noninflammatory?

5. Is there any associated warmth or redness that would suggest inflammation?
6. Are there are any other systemic symptoms (e.g., fever, weight loss, fatigue) or other symptoms of other organ system dysfunction that suggest systemic illness?

Physical Examination

The physical examination is the most crucial element of the rheumatologic evaluation. The major goal of the examination is to identify the involved structure that is responsible for the patient's symptoms. Articular conditions are characterized by joint effusion, soft tissue or bony swelling, tenderness, pain on motion, or reduced range of motion. Tendinitis and bursitis cause localized tenderness and occasionally swelling and lead to pain when the tendon or bursa is palpated or stretched. Muscular problems may be associated with local muscular tenderness or weakness. The history and physical examination as it relates to the rheumatic diseases are fully described by Polley and Hunder [4].

Often a specific diagnosis can be made on the basis of a history and physical examination and therapeutic strategies initiated. Roentgenograms and laboratory tests are occasionally helpful in cases when the diagnosis is uncertain or when the extent of articular disease needs to be established.

Roentgenograms

Standard roentgenograms of joints are useful in assessing bone alignment, bone density, articular cartilage integrity, and soft tissue abnormalities. Roentgenograms are not sensitive methods in establishing articular diagnoses given that a significant amount of cartilage damage or bone damage or reaction have to be present before the radiographic findings of joint space narrowing, marginal bony erosions, or osteophyte formation appear. Occasionally, radiographs can distinguish between inflammatory and degenerative arthritis. For instance, in assessing knee arthritis, uniform joint space narrowing in the medial, lateral, and patellofemoral compartments and the absence of osteophyte formation strongly suggest an inflammatory arthritis, whereas isolated medial compartment joint space narrowing and osteophytosis suggest a degenerative arthritis.

A more useful application of roentgenograms is to determine the extent of articular damage in a setting where the diagnosis is known. The severity and chronicity of the articular process can be determined by the extent of the joint space narrowing and the presence or absence of bone deformity or destruction and osteophyte formation. Such knowledge might be important to plan further therapeutic strategies. Diagnosis of soft tissue abnormalities can occasionally be aided by roentgenograms. Inflamed tendons and bursae periodically calcify as part of the healing process. These calcium deposits can be detected on standard radiographs of the affected areas. Care should be made not to rely totally on these findings in making or ruling out the diagnosis of tendinitis or bursitis, because not all cases of tendinitis or bursitis lead to calcium deposits and not all radiographically detectable calcium deposits are symptomatic. Alterations in the normal bony alignment of a joint can also suggest soft tissue abnormalities. For example, subluxing shoulder, a common complication of stroke and upper motor neuron injuries, can be diagnosed with a standard shoulder film.

More detailed descriptions of the use of radiology in the rheumatic diseases can be found in textbooks of rheumatology and radiology [5–7].

Laboratory Tests

Although much research is ongoing that investigates the relationship between autoantibody production and specific rheumatic diseases or syndromes, the use of the clinical laboratory in the diagnosis and management of the vast majority of patients with rheumatic complaints is limited both in the number and usefulness of these tests. The erythrocyte sedimentation rate (ESR), rheumatoid factor (RF) test, antinuclear antibody (ANA) test, and HLA-B27 test are discussed here as well as the standard screening tests (complete blood cell count, chemistry screen, and urinalysis). More exhaustive discussions may be found in the textbooks and articles listed in the reference list.

The ESR is commonly used to help the clinician distinguish between inflammatory and noninflammatory conditions. It is a simple test that measures the speed of red blood cell sedimentation in an anticoagulated environment. Inflammatory states are usually associated with high ESR levels and noninflammatory states with low ESR levels. Guidelines for the rational use of the ESR have been discussed by Sox and Liang [8]. In general, the results of an ESR are most useful when the clinical situation is ambiguous as to whether a patient is suffering from an inflammatory or noninflammatory syndrome, e.g., when the pain and stiffness noted on history and physical examination are consistent with either polymyalgia rheumatica or osteoarthritis.

The RF and ANA tests detect autoantibodies in the serum. Originally the RF test was developed to aid in the diagnosis of rheumatoid arthritis and the ANA test in systemic lupus erythematosus (SLE). Indeed, the RF test result is positive in approximately 75% of cases of rheumatoid arthritis, and the ANA test result is positive in nearly 99% of all cases of SLE. However, these test results can be positive (usually in low titer, but not always) in normal subjects as well as in patients with a variety of other inflammatory conditions. As noted before, the interpretation of these tests depends on whether the clinical presentation strongly suggests, somewhat suggests, or does not suggest rheumatoid arthritis or SLE. The usefulness of the test will be maximized when the presentation suggests an intermediate chance of disease.

The HLA-B27 test has been used as a diagnostic aid when the seronegative spondyloarthropathies (ankylosing spondylitis, Reiter's syndrome, and the spondyloarthropathies associated with psoriasis and inflammatory bowel disease) are considered. The test result is positive in approximately 95% of white patients who have ankylosing spondylitis, 85% of those with Reiter's syndrome, and approximately 7% of the normal white population. Because physical findings are often difficult to elicit in these conditions, and because roentgenograms are not very sensitive in detecting early spondylitis and associated sacroiliitis, the HLA-B27 test can be useful in patients with a history suggestive of inflammatory back pain (e.g., significant back pain or stiffness on awakening).

The complete blood cell count, chemistry screen, and urinalysis are commonly ordered in patients presenting with musculoskeletal complaints for many reasons. From a diagnostic point of view, they can aid in ruling in or ruling out systemic diseases (e.g., infectious diseases, malignancies, metabolic diseases including gout) that could cause the symptoms. In addition, it is necessary to know the status of the patient's bone marrow, liver, and kidney function before initiating medical therapy.

Synovial Fluid Analysis

The most useful test in distinguishing between inflammatory and noninflammatory arthropathies is the analysis of joint fluid obtained by arthrocentesis. Noninflammatory fluids are a transparent straw or yellow color through which newsprint can be read. The synovial fluid white blood cell count is usually less than 2,000/mm^3. Inflammatory fluids are usually translucent or opaque. Fluids with white blood cell counts above 100,000/mm^3 should be considered septic until proven otherwise, although noninfectious inflammatory arthropathies can occasionally cause this level of inflammatory response. Inflammatory arthropathies generally cause synovial effusions with white blood cell counts between 20,000 and 50,000/mm^3 although the variability is quite wide.

Polarized light microscopy and Gram's staining and culture of synovial fluid can be useful in the diagnosis of gout, pseudogout, and infectious arthritis. The crystals responsible for gout (monosodium urate) and pseudogout (calcium pyrophosphate dihydrate) can be identified by an experienced observer under compensated polarized light microscopy. Obviously, the culture is useful for septic arthritis, although false-negative results exist in gonococcal arthritis and in patients who are taking antibiotics when the synovial fluid is sampled.

Conclusions

The approach to the evaluation of musculoskeletal complaints always involves a careful history and physical examination, occasionally supplemented with roentgenograms and laboratory tests. The diagnostic process can be directed by attempting to categorize each patient presentation by the variables listed in Table 18-1. For instance, a chronic, generalized, articular, and inflammatory syndrome leads to the differential diagnosis of rheumatoid arthritis, not osteoarthritis. An acute, localized, nonarticular, noninflammatory syndrome suggests a traumatic tendinitis rather than an adhesive capsulitis. Further descriptions of the diagnostic process relevant to a rheumatology practice are discussed elsewhere [5, 6, 9]. What follows are descriptions of rheumatologic problems that have been described in the context of stroke, head injury, and spinal cord rehabilitation.

Common Rheumatologic Problems

Localized Soft Tissue Disorders

The most common musculoskeletal problems encountered in rehabilitation practice are subacute, localized, and nonarticular soft tissue conditions affecting the tendons and bursa. Most often these result from the overstress of particular structures mandated by the rehabilitation process. Initially, these problems are traumatic and noninflammatory, but they can become inflammatory as a secondary phenomenon.

Olecranon Bursitis

Chronic, repetitive pressure on the elbow is a frequent consequence of the independent transfer effort in patients with stroke and spinal cord injury. This can lead to irritation of the olecranon bursa at the elbow with fluid formation and occasionally profound swelling. Most of the time, olecranon bursitis is asymptomatic and does not interfere with elbow function because the bursa does not normally communicate with the elbow joint space. Elbow range of motion is usually not impaired. However, the bursa can become infected; thus, the major clinical consideration is whether the initial signs and symptoms justify a bursal aspiration to obtain fluid for culture. If infection is not a consideration, treatment of a large bursal swelling with a nonsteroidal anti-inflammatory drug or a local corticosteroid injection is generally initiated in order to forestall future infection.

Subacromial Bursitis, Rotator Cuff Injuries, and Subluxing Shoulder

Because most of the shoulder's stability is determined by the tonic contraction of approximately 20 muscles crossing the shoulder girdle, it is small wonder that patients with upper motor neuron lesions such as stroke or high cervical spinal cord injury are predisposed to shoulder instability. This instability can lead to a variety of shoulder syndromes. The most common, subacromial (or subdeltoid) bursitis, results from the trauma imparted to the rotator cuff and adjacent bursa by the humerus and acromial process coming together during abduction of the shoulder. Common symptoms include pain at the lateral aspect of the shoulder, which occasionally radiates down the arm. The pain occurs at rest and commonly interferes with sleep. The pain is also made worse by motion, especially abduction. Physical findings include local tenderness in the subacromial area. Occasionally swelling of the bursa can be detected. Range of motion, both passive and active, may be limited because of pain.

Shoulder roentgenograms are obtained to rule out other bone or joint pathologic entities such as a concomitant arthritis. Usually there are no radiographic findings associated with subacromial bursitis. Occasionally, calcification can be observed in the subacromial area that is due to calcification tendinitis of the rotator cuff. Treatment consists of ice application for acute attacks and heat for subacute or chronic syndromes, nonsteroidal anti-inflammatory analgesia, and local corticosteroid injections.

The shoulder instability associated with upper motor neuron lesions can lead to frank injury and dysfunction of the rotator cuff. This condition is often difficult to distinguish from subacromial bursitis in that it can cause chronic shoulder pain at rest as well as pain on motion and similar physical findings. Weakness of resisted shoulder abduction, especially when the arm is fully internally rotated, is highly suggestive of a cuff tear, but this is difficult to assess when the patient is in pain.

Again, the diagnosis is generally made on the basis of the physical examination, but an arthrogram can be helpful when the cause of the patient's shoulder pain or dysfunction is in doubt. The arthrographic finding diagnostic of a rotator cuff tear is dye appearing in the subacromial and sub-deltoid area after being injected into the gleno-humeral joint. Because the joint and the bursa are normally separated by an intact cuff, any dye that escapes into the bursa is a result of a discontinuity of the cuff. Initial treatment of a cuff injury is generally immobilization and analgesia. If the tear heals, then range of motion and strengthening exercises are prescribed.

The extreme result of shoulder instability is subluxation. Clinically this leads to pain and abnormal joint mechanics, which in turn can lead to osteoarthritis. Shoulder instability associated with frank subluxation nearly always can be detected on physical examination if there is excessive motion in all planes (e.g., anteroposterior, superoinferior).

Standard roentgenograms often show that the joint is subluxed in the resting position, most commonly inferiorly in stroke patients. The treatment in neurologically intact patients is strengthening exercises of the supporting shoulder muscles. Surgery is performed in extreme cases. The treatment in stroke or spinal cord patients is generally unsatisfactory but might include passive constraints such as slings, braces, and other orthotics.

When caring for a stroke or spinal cord patient, measures should be considered to prevent these shoulder syndromes. The simplest of these is to avoid active or passive abduction in performing functional tasks and in physical and occupational therapy sessions. Because of the inherent tendency of an unstable shoulder to lead to humeroacromial impingement with associated trauma to the rotator cuff and the subacromial bursa, theoretically it should be possible to prevent the bursitis and cuff tear conditions so commonly seen in these patients. Passive constraints should be considered early in the course if recovery of muscle control is considered to be limited.

Reflex Sympathetic Dystrophy

The etiology of reflex sympathetic dystrophy, which is a complication of stroke and trauma patients, is not clear (see also Chapter 16). Some believe the disruption of the automatic nervous system is responsible for the pain and vasomotor abnormalities that characterize this syndrome. Symptoms

include pain, often severe, in the distal part of an extremity (e.g., hand or foot), which may extend proximally (as in shoulder-hand syndrome). Physical findings include swelling, tenderness, and occasionally coolness and a lack of sweating of a distal extremity, which may also extend proximally.

The differential diagnosis includes cellulitis and gout of the affected limb. Roentgenograms may show patchy osteopenia of the hand or foot. Bone scans generally reveal decreased technetium-99m uptake distally in the affected limb. The diagnostic usefulness of these tests has been studied by Kozin and colleagues [10], but it is unclear how common these findings occur in other conditions that may be confused with reflex sympathetic dystrophy or with the disuse that accompanies this syndrome. Treatment efforts include mobilization, compression, analgesia, and occasionally corticosteroid therapy or stellate ganglion blocks. In general, the effectiveness of therapy is limited.

Generalized Soft Tissue Disorders

Although there are no etiologic links between stroke, brain trauma, or spinal cord injury and generalized soft tissue problems, fibromyalgia syndromes and polymyalgia rheumatica are commonly encountered with these disorders and deserve mention here.

Fibromyalgia (Fibrositis) Syndromes

Fibromyalgia syndromes are poorly understood but common noninflammatory conditions that can affect persons of any age and are characterized by stiffness and pain in localized areas known as trigger points. Several investigators have proposed diagnostic criteria for fibromyalgia, and others have documented the diagnostic usefulness of particular trigger points in distinguishing this syndrome from other musculoskeletal conditions. Common sites of discomfort include the neck and shoulder girdle, the epicondyles of the elbow, the greater trochanter about the hip, and the anserine area of the knee. Often several of the sites are affected. There is generally an absence of prolonged morning stiffness, and exercise or use of the painful area tends not to affect the symptoms adversely or beneficially. In addition, patients often complain of fatigue, and sleep disorders (which may be important in etiology) are common. Physical findings include tenderness in discrete areas around the previously mentioned sites. The tenderness may radiate in a specific direction (e.g., from a trigger point in the neck up to the occiput) but is not generalized to the entire joint or periarticular area.

The differential diagnosis includes localized myofascial syndromes and occasionally early systemic rheumatic diseases such as rheumatoid arthritis or systemic lupus erythematosus. Laboratory tests and roentgenograms are only useful in ruling out other diseases because fibromyalgia is not associated with any abnormality.

Treatment is symptomatic. Exercise such as slow stretching and strengthening is recommended. Aerobic conditioning can be useful in some patients. Pharmacologic treatments include nonsteroidal anti-inflammatory analgesia, muscle relaxants, and tricyclic antidepressants. An important part of the therapy for fibromyalgia syndrome is the reassurance that there is no crippling arthritis causing the symptoms and that normal and even therapeutic and recreational activity is not contraindicated.

Polymyalgia Rheumatica

Polymyalgia rheumatica is a subacute chronic inflammatory condition that affects the elderly. It is as common a new diagnosis as rheumatoid arthritis in the population aged 70 years and above. Symptoms include prolonged morning stiffness and proximal myalgias (i.e., shoulder and hip girdle). In addition, there may be systemic symptoms such as fatigue, weight loss, generalized weakness, and even low-grade fever. Because polymyalgia rheumatica is associated with giant cell arteritis, there may be headache, scalp pain, and jaw claudication. Physical findings may be absent, or there may be muscle tenderness in the periarticular areas of the shoulder and hip (usually in the anterior thigh). Scalp tenderness suggests giant cell arteritis.

The differential diagnosis of polymyalgia rheumatica includes early rheumatoid arthritis, systemic infections such as subacute bacterial endocarditis, hypothyroidism, and malignancy. The only laboratory abnormality associated with this syndrome is an elevated ESR. Other laboratory and radiologic tests are useful in ruling out other diseases. A temporal artery biopsy should be considered if giant cell arteritis is suspected.

Treatment for polymyalgia rheumatica is controversial. Low doses of corticosteroids (e.g., 20 mg of prednisone daily) are prescribed by most rheumatologists, with predictable beneficial response. Nonsteroidal anti-inflammatory agents also can be used but are less effective. Some recommend high-dose corticosteroids (e.g., 40–60 mg of prednisone a day) to prevent blindness due to concurrent giant cell arteritis. Some rely on the results of a temporal artery biopsy to determine the treatment strategy. Chang and Fineberg [11] have argued that the decision to perform a biopsy or to treat with low- or high-dose corticosteroids depends on whether there are any cranial symptoms suggesting giant cell arteritis and how many cases of severe corticosteroid side effects the decision maker is willing to accept to prevent blindness, the most devastating complication of the arteritis.

Localized Articular Problems

The added stresses and strains on the musculoskeletal system that occur as a result of the rehabilitation of stroke, brain trauma, and spinal cord injury can lead to frank arthritis of one joint manifested by joint pain, swelling, and loss of motion. Three such arthropathies are discussed here. A more complete differential diagnosis of monarthritis can be found in rheumatology textbooks [12].

Traumatic Arthritis

As stated previously, muscular tone is responsible for a great deal of stability in many joints. Thus, in the neurologically disabled patient, it is not uncommon to traumatize intra-articular structures such as the synovium, menisci, tendons, and even articular cartilage. The most common symptoms in these acute, subacute, or chronic syndromes are swelling and pain in the joint, with the knee being most frequently affected. A cool effusion is often detected on physical examination, and instability of the joint is occasionally demonstrated during stress maneuvers (such as varus, valgus, anterior, or posterior stress on the knee). The range of motion may be limited by the effusion, and the supporting muscles may be found to be weak.

Standard roentgenograms cannot detect intra-articular derangements. Thus, roentgenograms are obtained to determine whether there is evidence for chronic arthritis, fracture, or osseous lesions that might cause a joint effusion (e.g., bone metastases). If surgical therapy is contemplated, arthrography, computed tomography, or magnetic resonance imaging may be helpful in documenting the internal derangement preoperatively. The synovial fluid is usually noninflammatory or hemorrhagic.

Treatment is aimed at minimizing the pain and swelling of the arthritic condition. Nonsteroidal anti-inflammatory drugs are normally tried first. If the symptoms persist, reaspiration and local corticosteroid injection are then considered. A supporting brace or orthosis may be useful if the joint symptoms persist or return despite trials of nonsteroidal anti-inflammatory drugs and local corticosteroid injections. Arthroscopic surgery might be considered if conservative measures fail to control functionally significant symptoms. Every effort should be made to minimize the effusion because of its known deleterious effect on joint pressure and supporting muscle function, which may lead to further instability, pain, and swelling.

Crystal-Induced Monarthropathies

The pathophysiology of gout and pseudogout, the two most commonly encountered crystal-induced acute joint conditions, involves a metabolic abnormality that leads to an overabundance of a substance (monosodium urate in gout, calcium pyrophosphate dihydrate in pseudogout) in the cartilage matrix, synovium, and synovial fluid. Normally these substances remain in solution, but when they precipitate out of the solution, the clinical syndrome of acute pain and swelling in the affected joint(s) occurs. Initiating factors include trauma, surgical procedures, severe medical illness, and (in gout) rapid change in the concentration of uric acid.

Gout most commonly affects the first metatarsophalangeal joint, ankle, tarsal joints, and knee. The majority of pseudogout attacks occur in the knee. Physical examination reveals an inflamed joint characterized by warmth, swelling, and tenderness, which at times is exquisite. Occasionally the surrounding soft tissues become inflamed, which leads to a cellulitis-like presentation.

The differential diagnosis includes a septic joint and cellulitis. Thus, aspiration should be strongly considered in patients with an acute inflammatory monarthritis and mandatory when infection is a consideration, even in patients with a previous history of gout or pseudogout. The serum uric acid level is usually elevated in gout. There are no laboratory abnormalities associated with pseudogout unless it is secondary to hyperparathyroidism. The key laboratory test is examination of the synovial fluid for crystals. This requires analysis with a polarizing microscope. Specific diagnosis can be made if monosodium urate or calcium pyrophosphate dihydrate crystals are seen within synovial fluid white blood cells.

Reduction of the joint pain and swelling often begins with the diagnostic arthrocentesis. Pharmacologic treatments include nonsteroidal anti-inflammatory drugs or colchicine. When there are contraindications to these medicines or when they cause adverse effects, intra-articular, parenteral, or oral corticosteroids can be used provided infection has been ruled out. Allopurinol, although useful in the prevention of gout, should not be used in the acute situation because it may predispose the patient to more frequent attacks.

Infectious Monarthritis

Neurologically impaired patients are commonly afflicted with pressure sores, urinary tract stasis, and other conditions that predispose to local and systemic infection (see Chapter 12). The most common pathophysiologic mechanism for a septic joint is blood-borne spread to an already diseased joint. Thus, when a chronically ill patient becomes septic and presents with an acutely inflamed joint, the joint should be presumed infected until proven otherwise. An alternative mechanism for a septic joint is direct inoculation from the skin overlying the joint. This may occur when skin trauma goes unnoticed because of loss of sensation.

The clinical presentation of an infected joint, most commonly a hip or knee, may be acute, as in gout or pseudogout, but also may be insidious. Pain, swelling, and loss of motion are common symptoms, and warm effusions are detectable in accessible joints. Because the hip joint is difficult to assess on physical examination, suspicion of infection must be inferred from indirect evidence, such as pain on motion, resting flexion contracture, and signs and symptoms of a generalized inflammatory process.

Although the white blood cell count is usually elevated in septic arthritis, on occasion this falls within the normal range. Furthermore, inflammatory conditions such as gout are associated with a high white blood cell count. Standard roentgenograms can show cortical and subcortical destruction after weeks of joint infection, but they usually are not helpful in the initial stages. Again, it is mandatory to collect synovial fluid for Gram's stain and culture when septic arthritis is suspected. Specific bacteriologic identification leads to appropriate antibiotic treatment. If the patient is being treated with antibiotics for another reason when synovial culture is obtained, the decision on which antibiotic to use rests with the suspected site of origin of the bacteremia. Urinary tract and skin pathogens need to be considered in this setting.

An important adjunct to antibiotic treatment is drainage of the joint. This can be accomplished surgically (usually arthroscopically) and nonsurgically (repeated closed needle aspiration). There is controversy over which method is preferred (see the Broy and Schmid review [13]). Whichever method is chosen, it is important not to delay the procedure because the potential for cartilage destruction in a septic joint is great and the prevention of further structural damage in these already functionally impaired patients is most important.

Polyarthritis

Detailed discussion of the differential diagnosis of polyarthritis may be found in rheumatology textbooks. In the chronically disabled, the syndrome most directly related to neurologic impairment is polyarticular gout.

Polyarticular Gout

Although gout usually manifests as a monarticular syndrome, acute polyarticular syndromes are well described [14]. These occur more frequently in patients with previous gouty attacks; thus, it is unusual for a patient to initially present with this syndrome. Tophi are commonly detected on physical examination, and the uric acid level is usually elevated. The diagnosis and treatment of polyarticular gout is similar to that for monarticular gout.

Other Syndromes

Stover [15] reviewed the rheumatologic conditions associated with spinal cord injury detected by the National Spinal Cord Injury Statistical Center. The three categories described were heterotopic ossification, joint changes (specifically hip and sacroiliac joint changes), and dermal fibrosis. Heterotopic ossification is discussed in Chapter 5 of this book. The unusual joint and skin syndromes are briefly mentioned.

Hip Joint Changes

Seven cases of a radiologic syndrome characterized by slowly progressive fragmentation and resorption of the femoral head have been described. Subluxation and complete dislocation have also been reported. The pathophysiology of this condition is not clear, although avascular necrosis and neuroarthropathy have been suspected.

Sacroiliac Fusion

Khan and colleagues [16] reported radiographic changes of the sacroiliac joint in 40% of 186 spinal cord injured patients studied. The changes were found more commonly in patients with high levels of spinal cord injury and in those patients with a longer duration of injury. Again, the cause of these abnormalities is unknown. Decreased trunk mobility secondary to paralysis and a vascular component secondary to disruption of the autonomic nervous system have been suggested [16, 17].

Dermal Fibrosis

Stover and colleagues [18] reported 18 patients with spinal cord injuries (all with injuries above the T6 level) with brawny induration of the skin. The syndrome was insidious in onset in some and sudden in others. It was noted as early as 6 months after injury but more commonly reported during the next several years after injury. Pathologic studies indicate that the collagen distribution resembled that of scleroderma. Involvement by the autonomic nervous system is suspected because no patient with a lesion lower than at the T6 level has been described.

Conclusion

Musculoskeletal problems are commonly seen in the chronically disabled patient. Classification of these syndromes into categories describing the rapidity of symptom onset, the site (articular versus periarticular), the number of sites involved, and the amount of inflammation can lead to appropriate diagnosis and treatment. Most of the conditions seen in practice are local soft tissue problems. The appreciation of articular problems, however, especially the crystal-induced arthropathies and septic arthritis, is important because delay in initiating specific therapy may lead to joint damage, which could lessen the probability of successful rehabilitation. Finally, the study of musculoskeletal abnormalities in this population may shed light on the pathogenesis of the more commonly seen rheumatic diseases.

References

1. Chang RW (ed). Rehabilitation of Persons with Rheumatoid Arthritis. Gaithersburg, MD: Aspen, 1996.
2. Ehrlich GE (ed). Rehabilitation Management of Rheumatic Conditions (2nd ed). Baltimore: Williams & Wilkins, 1986.
3. Riggs GK, Gall EP (eds). Rheumatic Diseases: Rehabilitation and Management. Stoneham, MA: Butterworth, 1984.
4. Polley HF, Hunder GG. Rheumatologic Interviewing and Physical Examination of the Joints. Philadelphia: Saunders, 1978.
5. Kelley WN, Harris ED, Ruddy S, Sledge CB (eds). Textbook of Rheumatology (4th ed). Philadelphia: Saunders, 1993.
6. McCarty DJ, Koopman WJ (eds). Arthritis and Allied Conditions (12th ed). Philadelphia: Lea & Febiger, 1993.
7. Resnick D, Niwayama G (eds). Diagnosis of Bone and Joint Disorders (3rd ed). Philadelphia: Saunders, 1993.
8. Sox HC, Liang MH. The erythrocyte sedimentation rate: Guidelines for rational use. Ann Intern Med 1986;104:515.
9. Fries JF, Mitchell DM. Joint pain or arthritis. JAMA 1976;235:199.
10. Kozin F, Ryan LM, Carerra GF, Soin JS, et al. The reflex sympathetic dystrophy syndrome (RSDS): III. Scintigraphic studies, further evidence for the therapeutic efficacy of systemic corticosteroids, and proposed diagnostic criteria. Am J Med 1981;70:23.
11. Chang RW, Fineberg HV. Risk-benefit considerations in the management of polymyalgia rheumatica. Med Decis Making 1983;3:459.
12. McCune WJ. Monarticular arthritis. In WB Kelley, et al (eds), Textbook of Rheumatology (4th ed). Philadelphia: Saunders, 1993;368.
13. Broy SB, Schmid FR. A comparison of medical drainage (needle aspiration) and surgical drainage (arthrotomy or arthroscopy) in the initial treatment of infected joints. Clin Rheum Dis 1986;12:501.
14. Hadler NM, Franck WA, Bress NM, et al. Acute polyarticular gout. Am J Med 1974;56:715.
15. Stover SL. Arthritis related interests in spinal cord injury. J Rheumatol 1987;14(Suppl 15):82.
16. Khan MA, Kushner I, Freehafer AA. Sacroiliac joint abnormalities in paraplegics. Ann Rheum Dis 1979;38:317.
17. Abel MS. Sacroiliac joint changes in traumatic paraplegics. Radiology 1950;7:235.
18. Stover SL, Gay RE, Koopman W, et al. Dermal fibrosis in spinal cord injury patients: A scleroderma variant? Arthritis Rheum 1980;23:1312.

Index

Acid-base disorders, 15–17. *See also* Fluids and elec-
 trolytes, disorders of, acid-base disorders
Acidosis, metabolic, 15–16
 treatment, 17
Acute tubular necrosis (ATN), and acute renal failure, 10,
 12
Adrenal insufficiency, 126–128
 causes, 126–127
 diagnosis, 127–128
Afterload, 45
AIDS. *See* Infections, human immunodeficiency virus
Alcohol, and osteoporosis, 70
Aldosterone. *See* Hormonal levels
Aldosterone antagonists, in treatment of heart failure, 48
Alimentation and bowel motility, disorders of, 149–178.
 See also Colon and anorectum, disorders of
 diabetic gastroparesis, 163–164
 esophageal peristalsis, 158–159
 gastric emptying disorders, postsurgical, 164
 normal swallowing, 149–154
 functional elements of, 158
 mechanics of, 151–154
 medullary swallowing center, 150
 dysphagia
 esophageal, 159–160
 resulting from vagotomy, 159–160
 oropharyngeal, 154–157
 cricopharyngeal myotomy for, 157
 patient history, 155
 propulsive causes, 156–157
 structural causes (hyperpharyngeal diverticula), 156
 gastroesophageal reflux disease, 160–163
 and hiatal hernia, 160–162
 pharmacologic therapy, 162
 surgery for, 162–163
 idiopathic intestinal pseudo-obstruction, 165–166

superior mesenteric artery syndrome, 165, 166
Alkalosis, metabolic, 16
 treatment, 17
Alpha-adrenergic blocking agents, for autonomic dysreflexia, 295, 297
Aminoglycosides
 and nephrotoxic acute tubular necrosis, 10, 14
 for treatment of urinary tract infections, 239
Amphotericin B, and nephrotoxic acute tubular necrosis,
 10, 14
Amputees, hypertension in, 38
Anal sphincter, 167–168
Anemia of chronic disease, 217–229
 case studies, 224–227
 characteristics of, 217
 differential diagnosis of, 221–223
 anemia of hepatic and renal disease, 223
 hemolytic anemias, 223
 hypoplastic anemias, 222–223
 iron-deficiency anemia, 221–222, 225–226
 macrocytic anemias, 223
 evaluation of, 222
 ferritin levels, 226
 red blood cell indices, 225
 frequency of in the chronically disabled, 217
 iron metabolism, 218–219, 220
 laboratory values with chronic disease, 219
 pathophysiology, 219–221
 treatment, 223–224
 blood transfusions, 226
 erythropoietin, 224
Anemia of hepatic and renal disease, vs. anemia of chronic
 disease, 223
Angiography, pulmonary, for diagnosis of pulmonary embolism, 204
Angiotensin-converting enzyme inhibitors